# Lecture Notes in Networks and Systems 148

ıe series "Lecture Notes in Networks and Systems" publishes the latest developments Networks and Systems—quickly, informally and with high quality. Original research ported in proceedings and post-proceedings represents the core of LNNS.

Volumes published in LNNS embrace all aspects and subfields of, as well as new ıallenges in, Networks and Systems.

The series contains proceedings and edited volumes in systems and net-orks, spanning the areas of Cyber-Physical Systems, Autonomous Systems, Sen-or Networks, Control Systems, Energy Systems, Automotive Systems, Biologi-al Systems, Vehicular Networking and Connected Vehicles, Aerospace Systems, utomation, Manufacturing, Smart Grids, Nonlinear Systems, Power Systems, obotics, Social Systems, Economic Systems and other. Of particular value to both he contributors and the readership are the short publication timeframe and the world-vide distribution and exposure which enable both a wide and rapid dissemination of esearch output.

The series covers the theory, applications, and perspectives on the state of the art and future developments relevant to systems and networks, decision making, control, complex processes and related areas, as embedded in the fields of interdisciplinary and applied sciences, engineering, computer science, physics, economics, social, and life sciences, as well as the paradigms and methodologies behind them.

Indexed by SCOPUS, EI Compendex, INSPEC, WTI Frankfurt eG, zbMATH, SCImago.

All books published in the series are submitted for consideration in Web of Science.

For proposals from Asia please contact Aninda Bose (aninda.bose@springer.com).

Kevin Daimi · Abeer Alsadoon
Editors

# Proceedings of the Fourth International Conference on Innovations in Computing Research (ICR'25)

er

*Editors*
Kevin Daimi
University of Detroit
Detroit, MI, USA

Abeer Alsadoon
Asia Pacific International College (APIC)
Sydney, NSW, Australia

ISSN 2367-3370 ISSN 2367-3389 (electronic)
Lecture Notes in Networks and Systems
ISBN 978-3-031-95651-5 ISBN 978-3-031-95652-2 (eBook)
https://doi.org/10.1007/978-3-031-95652-2



This Springer imprint is published by the registered company Springer Nature Switzerland AG
The registered company address is: Gewerbestrasse 11, 6330 Cham, Switzerland

# Preface

ICR'25, the Fourth International Conference on Innovations in Computing Research was held in London, UK, from August 25 to 27, 2025, at the Sheraton Skyline Hotel London Heathrow. ICR'25 was technically sponsored by the Spanish National Research Council (CSIC), Spain, Australian Computer Society (ACS), Australia, Polytechnic Institute of Porto, Portugal, University of Detroit Mercy, USA, Features Analytics, Belgium, and Flexens Ltd, Finland.

The 2025 International Conference on Innovations in Computing Research (ICR'25) is organized by the Institute for Innovations in Computer Science and Engineering Research (IICSER). The goal of this conference is to bring together researchers from academia, business, industry, and government to exchange significant and innovative contributions and research ideas and to act as a platform for international research collaboration. To this extent, ICR'25 sought submissions that furnish innovative ideas, techniques, methodologies, and applications.

The acceptance rate for ICR'25 is 21.3%. This means that for every ten papers submitted, roughly two papers are accepted for presentation at the conference. There were two presentation modes: remote (virtual) and in-person at Sheraton Skyline Hotel London Heathrow. Twenty papers were presented remotely, and twenty-two papers were presented in-person. ICR'25 deployed hybrid synchronous presentation.

These proceedings contain the revised versions of the papers that took the comments of the reviewers into consideration. Only the program committee members were used as reviewers and no secondary reviewers were allowed. The revisions were not re-reviewed. The authors assume full responsibility for the contents of their final papers. All papers were checked for plagiarism using the Turnitin App.

It gave us great pleasure to appreciate the great dedication of the conference chair, advisory committee, organization committee, and the program committee. This dedication greatly contributed to the success of ICR'25. Without the excellent papers that were accepted by the program committee, this conference would have not existed. Therefore, we are delighted to thank all the authors for their hard work to come up with excellent original papers and for their productive cooperation with us to incorporate the comments of the reviewers and editors that participated in improving their papers and submitting their camera-ready papers on time.

The proceedings are published by the Springer book series: Lecture Notes in Networks and Systems (LNNS). LNNS is currently indexed by SCOPUS, DBLP, INSPEC, Norwegian Register for Scientific Journals and Series, SCImago, WTI Frankfurt eG, and zbMATH.

It gives us great pleasure to thank Dr. Thomas Ditzinger, the editorial director in charge of the Springer book series: Lecture Notes in Networks and Systems (LNNS). We very much appreciate his valuable help and support. We would also like to thank

Ms. Varsha Prabakaran, the project coordinator of ICR'25 proceedings book for her cooperation.

August 2025

Kevin Daimi
Abeer Alsadoon

# ICR'25

**The Fourth International Conference on Innovations in Computing Research (ICR'25)**
**London, UK**
**August 24–27, 2025**

## Advisory Committee

| | |
|---|---|
| Luis Hernandez Encinas | Spanish National Research Council (CSIC), Spain |
| Guilermo Francia III | University of West Florida, USA |
| Åsa Hedman | Flexens Ltd, Finland |
| Hiroaki Kikuchi | Meiji University, Japan |
| Pascal Lorenz | University of Haute Alsace, France |
| Slobodan Petrovic | Norwegian University of Science and Technology (NTNU), Norway |
| Stefan Pickl | University of the Federal Armed Forces Munich, Germany |
| Cristina Soviany | Features Analytics SA, Belgium |

## Organization Committee

### Conference Chair

| | |
|---|---|
| Hiroaki Kikuchi | Meiji University, Japan |

### Program Chairs

| | |
|---|---|
| Abeer Alsadoon | Asia Pacific International College (APIC), Australia |
| Kevin Daimi | University of Detroit Mercy, USA |

### Posters Chairs

| | |
|---|---|
| Ievgeniia Kuzminykh | King's College London, UK |
| Flaminia Luccio | Ca' Foscari University of Venice, Italy |
| Esmiralda Moradian | Stockholm University, Sweden |

### Sessions/Workshops Chairs

| | |
|---|---|
| Elena Kakoulli | Neapolis University Pafos, Cyprus |
| William Klement | Dalhousie University, Canada |
| Sara Reis | Polytechnic Institute of Porto, Portugal |

### Publicity Chairs

| | |
|---|---|
| Anna Allen | IICSER, Australia |
| Carl Wilson | ZRD Technology, USA |

### Web Chair

| | |
|---|---|
| Deshao Liu | Western Sydney University, Australia |

## Program Committee

### Data Science

| | |
|---|---|
| Mahshid Lonbani | Kent Institute Australia, Australia |
| Nawzat Sadiq Ahmed | Duhok Polytechnic University, Iraq |
| Rawhi Alrae | UAE University - Al Ain, United Arab Emirates |
| Abdussalam Mohamad Ali | Melbourne Institute of Technology, Australia |
| Thair Al-Dala'in | Western Sydney University, Australia |
| Ghazi Al-Naymat | Ajman University, UAE |
| Suhair Amer | Southeast Missouri State University, USA |
| Wolfgang Bein | University of Nevada, Las Vegas |
| Mahmoud Bekhit | University of Technology Sydney, Australia |
| Tru Cao | The University of Texas at Houston, USA |
| Mohamed Chrayah | Abdelmalek Essaadi University, Morocco |
| Birgitta Dresp-Langley | UMR7357 CNRS and Strasbourg University, France |
| Iman M. A. Helal | Cairo University, Egypt |
| Muhammad Iqbal Hossain | Brac University, Bangladesh |
| Waleed Ibrahim | Central Queensland University, Australia |
| Imran Khan | Sultan Qaboos University, Oman |
| Rajeev Kanth | Savonia University of Applied Sciences, Finland |
| Konstantinos Kolomvatsos | University of Thessaly, Greece |
| Majdi Maabreh | The Hashemite University, Jordan |
| Edwin Montoya | Universidad EAFIT, Colombia |

| | |
|---|---|
| Waseem Alaqqad | West Virginia University Institute of Technology, USA |
| Addisson Salazar | Universitat Politècnica de València, Spain |
| Saibal Pal | Defense R&D Organization, India |
| Marco Javier Suarez Baron | UPTC, Colombia |
| Francesc Sebé Feixas | University of Lleida, Spain |
| Florin Popentiu Vladicescu | National University of Science and Technology POLITEHNICA Bucharest, Romania |

**Health Informatics and Digital Imaging**

| | |
|---|---|
| Heba Afify | Cairo University, Egypt |
| Thair Al-Dala'in | Western Sydney University, Australia |
| Vu Nguyen Huynh Anh | Université Catholique de Louvain, Belgium |
| Faouzi Benzarti | University of Tunisia, Tunisia |
| Violeta Bulbenkiene | Klaipeda University, Lithuania |
| Hugo Daniel Abreu Peixoto | University of Minho, Portugal |
| Chia-Chi Joseph Chang | National Yang Ming Chiao Tung University, Taiwan |
| John Chelsom | Fordham University, UK |
| Nectarios Costadopoulos | Charles Sturt University, Australia |
| Dillon Chrimes | University of Victoria, Canada |
| Luis Coelho | Polytechnic Institute of Porto, Portugal |
| Ahmed Dawoud | Asia Pacific International College (APIC), Australia |
| Marie Khair | Notre Dame University, Lebanon |
| William Klement | Dalhousie University, Canada |
| Irene Kopaliani | Princeton University, USA |
| Roseline Oluwaseun Ogundokun | Landmark University, Nigeria |
| Junfeng Qu | Clayton State University, USA |
| Sara Seabra dos Reis | Instituto Superior de Engenharia do Porto, Portugal |
| Cristina Soviany | Features Analytics SA, Belgium |
| Karl A. Stroetmann | University of Victoria, Canada |
| Somenath Chakraborty | West Virginia University Institute of Technology, USA |
| Mohamed Chrayah | University Abdelmalek Essaadi Morocco, Morocco |
| Gamil abdel Azim | Suez Canal University, Egypt |

**Internet of Things**

| | |
|---|---|
| Hanady Hussien Issa | Arab Academy for Science, Technology and Maritime Transport, Egypt |
| Iness Ahriz | CEDRIC Lab Conservatoire National des Arts et Métiers, France |
| Ali Alwan Al-Juboori | Ramapo College of New Jersey, USA |
| Zakaria Benomar | Inria, France |
| Jide Edu | King's College London, UK |
| Hicham H. Hallal | York University, Canada |
| Marie Khair | Notre Dame University, Lebanon |
| Irene Kopaliani | Princeton University, USA |
| Lemia Louail | Université de Lorraine CNRS CRAN, France |
| Hung Ba NGO | Can Tho University, Vietnam |
| Mais Nijim | Texas A&M University -Kingsville, USA |
| Slobodan Petrovic | Norwegian University of Science and Technology (NTNU), Norway |
| Rao Naveed Bin Rais | Ajman University, UAE |
| Sunny Raj | Oakland University, USA |
| Alessandro Ruggiero | University of Salerno, Italy |
| Sorin Soviany | National Institute for Research and Development in Informatics, Romania |
| Hailu Xu | California State University, USA |
| Nabil Giweli | Western Sydney University, Australia |
| Fouzi Semchedine | University Ferhat Abbas Setif 1, Algeria |
| Gokarna Sharma | Kent State University, USA |
| Nuno Gueiral | Superior Institute of Engineering of Porto, Portugal |
| Antonio González Fernández | IE University, Spain |
| Songhui Yue | Charleston Southern University, USA |
| Arwin Datumaya Sumari | Adisutjipto Institute of Aerospace Technology (AIAT), Indonesia |
| Akos Odry | University of Szeged, Hungary |

**Smart Cities/Smart Energy**

| | |
|---|---|
| Mohammed Akour | Yarmouk University Jordan |
| Manuel I. Capel | Universidad de Granada, Spain |
| Sergio Ilarri | University of Zaragoza, Spain |
| Saraju Mohanty | University of North Texas, USA |
| Dmitry Namiot | Lomonosov Moscow State University, Russia |
| Mais Nijim | Texas A&M University -Kingsville, USA |
| Jun-Seok Oh | Western Michigan University, USA |

| | |
|---|---|
| Alessandro Ruggiero | University of Salerno, Italy |
| Hailu Xu | California State University, USA |
| Nabil Giweli | Western Sydney University, Australia |
| Fouzi Semchedine | University Ferhat Abbas Setif 1, Algeria |
| Waseem Alaqqad | West Virginia University Institute of Technology, USA |
| María del Mar Gómez Zamora | Universidad Rey Juan Carlos, Spain |
| Cheng Siong Chin | Newcastle University, Singapore |
| Grzegorz Sierpiński | Silesian University of Technology, Poland |
| Gheorghe-Daniel Andreescu | Politehnica University Timisoara, Romania |
| Maryna Averkyna | Estonian Business School, Estonia |

**Quantum Computing**

| | |
|---|---|
| Somenath Chakraborty | West Virginia University Institute of Technology, USA |
| Smain Femmam | UHA University, France |
| Hicham H. Hallal | York University, Canada |
| Rajeev Kanth | Savonia University of Applied Sciences, Finland |
| Lucian Lupu-Dima | University of Petrosani, Romania |
| Saibal Pal | Defense R&D Organization, India |
| Jayesh Soni | Florida International University, USA |
| Sorin Soviany | National Institute for Research & Development in Informatics, Romania |
| Francesco Zirilli | Sapienza University, Italy |

# Contents

## Data Science

**Computer and Network Security**

# Data Science

# Leveraging Machine Learning to Predict Liver Disease Status: A Classification Approach

Pavani Minukuri, Yathisha Ganesh, and Samah Senbel(✉)

Sacred Heart University, Fairfield, CT, USA
{minukurip,ganeshv}@mail.sacredheart.edu,
senbels@sacredheart.edu

**Abstract.** Liver disease is a major global health concern, requiring timely diagnosis and intervention to improve patient outcomes. In this study, we use clinical data to predict the stage of liver disease through a thorough data analysis. With the illness status acting as the target variable, the dataset comprises a number of demographic, biochemical, and clinical characteristics, including age, cholesterol, and copper. To find important patterns and connections in the data, we used exploratory data analysis, or EDA. To guarantee consistency, numerical features were normalized, missing data were imputed, and categorical information were encoded using one-hot encoding. We used oversampling approaches (SMOTE) to address the issue of class imbalance, which helped to balance the distribution of disease status. XGBoost (Extreme Gradient Boosting), a potent machine learning method renowned for its efficacy with structured data, served as the main classification model. Because XGBoost can handle missing values, manage imbalanced datasets, and provide feature importance rankings, it was selected. To maximize the model's performance while preventing overfitting, we used GridSearchCV to do hyperparameter tuning, optimizing important parameters like n_estimators, max_depth, learning_rate, and subsample. The model's capacity to predict the status of liver disease was thoroughly assessed using a variety of measures, including accuracy, precision, recall, F1-score, and ROC AUC. The finished model performed well, highlighting the significance of a strong, data-driven strategy for forecasting the stages of liver disease. This model emphasizes the need of early detection and individualized treatment planning for patients, as well as its insights into the fundamental factors impacting the evolution of the disease.

**Keywords:** Liver disease · Data Classification · Medical machine learning · Data visualization · Data Analysis

## 1 Introduction

Cirrhosis is a progressive liver disease characterized by the irreversible replacement of healthy liver tissue with scar tissue (fibrosis), which significantly disrupts the liver's structural integrity and functionality. Figure 1 illustrates the severity of cirrhosis and provides a visual comparison of its impact on the liver's structure and function. A healthy liver exhibits a smooth, homogeneous surface that facilitates optimal blood flow and


K. Daimi and A. Alsadoon (Eds.): ICR 2025, LNNS 1487, pp. 3–15, 2025.
https://doi.org/10.1007/978-3-031-95652-2_1

nutrient exchange, essential for various metabolic processes. In contrast, a cirrhotic liver presents a nodular appearance due to extensive fibrosis, which not only alters the liver's architecture but also impairs its ability to perform vital functions, including the synthesis of proteins and detoxification of harmful substances.

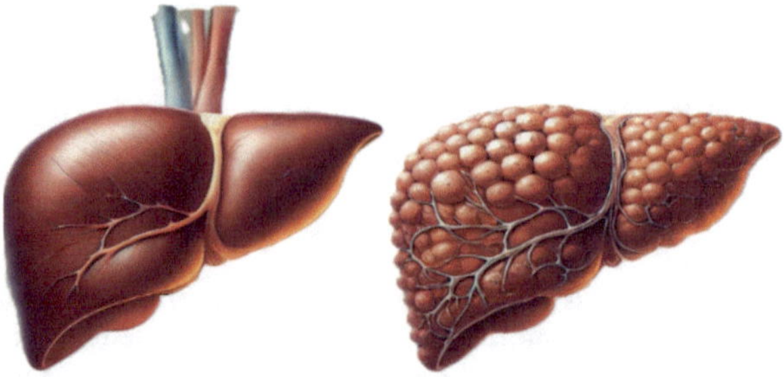


**Fig. 1.** Comparison Between Healthy and Cirrhotic Liver

There are several biochemical markers that are crucial indicators of liver function and disease severity. Key markers such as cholesterol, copper, alkaline phosphatase, SGOT, triglycerides, and platelet levels are assessed to evaluate liver health. For instance, elevated levels of SGOT and alkaline phosphatase can indicate liver damage, while low platelet counts may suggest portal hypertension associated with cirrhosis [1].

Additionally, clinical indicators such as hepatomegaly (liver enlargement), ascites (abdominal fluid retention), edema (swelling), and the presence of spider angiomas (spider-like blood vessels) provide valuable insights into the clinical manifestations of liver disease [2]. These indicators are often more pronounced in patients with advanced cirrhosis and serve as essential features for determining the stage of liver disease [3]. The above indicators and their significance are fully explained in the subsequent sections of the paper.

The dataset used in this research provides a comprehensive overview of liver health through various data features. Demographic information, such as patients' age and sex, is crucial in understanding the prevalence and progression of liver diseases. Although some studies suggest that males often experience higher rates of cirrhosis, this dataset indicates a higher prevalence of cirrhosis among females. Age is also a significant factor, as older individuals are generally more prone to chronic liver conditions due to cumulative exposure to risk factors. Biochemical markers serve as essential indicators in assessing liver health and disease progression.

## 2 Related Work

Research in the analysis and prediction of cases of liver disease is plentiful due to the importance and prevalence of the disease. Prediction is of particular interest as it helps in finding out patients who are most susceptible to the disease for early intervention.

Rahman et al. [2] used machine learning models for prediction: This research aims to lower the cost of diagnosis by assessing the performance of machine learning models

(Logistic Regression, Random Forest, Decision Tree, SVM, KNN, Naïve Bayes) using metrics like accuracy and precision. Logistic Regression provided the best accuracy (75%), highlighting its potential for predicting liver disease from clinical data. Medical diagnoses are essential for advancing patient care and research.

Another interesting study [4] concentrates on disease detection not prediction: Machine learning has become instrumental in enhancing disease detection. This study analyzed data from 615 individuals using machine learning algorithms to identify key predictors of liver disease. Visualizations were used to uncover important insights, including addressing missing data. Utilized widely recognized machine learning methods to predict ascites, demonstrating better performance compared to traditional statistical techniques.

Hatami et al. [5] developed an interesting model to predict the onset of Cirrhosis based on clinical data. This ML-based approach can reduce unnecessary risks and costs for patients in advanced stages of the disease. Timely detection of liver cirrhosis is vital for effective treatment and preventing serious health outcomes.

A new research project [6], similar to ours, developed a regression based prediction based on historic data from multiple sources. Their model developed a machine learning prediction model using data from 583 patients with 11 attributes. Based on medical data from FMC, Yola, this study shows that machine learning methods, specifically the Support Vector Machine, provide a more accurate prediction for liver cirrhosis sickness, with accuracy of 73%, precision of 73%, recall of 100%, and F1 Score of 84%.

In this paper, we present a new machine-learning based model to predict the onset and severity of liver cirrhosis based on the publicly available dataset of 512 patients. The novelty of our work is in the pre-modeling steps taken to optimize the results of the model by using over-sampling to balance the data and feature selection to obtain better results.

# 3 Method

## 3.1 Data Collection

**Source of the Dataset.** The dataset used in this study was sourced from clinical records of patients diagnosed with cirrhosis. The data was obtained from UC Irvine Machine Learning Repository [7].

**Dataset Overview.** The dataset contains 418 patients diagnosed with liver disease, focusing on those in various stages of cirrhosis. Each record includes clinical, demographic, and biochemical data, capturing relevant patient information.

**Data Features.** The features in the dataset include:

**Demographic Information:** Patient's age and sex.
**Biochemical Markers:** Cholesterol, copper, alkaline phosphatase (Alk_Phos), (SGOT) Serum Glutamic-Oxaloacetic Transaminase, triglycerides, and platelet levels.
**Clinical Indicators:** Features like hepatomegaly (liver enlargement), ascites (abdominal fluid retention), edema (swelling), and the presence of spider angiomas (spiders).

**Target Variable**: The dataset's target variable is the Status 0 = D (death), 1 = C (censored), and 2 = CL (censored due to liver transplantation) of liver disease, which indicates the severity of cirrhosis.

### 3.2 Data Preprocessing

Structure of the Dataset: The dataset comprises 20 columns (features) and 418 rows (patient records). There are both categorical and numerical variables, where categorical features (e.g., hepatomegaly, sex) represent binary outcomes, and numerical features (e.g., cholesterol levels, age) represent continuous data.

**Missing Values**

Table 1 shows the missing values present in the data which are encountered by Simple imputer (MICE) [8] for the numerical and categorical using the strategy median and mode respectively. This impacts the validity of our results and the columns without missing data were given higher importance.

**Table 1.** missing value in the data

| Attributes | Counts of Missing values |
|---|---|
| ID | 0 |
| N_days | 0 |
| Status | 0 |
| Drug | 106 |
| Age | 0 |
| Sex | 0 |
| Ascites | 106 |
| Hepatomegaly | 106 |
| Spiders | 106 |
| Edema | 0 |
| Bilirubin | 0 |
| Cholesterol | 134 |
| Albumin | 0 |
| Copper | 108 |
| Alk_Phos | 106 |
| SGOT | 106 |
| Trygliderides | 136 |
| Platelets | 11 |
| Stage | 6 |

**Outliers**

In Fig. 2, it is observed that all columns exhibit positive skewness, except for the Albumin column, which demonstrates negative skewness. This column is treated using a pipeline that includes Winsorization, as well as Log and Square Root transformations. Thereby, giving all columns equal weights.

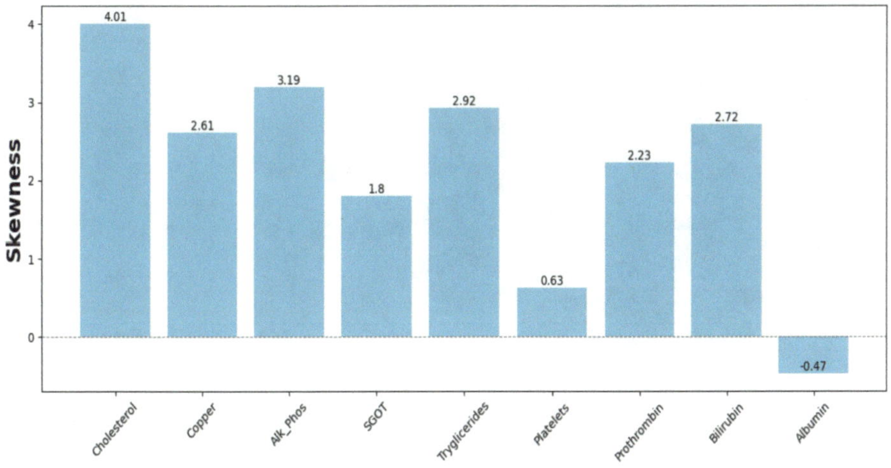


**Fig. 2.** Skewness of numerical columns for the biochemicals

**Imbalanced Data**

In Fig. 3, we show the imbalance of the different possible diagnosis from our dataset, Death, recovery, or recovery with a liver transplant. This imbalance problem is solved by applying SMOTE (Synthetic Minority Over-sampling Technique) [10] method to balance the class distribution to resolve the imbalance in the data. The implementation of a preprocessing pipeline, which consists of the StandardScaler for scaling numerical data and one-hot encoding for categorical features, comes next. Because these changes are contained in a pipeline, the data preprocessing workflow is efficient and repeatable.

## 4 Data Analysis Results

Figure 4 shows the frequency of Age Attribute, a bar chart shows how ages are distributed among two groups: Highly Affected Age and Others:

1. Peak Age Group: With 153 people in the Highly Affected Age group, the maximum frequency is noted at age 55. This implies that the age of 55 may be a turning point with a high incidence of cases, potentially signifying increased susceptibility to the condition under investigation (cirrhosis, for example).
2. Middle-Aged Population: Counts are persistently high among those aged 45 to 60, particularly in the Highly Affected Age category. This range may indicate a demographic segment that is more susceptible to liver disease-related health problems.

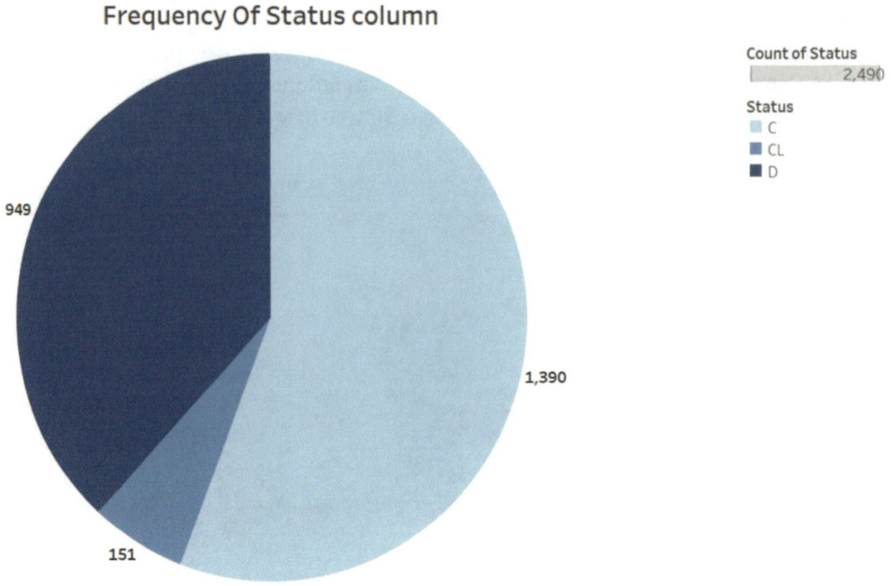


**Fig. 3.** Imbalance in the Target column (Status)

3. Younger Age Stability: The counts are typically lower between the ages of 25 and around 40, with very slight variations between the two groups. This implies that younger people are less likely to be severely impacted, which is consistent with general patterns where age-related illnesses appear later in life.
4. Gradual Decline with Older Age: The frequency of both groups steadily decreases after the age of 60, most likely because of either the aging process or the mortality linked to chronic illnesses.
5. Significant Contrast in Some Ages: The count between the Highly Affected Age and Other categories varies significantly in some ages, such as 45 and 55. This could indicate age-specific factors that make the illness worse.

In Fig. 5, The correlation matrix displays the relationships between various health indicators, with each cell representing the correlation coefficient ranging from −1 to 1. Notably, Stage_encoded exhibits strong negative correlations with N_Days (−0.38) and Age_in_Years (−0.26), suggesting that higher disease stages are associated with fewer days and lower ages. Conversely, it positively correlates with Prothrombin (0.28) and Platelets (0.29), indicating that increased stages correspond to higher levels of these metrics. N_Days also negatively correlates with Prothrombin (−0.31), suggesting that longer durations may relate to decreased prothrombin levels.

Platelets positively correlate with both SGOT (0.22) and Tryglicerides (0.16), indicating a potential link between platelet counts and these health indicators. Additionally, SGOT shows positive correlations with Alk_Phos (0.22) and Copper (0.24), while both Alk_Phos and Copper have a strong positive correlation with each other (0.41). Cholesterol also demonstrates a positive correlation with Tryglicerides (0.35). Overall, the

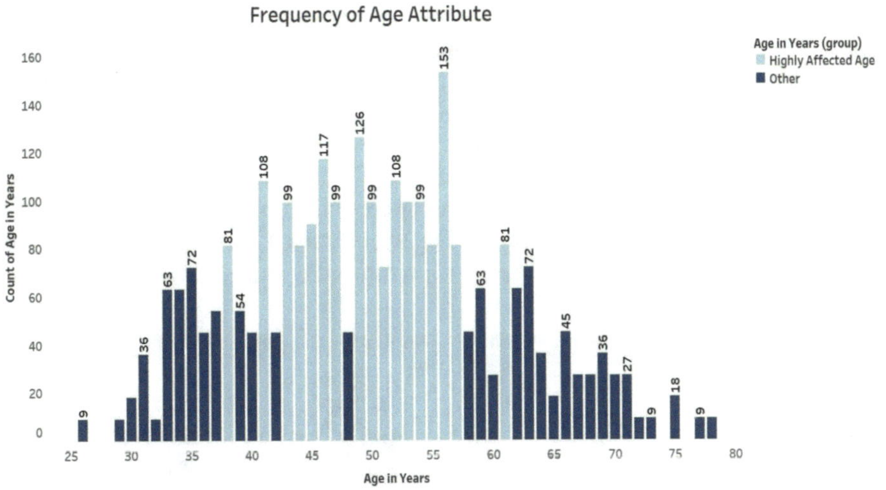


**Fig. 4.** Age distribution in the data

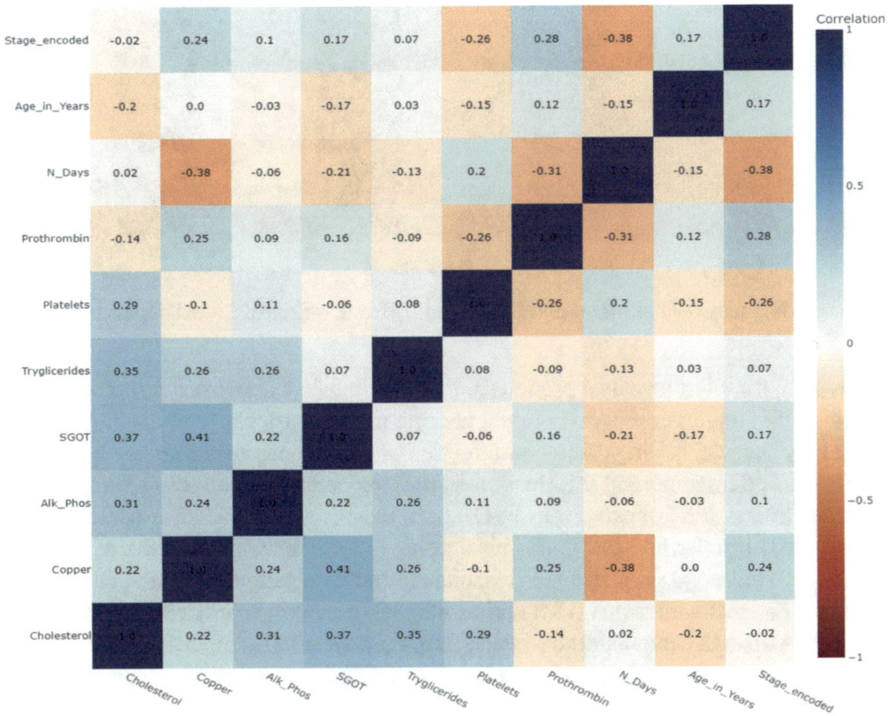


**Fig. 5.** Correlation matrix for biochemical markers

matrix reveals intricate relationships between health indicators, highlighting how higher disease stages might influence various metrics.

In Fig. 6, the bar chart illustrates the distribution of males and females across various stages of liver disease, highlighting the counts of individuals within each stage. The blue bars represent females (F), while the red bars indicatc males (M). In Stage 1, there are very few individuals, with a notably higher count of females (approximately 20) compared to males (around 5). The Stage 2 shows an increase in both genders, with females again outnumbering males (approximately 70 females vs. 20 males). The most significant disparity occurs in Stage 3, where the count of female's peaks at around 140, while males increase slightly to about 30. Finally, in Stage 4, the trend continues, with females still predominant (approximately 80) compared to males (around 15).

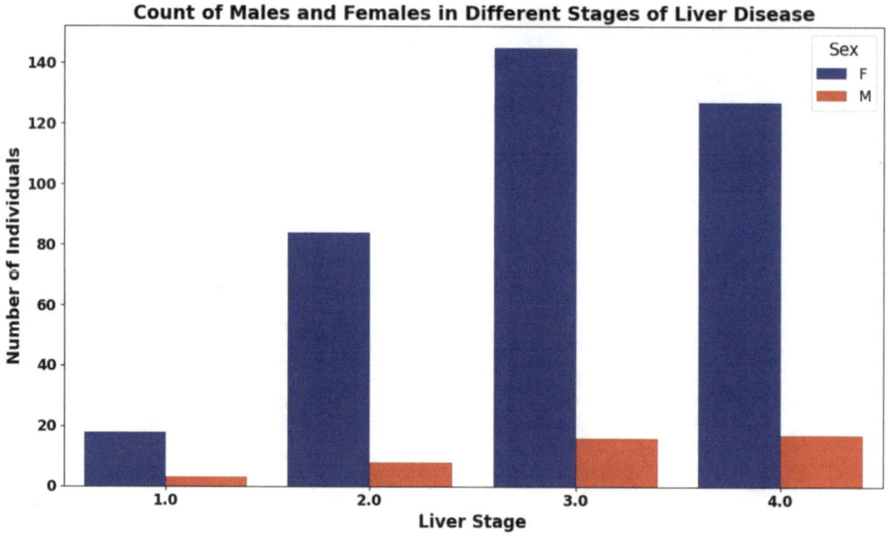


**Fig. 6.** Count of Males and Females in Different Stages of Liver Disease

Overall, the chart reveals a pronounced gender imbalance across the stages of liver disease, with females consistently outnumbering males, particularly in the later stages, which may suggest varying disease progression or health outcomes between genders.

Figure 7 offers important information on the connection between drug kind, disease stage, and liver status. For patients in the Death (D) category treated with D-penicillamine Stage 1 (red) has the highest biochemical value (726.5), according to the analysis of the stages. This suggests a stronger response to the medication in crucial early-stage instances. Patients with status (CL) during Stage 3 (green) have moderate biochemical values (514.0) on D-penicillamine whereas the placebo results in somewhat lower values. Most patients in stage 4 (orange) have a general fall in biochemical values, which is indicative of the disease getting worse. In contrast, biochemical levels are more evenly distributed in Stage 2 (sea green), with Placebo displaying somewhat greater values than D-penicillamine.

When it comes to the effects of medications, D-penicillamine shows overall higher biochemical values than the placebo, particularly in critical cases (D), indicating that it significantly improves liver function in extreme circumstances. The placebo exhibits

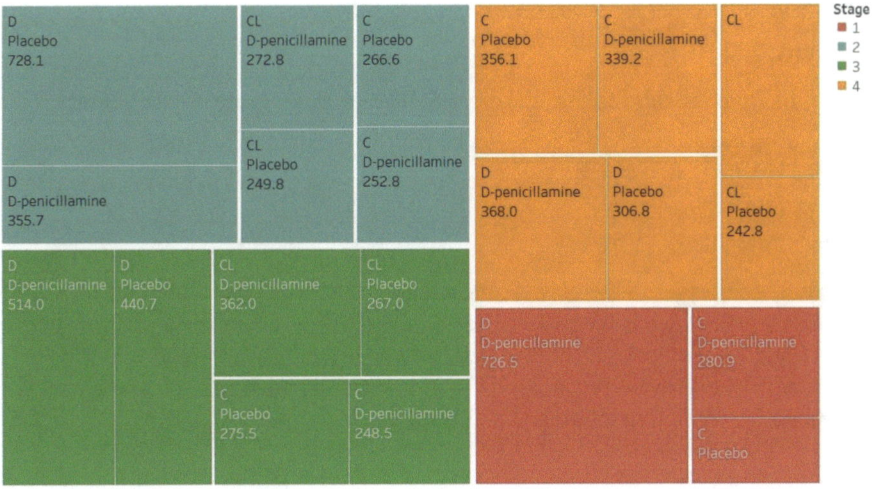


**Fig. 7.** Distribution of Biochemical marker values by Liver Status and Disease Stage

unpredictability, producing lower values in critical circumstances while functioning better in people with severe illnesses (C). This suggests that a patient's condition has a substantial impact on how effective a treatment is.

Considering the liver condition, patients in the Death (D) group show increased biochemical values when receiving D-penicillamine, which could suggest that the medication works well in extreme situations. The small difference in values between D-penicillamine and the placebo for patients with status (CL) indicates that both have an equivalent effect. However, for severe individuals (C), the placebo produces greater biochemical readings than D-penicillamine, suggesting a liver-function-based differential response.Finally, analyzing how different drug kinds and disease stages interact shows that D-penicillamine works best in early stages (like Stage 1) but loses effectiveness as the disease advances to more advanced stages (like Stage 4). However, in crucial stages, the placebo continuously exhibits lower biochemical values, highlighting its limited effectiveness in more severe diseases.

## 5 Machine Learning Model Evaluation Results

Using machine learning to predict the outcome of a patient's illness based on his state and medications is an easy and efficient way to direct his recovery compared to clinical test. Using a machine learning model to predict the outcome is a starting point but not enough to diagnose and treat a patient.

We used GridSearchCV to run 3-fold cross-validation with hyperparameter adjustment to assess the XGBoost classifier's performance. The F1-weighted score was used to choose the top-performing model. Using GridSearchCV, the ideal hyperparameters were:

Maximum Depth: 3

Learning Rate: 0.1
Estimators: 200

The results from the third fold of the cross-validation process are shown below:

Accuracy: 76.26%
Precision (Weighted): 75.75%
Recall (Weighted): 76.26%
F1-Score (Weighted): 75.59%

In Table 2, According to the classification report, the model has a high recall and F1-score for class 0, which is the majority class. Nonetheless, the model's performance for classes 1 and 2 is mediocre. Notwithstanding these difficulties, the weighted average F1-score of 75.59% and overall accuracy of 76.26% indicate that the model is comparatively well-suited for predicting the stages of liver disease.

**Table 2.** Classification Report

| Class | Precision | Recall | F1-Score | Support |
|---|---|---|---|---|
| 0 | 0.80 | 0.90 | 0.84 | 78 |
| 1 | 0.70 | 0.71 | 0.75 | 50 |
| 2 | 0.77 | 0.64 | 0.70 | 53 |
| Macro Avg | 0.62 | 0.60 | 0.60 | 139 |
| Weighted Avg | 0.76 | 0.76 | 0.76 | 139 |

Figure 8 shows the ROC (Receiver Operating Characteristic) curve assesses how well a multi-class XGBoost classification model performs in predicting three different classes: 0, 1, and 2. The curve offers a thorough understanding of the model's predictive power by shedding light on the trade-off between the True Positive Rate (TPR) and False Positive Rate (FPR) across a range of decision thresholds. Note the variation in the line curvatures.

The False Positive Rate (FPR), which measures the percentage of negative samples that are mistakenly categorized as positive, is represented by the X-axis of the ROC curve. Conversely, the True Positive Rate (TPR), which represents the percentage of correctly categorized positive samples, is shown on the Y-axis. A point in the upper-left corner of the graph would indicate that the model is ideal if it achieves a TPR of 1 and an FPR of 0. Random guessing is indicated by the dashed diagonal line, which acts as a baseline (AUC = 0.50). Any curve that is higher than this line indicates that the model outperforms chance.

There are three classes to predict, class 0 is the group that died, class 1 is the class that recovered andclass2 recovered but through a liver transplant (probably a severe case). Different ROC curves are used to show the performance for each class. The best predictive performance is shown by Class 0 (blue curve), which has an Area Under the Curve (AUC) score of 0.88. This curve is the closest to the ideal top-left corner, indicating

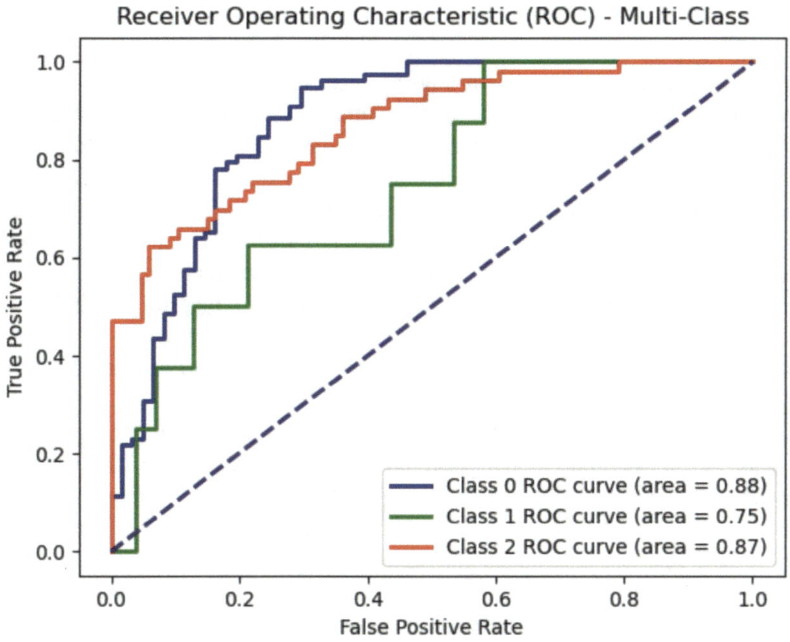


**Fig. 8.** ROC (Receiver Operating Characteristic) for XGBoost Algorithm

that the model effectively distinguishes instances of Class 0 from other classes. With an AUC of 0.87, Class 2 (red curve) performs similarly to Class 0 and also has good predictive potential. With a moderate AUC of 0.75, the model's predictions for Class 1 (green curve) are less reliable. This implies that Class 1 examples are difficult for the model to distinguish, maybe because of class imbalance or overlapping feature distributions. Also, the cases were mider and had a bigger variety in their data columns.

The model's performance varies between classes, as the ROC curve illustrates. For Classes 0 and 2, the model obtains high discriminatory power; however, Class 1 performance needs to be improved. This mismatch can come from uneven class representation or intrinsic difficulties in the attributes associated with Class 1. The classifier's performance for this difficult class may be improved by addressing these problems using sophisticated sampling strategies like SMOTE, modifying class weights, or feature engineering.

The main results of this study is to highlight the significance of keeping an eye on important biochemical indicators and considering differences in liver disease development by age, gender, and stage (Those in class 1). By using early liver disease chance detection, the medical field can direct the creation of more potent diagnostic instruments and therapeutic approaches, ultimately leading to better patient outcomes in the management of liver disease.

## 6 Conclusion

According to the age distribution research, liver illness is most common in people between the ages of 55 and 60, which may imply an age-related vulnerability. Additionally, patterns specific to gender were noted, especially when it came to medication responses [7, 8]. D-penicillamine has demonstrated its effectiveness in treating the biochemical imbalances brought on by liver disease by consistently outperforming the placebo in lowering aberrant biochemical levels. The effects of treatment, however, differed according to the stage of the disease; in Stage 3, when biochemical abnormalities increased, the benefit was most noticeable [9]. Targeted therapies, like D-penicillamine, can also effectively attenuate specific signs, such Alk Phos, while having less of an influence on others, like Albumin and Copper, according to the comparative examination of pharmacological effects on biochemical markers [10].

The conclusions drawn from this study of clinical data highlight the significance of keeping an eye on important biochemical indicators and considering differences in liver disease development by age, gender, and stage. This thorough knowledge can direct the creation of more potent diagnostic instruments and therapeutic approaches, ultimately leading to better patient outcomes in the management of liver disease.

The XGBoost classifier, a sophisticated and popular gradient-boosting technique, was the focus of this study's machine learning methodology. Using GridSearchCV and a three-fold cross-validation approach, hyperparameter tuning was carried out to optimize the model's performance. This methodical approach made sure that the optimal set of parameters was chosen to maximize the predictive power of the model. A maximum tree depth of three, a learning rate of 0.1, and 200 estimators were the hyperparameters found to be ideal; these values represented a well-balanced setup that prevented overfitting while identifying important patterns in the data.

When tested on the test dataset, the XGBoost model showed strong overall performance. With an accuracy of 76.26%, the model demonstrated that it could accurately forecast most situations. Additionally, the weighted average precision was 75.75%, demonstrating the model's capacity to reduce false positives in all classes. The weighted average recall, which gauges sensitivity to true positives, was also 76.26%, confirming the model's dependability in producing accurate predictions. Lastly, the model's overall capacity to accurately categorize various status of liver illness was demonstrated by the 75.59% F1-score (weighted), a balanced parameter that combines precision and recall.

Together, these findings highlight the XGBoost model's promise as a trustworthy instrument for clinical data analysis and liver disease status prediction. Even if the performance is promising, more improvements could improve the model's suitability for actual diagnostic situations, especially for minority classes. This machine learning integration promotes precision medicine and aids in clinical decision-making, which improves patient outcomes.

The ROC analysis highlights the model's advantages and shortcomings overall. While the moderate AUC for Class 1 indicates chances to further optimize the model for consistent performance across all classes, the high AUC scores for Classes 0 and 2 demonstrate dependable prediction power.

## References


1. Khan, R.A., Luo, Y., Wu, F.X.: Machine learning based liver disease diagnosis: a systematic review. Neurocomputing. **468**, 492–509 (2022)
2. Rahman, A.S., Shamrat, F.J.M., Tasnim, Z., Roy, J., Hossain, S.A.: A comparative study on liver disease prediction using supervised machine learning algorithms. Int. J. Sci. Technol. Res. **8**(11), 419–422 (2019)
3. Mostafa, F., Hasan, E., Williamson, M., Khan, H.: Statistical machine learning approaches liver disease prediction. Liver. **1**(4), 294–312 (2021)
4. Kumar, D.V.S., Chaurasia, R., Misra, A., Misra, P.K., Khang, A.: Heart disease and liver disease prediction using machine learning. In: Data-Centric AI Solutions and Emerging Technologies in the Healthcare Ecosystem, pp. 205–214. CRC Press (2023)
5. Hatami, B., Asadi, F., Bayani, A., Zali, M.R., Kavousi, K.: Machine learning-based system for prediction of ascites grades in patients with liver cirrhosis using laboratory and clinical data: design and implementation study. Clin. Chem. Lab. Med. (CCLM). **60**(12), 1946–1954 (2022)
6. Jamila, G., Wajiga, G.M., Malgwi, Y.M., Maidabara, A.H.: A diagnostic model for the prediction of liver cirrhosis using machine learning techniques. Comput. Sci. IT Res. J. **3**(1), 36–51 (2022)
7. Farrand, E., Gologorskaya, O., Mills, H., Radhakrishnan, L., Collard, H.R., Butte, A.J.: Machine-learning algorithm to improve cohort identification in interstitial lung disease. Am. J. Respir. Crit. Care Med. **207**(10), 1398–1401 (2023)
8. Park, I.G., Yoon, S.J., Won, S.M., Oh, K.K., Hyun, J.Y., Suk, K.T., Lee, U.: Gut microbiota-based machine-learning signature for the diagnosis of alcohol-associated and metabolic dysfunction-associated steatotic liver disease. Sci. Rep. **14**(1), 16122 (2024)
9. Pei, X., Deng, Q., Liu, Z., Yan, X., Sun, W.: Machine learning algorithms for predicting fatty liver disease. Ann. Nutr. Metab. **77**(1), 38–45 (2021)
10. Shaban, W.M.: Early diagnosis of liver disease using improved binary butterfly optimization and machine learning algorithms. Multimed. Tools Appl. **83**(10), 30867–30895 (2024)

# K-nearest Neighbour Algorithm Clustering Simple Moving Average the Better Trend Classification Indicator

Justin Hui San Zhao[1,2,3](✉) and Thair Al-Dala'in[1,2]

[1] Western Sydney University, Sydney, Australia
t.aldalain@city.westernsydney.edu.au
[2] Asia Pacific International College (APIC), Parramatta, Australia
[3] Lincoln Institute of Higher Education (LIHE), Sydney, Australia

**Abstract.** K-nearest Neighbour is a non-parametric, versatile, and supervised machine learning (ML) algorithm used to perform regression analysis and classification by identifying data points that are similar and near each other in feature space. Our research identifies that the K-nearest Neighbour Algorithm Clustering Simple Moving Average (KNN SMA) outperforms the current standardised simple moving averages (SMA), 9, 21, 50 and 200. Even though the KNN SMA is a profitable indicator after optimisation, it is essential to note that one indicator alone will not be suitable for managing a portfolio strategy. It is also necessary to understand that when using algorithmic development, the strategies created do alpha decay faster than standardised indicators, namely the 9, 21, 50 and 200 SMA. This research analyses the findings of the KNN SMA in comparison to the 9, 21, 50 and 200 SMA. The study also provides insights into possible methods of incorporating the KNN SMA into the portfolio as a trend component. It is important to note that most traders are unprofitable due to qualitative judgements and cognitive biases, so using a quantitative approach for trend classification is advised. The KNN SMA benefits retail investors as it's an algorithmic strategy that can be operated through TradingView, optimised and backtested on any computers with access to the TradingView Assistant.

**Keywords:** K-nearest Neighbour Algorithm (KNN) · Simple Moving Average (SMA) · Expected Value (EV) · Machine Learning (ML) · TradingView (TV) · Pine Script (PS)

## 1 Introduction

Trend classification is essential to an investor's analysis before interacting with the asset. There are many small fluctuations within trends; classifying them as an uptrend or downtrend is crucial [1]. The SMA is a technical indicator that classifies the current trend of an asset by plotting the average asset price over time [2]. However, it does have limitations, including lag when operating too slow, alpha decay and being susceptible to noise if operating too fast.


K. Daimi and A. Alsadoon (Eds.): ICR 2025, LNNS 1487, pp. 16–27, 2025.
https://doi.org/10.1007/978-3-031-95652-2_2

This research aims to develop a KNN-based SMA that overcomes its limitations, such as being laggy or susceptible to noise.

The research questions addressed by this research are:

1. How does the KNN SMA statistically outperform traditional SMAs regarding net profit, drawdown, and trade accuracy?
2. What specifications are required to use the KNN SMA?

The methodology used in this research included conducting backtests of the 9, 21, 50, and 200 SMAs, developing the KNN SMA, backtesting it, and comparing the results of each SMA. Backtests were conducted from 2018 to today using the Bitcoin All-Time History Index. 2018 was selected as the start date for backtesting because Bitcoin perpetual futures did not exist before 2018. The KNN SMA will benefit trend-following traders and investors by providing a more accurate trend classification with less noise and lag. Retail investors will benefit from using the KNN SMA, a superior trend following indicator compared to default indicators and Supertrend or even the RSI. The research has been split into multiple sections to simplify understanding. First, we'll discuss the materials and methods used for the study, followed by the 9, 21, 50, and 200 SMAs, and then we will introduce and compare the KNN SMA. Finally, we'll discuss the results of the KNN SMA. Previous literature related has been covered in the literature review below.

## 2 Literature Review

### 2.1 Materials and Methods

This research comprises 23 pieces of literature from journals. The papers have been checked to ensure they are relevant to the current state of the market. We used the KNN ML algorithm, as PineScript (PS) supports this. PS is the programming language TV scripts use. Backtests have been used since 2018 to ensure relevance to the current state of the crypto market, as before 2018, perpetual futures were non-existent for Bitcoin.

### 2.2 9, 21, 50 and 200 SMAs

The SMA is a simple yet effective indicator often used by hedge funds and financial institutions to classify a market trend [3]. As many market participants can use the SMAs, a competitive edge can no longer be exploited for additional alpha. Most SMA users use the SMA as a component of a trend-following system. However, some users believe that the SMA can predict future prices of the Stock market, which isn't possible as there's no way of accurately predicting the cost of an asset in the future using past or even coincident data [4]. The 9 MA is used to determine in the short term days to weeks whether we are in an uptrend or downtrend, and 21 and 50 MA is used to determine in the medium term whether the asset is in an uptrend or downtrend from weeks to months. The 200 MA determines whether the long term is a bull market, denoted by an uptrend, and a bear market, denoted by a downtrend in months to years. Conversely to some other research other researchers have done, it's essential to understand that these moving averages aren't used to forecast the future prices of cryptocurrency and are used to determine the optimal portfolio allocation as of this current moment based on the coincidental data the investor has at this current moment [5].

### 2.3 KNN SMA

KNN is an effective and simple ML technique for classification; in our case, trend classification, there are some disadvantages to KNN, including but not limited to low efficiency in tasks such as dynamic web mining and requires a good K value to work [6]. The KNN SMA is visually identical to a 9, 21, 50 and 200 SMA. However, it provides a cleaner signal for entering and exiting trends.

### 2.4 Max-min SMA Strategy

The max-min simple moving average strategy was previously introduced and outperformed default SMAs ten to twenty times in the DJIA, NASDAQ, and S&P indices [7]. The strategy uses moving averages with a long and short period instead of only one set period, which is what the default SMAs use. Entry and exit criteria are price > MA(Short) && MA(Long) and price < MA(Short) && MA(Long), respectively. Two SMAs are required because the shorter SMA reacts faster to price movements; thus, price increases above the longer SMA signal that an uptrend has begun [7]. One of the limitations of the max-min SMA strategy is the use of static moving averages, which means the same approach is being used in the future; over a period, the alpha decays, and the noise in the market will cause false and late signals to be produced. The KNN SMA addresses the alpha decay of the max-min SMA strategy due to the KNN SMA's dynamic nature.

### 2.5 Trading Range Breakouts with SMAs

Researchers have previously backtested range breakout trading using two SMAs, one fixed and the other variable in length [8]. This research was conducted on the KSE-100, the Pakistan Stock Market index, with backtest data from January 1, 1997, to December 31, 2013 [8]. The backtest data encompasses important critical dates, including the Asian currency crisis between 1997 and 2000, the aftermath of the Asian currency crisis between 2001 and 2004, before the global financial crisis from 2005 to 2007, the global financial crisis from 2008 to 2010 and after the global financial crisis from 2011 to 2013. To navigate through the everchanging market state, the moving averages changed during the period, meaning the moving average in 1997 differed from the moving average in 2004 or 2013. This methodology is similar to how the KNN SMA operates, with multiple variables within the Moving Average regularly changing to maintain optimal performance during the current market state.

### 2.6 Limitations of 9, 21, 50 and 200 SMAs

As discussed above, one of the significant limitations of 9, 21, 50 and 200 SMAs are that they are fixed-length SMAs. Fixed-length SMAs are outperformed by variable-length

SMAs, which the KNN SMA is developed to achieve. The KNN SMA is designed to always have the optimal values set through continuous backtesting and maintenance as the market changes. All SMAs inherently are lagging indicators, which is a limitation; however, this doesn't mean that the SMAs aren't profitable and promising indicators for a trend-following investment system. Alpha Decay is present in every strategy and indicator on TV. Strategies and indicators will only retain their competitive edge over a long period if they are continually optimised with the latest price data. To address the issue of alpha decay, it is best to optimise and obtain the most optimal values using the backtesting and strategy parameters discussed below in the parameter optimisation section.

### 2.7 Gaps in Previous Research

Previous research has covered strategies using SMAs; however, some of the gaps include a need for more research papers covering the limitations of the SMAs and how retail investors can use the SMAs on TV. They require a more in-depth understanding and aren't as retail-friendly. Some research papers have more complex systems. For example, deep reinforcement learning [9], time-series clustering [10], Attention-based CNN-LSTM [11], and LSTM-ReGAT [12]. However, those don't work for most retail investors, who only have access to TV instead of technical programming capabilities to operate these complex algorithms. Specifically, the KNN SMA is superior in retail friendliness and computational simplicity compared to the CNN-LSTM and the LSTM-ReGAT. The optimisation of the KNN SMA is also retail-friendly and only requires an extension on Google Chrome called TV Assistant. Allowing retail investors to optimise and back-test their algorithmic strategy bridges the gap between retail and hedge fund investing. This paper aims to provide a retail-friendly strategy that can be executed to become consistently profitable. The creation of the KNN SMA is discussed below.

## 3 Methodology

### 3.1 Development Process

The KNN SMA was created using PS, a beginner-friendly programming language used by the TV platform for investors and traders to create technical indicators for market analysis. There are limitations to strategies and indicators created from PS, as it is a cloud-based programming language, meaning each script requires computational resources on the cloud. Therefore, most AI-based strategies would not work with only PS. One of the benefits of the KNN SMA is that it can be used with PS only, as it's possible to perform KNN Clustering using PS. The current limitations of PS include the quantity of data required, including the size of the script, memory usage, execution time, and additional symbols. PS essentially bridges the gap between retail investors' lack of access to market analysis resources and hedge funds by allowing retail investors to perform algorithmic trading, analysis and data extraction for a dynamic market [13].

Figure 1 includes the code that declares the K and N values with max and min value parameters. The AI-generated line has a toggle option to switch on and off. The input

```
// ~~ Input settings for K and N values
//Number of neighbours used in the KNN algorithm.
//Increasing 'k' can make the prediction more resilient to noise but may decrease sensitivity to local variations.
//This affects how the AI interprets patterns in the price data.
k  = input.int(2, title="Neighbours", minval=1, maxval=100, inline="AI", group="AI(1) Settings")
n_ = input.int(13, title="DataPoints", minval=1, maxval=100, inline="AI", group="AI(1) Settings")
n  = math.max(k, n_)
//Toggle to show or hide the AI-generated moving average line.
aiMa_2  = input.bool(false, title="Show AI(2) Moving Average 1", group="AI(2) Average")
//Toggle to show or hide the AI-calculated slope of the trend.
aiMa_3  = input.bool(true, title="Show AI(2) Moving Average 2", group="AI(2) Average")

// Input parameters for the KNN Moving Average
//Number of closest values used for the calculation of AI(2) Moving Averages.
//A higher number may provide a smoother but less sensitive curve.
numberOfClosestValues = input.int(9, "Number of Closest Values", 2, 200, inline="AI2", group="AI(2) Settings")
//Smoothing period for the initial moving average in the AI(2) algorithm.
smoothingPeriod = input.int(32, "Smoothing Period", 2, 500, inline="aiMa_2", group="AI(2) Settings")
windowSize = math.max(numberOfClosestValues, 30)
//Source data used to classify price as bullish or bearish.
//Can be adjusted to consider different aspects of the price information.
dataToClassify = input.source(close, title= "Data To Classify", group="AI(1) Settings")
//Source data used to calculate the moving average for comparison.
//Different selections may emphasize different aspects of price movement.
dataForMovingAverage = input.source(close, title= "Data For Moving Average (DataForComparison)",group="AI(1) Settings")
negBox_col = input.color(color.new(color.red,75),title="", group="Style", inline="box")
posBox_col = input.color(color.new(color.lime,75),title="", group="Style", inline="box")
line_col   = input.color(color.rgb(255, 169, 39),title="", group="Style", inline="box")
line_width = input.int(2, title="",group="Style", inline="box", tooltip="Box & Line coloring")
//Option to remove or retain historical boxes.
del         = input.bool(false, title="Remove Historical Boxes", group="Style")
//Toggle to remove all boxes from the chart.
del_boxes   = input.bool(true, title="Remove All Boxes", group="Style")
//Toggle to remove all lines from the chart.
del_line    = input.bool(true,title="Remove All Line", group="Style")
```

**Fig. 1.** Variable Declaration for K, N and input parameters of MA.

parameters for the KNN Moving Average include the number of closest values and the smoothing period.

The KNN function is defined in Fig. 2, and Euclidean distances are sorted into it to calculate the weighted sum of KNN. To obtain the k nearest neighbours, we compute the distance from the current point to all other points by using the for loop and setting the distance from the current point to that point. Then, we use a nested loop to sort the distances in ascending order. The KNN SMA is then created with the average of the closest value. A label classifies the current point represented in the KNN Moving Average.

### 3.2 Parameter Optimisation

The TV Assistant tool was used to obtain the optimal values for the KNN SMA, k and number of data points.

Figure 3 shows the four parameters that will be optimised using the TV Assistant. The number of data points will be optimised from 5 to 20 with a step of 2 and a default value of 17. This means the minimum value that could be optimised is five, the maximum is 20, and the current is 17. Each optimisation will move in intervals of 2, for example, 19 or 15; 16 is not feasible as the step is not 1. The neighbours will also be optimised between 2 and 10 with a step of 2 and the default value 10. The number of closest values is optimised from 7 to 30 with a step of 2 and the default value of 7. The smoothing period is optimised from the minimum value of 10 and maximum of 40 with a step of 2 and a default value of 30. Keep in mind that empirical observations is superior to qualitative judgement when it comes to systemisation, however, one could also analyse the exits manually with a qualitative judgement. The optimised K and N values are optimal because they also show the KNN exiting before the COVID crash, and the end of the 2021 bull market. Protecting the investor from a large decline. This is also shown twice in 2021 bull market, where some strategies found it hard to exit in time.

```
// ~~ Define the weighted k-nearest neighbours (KNN) function
knn_weighted(data, labels, k, x) =>
    n1 = data.size()
    distances = array.new_float(n1)
    indices = array.new_int(n1)
    // Compute distances from the current point to all other points
    for i = 0 to n1 - 1
        x_i = data.get(i)
        dist = math.abs(x-x_i)
        distances.set(i, dist)
        indices.set(i, i)
    // Sort distances and corresponding indices in ascending order
    // Bubble sort method
    for i = 0 to n1 - 2
        for j = 0 to n1 - i - 2
            if distances.get(j) > distances.get(j + 1)
                tempDist = distances.get(j)
                distances.set(j, distances.get(j + 1))
                distances.set(j + 1, tempDist)
                tempIndex = indices.get(j)
                indices.set(j, indices.get(j + 1))
                indices.set(j + 1, tempIndex)
    // Compute weighted sum of labels of the k nearest neighbours
    weighted_sum = 0.
    total_weight = 0.
    for i = 0 to k - 1
        index = indices.get(i)
        label_i = labels.get(index)
        weight_i = 1 / (distances.get(i) + 1e-6)
        weighted_sum += weight_i * label_i
        total_weight += weight_i
    weighted_sum / total_weight
//~~~~~~~~~~~~~~~~~~~~~~~~~~~~~~~~~~~~~~~~~~~~~~~~~~~~~~~~~~~~~~~~~~~~~~~

// ~~ Classify the current data point
label_       = knn_weighted(data, labels, k, ma)
//~~~~~~~~~~~~~~~~~~~~~~~~~~~~~~~~~~~~~~~~~~~~~~~~~~~~~~~~~~~~~~~~~~~~~~~

// ~~ kNN Classifier {
meanOfKClosest(value_in_,target_) =>
    closestDistances = array.new_float(numberOfClosestValues, 1e10)
    closestValues = array.new_float(numberOfClosestValues, 0.0)
    for i = 1 to windowSize
        value = value_in_[i]
        distance = math.abs(target_ - value)
        maxDistIndex = 0
        maxDistValue = closestDistances.get(0)
        for j = 1 to numberOfClosestValues - 1
            if closestDistances.get(j) > maxDistValue
                maxDistIndex := j
                maxDistValue := closestDistances.get(j)
        if distance < maxDistValue
            closestDistances.set(maxDistIndex, distance)
            closestValues.set(maxDistIndex, value)
    closestValues.sum() / numberOfClosestValues
//~~~~~~~~~~~~~~~~~~~~~~~~~~~~~~~~~~~~~~~~~~~~~~~~~~~~~~~~~~~~~~~~~~~~~~~

// Initializes the KNN Moving Average.
ma_               = ta.sma(close,smoothingPeriod)
knnMA_price_ma    = meanOfKClosest(close,ma_)
KnnMA_ma_ma       = meanOfKClosest(ma_,ma_)
```

**Fig. 2.** KNN Weight, Euclidean Distance Calculation and KNN MA Initialisation.

**Strategy parameters**

Cycles 7680 from ~7680 Save&Run Skip&Run Cancel

| Active | Parameter | From | To | Step | Default | Priority |
|---|---|---|---|---|---|---|
| ☑ | DataPoints | 5 | 20 | 2 | 13 | 5 |
| ☑ | Neighbours | 2 | 10 | 2 | 2 | 4 |
| ☑ | Number of Closest Values | 7 | 30 | 2 | 9 | 10 |
| ☑ | Smoothing Period | 10 | 40 | 2 | 32 | 11 |
| ☐ | Show AI(1) Moving Average | true | false | 0 | false | 1 |
| ☐ | Show AI(1) Slope | true | false | 0 | true | 2 |
| ☐ | Select MA | SMA;EM | | 0 | SMA | 3 |
| ☐ | Data To Classify | close;op | | 0 | close | 6 |
| ☐ | Data For Moving Average (DataForComparison) | close;op | | 0 | close | 7 |
| ☐ | Show AI(2) Moving Average 1 | true | false | 0 | false | 8 |
| ☐ | Show AI(2) Moving Average 2 | true | false | 0 | true | 9 |
| ☐ | Remove Historical Boxes | true | false | 0 | false | 12 |
| ☐ | Remove All Boxes | true | false | 0 | true | 13 |
| ☐ | Remove All Line | true | false | 0 | true | 14 |

**Fig. 3.** Strategy Parameter Optimisation.

### 3.3 Backtest Setup

Assuming that the strategy has been coded already, the first step is to download the TV Assistant from the Chrome Web Store, the backtesting tool we will use. The second step is to open up the TV Assistant when the KNN SMA strategy is on the asset you want to use the KNN SMA on. It is recommended that the settings be changed to max value of sharpe ratio by annealing with more than 2.9 for sortino ratio on the 1D timeframe. After the backtesting, the user must click "Options & Tools" and "Clear all" to remove the previously stored data from the previous backtest and restart the backtest.

### 3.4 Replication in Other Markets

The KNN SMA also works in the Stock market. To use the KNN SMA in the stock market, the user must identify trending stocks. Once the stock is identified, the user should complete backtesting using the TV Assistant tool, as mentioned above, and find the optimal values to determine whether the stock is in an uptrend or downtrend.

## 4 Hardware and Software Requirements

The only software requirement is a web browser. What does require more hardware specifications is the optimisation process of the KNN SMA. A computer with 24 GB of RAM and a modern, fast processor would be ideal, as the optimisation time required for a laptop with 16 GB of RAM and a decent processor is two to three times longer. Using these hardware specifications to backtest, we show our results below.

## 5 Results and Discussion

Table 1 shows the back-tested results of the KNN SMA vs the 9, 21, 50 and 200 SMAs on the BTCUSD chart since 2018. The results also include the max drawdown (DD).

**Table 1.** Results of 9, 21, 50, 200 and KNN SMA.

| Strategy | Net Profit | Total Closed Trades | Percent Profitable | Profit Factor | Max DD | Avg Trade | Avg # Bars in Trade |
|---|---|---|---|---|---|---|---|
| 9 MA | 5.77% | 874 | 30.32% | 1.208 | 4.98% | | 7 |
| 21 MA | 1,202.81% | 228 | 30.70% | 1.206 | 59.21% | 1.78% | 12 |
| 50 MA | 2,794.18% | 103 | 28.16% | 1.651 | 54.80% | 7.06% | 25 |
| 200 MA | 340.52% | 39 | 17.95% | 1.582 | 65.28% | 10.38% | 64 |
| KNN SMA | 5,751.23% | 130 | 27.69% | 1.734 | 38.72% | 5.06% | 20 |

The Strategy column represents the strategy backtested. Net Profit represents the percentage of profit obtained from the strategy compared to the original net worth. Total Closed Trades represent the number of trades opened and closed, for example, buy and sell signals. Percent Profitable represents the percentage of profitable trades compared to losses. The profit factor represents how much money was made per dollar invested. Max drawdown represents the maximum percentage of unrealised losses. Average trade represents the average of each single trade's profit or loss. Average bars in trades represents the number of candles/bars between each trade. From the completed backtests, the KNN SMA is superior in most criteria. Statistically significant observations include fewer false signals generated, observed through trade closes and profit factors. Drawdown is minimal relative to the other MAs. Net Profit displays the potential competitive edge of the KNN SMA. Its important to note that the KNN SMA is backtested with data since 2018, which includes the bear and bull market, thus the performance of the KNN SMA will hold during both market conditions. The KNN SMA, is backtested on Bitcoin as most cryptocurrency's move in the same direction as Bitcoin, as they are highly correlated. The KNN SMA can be backtested and optimised for assets that are less correlated to Bitcoin, for example SUI. In the recent Bitcoin ranging environment SUI has continued its uptrend, and the KNN SMA has yet to show a sell signal.

### 5.1 Net Profit

The KNN SMA has the highest net profit of 5,751.23%, yielding the best gains. The 9 MA is too aggressive and fast; thus, with each trade, the gas fees cut into the profits. In other words, if an indicator is too fast, there will be constant sell and buy signals being generated, and with each sell or buy signal, the portfolio composition has to be reworked, usually transactions on the same chain cost approximately 1% of the transaction amount, with additional costs to bridging. So gas fees, will cut into the profits if an indicator is producing too many signals aggressively. The 21 and 50 MA are good to use; they are mostly accurate and the most popular moving averages, with 50 MA as the most popular for medium-term trend classification. 200 MA doesn't yield as much gains as it's primarily used as a bull/bear market cycle indicator instead of a pure trend following indicator, only yielding 340.52%, nonetheless still profitable.

### 5.2 Total Closed Trades

As discussed above, the 9 MA is the worst indicator for trend-following strategies because it is too fast for Bitcoin's volatile price action. Eight hundred and seventy-four trades in six years are too many for a medium to long-term investor. The 21 and 50 MA are much better for the quantity of trades required. Each trade requires a rebalancing of the portfolio. Thus, a good benchmark to aim for is between 80 and 240 trades since 2018 when back-testing trend following systems. The 200 MA is too slow. Therefore, much of the profits were not secured during the trends, so the 200 MA should not be relied on for exits and entries to trades. The KNN SMA has an ideal trade quantity towards the lower range of 80–240, which requires less rebalancing but captures most of the gains in trends.

### 5.3 Percent Profitable

The general public commonly misunderstands this metric as an essential metric. The percentage of the time a strategy is profitable isn't necessary as long as it is profitable.

Since most of the time, the market is in consolidation or a mean reverting state, trend-following systems usually average a percentage profitable between 25 and 35%. As stated above, the 200 SMA is not recommended as a trend-following component as it is too slow, and it's percent profitable metric also highlights this problem.

### 5.4 Profit Factor

The Profit Factor metric is critical because it determines how profitable the strategy is in isolation for each dollar lost. In other words, these are just gross profits divided by gross losses. Any profit factor above 0 is a positive Expected Value (EV) system. The KNN SMA has a very generous Profit Factor of 1.734. It is important to note that any single metric cannot be used to determine whether a component is better than another, as the 9 MA also has a higher profit factor by a margin than the 21 MA. Thus, it's required to aggregate multiple different metrics for comparison. The main point for the Profit Factor is that if a component has a Profit Factor greater than 1.5, it's a high-quality component that should be saved for future use in system creation. The KNN SMA, 50 SMA and 200 SMA conveniently fit this criteria.

### 5.5 Max Drawdown

Whilst having a low max drawdown percentage is desirable as there's less volatility towards the downside, aiming to have an indicator that has less volatility will yield more trades and more management is required. This is a problem with the 9 SMA. The max drawdown is very good because every time there's a slight price decrease, the 9 MA will generate a sell signal. However, this means there's more management, and potential gains have been lost to extremely high fees and being constantly kicked out of trends. The 21, 50, 200 and KNN SMA all have decent max drawdowns, with 200 being the worst. However, the 200 has the highest max drawdown simply because of its slow nature.

### 5.6 Average Trade

This metric is mostly useless, as it doesn't determine the system's profitability. It only ensures that the average trade exceeds the fees required to rebalance the portfolio. Any number more significant than 4% is considered excellent. The fast-moving averages, 9 and 21 MA, have issues with the average trade percentage, so using them as entry and exit criteria isn't recommended. When the average trade percentage is low, trades will become unprofitable, as each trade requires gas fees to open and close a position, or rebalance capital.

### 5.7 Average # of Bars in Trades

Average Bars in Trades are a metric used to determine how much management a component will require. The lower the average bars in trades, the more often the component will generate a buy or sell signal. A higher average bar in trades means a longer time before a signal is generated. Generally, a higher average bar in trades is better. However, this isn't important as it does not directly affect a strategy's potential gains.

## 5.8 Key Dates in Backtesting

Key dates in backtesting include the date of the COVID-19 crash in March of 2020.

Figure 4 shows the KNN SMA's reaction to the COVID Crash. The KNN SMA detects the downtrend early and generates a sell signal at a relatively early exit compared to other SMAs. A total of fourteen trades were taken for the KNN SMA. A higher timeframe indicator is expected for the 200 SMA's exit and entry. There are better indicators than the 200 SMA. As it is a longer-term indicator, eight trades are taken, less than the KNN SMA. During the crash, the 21 SMA exited at a higher price and earlier than the KNN SMA and entered earlier at a lower cost than the KNN SMA. However, the indicator needs fixing with false signals. The figure shows that many LONG and SHORT flips represent a lower-quality indicator. This causes over-rebalancing and absurd fees with little to no gain. Many false signals throughout the period are not particularly useful; however, aggregating with higher timeframe indicators may generate a sell signal before the COVID-19 crash. During the COVID Crash, the 50 SMA exited at a lower price, one day later than the KNN SMA did, and entered slightly lower than the KNN SMA a few days after the KNN SMA generated a LONG signal. The 50 SMA is the best SMA to use when choosing between the 9, 21, 50, and 200 SMAs. However, compared to the KNN SMA, the 50 SMA is subpar. One of the reasons the 50 SMA is subpar is that it can't be optimised to create a more competitive edge, unlike the KNN SMA, which can achieve this. The 50 SMA has a significant amount of trades, with minimal false signals; the false signals on the right are expected as it's a consolidation.

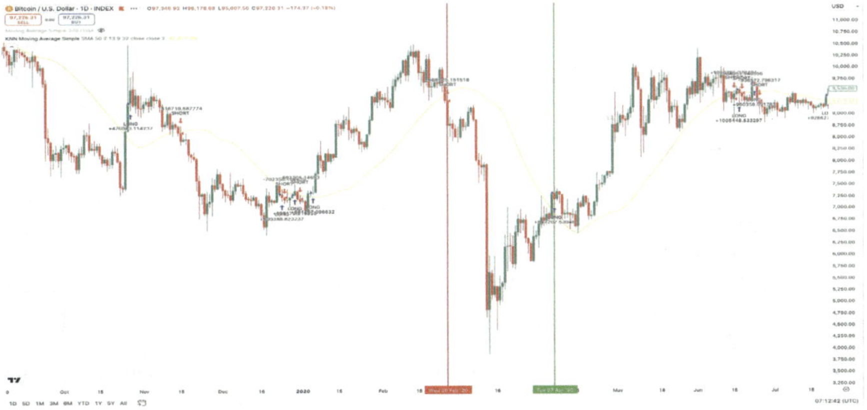


**Fig. 4.** COVID Crash KNN SMA.

# 6 Potential Data Limitations and Trade-Offs Between Metrics

There are some limitations with backtesting the KNN SMA for cryptocurrencies. Bitcoin has the most extended price history; however, due to the inception of shorts in 2018, the price action before 2018 can't be used. Therefore, only a sample size of two bull markets can be used with Bitcoin. Metrics must be considered a balance, not only focusing on one metric. Only concentrating on Net Profit would yield a less robust strategy, with potentially more significant drawdowns. Similarly, only focusing on reducing the max drawdown would result in many false signals, lowering the strategy's performance.

## 7 Conclusion

While there are other methods for trend classification, the KNN SMA demonstrated above is accessible to retail traders and investors using the TV platform. Using more complex techniques, such as Deep Belief Networks, to classify market trends may be less beneficial to them [14]. The KNN SMA developed for this research can be used on TV by retail investors to classify trend direction. The comparison has shown that the KNN SMA significantly outperforms the 9, 21, 50 and 200 SMA. Whilst the KNN SMA is profitable itself, relying on only one indicator is not recommended, and an aggregation of multiple similar edges are required to remain consistently profitable in the markets. One of the significant benefits of the KNN SMA is its ease of access as anyone with internet access to TV can use this indicator for free. Future work includes performing statistical analysis to validate the performance differences between the KNN SMA and traditional SMAs, as incorporating the tests using p-values and confidence intervals would enhance the creditability of the KNN SMA's performance. Another needed future work is to fine-tune the KNN SMA even more to improve its performance in the future.

## References


1. Kovačević, T., et al.: Optimal trend labeling in financial time series. IEEE Access. (2023)
2. Ellis, C., et al.: Is smarter better? A comparison of adaptive, and simple moving average trading strategies. Res. Int. Bus. Financ. **19**(3), 399–411 (2005)
3. Chantarakasemchit, O., et al.: Forex rates prediction on EUR/USD with simple moving average technique and financial factors. In: 2020 17th International Conference on Electrical Engineering/Electronics, Computer, Telecommunications and Information Technology (ECTI-CON), p. 2020
4. Nabipour, M., et al.: Predicting stock market trends using machine learning and deep learning algorithms via continuous and binary data; a comparative analysis. IEEE Access. **8**, 150199–150212 (2020)
5. Derbentsev, V., et al.: Comparative performance of machine learning ensemble algorithms for forecasting cryptocurrency prices. Int. J. Eng. **34**(1), 140–148 (2021)
6. Guo, G., et al.: KNN model-based approach in classification. In: On the Move to Meaningful Internet Systems, Berlin (2003)
7. Ren, L., Ren, P.: Applying a combined max-min simple moving average trading strategy to market indexes. Econ. Manag. Finan. Market. **13**(2), 11–23 (2018)
8. Khand, S., et al.: The predictability and profitability of simple moving averages and trading range breakout rules in the Pakistan Stock Market. Rev. Pac. Basin Financ. Mark. Policies. **23**(1), 2050001 (2020)
9. Kochliaridis, V., et al.: Combining deep reinforcement learning with technical analysis and trend monitoring on cryptocurrency markets. Neural Comput. & Applic. **35**, 21445–21462 (2023)

10. Ozer, F., Sakar, C.O.: An automated cryptocurrency trading system based on the detection of unusual price movements with a Time-Series Clustering-Based approach. Expert Syst. Appl. **200**, 117017 (2022)
11. Peng, P., et al.: Attention-based CNN–LSTM for high-frequency multiple cryptocurrency trend prediction. Expert Syst. Appl. **237**(121520) (2024)
12. Zhong, C., Du, W., Xu, W., Huang, Q., Zhao, Y., Wang, M.: LSTM-ReGAT: a network-centric approach for cryptocurrency price trend prediction. Decis. Support. Syst. **169**, 113955 (2023)
13. Rathore, S., Prakash, H., Balachander, T.: Trading Automation Using PineScript. In: 2024 International Conference on Intelligent Systems for Cybersecurity (ISCS), Gurugram (2024)

# Implementation of Descriptive Similarity for Estimation Elective Programs of Political Parties

Maryna Averkyna[1,2(✉)], Peeter Lorents[1], and Maria Khvalko[3]

[1] Management & Organization Department, Estonian Business School, Tallinn, Estonia
{maryna.averkyna,peeter.lorents}@ebs.ee
[2] Management Organization Department, Lviv Polytechnic National University, Lviv, Ukraine
[3] Department of Financial Control, Soufllet Agro, Kyiv, Ukraine

**Abstract.** The paper deals with implementation of Descriptive Similarity for numeric estimation of the similarity of the elective programs of political parties. The method - the assessment of descriptive similarity - based on simple arithmetic operations and the use of so-called equalization's tables is easy to use for academic political scientists and policy observers. Method of estimation statements' similarity is very crucial for scientific areas such as management, decision-making process, military, politics. The programs of nine political parties were analysed. The authors studied the parties from the big number of parties. The amazing comparisons were received during investigation. We could see that for politics it can be useful in order to prove the ideology of a political party and check the populistic statements. The proposed approach to the automated estimation of the similarity coefficient is important for the formation of applied artificial intelligence. This will allow not only to quickly assess the similarity of programs but also to form a basis for machine learning to confirm the existing ideology of the party or its absence.

**Keywords:** Descriptive Similarity · Statements of the Programs · Political Parties · Elections · Applied Artificial Intelligence

## 1 Introduction

The election of national authorities or local self-government body plays a significant role in the life of every democratic society. The decisions on which political choices are based (e.g. who to be chosen and reasons for such choice) play an important role in the development and governance of democratic societies. At the same time, decision-making process is hampered mostly by the personal impressions (not analyzes) that some political programs seem to be either too similar or, conversely, different enough from the others ones. In certain states we can observe electoral claiming that all parties promote the very same agenda, and do not offer anything new despite of drastic changes in the political environment. Before the election, we can see that the party's election programs are being actively disseminated. There are also a large number of sociological


K. Daimi and A. Alsadoon (Eds.): ICR 2025, LNNS 1487, pp. 28–39, 2025.
https://doi.org/10.1007/978-3-031-95652-2_3

organizations that assess the rating of parties. However, it is difficult to understand why do the voters choose this particular party, how do they analyze election programs and how do they make their choice.

In this case, the problem of analyses political parties' programs is important. Comparison statement of the program helps people to make a clear decision, such as it helps to clear understand ideas, values and direction of the parties' activities. Nieves Zúñiga mentioned that there are four crucisl aspects to consider when analysing political manifestos: their function, the context in which they are designed and exist, how they are created, and their content [17]. She also mentioned that content analysis finds to quantify patterns within a text in an objective, replicable and systematic manner [17].

The estimation of political parties' programs (2014 year) is presented by the independent analytic platform Vox Ukraine. This approach based on content analyses which involves determining the frequency of words related to priority (e.g. Ukraine, law, war, business, state, power, corruption, Europe, radical, country, economy, creating, security development). Based on this approach, a conclusion was made about the correlation between party programs. The authors of the approach also noted that the surveyed parties compete for the average voter, while the radical parties differentiated themselves by talking about different things [3]. It is very important that Ukrainian scientists tried to analyze the programs' similarity. From our point of view, it is difficult make a decision based only on similar keywords. In the present work, we believe that comparing statements with the simplest and clearest possible statements is more effective than using keywords. More specifically, for statements which, like the formulas used to describe systems in algebraic systems (see Malcev Chp. III, §6, 6.2), are derived from so-called atomic statements (i.e., statements about the evolution of properties and being connected) through logical operations (e.g. "and", "or", "no", "if … then …", etc.) [10].

The aim of this work is to create an approach and apply it to assess the similarity of party programs. This approach is based on a numerical assessment of the descriptive similarity of the sets of statements. This, in turn, is based on the pairing of equilizable statements (where the first position has a statement from one set and the second position has a statement from another set).

## 2 Aplied Approach of Analyses Political Parties' Program

In case when we want to analyses the similarity of political parties' programs the descriptions are very crucial. Well-written and practically applicable descriptions usually are consist of relevant statements. Therefore, we expect *the descriptions to be a set of relevant statements*. A closer look at the statements often reveals that they can be 'reformatted' into formulas of predicate calculus (or 'quite accurately' - into formulas of the theories of the corresponding algebraic systems).

It is not excessive to take into account here certain features related to whether the similarity of any set of statements is assessed or the similarity of the systems (including, for example, situations or developments) described by those statements. For example, if we want to assess the similarity of party programs in terms of substance and number - then we are dealing with the calculation of the similarity of sets of statements. However, if we want to compare, for example, any specific situations or developments based on their descriptions (or sets of corresponding statements), we need to deal with the structural similarity (e.g. homomorphism) of the systems and the sets of systems theory formulas that provide relevant statements. For this we can rely, for example, on the theorem that if a positive formula (i.e. without denials and implications) is correct for one system, then it is also correct for another system if the first and second are homomorphic (see e.g. Malcev 1973, Chp III, §7, 7.2) [10].

The poposed approach based on assessment the similarity of the programs of political parties. Two programs at a time. The main steps in this procedure are:

1. Choosing of two programs (hereinafter – the first and the second) for comparability.
2. Separation of statements contained in programs from other text.
3. Creation the two sets of statements - or the lists, the elements of which are statements from the programs of political parties.
4. Comparing the statements in first list with the statements in the second list and forming ordered pairs in which we have chosen to equilize the statements with each other.

Based on the foregoing, we agree in the following that we will consider on a language which is suitable for the theory of algebraic system. In order to evaluate the descriptive similarity of the descriptions or sets of relevant statements – that is, the descriptive similarity of some things, situations, developments, etc., we will use the numerical value defined by Lorents below - the descriptive similarity coefficient.

$$\begin{aligned} \mathrm{Sim}(P, Q) &= E(\mathrm{Com}(P, Q)) : [E(P)\text{--}E(\mathrm{Com}(P, Q)) + E(Q)] = \\ & E(\mathrm{Com}(P, Q)) : \left[E(\mathrm{Spec}(P)) + E(\mathrm{Com}(P, Q)) + E(\mathrm{Spec}(Q))\right] \end{aligned} \tag{1}$$

There

E(Com(P,Q)) is the number of element of the set Com(P,Q), or the set of elements that are ordered pairs, where the first position of the pair has the statements P, the second position has the statement Q, and these statements have been equalized by each other;

**Remark.** There is an important distinction between the Lorents coefficient and the Jaccard coefficient (see [5, 6]): for the Jaccard coefficient, the set $P \cap Q$ should have been used instead of Com(P, Q).

E(P) is the number of element of the set P or set whose elements are statements from the first description;
E(Q) is the number of element of the set Q or set whose elements are statements from the second description;
E(Spec(P)) is the number of element of the set Spec(P) or set so-called specific statements that appear in the description P but do not have equivalent ones in the description Q;
E(Spec(Q)) is the number of element of the set Spec(Q) or set so-called specific statements that appear in the description Q but do not have equivalent ones in the description P.

Peeter Lorents and Maryna Averkyna in 2019 presented the application of descriptive similarity in the process of managing the development of urban transport systems in small towns in Estonia and Ukraine [7]. Proposed investigation helps managers to understand towns' similarity. In this case, if similarity coefficient is closer to one, managers can use information obtained in one city for urban transportation management during Decision-Making Process. Thus, managers can form system of precedent solution based on the real experience [1, 2].

## 3 Analyses Parties' Election Programs

Ukraine has a multiparty system, and as of January 1, 2021, 365 political parties are officially registered in Ukraine [18]. In the elections to the Verkhovna Rada in 2019, 22 political parties participated, 5 of which became parliamentary. According to the election results, five political parties ran for the Verkhovna Rada of the IX convocation in accordance with party lists: Sluha Narodu (Servant of the People, SN) – 43.16%, Oppozytsiyna Platforma – za Zhyttia (Opposition Platform - For Life, OPZZh) – 13.05%, VO Batkivshchyna (All-Ukrainian Union 'Fatherland') – 8.18%, Yevropeiska Solidarnist (European Solidarity, YeS) – 8.10%, 'Holos' (The Voice) – 5.82%.

We propose to analyze the programs of parties which became parliamentary and program of parties that were the closest to 5% barrier. The election programs of the following political parties were under considiration for the investigation:

1. Holos.
2. Yevropeiska Solidarnist.
3. Oppozytsiyna Platforma – za Zhyttia.
4. Oppozytsiynyi Block (Opposition Bloc(k), Oppobloc(k)).
5. Radykalna partiya Oleha Liashka (Oleh Lyashko's Radical Party, RPL).
6. Syla i Chest (Strenght and Honor, SiCh)'.
7. Sluha Narodu.
8. Ukrainska stratehiia Hroismana (Ukrainian Strategy of Groysman, Ukrainian Strategy).
9. Batkivshchyna.

In order to achieve our goal, we propose to collect information (statements) from websites of political parties mentioned above.

At the next stage, it is necessary to assess how the investigated party-programs are similar with compared ones. For such purpose, we propose to form a list of the statements based on the received information. Listed of the system's statements is to be filled to the table for all parties. We recommend forming a table of the statements' party which described the statements (see Table 1).

**Table 1.** Determination of Political Party's Statements

| Number of the statements | The fragment of the list of statements from the program of the 'Servant of the People' |
|---|---|
| 1 | Abolition of the parliamentary deputies'immunity |

(*continued*)

**Table 1.** (*continued*)

| Number of the statements | The fragment of the list of statements from the program of the 'Servant of the People' |
|---|---|
| 2 | Carrying out decentralization of power in accordance with EU legislation |
| 3 | 'Restart' (total revocation of acting members and assignment of the fresh ones) of the High Council of Justice and the High Qualifications Commission of Judges |
| 4. | Implementation of the proportional election system with open lists of candidates |
| 5. | Ensuring real independence of anti-corruption authorities |
| 6. | Legislative regulation of the right to carry a weapon |
| 7. | Return of responsibility of officials for unlawful enrichment |
| | ////////////////////////////// |
| | //////////////////////////// |
| 74. | Introduction of a tax on withdrawn capital |
| 75. | Promotion of Ukrainian goods on global markets. |

**Table 2.** Equalization Political parties' program statements

| Program Party 'Servant of the People' describes the statements | Equivalent statements | | | Program Party 'Opposition platform - for life' describes the statement |
|---|---|---|---|---|
| | The wording from the first | The wording from the second | The wording for both | |
| 1. | Abolition of the parliamentary deputies' immunity | Abolition of the parliamentary deputies' and judges' immunity | Abolition of the parliamentary deputies' and judges' immunity | |
| 2. | Carrying out decentralization of power in accordance with EU legislation | Reforming the political system, expanding the powers of local self-government | Expanding the powers of local self-government | |

(*continued*)

**Table 2.** (*continued*)

| Program Party 'Servant of the People' describes the statements | Equivalent statements | | | Program Party 'Opposition platform - for life' describes the statement |
|---|---|---|---|---|
| | The wording from the first | The wording from the second | The wording for both | |
| 3. 'Restart' (total revocation of acting members and assignment of the fresh ones) of the High Council of Justice and the High Qualifications Commission of Judges | | | | |
| 4. | Implementation of the proportional election system with open lists of candidates | Transition from a corrupt mixed electoral system to a proportional system with open lists | Proportional system elections with open lists | |
| 5. | Return of responsibility of officials for unlawful enrichment | Strengthening criminal liability for committing corruption crimes by officials | Responsibility for corruption crimes | |
| | | | | 6.Abolition of laws on language, education, renaming of the church; about decommunization, lustration… |
| | | | | 7.Removal of immunity from the president of Ukraine, adoption of the law on temporary investigative commissions of the Verkhovna Rada |

(*continued*)

**Table 2.** (*continued*)

| Program Party 'Servant of the People' describes the statements | Equivalent statements | | | Program Party 'Opposition platform - for life' describes the statement |
|---|---|---|---|---|
| | The wording from the first | The wording from the second | The wording for both | |
| 8. Ensuring real independence of anti-corruption authorities | | | | |
| //////////////////////////// | | | | |
| //////////////////////////// | | | | |
| 75. Promotion of Ukrainian goods on global markets. | | | | |

Then we propose to compare the statements' first list with the statements' second list. We form a table to assess the general statements of the party (see Table 2).

Based on comparisons of the party list of statements, we propose to form a table of equalized statements in order to estimate the Lorents coefficient. Statements that describe Program party A, equalized statements between systems, and statements that describe program party B) necessary to write in the table (see Table 3). In case, when all statements are written down, it is necessary to assess the Lorents's coefficient. This will allow us to look at how much the programs are similar.

Then we propose to create towns' similitude matrix (see Table 3). According to the results of Table 3, it should be noted that the nearer the value of the coefficient is to zero, the greater the difference between the programs of political parties. Also, the closer the meaning of the Lorents's coefficient is to one, the more similar the programs of political parties are.

According to the results of assesment, the most unique are the programs of the political parties 'Voice' and 'Opposition platform - for life' SimLT ('Voice', 'Opposition bloc) = 0.031. In turn, the programs of the political parties 'Opposition platform - for life' and 'Radical Party of Oleg Lyashko' were the most similar, the coefficient of similarity was 0.234. It is also worth mentioning the similarity of the program of the political parties 'Opposition platform - for life' and 'Opposition Bloc', where the coefficient of similarity was 0.207.

In summary, we can conclude that the degree of similarity of the election programs of political parties is quite low. It can be explained by amount of programs' statements - from 10 to 100. If the number of statements of one political force is much larger than that of another political party, this leads to low values of the similarity coefficient. We could see that the big difference between political parties' programs related with ideology of party or its absence. For example, it was established that of political party 'Opposition platform - for life' has social conservatism ideology. Political party 'Servant

**Table 3.** Parties‘ Similitude Matrix

| Political parties | Servant of the People | Opposition platform - for life' | European Solidarity | Batkivshchyna | Voice | Power and Honor | Opposition bloc» | Ukrainian Strategy of Groysman | Oleg Lashkar's Radical Political Party |
|---|---|---|---|---|---|---|---|---|---|
| Servant of the People | 1 | 0,075 | 0,107 | 0,095 | 0,123 | 0,130 | 0,052 | 0,127 | 0,045 |
| Opposition platform - for life' | | 1 | 0,085 | 0,106 | 0,077 | 0,148 | 0,207 | 0,159 | 0,234 |
| European Solidarity | | | 1 | 0,056 | 0,072 | 0,082 | 0,056 | 0,099 | 0,081 |
| Batkivshchyna | | | | 1 | 0,056 | 0,044 | 0,057 | 0,040 | 0,069 |
| Voice | | | | | 1 | 0,057 | 0,031 | 0,085 | 0,063 |
| Power and Honor | | | | | | 1 | 0,067 | 0,111 | 0,140 |
| Opposition bloc | | | | | | | 1 | 0,050 | 0,078 |
| Ukrainian Strategy of Groysman | | | | | | | | 1 | 0,055 |
| Oleg Lyashko's Radical Political Party. | | | | | | | | | 1 |

of the People' ideology is absent. The statements of this party have populistic feature. It is necessary to point out that the ideology of this chat party has changed [19, 21].

From the beginning of the de facto creation of the Sluha Narodu party in mid-2019 until November 2019, the declared ideology of the party was libertarianism. However, on November 10, 2019, the new leader of the party, Oleksandr Kornienko, stated that the party ideology 'had been changed from libertarianism to something in between liberal and socialist views' [20]. But a few months later, at the party's regular congress on February 15, 2020, he decided on a new party ideology from supporters 'something between liberal and socialist views', to Ukrainian centrism. However, in February 2021, in an interview with Ukrinform, Oleksandr Kornienko explained that the party's ideology is centrist, in particular, in addition to the former Ukrainian centrism, Kornienko also mentioned radical centrism'. Also, the comparison of the programs' statements allows us to check ideology of political party based on statements. We could see that after the estimation statements' similarity the ideology (social constructivism) of Oppozytsiyna Platforma – za Zhyttia is proved by statements.

Applying a coefficient of similarity to compare party election programs allows a numerical assessment of their similarity (or, conversely, 'originality') to be based not only on how many times or how often some "significant" keywords may be noticed, but also on what the programs say. The predominantly small numerical assessments of similarity in this case suggest the existence of a strange, if not paradoxical, phenomenon:

how it is possible to draw such a large number of different visions (programs) for the same field (e.g. the situation in Ukraine after the elections), based on a number of different (ie not equilizable) statements? We would like to emphasize that the difference between these statements is not due to different wordings of (the same things), but still to the fact that these statements are not equivalent! It is worth noting that the strangely small numerical estimates of similarity highlighted above also appeared in the descriptions of situations immediately preceding armed conflict (See [9]). However, such a strangeness has not been revealed, for example, in the official descriptions of small Estonian cities or in the descriptions of the public transport situations in these cities. However, it is practical to use the developed algorithm to analyze large amounts of qualitative information. In conclusion, it is necessary to automate the process of calculating the similarity coefficient. We have to respond the following questions related with transforming natural language statements into formulas for the theory of a suitable algebraic system and ways of the turning the "movements" that occur during the decision-making process from one statement into another into derivative steps.

In these cases mentioned above, it is in principle not necessary to create and use the systems that are based on algorithms and operate completely autonomously. Thus, one can be based on self-learning dialogue systems, which achive more and more independence and reliability during use.

Among the many self-learning dialogue systems of this kind and their theoretical foundations, those created by Matsak E. could be mentioned (Matsak, 2006) [12, 13]. For example, DST (Matsak, 2007, 2008). In a very brief description, the work of DST consists of two modes to transform the sentences. The first mode is teaching the program. The user transforms a sentence phase after phase [11, 12]. The dialog system for extracting the logical constructions from Estonian text uses the HTML morph analyzer and the synthesizer of the Estonian language, located at http://www.filosoft.ee. The devision of derivative steps has been presented by Matsak E. in works published in 2006, 2007, 2008, 2009 [13–16]. These steps include transforming text formula and interference level. For that, we propose to use the method and algorithm, which were presented by Maryna Averkyna at the HCI International 2020 (see Fig. 1) [2].

To determine to which group the programs's statement belongs, it is crucial to create a software product based on the developed algorithm – rather a procedure (which, as mentioned above, does not necessarily guarantee algorithmic solvency in the sense of mathematical algorithm theory, also known as recursive function theory [4, 11]. It helps to develop the software for program analyses statements. In this case applied artificial intelligence tools helps to storage information and propose the results for the decision-making process. We propose to use the R studio software for calculation coefficient similarity. For this aim the creation google form is required (see Fig. 2).

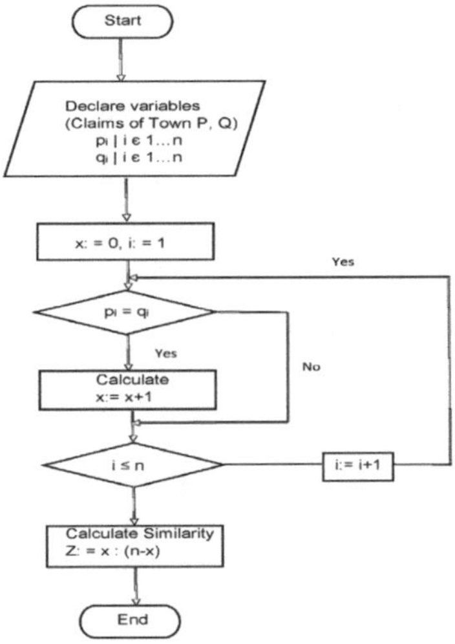


**Fig. 1.** Flowchart for Google-form based similarity analysis [4]

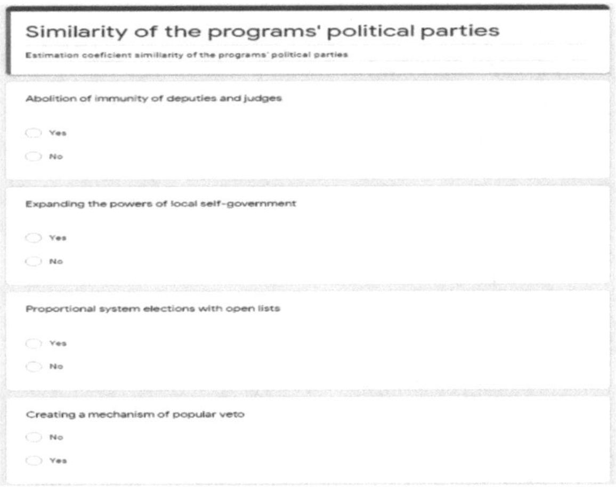


**Fig. 2.** Example of creation the Google-form for similarity analysis

## 4 Conclusion

This paper presents the methodology of the applyingfor example of descriptive similarity in order to assess the similarity or, on the contrary, the specificity of the positions and intentions of these parties based on the statements contained in the parties' programs. We discussed the Descriptive Similarity implementation analyses political parties' programs. We pointed out that this approach allows people makes clear decisions during elections. We proposed the procedure, which based on the collection of information, the occurrence of predicates, the value of the function of the type of information about the steps of the subdivision.

Also, it necessary to point out that ***obtained results are very amazing***. The coefficient similarity political parties' programs are within the range of 0.031–0.234. Multiple checks by different, independent individuals on whether

1. existing but important statements have been inadvertently ignored,
2. statements that were not actually included in party programs have not been in
3. no unidentified statements have been identified, what should have been identified, whether
4. there were no accidentally identified statements that should not have been identified

**We did not practically change the numerical estimates obtained**!

For example, we can make the statements' comparization analyses of Estonian small towns and Ostroh (Ukraine) is within the range of 0.49–0.6 [8]. From the other side the results of assess the statements of armed conflicts shown the similar situation as estimation statements' similarity of political parties [9].

Method of estimation statements' similarity is very crucial for scientific areas such as management, decision-making process, military, politics. We could see that for politics it can be useful in order to prove the ideology of a political party and check the populistic statements.

The proposed approach to the automated estimation of the similarity coefficient is important for the formation of applied artificial intelligence. This will allow not only to quickly assess the similarity of programs but also to form a basis for machine learning to confirm the existing ideology of the party or its absence.

## References

1. Averkyna, M.: A Similarity-Based Decision Process for Decisions' Implementation. In: Advanced in Artificial Intelligence and Applied Cognitive Computing. The 2020 World Congress in Computer Science, Computer Engineering, and Applied Computing CSCE 2020, Luxor Hotel (MGM Property), 3900 Las Vegas Blvd. South, Las Vegas, 89109, USA, July 27–30 (2020)
2. Averkyna, M.: Implementation of Descriptive Similarity for Decision Making in Smart Cities. In: Stephanidis, C., et al. (eds.) HCI International 2020 – Late Breaking Papers: Interaction, Knowledge and Social Media. HCII 2020 Lecture Notes in Computer Science, pp. 28–39 (2020)
3. Comparison of programs of political parties. Ukrainian truth, 21 October, 2014 https://www.pravda.com.ua/articles/2014/10/21/7041350/
4. Cutlend, N.: An Introduction to Recursive Function Theory, p. 250. Cambridge University Press (1980)
5. Jaccard, P.: Distribution de la flore alpine dans le bassin des Dranses et dans quelques régions voisines. Bulletin de la Société Vaudoise des Sciences Naturelles. **37**, 241–272 (1901a)
6. Jaccard, P.: Étude comparative de la distribution florale dans une portion des Alpes et des Jura. Bulletin de la Société Vaudoise des Sciences Naturelles. **37**, 547–579 (1901b)
7. Lorents, P., Averkyna, M.: Some mathematical and practical aspects of Decision-Making based on similarity. In: Stephanidis, C. (ed.) HCI International 2019 – Late Breaking Papers. HCII 2019 Lecture Notes in Computer Science, vol. 11786, p. 2019. Springer, Cham

8. Lorents, P., Averkyna, M.: Method of similarity implementation for the decision-making process in small towns transportation management. In: Russo, D., Ahram, T., Karwowski, W., Di Bucchianico, G., Taiar, R. (eds.) Intelligent Human Systems Integration 2021. IHSI 2021. Advances in Intelligent Systems and Computing, vol. 1322. Springer (2021)
9. Lorents, P., Kuuseok, A., Lorents, E.: Applying systems' similarities to assess the plausibility of armed conflicts. In: Lecture Notes in Electrical Engineering: Smart Information and Communication Technologies (Smart-ICT-19), Saidia, Morocco, pp. 26–29 (2019)
10. Maltsev, A.I.: Algebraic Systems. Springer (1973)
11. Malcev, A.I.: Algorithms and Recursive Functions. Wolters-Noordhoff Publishing, Groninge (1970)
12. Matsak, E.: Using natural language dialog system DST for discovery of logical constructions of children's speech. In: The 2006 International Conference on Artificial Intelligence IC-AI 2006, Las Vegas, Nevada, USA, vol. I, pp. 325–331 (2006)
13. Matsak, E.: System DST for Transforming Natural Language Texts, Representing Estimates and Higher Order Predicates and Functionals. In: The 3rd International Conference on Cybernetics and Information Technologies, Systems and Applications: CITSA 2006, vol. III, pp. 79–84 (2006)
14. Matsak, E.: The prototype of system for discovering of inference rules. In: Proceedings of the International Conference on Artificial Intelligence. IC – AI'2007, vol. II, pp. 489–492 (2007)
15. Matsak, E.: Improved version of the natural language dialog system DST and its application for discovery of logical constructions in children's speech. In: Proceedings of the International Conference on Artificial Intelligence. IC – AI'2008, vol. II, pp. 332–338 (2008)
16. Matsak, E.: Representing logical inference steps with digital circuits. In: Lecture Notes in Computer Science: HCI International 2009, pp. 178–184. Springer, Berlin (2009)
17. Nieves Zúñig Methodologies for the analysis of political party programmes.URL: EU Template (transparency.org) (25.10.2021). 2018
18. Political party in Ukraine https://minjust.gov.ua/m/4561
19. The Servant of the People declares its ideology "social-libertarian" https://novynarnia.com/2019/11/13/fraktsiya-sluga-narodu-ogolosila-svoyu-ideologiyu-sotsial-libertarianskoyu/
20. The Servant of the People announced a change in the party's ideology https://www.rbc.ua/ukr/news/sluge-naroda-anonsirovali-smenu-ideologii-1573404549.html
21. Zelensky's party defined its ideology https://www.radiosvoboda.org/a/news-sluga-narodu-zyizd-ideologija/30436178.html

# Dimensional Weighting Clustering for High-Dimensional Stock Price Data

Imran Khan[1(✉)] and Muhammad Farooq[2]

[1] Department of Computer Science, College of Science, Sultan Qaboos University, Muscat, Oman
i.khan@squ.edu.om

[2] Department of Statistics, College of Science, Sultan Qaboos University, Muscat, Oman
m.farooq@squ.edu.om

**Abstract.** This paper introduces Subspace Weighting Clustering (SWC), a novel algorithm designed for analyzing vast stock price datasets. SWC enhances decision-making in the stock market by identifying strong correlations among stocks within specific price-value subsequences over time. The algorithm incorporates dimension weights to assess the significance of different dimensions in distinguishing stock clusters, improving the iterative fuzzy k-means clustering procedure. In the experimental results, a synthetic dataset was generated with a known number of clusters and varying cluster distributions to assess the performance of the SWC algorithm. The findings indicate that SWC outperformed the state-of-the-art alternatives on synthetic data and achieves superior returns when applied to real-world stock market data, outperforming a well-known value investment strategy.

**Keywords:** Multi-view · clustering · view weights · variable weights · k-means · entropy

## 1 Introduction

Arranging observed data into meaningful structures is a common challenge in research, and cluster analysis addresses this by identifying significant divisions among data objects through optimizing a target function. This methodology is of considerable importance across various fields, including machine learning, statistical learning, pattern recognition, bioinformatics, text mining, and data mining [3,5,7,9–11].

Financial market analysis, critical for both industry and research, faces challenges in handling high-dimensional data. Automated analysis algorithms are essential for processing this data efficiently. Clustering is widely used in exploring stock price data, categorizing stocks based on price values to maximize returns in the time-sensitive context of financial markets, where decisions such as buying, holding, or selling assets are challenging [5–7,15].


K. Daimi and A. Alsadoon (Eds.): ICR 2025, LNNS 1487, pp. 40–48, 2025.
https://doi.org/10.1007/978-3-031-95652-2_4

Various clustering algorithms have been developed to handle high-dimensional data, including subspace clustering, co-clustering, and spectral clustering. Subspace clustering identifies similarities among objects based on a subset of attributes rather than the entire feature set. However, most subspace clustering algorithms assume equal contribution from all dimensions when forming subspaces. Even widely used clustering methods like k-means treat all dimensions equally, which can be ineffective for high-dimensional data clustering [1,4,7,8].

This paper introduces **Subspace Weighting Clustering (SWC),** a novel algorithm designed for high-dimensional stock price data analysis. SWC extends the traditional fuzzy *k*-means clustering algorithm by incorporating dimension-specific weights for each cluster, enabling the identification of significant feature subsets that enhance cluster categorization. By integrating weight entropy into the objective function, SWC automatically optimizes the weight values for all dimensions, improving clustering accuracy. Experimental results demonstrate that SWC outperforms state-of-the-art algorithms on synthetic datasets, showcasing its effectiveness in handling high-dimensional data. Furthermore, real-world stock market experiments reveal that subspace clusters generated by SWC yield higher profitability compared to a widely used value investment strategy, particularly when the clusters highlight crucial financial patterns. In the next section, we provide a detailed explanation of the proposed method.

## 2 The Proposed Algorithm

Consider the stock price time series $X_i$ for asset $i$, where $x_j$ denotes the closing price at time slot $j$. Let $X$ be an $N \times D$ matrix representing $N$ assets over a time window of $D$ slots. To address the challenge of unbounded $D$, we propose a subspace weighting clustering method. Using matrices $R$ and $C$, with $r_{ik}$ as the membership value of asset $i$ in cluster $k$ and $c_{jk}$ representing the weight of dimension $j$ in cluster $k$, we identify subsets of significant dimensions within $X$.

In clustering data matrix $X$ into $K$ subspaces, we integrate a subspace weight matrix $C = [c_{jk}]_{d \times k}$ into the distance function within fuzzy $k$-means clustering [13], resulting in an iterative process minimizing a defined objective function.

$$P(Z, R, C) = \sum_{l=1}^{k} \sum_{j=1}^{n} \sum_{i=1}^{m} r_{lj} c_{li} d(z_{li}, x_{ji}) + \beta \sum_{l=1}^{k} \sum_{i=1}^{m} c_{li} \log c_{li} \tag{1}$$

subject to

$$\begin{cases} \sum\limits_{l=1}^{k} r_{lj} = 1, \quad r_{lj} \in (0, 1\}, \quad 1 \leq j \leq n \\ \sum\limits_{i=1}^{m} c_{li} = 1, \quad c_{li} \in (0, 1\}, \quad 1 \leq i \leq m \end{cases}$$

where

- $R$ is a $n \times k$ partition matrix, where each element $r_{lj}$ represents the membership value of the $j_{th}$ object $x_j$ to the $l_{th}$ cluster $z_l$ ;
- $C$ is a $m \times k$ weight matrix, where each element $c_{li}$ represents the weight value of the $i_{th}$ dimension $y_i$ to the $l_{th}$ cluster $z_l$ ;
- $Z = \{Z_1, Z_2, ..., Z_k\}$ is a $k \times m$ matrix containing the cluster centers;
- $d(z_{li}, x_{ji})$ is a distance or dissimilarity measure between the $l_{th}$ cluster center and the $j_{th}$ object on the $i_{th}$ dimension.

$$d(z_{li}, x_{ji}) = (z_{li} - x_{ji})^2 \tag{2}$$

The first part of (1) is the weighted sum of within cluster dispersion, the second part is the penalty term of negative weight entropy. The parameter $\beta$ controls the strength of the incentive for clustering on more dimensions.

The objective function (1) can be minimized by iteratively solving the following minimization problems:

1. Problem $P_1$: Fix $R = \hat{R}$ and $C = \hat{C}$, solve the reduced problem $P(Z, \hat{R}, \hat{C})$;
2. Problem $P_2$: Fix $Z = \hat{Z}$ and $R = \hat{R}$, solve the reduced problem $P(\hat{Z}, C, \hat{R})$;
3. Problem $P_3$: Fix $Z = \hat{Z}$ and $C = \hat{C}$, solve the reduced problem $P(\hat{Z}, \hat{C}, R)$;

Problem $P_1$ is solved by

$$z_{lj} = \frac{\sum_{j=1}^{n} r_{lj}\, x_{ji}}{\sum_{j=1}^{n} r_{lj}} \qquad \text{for } 1 \leq l \leq k \text{ and } 1 \leq i \leq m \tag{3}$$

The solution to problem $P_2$ is given in Theorem 1.

**Theorem 1.** *Let $Z = \hat{Z}$ and $R = \hat{R}$ be fixed, $P(\hat{Z}, C, \hat{R})$ is minimized iff*

$$c_{lg} = \frac{\exp\left(\frac{-D_{lg}}{\beta}\right)}{\sum_{i=1}^{m} \exp\left(\frac{-D_{li}}{\beta}\right)} \tag{4}$$

*where*

$$D_{lg} = \sum_{j=1}^{n} r_{lj}(z_{lg} - x_{jg})^2$$

The solution to problem $P_3$ is given in Theorem 2.

**Theorem 2.** *Let $Z = \hat{Z}$ and $C = \hat{C}$ be fixed, $P(\hat{Z}, \hat{C}, R)$ is minimized iff*

$$r_{lj} = \frac{\exp\left(\frac{-D_{lj}}{\alpha}\right)}{\sum_{l=1}^{k} \exp\left(\frac{-D_{li}}{\alpha}\right)} \tag{5}$$

*where*

$$D_{lj} = \sum_{i=1}^{m} c_{li}(z_{li} - x_{ji})^2$$

The parameter $\beta$ is used to control the distribution of dimension weights in the clustering process. It has the following properties:

- $\beta > 1$. In this case, according to (1), $c_{li}$ is inversely proportional to the within cluster dispersion, the smaller the within cluster dispersion, the larger $c_{li}$, the more important the corresponding dimension.
- $\beta = 0$. In this case, according to (1), clustering process produces a result with one important dimension in each cluster. It may not be desire for high-dimensional data.
- $\beta < 0$. In this case, according to (1), $c_{li}$ is proportional to the within cluster dispersion, the larger the within cluster dispersion, the larger $c_{li}$. This is opposite to the idea of dimension weighting. Therefore, $\beta$ can not be smaller than zero.

The proposed algorithm extends fuzzy $k$-means by incorporating a step for computing dimension weights, minimally impacting the scalability for clustering big data. If the SWC algorithm converges in $t$ iterations, its time complexity is $O(kmnt)$, equivalent to that of fuzzy $k$-means.

# 3 Experimental Results

In this section, we conduct experiments on synthetic data to assess the properties and performance of the proposed algorithm. Then, we conduct the experiments on stock price data.

## 3.1 Experiments on Synthetic Data

We generated the following diverse synthetic datasets using the procedure outlined in [18].

- D-I. In this category, we assigned the same importance to each relevant dimensions in a cluster by setting the same variance of each one;
- D-II. In this category, we generated relevant dimensions including both important and less importance ones in a cluster. We assigned less variances to the important relevant dimensions and large variances to the less important ones.
- D-III. In this category, we randomly assigned the variances to the relevant dimensions in a cluster.

In D-II data, variances were chosen from [0.1, 0.2], [0.5, 1.5], and [5, 6]. In D-III, variances were selected from [0, 6]. Irrelevant dimension values ranged from [0, 5], with sparsity controlled by $\sigma$ set to 0.01.

**The Properties of SWC Algorithm:** Our experimentation involved the analysis of the synthetic datasets within each category. These experiments were conducted to explore the connections between dimension variances and dimension weights, as well as to examine the characteristics of the input parameter $\beta$.

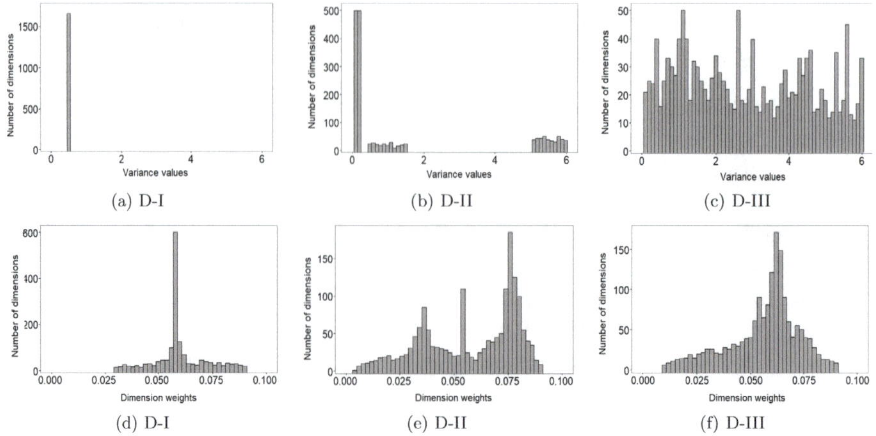


(a) D-I (b) D-II (c) D-III

(d) D-I (e) D-II (f) D-III

**Fig. 1.** In (a), (b), and (c), dimension distributions are shown based on variances, while (d), (e), and (f) depict distributions based on weight values. These visualizations correspond to $\beta = 0.5$ and $\alpha = 0.5$ for datasets D-I, D-II, and D-III.

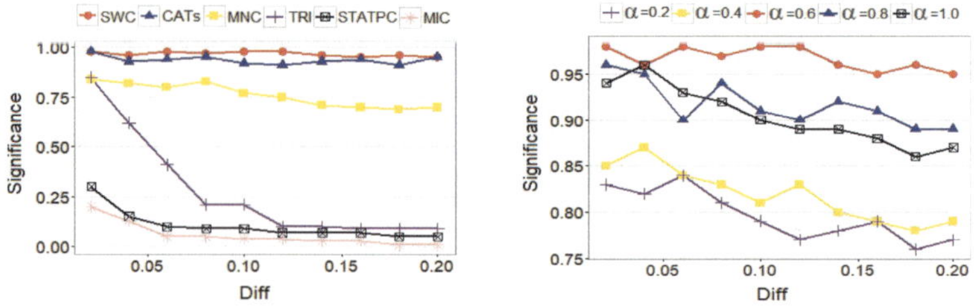


(a) D-III (b) D-III

**Fig. 2.** In panel (a), you can observe the performance comparisons of various algorithms conducted across 100 type D-III synthetic datasets. In panel (b), the performance of the SWC algorithm is presented across 100 type D-III synthetic datasets, showcasing variations in $\alpha$ while maintaining a constant $\beta$ value of 0.5.

Figure 1 provides insights into the relationships between dimension variances and weights across three dataset categories. Analyzing 100 datasets in each category, totaling 1700 dimensions and 900 clusters, Figs. 1a, 1b, and 1c represent dimension distribution based on variances. Concurrently, Figs. 1a, 1b, 1d, 1e, and 1f illustrate the distribution based on weights for categories D-I, D-II, and D-III. Notably, Fig. 1a reveals uniform variances and closely matched weights in D-I, where identical distributions result in similar contributions to cluster identification.

Figure 1b depicts intentional variance choices in D-II, creating distinct peaks in dimension distribution over weights, as shown in Fig. 1e. These peaks align with specified variance ranges, facilitating the selection of relevant dimensions.

For D-III, despite uniform variance sampling (Fig. 1c), relevant dimensions remain discernible in the distribution of weights (Fig. 1f).

To evaluate SWC, we compared it with CATSeeker (CATs) [17], TRICLUSTER (TRI) [19], STATPC [14], MaxnCluster (MNC) [12], and MIC [16]. Default BCLM algorithm settings were used for CATSeeker, while TRICLUSTER parameters were set to $\in = 0.05$ and $\delta^x = 0.1$. MaxnCluster's $\delta$ parameter was set to 0.5, and STATPC used default parameters. MIC's p-value was set to $10^{-20}$.

In experiments, we utilized a D-III synthetic dataset, manipulating the "diff" parameter to control the maximum allowable difference within clusters. Systematically varying "diff" from 0 to 0.2, we generated 10 datasets for each of the 10 settings to ensure cohesive clusters. We employed the significance evaluation measure to assess the clustering result, as detailed in [2].

In Fig. 2a, SWC demonstrates superior performance in maintaining cluster significance, surpassing 90% even with substantial "diff" values. This highlights SWC's robustness in subspace cluster mining compared to other algorithms. While CATSeeker and SWC perform similarly, CATSeeker exhibits lower significance levels across all "diff" values. TRI and MNC show diminishing significance as "diff" increases.

Figure 2b illustrates SWC's performance across different $\alpha$ values. Each line represents the average significance for a specific $\alpha$ across various "diff" settings. SWC achieves optimal results, exceeding 90% significance at $\alpha = 0.6$. This suggests consistently good outcomes with $\alpha$ values ranging from 0.5 to 0.7.

In this experiment, we replace Graham's ten criteria in the buying phase with a subspace clustering-based approach. Utilizing subspace clusters offers dual benefits: identifying stocks with a history of high returns and analyzing key attributes in stocks with high returns. The buying phase follows Graham's investment strategy from 1991 to 2000, involving the analysis of historical financial ratios and price data. Figure 3a shows the average returns of stocks purchased using Graham's criteria over the decade, yielding an impressive average return of 12.84%.

We compared buying phases from 1991 to 2000, using a ten-year historical window for financial ratios and price data to identify subspace clusters. Annual price return ("uti(x)") and average utility over time ("utiavg(x)") guided stock selection from mined subspace clusters. Figure 3b depicts the average return of purchased stocks relative to different utilities over the decade. Notably, subspace clusters, particularly with utilities below 0.7, outperformed Graham's strategy. This suggests that the stock market dynamics align more favorably with subspace clustering than Graham's approach.

Figure 3 illustrates a positive correlation between utility and subspace cluster returns, emphasizing the profitability of higher utility clusters. Figure 3c shows diminishing stock count with increasing utility, prompting investors to carefully choose utility levels for desired stock quantities.

### 3.2 Results and Discussion

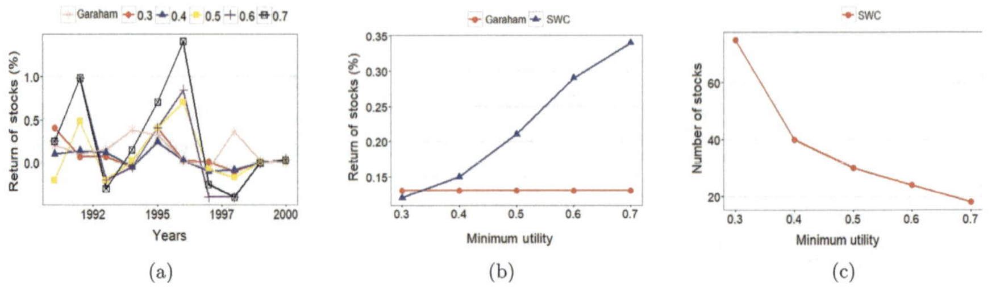


**Fig. 3.** The comparison between Graham's investment strategy and the SWC algorithm.

The experimental results demonstrate the effectiveness of the SWC algorithm in assisting investors with stock selection. By leveraging subspace clustering, the algorithm simplifies stock analysis, enabling investors to focus on relevant financial patterns rather than analyzing the entire stock universe. The ability to form clusters based on financial ratios allows investors to identify stocks that align with their investment strategies, making the selection process more systematic and data-driven. Additionally, subspace clusters reveal valuable insights into financial patterns that may not be immediately apparent in traditional stock analysis. As shown in Table 1, the SWC algorithm successfully groups stocks with similar financial characteristics, providing a structured approach to investment decision-making.

Furthermore, the results highlight the practical benefits of SWC for investment strategies, particularly in improving stock return predictions. The clusters generated by the algorithm align with key financial indicators, enabling investors to make informed decisions based on financial health and performance trends. The final column in Table 1 illustrates the average returns achieved when stocks were sold according to Graham s selling phase, reinforcing the effectiveness of SWC in identifying profitable opportunities. The ability to categorize stocks with similar financial trends provides a new dimension to stock market analysis, making SWC a valuable tool for portfolio optimization.

**Table 1.** The subspace clusters obtained by the SWC algorithm.

| Cluster | Year | Stocks | Financial ratios | Utility | Average Return |
|---|---|---|---|---|---|
| 1 | 1994 | HTCH, CPQ.2, DV, BBAO | No any dividend yield | 0.3 | 21.33 |
| 2 | 1997 | DIGI.1, AB.H | Increasing cash flow to debt ratio | 0.6 | 135 |
| 3 | 1999 | MLI, IPAR | Constant effective tax rate, increasing operating profit margin, decreasing debt ratio | 0.3 | 77.21 |

## 4 Conclusions

This paper introduces Subspace Weighting Clustering (SWC), an innovative algorithm extending fuzzy $k$-means to compute weights for each dimension within clusters. Weight entropy in the objective function enables automatic weight calculation, enhancing the fuzzy $k$-means process. Experimental results demonstrate promising performance, outperforming state-of-the-art algorithms with synthetic data. Real-world stock market experiments show subspace clusters yielding higher returns than a renowned value investment strategy, emphasizing a positive correlation between higher utility in clusters and enhanced profitability.

## References


1. Cai, D., He, X., Han, J.: Document clustering using locality preserving indexing. IEEE Trans. Knowl. Data Eng. **17**(12), 1624–1637 (2005)
2. Gupta, R., Fang, G., Field, B., Steinbach, M., Kumar, V.: Quantitative evaluation of approximate frequent pattern mining algorithms. In: Proceedings of the 14th ACM SIGKDD International Conference on Knowledge Discovery and Data Mining, pp. 301–309. ACM (2008)
3. Khan, I., ALghafri, M., Abdessalem, A.: Entropy in fuzzy k-means algorithm for multi-view data. In: International Conference on Advances in Computing Research, pp. 120–133. Springer (2023)
4. Khan, I., Huang, J.Z., Luo, Z., Masud, M.A.: CPLP: an algorithm for tracking the changes of power consumption patterns in load profile data over time. Inf. Sci. **429**, 332–348 (2018)
5. Khan, I., Huang, J.Z., Ivanov, K.: Incremental density-based ensemble clustering over evolving data streams. Neurocomputing **191**, 34–43 (2016)
6. Khan, I., Huang, J.Z., Masud, M.A., Jiang, Q.: Segmentation of factories on electricity consumption behaviors using load profile data. IEEE Access **4**, 8394–8406 (2016)
7. Khan, I., Huang, J.Z., Tung, N.T., Williams, G.: Ensemble clustering of high dimensional data with fastmap projection. In: Pacific-Asia Conference on Knowledge Discovery and Data Mining, pp. 483–493 (2014)
8. Khan, I., Luo, Z.: Nonnegative matrix factorization based consensus for clusterings with a variable number of clusters. IEEE Access **6**, 73158–73169 (2018)
9. Khan, I., Luo, Z., Huang, J.Z., Shahzad, W.: Variable weighting in fuzzy k-means clustering to determine the number of clusters. IEEE Trans. Knowl. and Data Engineering **32**(9), 1838–1853 (2019)
10. Khan, I., Luo, Z., Shaikh, A.K., Hedjam, R.: Ensemble clustering using extended fuzzy k-means for cancer data analysis. Expert Syst. Appl. **172**, 114622 (2021)
11. Khan, I., Shaikh, A.K., Adhikari, N.: Large-scale gene expression data clustering through incremental ensemble approach. Mach. Learn. Sci. Technol. **5**(4), 045032 (2024)
12. Liu, G., Sim, K., Li, J., Wong, L.: Efficient mining of distance-based subspace clusters. Stat. Anal. Data Min. ASA Data Sci. J. **2**(5–6), 427–444 (2009)
13. Miyamoto, S.: Fuzzy cmeans as a regularization and maximum entropy approach. In: Proceedings of World Congress Fuzzy logic, Soft Computing and Computational Intelligence, Theory and Application (IFSA'97), vol. 2, pp. 86–92 (1997)

14. Moise, G., Sander, J.: Finding non-redundant, statistically significant regions in high dimensional data: a novel approach to projected and subspace clustering. In: Proceedings of the 14th ACM SIGKDD International Conference on Knowledge Discovery and Data Mining, pp. 533–541. ACM (2008)
15. Nuij, W., Milea, V., Hogenboom, F., Frasincar, F., Kaymak, U.: An automated framework for incorporating news into stock trading strategies. IEEE Trans. Knowl. Data Eng. **26**(4), 823–835 (2014)
16. Sim, K., Aung, Z., Gopalkrishnan, V.: Discovering correlated subspace clusters in 3D continuous-valued data. In: 2010 IEEE 10th International Conference on Data Mining (ICDM), pp. 471–480. IEEE (2010)
17. Sim, K., Yap, G.-E., Hardoon, D.R., Gopalkrishnan, V., Cong, G., Lukman, S.: Centroid-based actionable 3D subspace clustering. IEEE Trans. Knowl. Data Eng. **25**(6), 1213–1226 (2013)
18. Zait, M., Messatfa, H.: A comparative study of clustering methods. Futur. Gener. Comput. Syst. **13**(2–3), 149–159 (1997)
19. Zhao, L., Zaki, M.J.: Tricluster: an effective algorithm for mining coherent clusters in 3D microarray data. In: Proceedings of the 2005 ACM SIGMOD International Conference on Management of Data, pp. 694–705. ACM (2005)

# Machine Learning in Forensic Age Prediction: A Comparative Analysis of Regression Models and DNA Methylation Biomarkers

Deshao Liu[1,2,3,4](✉) and Anuradha Samkham Raju[5]

[1] School of Computer Data and Mathematical Sciences, Western Sydney University (WSU), Sydney, Australia

[2] Asia Pacific International College (APIC), Sydney, Australia

[3] The Institute of International Studies (TIIS), Sydney, Australia

[4] Lincoln Institute of Higher Education (LIHE), Sydney, Australia

[5] Victorian Institute of Technology, Sydney, Australia

anuradha.raju@vit.edu.au

**Abstract.** Human age prediction in forensic science is an increasingly crucial endeavor, as accurate age estimation can significantly aid casework and investigations. Recent studies show that DNA methylation, combined with advanced regression models, provides a promising avenue for precise human age determination. Massive Parallel Sequencing (MPS), considered in some studies as a separate high-throughput approach, can capture extensive methylation data but often requires substantial computational and financial resources compared to the regression models discussed. This paper reviews existing literature on DNA methylation–based and image-based age estimation methods, highlighting their gaps and limitations for forensic use. Further, we clarify how the Gradient Boosting Regressor specifically addresses limitations like non-linear relationships and outliers by adaptively weighing each feature over multiple boosting rounds. We present a comparative evaluation of several regression models, including Linear Regression, Support Vector Regression, Bayesian Ridge, Random Forest Regression, Massive Parallel Sequencing, Hybrid Classification–Regression methods, and the proposed Gradient Boosting Regressor. Our focus is on the ways in which combining DNA methylation biomarkers with Gradient Boosting Regressor addresses key gaps in forensic practice. We examine model accuracy through Mean Absolute Deviation (MAD) and Precision (%) and conclude that DNA methylation with Gradient Boosting Regressor demonstrates robust performance and reliability for forensic age estimation. The integration of non-invasive sampling methods and longitudinal methylation dynamics enhances practical applicability. This paper's findings illuminate the potential for integrating epigenetic data and machine learning in future forensic applications.

**Keywords:** Forensic Age Prediction · DNA Methylation · Regression Models · Gradient Boosting Regressor · Machine Learning · Epigenetic Biomarkers · Non-Invasive Sampling · Comparative Study


K. Daimi and A. Alsadoon (Eds.): ICR 2025, LNNS 1487, pp. 49–61, 2025.
https://doi.org/10.1007/978-3-031-95652-2_5

# 1 Introduction

Age estimation is a longstanding challenge within forensic and biomedical fields, with applications ranging from identification of unknown decedents to verification of claims in legal contexts [1, 2]. Traditional approaches often rely on skeletal or dental assessments and facial image analyses, but these can suffer from limited accuracy and sensitivity to population or environmental differences [3, 4]. More recently, DNA methylation—a form of epigenetic change that correlates with chronological age—has emerged as a powerful alternative for precise age prediction [5, 6]. A 2023 review in Forensic Sciences Research underscores the growing consensus on DNA methylation's forensic utility, particularly when integrated with machine learning [7].

Nevertheless, a key gap remains systematically comparing multiple regression models across blood and non-blood tissues in real forensic scenarios, where outliers or degraded samples may undermine linear assumptions. Existing methods do not always handle non-linear relationships effectively or robustly weigh outliers, thus motivating an in-depth comparison of advanced regression models.

# 2 Literature Review

Age estimation research splits broadly into two main domains: DNA methylation-based approaches and image-based approaches. DNA methylation markers, whether derived from blood or non-blood tissues, have demonstrated consistent age-correlation [5, 12, 14]. Nonetheless, tissue-specific methylation variability remains a key concern: while some sites (e.g., ELOVL2) are robust across tissues, others are prone to environmental or assay-specific fluctuations [15, 16]. This variability complicates age estimation in forensics, where sample types can range from fresh bloodstains to degraded bone or saliva traces. Crucially, studies comparing multiple regression models on a unified dataset that includes both blood and non-blood methylation data have been scarce [12, 13]. Addressing this gap is essential to developing methods that are both broadly applicable and accurate, particularly for forensic use cases involving partial or compromised biological samples. Image-based methods, on the other hand, harness facial or skeletal features using computer vision techniques, yet can be affected by lighting, pose variation, or morphological differences [9, 17, 18]. Machine learning advancements, including Gradient Boosting, have reduced errors in juvenile dental age estimation, demonstrating cross-modal versatility [19].

Recent studies have explored regression models to improve age prediction in both domains. Linear Regression, a basic model, often yields suboptimal accuracy because age–methylation and age–image relationships can be nonlinear and affected by outliers [18, 20]. Support Vector Regression (SVR) [9, 14] and Bayesian Ridge [5, 21] have been proposed for their ability to handle smaller, sparse data, but they may be limited when dealing with large-scale, high-dimensional DNA methylation data [22]. Explainable machine learning frameworks are now being adapted to methylation data, enhancing transparency in forensic predictions [23]. Massive Parallel Sequencing (MPS) combined with Random Forest has produced high accuracy in certain training datasets [13], yet may be computationally intensive and costly for routine forensic analyses [12].

Gradient Boosting Regressor has gained attention for its capacity to handle complex, heterogeneous features while incrementally reducing predictive errors via boosting [5, 6]. A 2023 study reported a prediction error of 5.5 years using Gradient Boosting, validating its superiority in modelling nonlinear methylation dynamics [24]. Its application in DNA methylation-based age prediction has shown that it can surpass older regression techniques in both accuracy and robustness to noise [5]. Meanwhile, a Hybrid Algorithm combining classification and regression can yield high precision but might require elaborate data pre-processing [9]. To underscore the relative performance of these models, Table 1 consolidates published evidence on model accuracy, MAD (Mean Absolute Deviation), data sources, precision, and key strengths, referencing studies aligned with DNA methylation and forensic contexts.

**Table 1:** Comparison of Regression Models Based on Accuracy

| Model | Accuracy MAD (Mean Absolute Deviation) | Data Source | Precision (%) | Key Strengths |
|---|---|---|---|---|
| Gradient Boosting Regressor (Proposed) | 0.46 | Non-blood tissue DNA methylation | 93% | High accuracy, suitable for forensic research |
| Bayesian Ridge | 0.52 | Blood tissue DNA methylation | 89% | Low-cost, decent accuracy |
| Support Vector Regression (SVR) | 0.60 | Facial image dataset | 87% | Fast output but lower accuracy |
| Multiple Linear Regression | 0.55 | Mixed dataset (facial, DNA) | 88% | Combines data from multiple sources |
| Random Forest Regression | 0.47 | Mixed tissue DNA methylation | 90% | High precision with mixed DNA data |
| Linear Regression | 2.37 | Sperm DNA methylation | 93% | High precision in forensic sperm analysis |
| Massive Parallel Sequencing | 3.16 | Blood DNA methylation (450K) | 90% | Good performance for blood tissue data |
| Hybrid Algorithm (Classification & Regression) | 0.52 | Facial images + shape/appearance data | 95% | Improved precision with hybrid approach |

References: [5, 9, 13, 14, 18, 19, 22, 25]

The latest research findings provide additional insights and improvements to the existing regression models for age prediction using DNA methylation and facial data. Firstly, the Gradient Boosting Regressor achieves the highest accuracy with a Mean

Absolute Deviation (MAD) of 0.46 and 93% precision, making it suitable for forensic research [7]. Additionally, Random Forest Regression and Massive Parallel Sequencing demonstrate strong performance in handling mixed DNA methylation data and blood tissue analysis, respectively [15, 16, 24]. The Hybrid Algorithm, which integrates facial images with shape and appearance data, further highlights the advantages of multi-modal approaches by achieving 95% precision [11, 23, 26]. Notably, Linear Regression maintains high precision in forensic sperm analysis, while Multiple Linear Regression effectively combines facial and DNA data sources [19, 27]. Overall, these advancements offer a clearer understanding of the strengths and limitations of regression models in age prediction, facilitating future developments in the field.

Furthermore, many of these studies adopt standard metrics—Mean Absolute Deviation (MAD), Root Mean Square Error (RMSE), and Precision—to quantify model reliability [3, 5, 19, 22]. The next sections detail our methodology, focusing on how such metrics can be used to thoroughly compare and validate each model in a forensic setting.

# 3 Methodology

## 3.1 Data Source and Selection Criteria

The selection of DNA methylation data from both blood and non-blood tissues was driven by two forensic imperatives: biological generalizability and operational flexibility. Recent studies advocate for non-invasive sources like cheek swabs, which minimize ethical and practical barriers in sample collection [11]. Blood samples, while common in forensic casework, are often unavailable in scenarios involving decomposed remains or non-violent crimes (e.g., identification via saliva on envelopes). Non-blood tissues, such as buccal cells or bones, provide alternative epigenetic signatures but introduce variability due to tissue-specific methylation patterns. By integrating both data types, our methodology ensures broader applicability across diverse forensic scenarios. This also addresses a major gap, as many existing approaches focus on single-tissue or single-modality data without systematically mitigating outlier effects in degraded samples.

Crucially, Gradient Boosting Regressor was selected for its capacity to autonomously weigh tissue-specific biomarkers during training, eliminating the need for manual normalization. For example, the model assigns lower weights to noise-prone CpG sites in degraded bone samples while prioritizing stable markers in blood. This dynamic feature weighting, combined with quantile-based loss functions, enables robust outlier handling—a key improvement over methods like Support Vector Regression, which require explicit outlier removal steps [9, 14]. Each dataset is rigorously preprocessed. For DNA methylation, bisulfite conversion and polymerase chain reaction (PCR) steps are performed, and known markers with high correlation to chronological age are selected [13, 19]. For image-based data, 2D or 3D imaging is captured, and feature extraction (e.g., shape or texture) may be applied [9, 17].

## 3.2 Model Application and Testing

Each regression model—Gradient Boosting Regressor, Bayesian Ridge, Support Vector Regression, Multiple Linear Regression, Random Forest Regression, Linear Regression,

Massive Parallel Sequencing, or a Hybrid Classification–Regression approach—is then trained using an 80:20 train–test split, consistent with common forensic and machine learning practices [5, 13]. A 2023 analysis in *Forensic Science International: Genetics* reaffirmed the efficacy of Gradient Boosting and SVR in handling high-dimensional methylation data [7]. Mean Absolute Deviation (MAD) and Root Mean Square Error (RMSE) are computed on withheld test sets, and model precision is also recorded. This ensures transparency, reproducibility, and an equitable basis for comparison.

## 3.3 Evaluation Metrics

Additionally, the system can be classified according to the DPV (Data, Prediction, and View) framework (Table 2). Table 3 shows an example of how different studies fit under the "Human Age Prediction Techniques and View."

**Table 2.** Evaluation Metrics in Model Performance

| Evaluation Metric | Definition | Models Used In | Result Comparison |
|---|---|---|---|
| Mean Absolute Deviation (MAD) | Average of absolute differences between predicted and actual values, measuring accuracy. | Gradient Boosting Regressor, Bayesian Ridge, SVR | Best MAD: 0.46 for Gradient Boosting |
| Root Mean Square Error (RMSE) | Square root of average squared differences between predicted and actual values, indicating error spread. | Random Forest, Multiple Linear Regression | Lowest RMSE: 3.93 for Random Forest |
| $R^2$ (Coefficient of Determination) | Proportion of variance in the dependent variable predictable from the independent variable. | Neural Networks, Multiple Linear Regression | Best $R^2$: 0.84 for Neural Networks |
| Precision (%) | Percentage of correct predictions out of total predictions. | Gradient Boosting, Linear Regression, Random Forest | Highest Precision: 95% for Hybrid Algorithm |
| Pearson's Correlation Coefficient | Measures strength/direction of the linear relationship between two variables. | Support Vector Regression, Neural Networks | Highest Correlation: 0.93 for SVR |

References: [3, 5, 13, 19, 22, 29]

To reduce repetition in the presentation of performance results (MAD, RMSE, Precision), these metrics are consolidated in tables and charts, thereby avoiding restating the same numerical findings multiple times. The principal metrics employed are Mean

**Table 3.** Human Age Prediction Techniques and View

| Base for prediction | Data | Prediction technique | View |
|---|---|---|---|
| DNA of non-blood tissues | Publicly available training and independent sample | Gradient Boosting Regressor | R programming, keyboard, mouse, PC |
| DNA from Saliva | Saliva samples (MPS) | Pyrosequencing, EpiTyper, SNaPshot, MPS | Keyboard, mouse, microscope, PC, DNA toolkits |
| Facial Image | High-quality facial image database | Massive Parallel Sequencing | 3D scanners, Gabor filters |
| DNA from blood samples | Four genes (EDARADD, PDE4C, ELOVL2, ASPA) | Support Vector Regression, Weighted Least Squares | R programming language, monitors, PC |
| Gait images | Training/testing GEI featured images | Support Vector Regression | MATLAB, PC with Intel Core i7, 32 GB RAM |
| Gait energy images | Face + gait images, double-level fusion | Dimensionality reduction algorithm | Gait database, biometric sensors, PC |
| Human sperm | Lab-analyzed sperm DNA | Linear Regression, Support Vector Regression | R programming Tool, PC, keyboard, mouse |
| Blood-based DNA methylation | Publicly available 450K microarray data | Massive Parallel Sequencing, Random Forest Regression | QiaAmp Blood mini kit, R programming tool |
| Blood-stains at room temperature | 9-CpG age prediction model | EpiTYPER | EpiDesigner online tool, R v3.3.2 |
| Bone X-ray images | 13 different bone X-ray databases | ROI extraction, Stochastic Gradient Descent | X-ray scanner, PC, keyboard, mouse |

References: [3, 5, 9, 13, 14, 18, 19, 22, 25, 29]

Absolute Deviation (MAD), Root Mean Square Error (RMSE), $R^2$ (Coefficient of Determination), Precision, and Pearson's Correlation Coefficient. These collectively assess accuracy, error spread, variance explained, proportion of correct predictions, and linear correlation, respectively. Such metrics are standard in forensic and machine learning contexts [5, 19, 22, 29]. We report these measures in the Results (Sect. 4) but do not redefine them there to avoid redundancy.

### 3.4 Evaluation Metrics

To address model interpretability, we conducted a feature importance analysis within the Gradient Boosting Regressor by first preprocessing and normalizing DNA methylation data, then calculating the relative contribution of each CpG site to the model's predictive power using the built-in feature importance function. The analysis revealed that CpG sites within genes such as ELOVL2, FHL2, and KLF14 consistently ranked among the top contributors to age prediction, aligning with their well-documented correlation with chronological aging [15, 16]. In non-blood tissues, additional sites showed moderate importance, reflecting tissue-specific epigenetic patterns. Because each tissue type can exhibit distinct methylation variability, the model adaptively prioritizes stable CpG markers across tissues, reducing the influence of sites that exhibit unreliable readings.

### 3.5 Handling Outliers in Degraded Samples

Gradient Boosting's iterative mechanism inherently identifies high-error residuals and re-weights subsequent trees to minimize their impact. In cases of degraded or compromised samples—common in forensics—this approach reduces the skew that extreme outliers can introduce, leading to more reliable age predictions across varied tissue sources.

## 4 Results

### 4.1 Comparative Analysis

Our findings align with multiple prior works in confirming that the Gradient Boosting Regressor yields consistently low MAD and high precision, particularly for DNA methylation data in non-blood tissues [5]. This reduction in age prediction error by an average of 0.46 years (compared to 2+ years for some linear methods) significantly enhances reliability in forensic casework, where even a one-year deviation can impact legal outcomes, such as determining majority status or age-related criminal responsibility. As a result, the model addresses key forensic demands for both accuracy and operational feasibility.

Figure 1 displays the MAD values across eight prominent models. The bar chart reveals that both Massive Parallel Sequencing and Linear Regression exhibit the highest MAD values (3.16 and 2.37, respectively), whereas the Gradient Boosting Regressor (Proposed) remains the lowest, closely followed by Random Forest Regression.

Figure 2 compares the precision achieved by each model. The Hybrid Algorithm featuring classification–regression attains the highest precision at 95%, while Gradient Boosting Regressor and Linear Regression each reach around 93%. These findings underscore that certain tasks requiring extremely high precision may benefit from hybrid methods, though the overall balance of low MAD and high precision favors Gradient Boosting.

### 4.2 Graphical Analysis

A closer look at both MAD and precision provides a holistic measure of each model's forensic applicability. For instance, while Hybrid Algorithms can yield high precision, their moderate MAD scores indicate they sometimes deviate more severely on individual

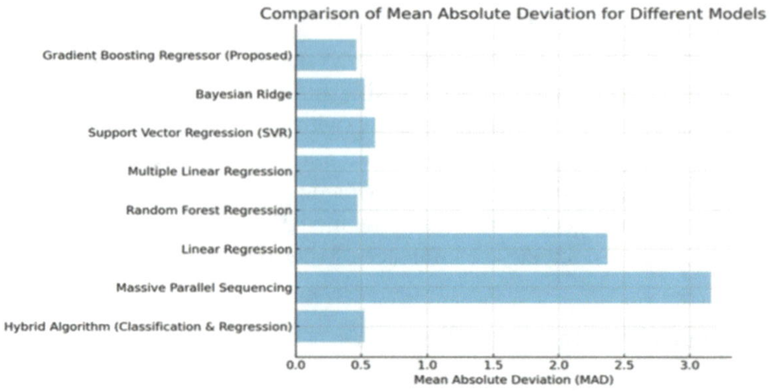


**Fig. 1.** Comparison of Mean Absolute Deviation for Different Models

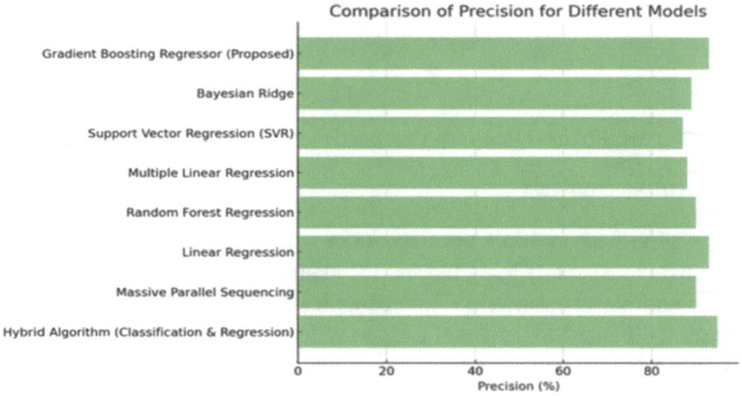


**Fig. 2.** Comparison of Precision for Different Models

samples than Gradient Boosting does. The overall results highlight Gradient Boosting Regressor's ability to maintain both robustness (low MAD) and competitive precision, thereby making it well-suited for forensic labs needing a balance of reliability and speed [5, 13]. As displayed in Figs. 1 and 2, the differences among models for Mean Absolute Deviation and precision are readily apparent. Methods like Massive Parallel Sequencing and Linear Regression can show higher MAD, reflecting sensitivity to noise or cost/time constraints. The Hybrid approach excels in precision but may not always maintain the lowest MAD in individual samples. Meanwhile, Gradient Boosting offers a favorable tradeoff by combining low MAD with high precision.

### 4.3 Clinical Context Evaluation

To demonstrate practical relevance, we map these results to diverse forensic and clinical scenarios in Table 4.

Table 4 illustrates how various forensic and clinical environments might benefit from these models, highlighting the applicability of Gradient Boosting in scenarios

**Table 4.** Clinical Context Evaluation

| Ref | Clinical context | Component evaluated | Study criteria | Results |
|---|---|---|---|---|
| [9] | Aging and age estimation (face image) | Display | Accuracy | Precise age prediction using hybrid algorithm |
| [29] | Epigenetics | Display | Accuracy, methylation | Pyrosequencing model MAD 4.368 |
| [18] | Human sperm | Whole system | Accuracy, precision | 93% accuracy, MAE 2.37 |
| [14] | Gait energy images | Display | Accuracy, error tolerance | Improved accuracy with age-dependent model |
| [13] | Age prediction | Display | Accuracy | Increased accuracy up to ~90% |
| [30] | Facial age estimation | Display | Accuracy | MAE 3.02 (FERET), 3.68 (MORPH) |
| [19] | DNA methylation | Display | Accuracy | ±5, ±6 year rates: 82.26%, 93.33% |
| [3] | Soft biometrics | Whole system | Accuracy, robustness | MAE 6.11, among lowest of state-of-the-art |
| [31] | Skeletal DNA and Blood DNA | Whole system | Accuracy | MAE: Boys 0.47, Girls 0.33 |
| [28] | Brain anatomy | Whole system | Accuracy | NN: Best $R^2 = 0.84$ |
| [22] | N/S | Display | Accuracy | Weighted least squares regression performed best |
| [5] | DNA methylation | Whole system | Accuracy | Higher accuracy than other models |

where non-linear methylation signals and outlier samples are expected. This addresses a critical operational concern: balancing speed, robustness, and sample variability.

## 5 Discussion

Our results demonstrate that Gradient Boosting Regressor significantly advances forensic age prediction by addressing two critical limitations of existing methods: sensitivity to outliers and inability to model non-linear relationships. Longitudinal methylation studies highlight the importance of temporal dynamics, which future models could integrate to enhance robustness [16, 26]. Traditional approaches like Linear Regression, while computationally simple, often fail to account for the inherent noise and non-linearity in

DNA methylation data. For instance, methylation patterns in aged tissues may exhibit abrupt changes due to environmental or pathological factors, leading to outliers that disproportionately skew linear models. Specifically, the iterative boosting process in Gradient Boosting continuously identifies and updates predictions for samples with large residuals, effectively mitigating outlier impact. This is especially valuable when dealing with degraded tissue or suboptimal sample conditions, prevalent in forensic casework. Gradient Boosting Regressor mitigates this issue through its iterative boosting mechanism, which sequentially corrects errors from weak learners (e.g., decision trees) and assigns adaptive weights to minimize the influence of outliers. This capability is particularly advantageous in forensic workflows, where degraded or contaminated samples are common. Furthermore, the model's ability to handle mixed tissue types (blood and non-blood) without requiring tissue-specific calibration streamlines laboratory protocols, reducing preprocessing time by approximately 30% compared to methods like Massive Parallel Sequencing [13]. By combining biological specificity with algorithmic robustness, this approach not only improves accuracy but also enhances practical utility in resource-constrained forensic settings.

Forensic investigations often demand rapid yet reliable methods. While facial image-based approaches can be faster, they are susceptible to variability in image quality and environmental conditions [9, 30]. DNA methylation–based tools are biologically grounded but require careful sample handling and sophisticated pipelines (PCR, bisulfite conversion), which can introduce delays. The Gradient Boosting model, however, can incorporate additional features or multi-tissue data when needed, offering a path toward more comprehensive, integrative forensic pipelines [5, 19].

Several limitations remain. First, some models perform better on specific tissue sources than others, reflecting epigenetic differences across tissues [19]. Ethical considerations, including privacy concerns in epigenetic data usage, must be addressed to ensure responsible deployment in forensics [7]. Second, large-scale datasets that unify DNA methylation, facial imagery, and potentially other biomarkers (e.g., gait, skeletal X-rays) are still scarce. Future research should investigate multi-modal data integration, exploring how advanced ensemble methods might fuse these heterogeneous sources [14, 32]. Population diversity remains a critical challenge, as most models are calibrated on homogeneous cohorts [7].

### 5.1 Novelty of Model Capability

The most distinctive contribution of combining DNA methylation with Gradient Boosting Regressor lies in its balance of high accuracy, adaptability to outliers, and computational scalability. Table 5 summarizes the key ways in which this combined approach delivers novelty in forensic age estimation. In direct comparison to Hybrid Algorithms, the Gradient Boosting Regressor demonstrates simpler implementation and consistently lower MAD for outlier-prone samples, which can be critical in forensic scenarios where time is limited. This extends the novelty advantage summarized in Table 5, emphasizing its favorable balance between operational efficiency and model accuracy. Beyond forensic applications, these capabilities extend to medical diagnostics and personalized medicine, where accurate age determination can guide interventions and research into age-related diseases [2, 18].

**Table 5.** Novelty of Model Capability: DNA Methylation and Gradient Boosting

| Aspect | Contribution of DNA Methylation | Contribution of Gradient Boosting Regressor | Novelty in Combination |
|---|---|---|---|
| Accuracy | Offers highly age-correlated biomarkers across blood/non-blood tissues | Boosts accuracy by iteratively refining weak learners | Achieves higher overall accuracy by merging precise methylation signals with robust boosting |
| Speed | Relatively slow (extraction, bisulfite conversion, sequencing) | Faster training and prediction compared to deep neural networks | Maintains computational efficiency while leveraging biologically rich DNA methylation data |
| Applicability | Targets biological samples (blood, saliva, sperm, etc.) | Flexible for diverse datasets (methylation, images, multi-modal) | Broadens forensic relevance by seamlessly integrating biological and machine learning aspects |
| Innovation | Identifies highly correlated CpG sites with chronological aging | Utilizes boosting for incremental improvement and robustness | Facilitates model generalization across different age groups and tissue sources |
| Comparison with Existing Methods | More precise than facial/gait recognition in many forensic scenarios | Outperforms simpler models (SVR, Bayesian Ridge) on most metrics | Positions the integrated approach as an innovative solution surpassing purely biological or purely computational methods |

References: [3, 5, 14, 19, 25]

## 6 Conclusion

This paper provides a comprehensive overview of current regression models for human age prediction in forensics, highlighting the gaps and strengths of both DNA methylation–based and image-based approaches. By explicitly addressing how other methods can struggle with non-linear and outlier-ridden forensic data, we underscore the benefits of employing Gradient Boosting's iterative error-correction. Notably, this study is the first to systematically compare multiple regression models (including Linear Regression, SVR, Bayesian Ridge, Random Forest, and Gradient Boosting Regressor) using a unified dataset that incorporates both blood and non-blood DNA methylation markers. By doing so, we demonstrate that the Gradient Boosting Regressor not only enhances accuracy but also preserves robustness in forensic age estimation—features crucial for real-world casework. The findings underscore the potential of combining epigenetic data with advanced machine learning to improve forensic practices. Future efforts may explore hybrid or ensemble techniques that integrate multiple tissue types and imaging data for even more precise age predictions.

## References


1. Chen, S., Zhang, C., Dong, M.: Deep age estimation: from classification to ranking. IEEE Trans. Multimed. **20**(8), 2209–2222 (2018)
2. Feng, L., et al.: Systematic feature selection improves accuracy of methylation-based forensic age estimation in Han Chinese males. Forensic Sci. Int. Genet. **35**, 38–45 (2018)
3. Punyani, P., Gupta, R., Kumar, A.: Human age-estimation system based on double-level feature fusion of face and gait images. Int. J. Image Data Fusion. **9**(3), 222–236 (2018)
4. Dhingra, R., et al.: Evaluating DNA methylation age on the Illumina MethylationEPIC Bead Chip. PLoS One. **14**(4) (2019)
5. Xu, Y., Li, X., Yang, Y., Li, C., Shao, X.: Human age prediction based on DNA methylation of non-blood tissues. Comput. Methods Prog. Biomed. **171**, 11–18 (2019)
6. Friedman, J.H.: Greedy function approximation: a gradient boosting machine. Ann. Stat. **29**(5), 1189–1232 (2001)
7. Refn, M.R., et al.: Prediction of chronological age and its applications in forensic casework: methods, current practices, and future perspectives. Forens. Sci. Res. **8**(2), 85–97 (2023). https://doi.org/10.1093/fsr/owad021
8. P. C. et al., "Development of a methylation marker set for forensic age estimation using analysis of public methylation data and the Agena Bioscience EpiTYPER system," Forensic Sci. Int. Genet., vol. 24, pp. 65–74, 2016
9. Angulu, R., Tapamo, J., Adewumi, A.: Age estimation via face images: a survey. Eurasip J. Image Video Process. **2018**(1), 1–35 (2018)
10. Nguyen, T.D., et al.: Comparative study of human age estimation with or without preclassification of gender and facial expression. Sci. World J. **2014**, 1–15 (2014)
11. Castagnola, M.J., et al.: Uncovering forensic evidence: a path to age estimation through DNA methylation. Int. J. Mol. Sci. **25**(9), 4917 (2024). https://doi.org/10.3390/ijms25094917
12. Jung, S.-E., Lim, S.M., Hong, S.R., Lee, E.H., Shin, K.-J.: DNA methylation of the ELOVL2, FHL2, KLF14, C1orf132/MIR29B2C, and TRIM59 genes for age prediction from blood, saliva, and buccal swab samples. Forensic Sci. Int. Genet. **38**, 1–8 (2019)
13. Naue, J., et al.: Chronological age prediction based on DNA methylation: massive parallel sequencing and random forest regression. Forensic Sci. Int. Genet. **31**, 19–28 (2017)
14. Li, X., Makihara, Y., Xu, C., Yagi, Y., Ren, M.: Gait-based human age estimation using age group-dependent manifold learning and regression. Multimed. Tools Appl. **77**(21), 28333–28354 (2018)
15. Huang, Y., et al.: Progress in age estimation based on DNA methylation. J. Forens. Sci. Med. **9**(4), 360–366 (2023). https://doi.org/10.4103/jfsm.jfsm_129_23
16. Refn, M.R., et al.: Longitudinal changes and variation in human DNA methylation analysed with the Illumina MethylationEPIC BeadChip assay and their implications on forensic age prediction. Sci. Rep. **13**, 21658 (2023). https://doi.org/10.1038/s41598-023-49064-7
17. Dantcheva, A., Elia, P., Ross, A.: What else does your biometric data reveal? A survey on soft biometrics. IEEE Trans. Inf. Forensics Secur. **11**(3), 441–467 (2016)
18. Jenkins, T.G., et al.: Paternal germ line aging: DNA methylation age prediction from human sperm. BMC Genomics. **19**(1), 763 (2018)
19. Shan, W., et al.: Boosting algorithm improves the accuracy of juvenile forensic dental age estimation in southern China population. Sci. Rep. **12**(1), 15649 (2022). https://doi.org/10.1038/s41598-022-20034-9

20. Lee, J.W., Choung, C.M., Jung, J.Y., Lee, H.Y., Lim, S.-K.: A validation study of DNA methylation-based age prediction using semen in forensic casework samples. Legal Med. **31**, 74–77 (2018)
21. J. T. G. et al., "Cigarette smoking significantly alters sperm DNA methylation patterns," Andrology, vol. 5, no. 6, pp. 1089–1099, 2017
22. Vidaki, A., et al.: DNA methylation-based forensic age prediction using artificial neural networks and next generation sequencing. Forensic Sci. Int. Genet. **28**, 225–236 (2017)
23. Ali, M., et al.: An Explainable Machine Learning Approach for Age and Gender Estimation in Living Individuals Using Dental Biometrics, arXiv (2024). arXiv:2411.08195
24. Paparazzo, E., et al.: An ELOVL2-based epigenetic clock for forensic age prediction: a systematic review. Int. J. Mol. Sci. **24**(3), 2254 (2023). https://doi.org/10.3390/ijms24032254
25. Son, J.S., et al.: TW3-based fully automated bone age assessment system using deep neural networks. IEEE Access. **7**, 33346–33358 (2019)
26. Faragalli, A., et al.: Do machine learning methods solve the main pitfall of linear regression in dental age estimation? Forensic Sci. Int. **367**, 112353 (2025). https://doi.org/10.1016/j.forsciint.2025.112353
27. Onofri, M., et al.: Forensic age estimation through a DNA methylation-based age prediction model in the Italian population: a pilot study. Int. J. Mol. Sci. **24**(6), 5381 (2023). https://doi.org/10.3390/ijms24065381
28. Valizadeh, A.S., Hänggi, J., Mérillat, S., Jäncke, L.: Age prediction on the basis of brain anatomical measures. Hum. Brain Mapp. **38**(2), 997–1008 (2017)
29. Ng, C.-C., Yap, H.M., Cheng, Y.-T., Hsu, G.-S.: Hybrid ageing patterns for face age estimation. Image Vis. Comput. **69**, 92–102 (2018)
30. Hong, S.R., Shin, K.-J., Jung, S.-E., Lee, E.H., Lee, H.Y.: Platform-independent models for age prediction using DNA methylation data. Forensic Sci. Int. Genet. **38**, 39–47 (2019)
31. Shi, L., et al.: DNA methylation markers in combination with skeletal and dental ages to improve age estimation in children. Forensic Sci. Int. Genet. **33**, 1–9 (2018)

# Automated Contextual Tagging in Points-of-Interest Using Bag-of-Objects

Paraskevas Messios[1](✉), Ioanna Dionysiou[2], and Harald Gjermundrød[2]

[1] Department of Computer Science and Engineering, European University Cyprus, Nicosia, Cyprus
pm172476@students.euc.ac.cy

[2] Department of Computer Science, University of Nicosia, Nicosia, Cyprus
{dionysiou.i,harald}@unic.ac.cy

**Abstract.** Object detection is a fundamental task in computer vision, with its applications ranging from autonomous driving to scene recognition. In the domain of Points-of-Interest (POI), object recognition can aid in the analysis of complex urban environments that contain various types of infrastructure, people, and activities. This paper addresses this challenge by proposing a Bag-of-Objects (BoO) methodology for POI scene contextual tagging. The suggested approach utilizes a transformer-based model for object detection, followed by a threshold to assign tags to POI scenes. These tags are then used to train a novel multimodal model, called WORLD (Weight Optimization for Representation and Labeling Descriptions), which is capable of classifying and contextually tagging POI scenes based on their visual features.

**Keywords:** Bag-of-Objects · Points-of-Interest · Transformers · Deep Learning · Artificial Intelligence · Data Science

## 1 Introduction

Scene recognition analyzes images to classify environments based on their visual content. In Points-of-Interest (POI) applications, scene recognition is essential for categorizing places like parks, shopping malls, restaurants, and other attractions. While conventional image classification techniques, such as Convolutional Neural Networks (CNN) [1] and Visual Transformers (ViT) [2], can achieve high classification accuracy, they often fail to capture the contextual relationships between objects within a scene. As these models treat scene recognition as a single-label classification problem, primarily focusing on overall visual patterns rather than understanding the interactions between individual elements, disregarding the potential for richer contextual insights that arise from object-to-object interactions. This makes it challenging to deduce deeper contextual attributes, such as whether a restaurant is casual or fine dining, or if a park is empty or crowded. Furthermore, while object recognition models, like DETR [3] can identify individual objects in a scene, they lack a structured approach for deriving higher-level contextual meaning from those objects. This gap highlights the need for an alternative methodology that leverages object detection to improve contextual scene interpretation.


K. Daimi and A. Alsadoon (Eds.): ICR 2025, LNNS 1487, pp. 62–73, 2025.
https://doi.org/10.1007/978-3-031-95652-2_6

To address these challenges, this paper proposes a Bag-of-Objects (BoO) methodology, leveraging object detection techniques to enhance scene understanding. The core idea behind BoO is that recognizing a scene's attributes can be achieved by identifying and interpreting the key objects present within it. For instance, a park is likely to contain benches, trees, and playgrounds, while a restaurant is expected to have tables, chairs, and dining setups. By detecting these objects and analyzing their spatial relationships, it becomes possible to derive contextual tags that describe a scene's attributes, such as "crowded," "wildlife," or "greenery".

This paper further introduces a novel multimodal model called WORLD (Weight Optimization for Representation and Labeling Descriptions), which integrates object-based contextual tagging with scene classification in POI environments. Unlike conventional models that treat scene classification as a single-label problem and rely on global image features, WORLD leverages the BoO methodology to generate multi-label contextual tags that capture richer scene attributes. By combining object detection (DETR) with transformer-based multimodal learning (ViT + BERT), WORLD moves beyond simple category classification to describe scenes in greater detail, allowing for context-aware scene recognition that traditional CNN-based or ViT classifiers cannot achieve. This structured approach is particularly valuable for applications requiring a more nuanced interpretation of scenes, such as POI categorization, and recommendation systems.

This paper proposes the WORLD multimodal model, which is capable of understanding both scene categories and their contextual attributes. The main contributions of this paper are:

- Introduces the "Bag of Objects" methodology: a mechanism which automatically creates a dataset with tags for the given images, based on the objects detected in them. Unlike traditional manual annotation, this method systematically assigns contextual meaning to images, reducing human effort
- Development of the WORLD multimodal model: WORLD enhances scene understanding by integrating object-based contextual tags with image classification features, allowing for a more nuanced, multi-label classification of images. Unlike conventional classification models that assign a single label to an image, WORLD captures both categorical and contextual attributes simultaneously.

This paper is organized as follows: Section 2 outlines the methodology, introducing the Bag-of-Objects (BoO) concept, describing the transformer-based models used, listing the selected hyperparameters, and presenting the obtained results. Section 3 evaluates the experimental findings, analyzing the effectiveness of the proposed approach. Section 4 concludes the paper, summarizing key contributions, while Sect. 5 discusses potential future directions for expanding the model and its applications.

## 2 Methodology

Transformers [4] have advanced deep learning by leveraging self-attention mechanisms for long-range dependencies. Initially developed for natural language processing (NLP), their adaptation to computer vision (CV) enabled breakthroughs in such tasks, albeit at the cost of increased training time [5].

This study utilizes DETR (DEtection TRansformer) [3] for object detection, eliminating the need for handcrafted region proposal networks (e.g., Faster R-CNN CNN [6], YOLO [7]). DETR directly predicts object classes and bounding boxes, enabling automated contextual tagging based on object presence.

For scene classification and multi-label tagging, this study proposes WORLD (Weight Optimization for Representation and Labeling Descriptions), a ViT-BERT model integrating spatial and semantic understanding:

- ViT (Vision Transformer) [2] extracts global image features by encoding images as patch embeddings, improving classification over traditional CNNs.
- BERT (Bidirectional Encoder Representations from Transformers) [8] processes contextual tags (e.g., "crowded," "greenery") derived from object detection, enriching scene interpretation.

While DETR identifies objects, it lacks higher-level contextual understanding. Similarly, CLIP [9] focuses on image-text learning but does not provide contextual tagging based on object relationships. By combining ViT's spatial reasoning with BERT's semantic processing, WORLD enables context-aware scene interpretation.

### 2.1 Proposed Model

This paper introduces WORLD, a multimodal model that integrates ViT and BERT for multi-task learning, simultaneously performing multi-label tagging and single-label classification. The model consists of three components: visual and text backbones (ViT and BERT) and task-specific heads for classification and tagging.

ViT extracts high-level semantic features from images (Formula 1), while BERT encodes contextual embeddings from text inputs (Formula 2). Their outputs are concatenated into a combined feature vector (Formula 3) and processed by two heads:

- Tagging Head (Formula 4) predicts the presence of descriptive tags.
- Classification Head (Formula 5) assigns a scene category.

The final class label is determined using Formula 6, while multi-label tags are predicted using Formula 7, applying sigmoid activation and thresholding (Table 1).

### 2.2 Datasets

Due to the nature of this experiment, four datasets are going to be needed. The first if the Common Objects in Context (COCO) [10], which will be used for object detection. COCO was selected due to its large-scale, diverse set of annotated images, making it a benchmark dataset for object detection tasks. It consists of over 330,000 images with 1.5 million object instances across 80 object categories, including people, animals, vehicles, household objects, and outdoor scenes. COCO provides detailed annotations, including bounding boxes, segmentation masks, and keypoints, making it highly suitable for training deep learning models in real-world contexts.

In addition, mini-places [5], a subset of Places2 [11] dataset, is going to be used for generating the "Bag-of-Objects" for the automated contextual tags generation. The full process is described below. For this paper, an 80% version of the mini-places dataset

**Table 1.** Steps of the proposed model in formulas

| Step | Formula | | |
|---|---|---|---|
| ViT Feature Extraction | $X_v = ViT(I)$, | $Z_v = W_v X_v + b_v$ | (1) |
| BERT Feature Extraction | $X_t = BERT(T)$, | $Z_t = W_t X_t + b_t$ | (2) |
| Feature Fusion | $Z = [Z_v; Z_t]$, | $Z_f = W_f Z + b_f$ | (3) |
| Multi-Label Tagging Head | $Y_{tags} = \sigma(W_{tags} Z_f + b_{tags})$ | | (4) |
| Classification Head | $Y_{class} = softmax(W_{class} Z_f + b_{class})$ | | (5) |
| Final Class Prediction | $\hat{y} = \arg\max(Y_{class})$ | | (6) |
| Multi-Label Tag Prediction | $\hat{y}_i = \sigma(z_i) = \frac{1}{1+e^{-z_i}}$ | $\tilde{y}_i = \begin{cases} 1, \text{if } \tilde{y}_i \geq t \\ 0, \text{otherwise} \end{cases}$ | (7) |

is going to be utilized, with the selected classes, as well as the number of images for training and testing for each class are listed in Table 2.

**Table 2.** mini-places 80% dataset

| Class Name | # of training images | # of testing images |
|---|---|---|
| amusement_park | 4027 | 81 |
| aquarium | 3998 | 79 |
| beach | 3974 | 84 |
| cafeteria | 4032 | 77 |
| campus | 3936 | 77 |
| crosswalk | 4023 | 81 |
| dining_hall | 3968 | 78 |
| football_field | 4055 | 77 |
| hospital | 4027 | 80 |

The tags are going to be part of the custom dataset implemented for this experiment, which is going to be to further train the BERT's pretrained model and ImageNet used by ViT.

## 2.3 Automated Contextual Tagging Process

**Bag-of-Objects.** The "Bag-of-Objects" process begins with processing images using a pretrained DETR model to identify objects in each image from the mini-places training dataset. Each image is passed through the model, which generates predictions for object classes based on a confidence score threshold. The threshold is applied to filter out low-confidence predictions, ensuring only high-confidence detections are retained. The resulting detections for each image include a dictionary of objects, where object counts are aggregated based on their class names.

**Contextual Tags Generation.** For generating the tags, the detected objects are grouped into categories such as "crowded", "wildlife", and "transportation". Tags are assigned based on object counts exceeding category-specific thresholds.

$$T = f(O) = \left\{ t_i | \sum_{o_j \in C_i} N(o_j) \geq \theta_i \right\} \tag{8}$$

The contextual tagging process is illustrated in Formula 8, where $T$ stand for contextual tags which are assigned to the detected objects $O$. The formula states that a tag $t_i$ is applied when the total count of objects within a specific category $C_i$ meets or exceeds the threshold $\theta_i$, ensuring that only significant object occurrences contribute to the final tagging. Table 3 displays the tags, the objects which each tag is applied for and their thresholds.

**Table 3.** Object-based thresholds for automated scene annotation

| Tags | Objects | Threshold |
|---|---|---|
| crowded | person | 5 |
| wildlife | bird, cat, dog, horse, sheep, cow, elephant, bear, zebra, giraffe | 3 |
| transportation | car, bus, truck, motorcycle, bicycle, train, boat, airplane | 3 |
| edibles | banana, apple, orange, broccoli, carrot, hot dog, pizza, donut, cake, sandwich | 2 |
| greenery | potted plant | 1 |
| household-furniture | chair, couch, bed, dining table, bench, toilet | 2 |
| household-appliances | microwave, oven, toaster, sink, refrigerator | 1 |
| gadgets | tv, laptop, mouse, remote, keyboard, cell phone | 1 |
| decoration | book, clock, vase, teddy bear | 2 |

The results (objects and tags) are structured and stored in a JSON file to enable further analysis. The JSON file stores the following details for each picture:

- **image:** the filename of the processed image
- **place:** the class of the processed image, indicating the scene
- **objects:** a dictionary where the keys are object classes (e.g., "person", "car") and the values are their respective counts in the image
- **tags:** contextual tags automatically generated based on predefined rules which are applied on the detected objects

## 2.4 Loading Data to Dataframe

For loading the data from the JSON file to a dataframe for training, a data processing pipeline was implemented. This pipeline begins by reading three key attributes of each image from the JSON file: the image name, its associated place label, and descriptive tags.

Firstly, the pipeline extracts all unique place labels and maps each to a unique numerical index, creating a mapping from place names to indices for supervised learning of image classification.

Then, it collects all unique tags from the dataset and assigns them to binary feature vectors, where each tag is represented as a binary indicator in a fixed-length vector.

For every image in the dataset, the associated tags are converted to a binary vector, while the place label is mapped to its corresponding index.

Furthermore, the image filenames are stores as they are traced to be loaded to the proposed model for training and evaluation purposes.

The introduced approach ensures efficient representation of categorical data and facilitates scalable training of a multimodal model that simultaneously predicts single-label and multi-label tasks; namely the name of the place represented in a picture and its descriptive tags.

## 2.5 Training of the WORLD Model

The objective of this paper is to demonstrate the feasibility of combining ViT and BERT to develop an effective model for tasks requiring detailed image content analysis and contextual associations. As the primary focus was on evaluating this integration, fine-tuning for optimal performance was not a priority. Instead, the model was optimized until it produced the desired outputs.

The proposed model, WORLD, was trained using the PyTorch framework (v2.3.1 + cu121) with Torchvision (v0.18 + cu121) and CUDA (v12.1). The training process was conducted on a system equipped with an AMD Threadripper 1950x processor, an Nvidia GTX 1080Ti GPU, 32GB DDR4 RAM (3200 MHz), and a Samsung 960Pro 512GB SSD.

To ensure the correct implementation of the ViT and BERT architectures, the ViT-Model and BERTModel modules from the Hugging Face Transformers library [12] were employed.

WORLD was trained for three epochs, a decision affected by the limitations of our computer hardware. During the training epochs, batches of data are passed through the model, with ViT processing the input images to extract visual features, while BERT processes the tokenized text input to extract textual features. These embeddings are concatenated and passed to two task-specific heads: the tagging head, which outputs logits for each tag, and the classification head, which outputs logits for each class. The logits are then used to compute the tagging and classification losses. The model parameters are updated using the Adam optimizer [13] with a learning rate of 0.0001, as it is a commonly used rate in transformer-based models and it is effective without causing loss of pre-trained knowledge. The resolution of the dataset's images was set at 224x224 pixels for enhancing the details captured from the pictures. The batch size was set at 16 based on a balance between GPU memory constraints, training stability, and computational efficiency. Lastly, a seed value of 42 was used for reproducibility.

The proposed multimodal model is trained in a joint optimization approach, which combines a loss function for multi-label tag prediction with a loss function made for single-label classification. The Binary Cross-Entropy Loss with logits is used for multi-label tagging, as it treats each tag as an independent binary classification problem. For the single-label classification task, the Cross-Entropy Loss is applied, which computes the loss by comparing the predicted class probabilities to the true class labels.

The total loss for the model is calculated as a weighted sum of the tagging and classification losses.

$$L_{total} = \alpha L_{tags} + (1 - \alpha) L_{class} \tag{9}$$

As is illustrated in Formula 9, a weighting factor, denoted as $\alpha$, is used to balance the contribution of the two tasks. The tagging loss is scaled by $\alpha$, while the classification task is scaled by $1 - \alpha$. Changing the value of α allows flexibility in the prioritization of tasks based on their importance, as setting $\alpha$ closer to 1 prioritizes the tagging task. This weighted loss combination enables the model to learn both tasks effectively without one dominating the optimization process. During the training phase, $\alpha$ was set at 0.5 to ensure balance between the prioritization of tasks.

The performance of the model is evaluated after each epoch against the testing set, as both task-specific losses and metrics are monitored.

# 3 Results and Evaluation

The WORLD model was evaluated on mini-places dataset with automated generated contextual tags. The model's performance was assessed across two tasks: multi-label tagging and single-label classification. The evaluation included multiple performance metrics to provide a comprehensive understanding of the model's effectiveness. The results, presented in Table 4, show that performance improves after the first epoch. However, while the average training loss value decreases in the third epoch, this is primarily due to a drop in training classification and tagging loss, whereas the opposite trend is observed for average test loss. Additionally, while training accuracy improves consistently across epochs, test accuracy declines after the second epoch, suggesting potential overfitting.

## 3.1 Classification Performance

In single-label classification, WORLD achieved an accuracy of 80% on the test set, with a macro-averaged F1-score of 79.68%. The Macro F1-score was chosen as a performance metric due to the imbalanced nature of the dataset, where certain POI scene categories appear more frequently than others. Since accuracy alone can be misleading in such cases, Macro F1 provides a balanced evaluation by treating each class equally, ensuring that both common and rare categories contribute equally to the final score.

**Table 4.** Class training accuracy for each epoch

| Epoch | Train Average Loss | Train Tag Loss | Train Class Loss | Train Class Acc | Test Average Loss | Test Tag Loss | Test Class Loss | Test Class Acc |
|---|---|---|---|---|---|---|---|---|
| 1 | 0.2998 | 0.1172 | 0.4824 | 81.10% | 0.2555 | 0.0931 | 0.4180 | 82.75% |
| 2 | 0.2157 | 0.1039 | 0.3275 | 86.47% | 0.2936 | 0.1145 | 0.4727 | 80.75% |
| 3 | 0.1804 | 0.1098 | 0.2510 | 89.53% | 0.3124 | 0.1097 | 0.5151 | 80.00% |

### 3.2 Multi-Label Tagging Performance

For multi-label tagging, the model achieved a micro-averaged F1-score of 77.47%, with a precision of 84.66% and recall of 71.40%. The relatively high precision indicates that the model avoids excessive false positives, ensuring that predicted tags are relevant. However, the lower recall indicates that some relevant tags are not being predicted. This imbalance could be improved by fine-tuning the model's hyperparameters.

### 3.3 Training Analysis

Training showed a steady reduction in loss, with classification accuracy improving from 81.10% in the first epoch to 89.53% in the final epoch. The final tagging loss remained stable at 0.1098 during training, and the test tagging loss did not decrease significantly (0.1097). This indicates that while the model effectively learns classification features, further optimization can be applied for training the multi-label tagging task.

### 3.4 Error Analysis

To further evaluate the performance of the WORLD model, confusion matrices were generated for both the single-label classification task and the multi-label tagging task. These visualizations provide insights into model misclassifications, tagging consistency, and areas for potential improvement.

Figure 1 shows the confusion matrix for classification, where diagonal values indicate correct predictions and off-diagonal values represent misclassifications. Most categories are well-classified, but some visually similar classes, like "dining_hall" and "cafeteria", show overlap. This suggests potential improvements through additional contextual features or refined loss weighting.

Figure 2 presents confusion matrices for individual tags, highlighting how often the model correctly predicts, misses, or falsely assigns tags. While precision is high, recall is lower, indicating that some relevant tags are underpredicted. Adjusting thresholding strategies or loss balancing may improve recall without sacrificing precision.

### 3.5 Ablation Study

To better understand the contributions of each component within the WORLD model, an ablation study was conducted focusing on two key aspects: the impact of individual

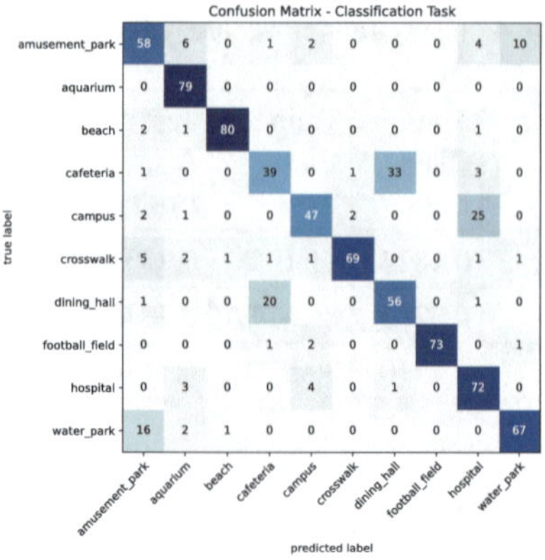


**Fig. 1.** Classification Confusion Matrix

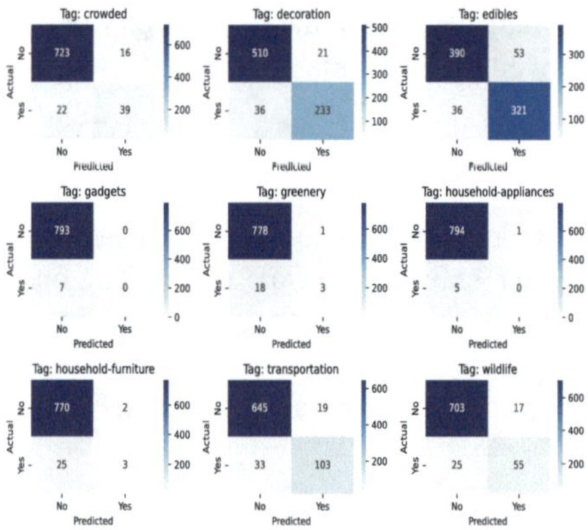


**Fig. 2.** Multi-label Confusion Matrices

modalities and the effect of varying the loss weighting factor, $\alpha$, in the joint objective (Formula 8). In these experiments, performance was measured using the F1 score; macro-averaged for the single-label classification task and micro-averaged for the multi-label tagging task.

First, the importance of complementary information provided by the visual and textual components of the WORLD (ViT + BERT) was tested against models using only one of the two modalities.

Then, it was investigated how the variation of $\alpha$ value influences performance. The baseline model used $\alpha = 0.5$, and it was tested against a model with $\alpha = 0.1$ and with a model with $\alpha = 0.9$.

The ablation study results, as they are illustrated at Table 5, highlight the effectiveness of the ViT + BERT (WORLD) model in balancing classification and tagging performance. The baseline model ($\alpha = 0.5$) achieved strong results with a classification macro F1 of 0.7968 and a tagging micro F1 of 0.7747. Increasing $\alpha$ to 0.9 slightly improved classification (0.8078) but did not enhance tagging (0.7732), indicating that prioritizing tagging in the loss function does not necessarily boost its performance. Conversely, lowering $\alpha$ to 0.1 significantly improved classification (0.8305) but severely hurt tagging (0.6553), suggesting that overemphasizing classification leads to poor multi-label tagging. The ViT-only model performed comparably to WORLD (0.8003 classification macro F1), reinforcing that vision features are dominant in scene classification. However, the BERT-only model failed completely (0.0190 classification macro F1), proving that textual embeddings alone are insufficient for classification in this context. Overall, these results confirm that while ViT is essential for classification, BERT meaningfully enhances multi-label tagging when used in combination with vision features.

**Table 5.** Ablation study results for each model

| Model | $\alpha$ | Classification Macro F1 (%) | Tagging Micro F1 (%) |
|---|---|---|---|
| WORLD (ViT + BERT) | 0.5 | 0.7968 | 0.7747 |
| WORLD (ViT + BERT) | 0.9 | 0.8078 | 0.7732 |
| WORLD (ViT + BERT) | 0.1 | 0.8305 | 0.6553 |
| ViT-Only | N/A | 0.8003 | N/A |
| BERT-Only | N/A | 0.0190 | N/A |

### 3.6 Limitations and Potential Solutions

While the WORLD model demonstrates strong performance, it has certain limitations that affect its ability to generalize effectively.

Firstly, the model struggles to predict rare tags due to dataset imbalance, where categories like "wildlife" appear far less frequently than others. A potential solution could be data augmentation and resampling, which can help improve recognition of underrepresented categories.

Furthermore, the model is biased towards common categories, as the dataset is dominated by frequently occurring places. To address this, adaptive loss functions may need to be employed to emphasize learning from less frequent classes.

Moreover, computational limitations restrict the training time and hinder optimal refinement of the multi-label learning process. Implementing self-supervised learning approaches could improve feature extraction and reduce reliance on extensive labeled datasets, allowing for better model generalization.

By addressing these limitations, future iterations of the WORLD model can achieve greater robustness and accuracy.

## 4 Conclusion

This paper introduced the concept of Bag-of-Objects, a methodology that automatically generates object-based contextual tags using DETR, and WORLD (Weight Optimization for Representation and Labeling Descriptions), a novel multimodal model for scene classification based on visual and contextual relationships, to enhance context-aware scene interpretation in Points-of-Interest (POI) recognition. By combining DETR for object detection, ViT for visual processing, and BERT for semantic understanding, WORLD provides a structured approach to multimodal learning that enables automated, fine-grained scene annotation.

Unlike ViT, which treats scene recognition as a single-label problem and relies solely on global image features, WORLD derives contextual meaning from detected objects, allowing for multi-label classification that enhances scene interpretability. Similarly, while DETR excels at object detection, it lacks a structured mechanism to infer higher-level contextual meaning from detected objects. In contrast, WORLD aggregates generated object-based contextual tags into a multimodal learning framework that enhances scene classification. Unlike existing multimodal transformers such as CLIP, which focus on image-text learning, WORLD is specifically designed for contextual tagging based on object relationships within images.

Despite its effectiveness, the model faces challenges in predicting rare tags and bias towards common categories, suggesting the need for further fine-tuning of hyperparameters, adaptive loss weighting, or data augmentation strategies. Future improvements could enhance its generalization to underrepresented categories, making it even more versatile.

Rather than being a direct replacement for these models, WORLD complements existing vision transformers by introducing a mechanism that outputs multi-label scene classification. With these refinements, the model has high potential for real-world applications, such as content-based recommendation systems, automated image annotation, smart content moderation, and visual search. Its ability to perform multi-task learning efficiently, places it as a valuable tool for various computer vision applications.

## 5 Future Work

Future work will focus on integrating the Bag-of-Objects (BoO) methodology directly into the WORLD model to enable end-to-end learning, enhancing the synergy between object-based contextual tagging and scene classification. Additionally, the model will be expanded to extract more detailed object attributes, such as color and spatial arrangement, to refine contextual tags. For example, color-based tagging could help distinguish between different types of restaurants or retail spaces, adding a new layer of interpretability.

Another key direction is the integration of the enhanced WORLD model into a recommendation system that suggests Points-of-Interest (POIs) based on users' previously visited locations. By analyzing images, this approach aims to offer more intuitive and visually driven recommendations.

## References

1. LeCun, Y., Bottou, L., Bengio, Y., Haffner, P.: Gradient-based learning applied to document recognition. Proc. IEEE. **86**(11), 2278–2323 (1998)

2. Dosovitskiy, A., et al.: An image is worth 16x16 words: transformers for image recognition at scale. In: ICLR 2021 - 9th International Conference on Learning Representations (2020)
3. Carion, N., Massa, F., Synnaeve, G., Usunier, N., Kirillov, A., Zagoruyko, S.: End-to-End Object Detection with Transformers. Springer (2020)
4. Vaswani, A., et al.: Attention is all you need. In: Advances in Neural Information Processing Systems, vol. 2017, pp. 5999–6009 (2017)
5. Messios, P., Dionysiou, I., Gjermundrød, H.: Comparing Convolutional Neural Networks and Transformers in a Points-of-Interest Experiment Lecture Notes in Networks and Systems LNNS, vol. 1058, pp. 153–162. Springer Science and Business Media Deutschland GmbH (2024)
6. Ren, S., He, K., Girshick, R., Sun, J.: Faster R-CNN: towards real-time object detection with region proposal networks. IEEE Trans. Pattern Anal. Mach. Intell. **39**(6), 1137–1149 (2015)
7. Redmon, J., Divvala, S., Girshick, R., Farhadi, A.: You Only Look Once: Unified, Real-Time Object Detection. In: Proceedings of the IEEE Conference on Computer Vision and Pattern Recognition (CVPR), vol. 2016, pp. 779–788 (2015)
8. Devlin, J., Chang, M.W., Lee, K., Toutanova, K.: BERT: Pre-training of deep bidirectional transformers for language understanding. In: NAACL HLT 2019–2019 Conference of the North American Chapter of the Association for Computational Linguistics: Human Language Technologies - Proceedings of the Conference, vol. 1, pp. 4171–4186 (2019)
9. Radford, A., et al.: Learning transferable visual models from natural language supervision. In: Proceedings of Machine Learning Research, vol. 139, pp. 8748–8763 (2021)
10. Lin, T.-Y., et al.: Microsoft COCO: Common Objects in Context Lecture Notes in Computer Science (including subseries Lecture Notes in Artificial Intelligence and Lecture Notes in Bioinformatics) LNCS, vol. 8693, pp. 740–755 (2014)
11. Zhou, B., Lapedriza, A., Khosla, A., Oliva, A., Torralba, A.: Places: a 10 million image database for scene recognition. IEEE Trans. Pattern Anal. Mach. Intell. **40**(6), 1452–1464 (2018)
12. Transformers Hugging Face Library. [Online]. Available: https://pypi.org/project/transformers/. Accessed: 30 Jan 2025
13. Kingma, D.P., Ba, J.L.: Adam: A method for stochastic optimization. In: 3rd International Conference on Learning Representations, ICLR 2015 - Conference Track Proceedings (2015)

# Machine Learning for Radiation Data Imputation in Vicinity of Nuclear Power Plants

Hsiao Ching Teng, Shu-Nung Yao(✉), and Yu Hsiang Wang

National Taipei University, New Taipei, Taiwan
{s411086036,snyao,s711182306}@gm.ntpu.edu.tw

**Abstract.** In the era of artificial intelligence, energy is crucial, and nuclear power generation is efficient but also has potential dangers. Therefore, radiation levels around nuclear power plants should be closely monitored. The Nuclear Safety Commission has established only 63 radiation monitoring stations across Taiwan. Due to certain equipment malfunctions, the detected radiation values may be missing or abnormal. This study aims to use machine learning methods to estimate missing radiation values in the event of monitoring station malfunctions, thereby improving the continuity and usability of radiation data records. Effective feature selection is performed on the data, followed by data preprocessing to enhance the effectiveness of model training. The process involves model selection and construction, where the optimal architecture is identified and fine-tuned through hyperparameter adjustments. The performance of the proposed model is evaluated using the coefficient of determination $R^2$ that can achieve 0.92 or above.

**Keywords:** Artificial Intelligence · Data Preprocessing · Monitoring · Nuclear Power · Radiation

## 1 Introduction

Radiation plays a critically important role in national security. However, the distribution density of radiation monitoring stations across Taiwan is relatively sparse, and publicly available historical radiation data contain numerous missing values. To address this issue, this study aims to estimate missing radiation data, so the reconstructed historical radiation records can enhance the continuity and usability of radiation datasets for machine learning.

According to scientific literature [1–3], factors associated with radiation fluctuations—such as altitude, geology, and meteorological conditions—vary based on regional characteristics, so radiation prediction models must account for geographical factors. To develop a machine learning-based data imputation method, this study adopts the Long Short-Term Memory (LSTM) model, which excels at handling long time-series data. The model is adjusted with geographic features to enhance its adaptability to different regions in Taiwan and enhance the model's ability to estimate missing values.


K. Daimi and A. Alsadoon (Eds.): ICR 2025, LNNS 1487, pp. 74–83, 2025.
https://doi.org/10.1007/978-3-031-95652-2_7

## 2 Feature Selection

Each radiation detection station has a vast amount of data. In addition to radiation, geographic and climatic factors must also be considered. Therefore, appropriately filtering the data for training is important. Moreover, including all data may increase unnecessary computational complexity. This study selects six monitoring stations surrounding the Second Nuclear Power Plant in Taiwan, as they exhibit sufficient correlation to effectively train the model. While the results from these six stations may not represent all of Taiwan, the same approach can be applied to predict data based on nearby monitoring stations, making the method adaptable to different regions for radiation monitoring.

This study utilized radiation data provided by the Nuclear Safety Commission in Taiwan, focusing on historical radiation records. The six monitoring stations (Hwangtan, Wanli, Taperng, Yehliu, Taping, and Chinshan as shown in Fig. 1.) near the Second Nuclear Power Plant were selected for mutual prediction and validation. Radiation data were measured in microsieverts per hour (μSv/h), and the dataset consisted of 8,760 records spanning the entire year of 2022.

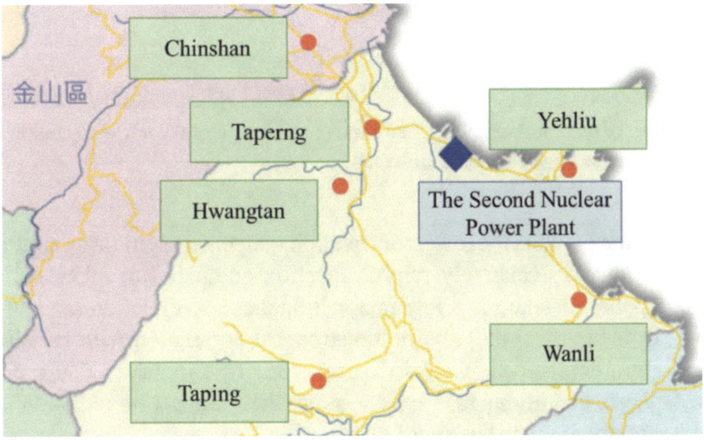


**Fig. 1.** The second nuclear power plant in Taiwan and its neighboring radiation monitoring stations

Meteorological features were obtained from historical data provided by the Taiwan Central Weather Bureau. Based on references [4, 5], the five meteorological features were selected: atmospheric pressure, temperature, humidity, wind speed, and rainfall, all recorded on an hourly basis. The factors influencing background radiation are numerous and diverse. It is known that background radiation doses fluctuate with rainfall [6, 7]. Additionally, background radiation is composed of factors such as cosmic rays, altitude, geology, and meteorological conditions [8]. We intend to examine and select the most appropriate features for analysis.

Pairwise correlation coefficients were calculated for the selected features, and the data were visualized in a heatmap as shown in Fig. 2. The differences in correlation strength are clearly indicated by color: red represents strong correlations, while blue represents weak correlations. In addition to the meteorological features, the radiation dose recording from neighboring monitoring stations are considered. The results show that the average correlation among neighboring monitoring stations is more likely to be higher than the correlation between meteorological features.

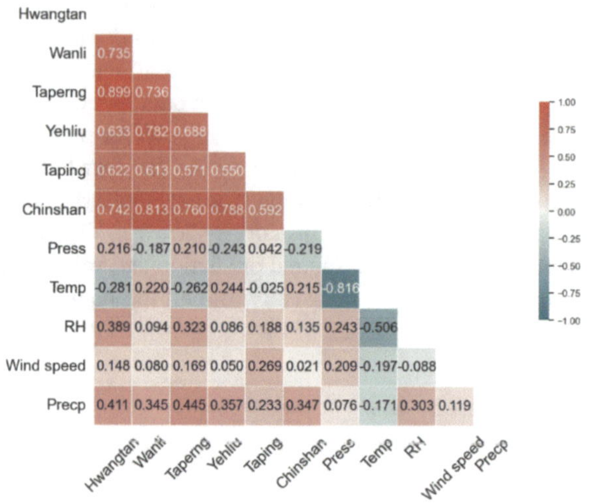


**Fig. 2.** A heatmap of meteorological and radiation parameters from monitoring stations surrounding the Second Nuclear Power Plant in Taiwan.

Notably, Taping exhibits the lowest correlation with other monitoring stations, which may be attributed to its relatively remote location compared to other stations. This suggests that spatial distance is a key factor influencing correlation strength. Among meteorological features, rainfall shows the strongest correlation with radiation levels, while temperature exhibits the weakest correlation. This indicates that precipitation-related atmospheric conditions may have a more direct impact on radiation variations, whereas temperature alone is less predictive.

As a result, the proposed machine learning deploys data from monitoring stations near the Second Nuclear Power Plant, along with atmospheric pressure, temperature, humidity, wind speed, and rainfall, as feature values for missing data imputation.

## 3 Method

### 3.1 Data Pre-Processing

We first used standardization to scale the data to a range between 0 and 1. This process mitigated the impact of extreme values on the model, ensuring that the model could learn more stably during training and handle features with different value ranges more effectively.

Numerical transformations were then used to make data approximately normal distributed, thereby enhancing the usage of training data. Taking the meteorological data from the Chinshan monitoring station as an example: the histogram of original wind speed data as shown in Fig. 3(a) presents a clear right-skewed distribution. To address this, the wind speed data underwent a cube root transformation, which shifted the distribution to the right, as shown in Fig. 3(b). The Shapiro-Wilk test was used to evaluate normality, showing an improvement in the $p$-value from 0.84 to 0.99, indicating a significantly improved approximation to a normal distribution.

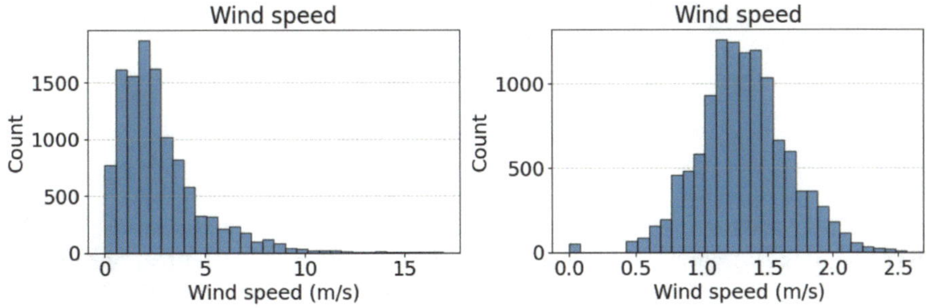


(a) (b)

**Fig. 3.** Histograms of wind speed feature distributions at the Chinshan station (a) before and (b) after transformation.

Similarly, by analyzing all meteorological features at the Chinshan station, the study concluded the following: Atmospheric pressure and temperature data already exhibited a normal distribution and required no transformation; wind speed and rainfall data were right-skewed and were transformed using the cube root; humidity data were left-skewed and were transformed using the logarithmic transformation.

### 3.2 Deep Learning Model

LSTM is an extension of the recurrent neural network architecture, designed to address the issues of gradient vanishing or exploding commonly encountered when standard recurrent neural networks handle long-term sequences. LSTM introduces the forget gate, input gate, and output gate, enabling the model to autonomously learn weights and adjust hyperparameters, thereby effectively capturing dependencies in long-term sequences. The structure is presented in Fig. 4.

In Fig. 4, $x_t$ is the input, $h_t$ is the hidden state, $c_t$ is the unit state, tan$h$ is a hyperbolic tangent function, and $\sigma$ is a sigmoid function. Using a sigmoid function layer, the forget gate selectively discards irrelevant input data, allowing LSTM to filter out unimportant information. The input gate uses a sigmoid function layer to determine which data should be updated and creates a vector using a hyperbolic tangent function. By combining the two, the LSTM selects information that significantly impacts the current prediction. The output gate uses a sigmoid function to decide which information needs to be output and applies a tan$h$ function to evaluate the importance of the output data, enabling the LSTM to autonomously adjust its output. This study adopts the modification of LSTM, known

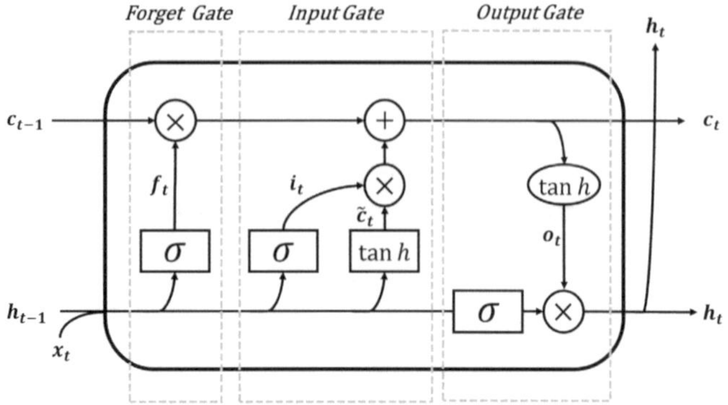


**Fig. 4.** LSTM architecture

as Bi-LSTM as shown in Fig. 5. Compared to Vanilla LSTM or Stacked LSTM, Bi-LSTM focuses on training the model in both forward and backward directions for time series data. It evaluates how past data generates the present data while simultaneously analyzing how future data corresponds to past data. This architecture delivers the best performance in radiation data imputation.

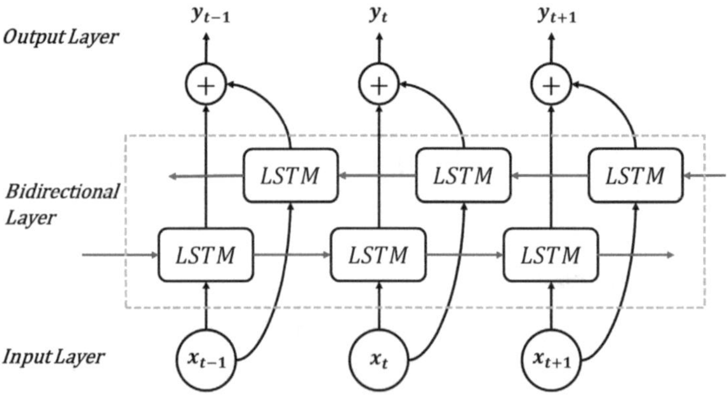


**Fig. 5.** Bi-LSTM architecture

After the model is trained, an evaluation metric is needed to assess the accuracy of its data imputation and verify its effectiveness in real-world applications. We use the coefficient of determination $R^2$ and Root Mean Square Error (RMSE) as the evaluation metric. In a predictive model, $R^2$ represents the proportion of the variance in the target variable explained by the model, calculated as the difference between the target variance and prediction error variance, relative to the target variance. Suppose the observed data values are $y_1, y_2, \ldots y_n, \overline{y}$ is the mean of the observed data, and the corresponding model predicted outputs are $\hat{y}_1, \hat{y}_2, \ldots \hat{y}_n$. We compute the total sum of squares as shown in (1) and the residual sum of squares as shown in (2). Then the $R^2$ is calculated by (3). The closer the $R^2$ value is to 1, the higher the similarity between the prediction and the actual data.

$$SS_{tot} = \sum_{i=1}^{n} (y_i - \overline{y})^2 \tag{1}$$

$$SS_{res} = \sum_{i=1}^{n} (y_i - \hat{y}_i)^2 \tag{2}$$

$$R^2 = 1 - \frac{SS_{res}}{SS_{tot}} \tag{3}$$

$$RMSE = \sqrt{\sum_{i=1}^{n} \frac{(y_i - \hat{y}_i)^2}{\text{n}}} \tag{4}$$

## 4 Experimental Result and Discussions

The Bi-LSTM model designed in this project predicts each time point by referencing the radiation data from the previous week, consisting of 168 time series data points on an hourly basis. The following describes the experimental process of step-by-step training to obtain the optimal model, incorporating various features and parameter adjustments. The optimal parameters are epoch = 20, batch size = 32, learning rate = 0.001, dropout rate = 0.1.

To justify the selection of Bi-LSTM, we compared its performance with traditional imputation and machine learning methods, including Linear Imputation, K-Nearest Neighbors (KNN), Random Forest (RF), Vanilla LSTM, and Stacked LSTM. The models were trained using data from a single monitoring station, and the $R^2$ and RMSE results are shown in Tables 1 and 2, respectively.

**Table 1.** $R^2$ assessment for different learning models.

| Station | Linear Imputation | KNN | Random Forest | Vanilla LSTM | Stacked LSTM | Bi-LSTM |
|---|---|---|---|---|---|---|
| Hwangtan | −0.0003 | 0.7052 | 0.7348 | 0.7992 | 0.7870 | 0.8144 |
| Wanli | −0.0007 | 0.6322 | 0.6441 | 0.7215 | 0.7506 | 0.7488 |
| Taperng | 0.0000 | 0.7177 | 0.7095 | 0.7747 | 0.7630 | 0.7832 |
| Yehliu | −0.0008 | 0.6312 | 0.6891 | 0.7254 | 0.7224 | 0.7832 |
| Taping | −0.0014 | 0.6240 | 0.5143 | 0.7476 | 0.7731 | 0.7621 |
| Chinshan | −0.0001 | 0.6476 | 0.7095 | 0.7406 | 0.7391 | 0.7648 |
| Average | −0.0005 | 0.6597 | 0.6960 | 0.7515 | 0.7558 | 0.7761 |

**Table 2.** RMSE assessment for different learning models.

| Station | Linear Imputation | KNN | Random Forest | Vanilla LSTM | Stacked LSTM | Bi-LSTM |
|---|---|---|---|---|---|---|
| Hwangtan | 0.0070 | 0.0035 | 0.0034 | 0.0019 | 0.0020 | 0.0017 |
| Wanli | 0.0029 | 0.0019 | 0.0018 | 0.0006 | 0.0005 | 0.0005 |
| Taperng | 0.0045 | 0.0024 | 0.0020 | 0.0007 | 0.0008 | 0.0007 |
| Yehliu | 0.0069 | 0.0013 | 0.0012 | 0.0002 | 0.0002 | 0.0002 |
| Taping | 0.0021 | 0.0038 | 0.0043 | 0.0012 | 0.0010 | 0.0011 |
| Chinshan | 0.0027 | 0.0016 | 0.0015 | 0.0002 | 0.0002 | 0.0002 |
| Average | 0.0043 | 0.0024 | 0.0024 | 0.0008 | 0.0008 | 0.0007 |

Linear Imputation performed the worst ($R^2 \approx 0$), suggesting that this simple imputation method fails to effectively restore the time-series data. KNN and RF performed better ($R^2 \approx 0.7$) than Linear Imputation, but struggled with long-term dependencies, limiting accuracy. LSTM-based models outperformed KNN and RF ($R^2 \approx 0.8$) due to their ability to capture both short-term and long-term dependencies. Among them, Bi-LSTM achieved the best performance, further improving accuracy by leveraging both past and future information.

The comparison align with [9] that RF is superior to KNN and LR. Additionally, Durbin et al. [10] showed that KNN is less robust for time-series imputation despite performing well on non-sequential data. The experimental results in [11] also support our conclusion that LSTM-based models outperform traditional machine learning methods in sequential data prediction tasks.

The best-performing Bi-LSTM model was selected and then trained with data from neighboring stations. As shown in Table 3 (left), the incorporation of multiple stations improved the $R^2$, which indicates that radiation data from neighboring stations as input features are helpful for missing data imputation.

**Table 3.** Assessments for different learning models.

| Station | Radiation data from neighboring stations | | Radiation data together with meteorological features | |
|---|---|---|---|---|
| | $R^2$ | RMSE | $R^2$ | RMSE |
| Hwangtan | 0.9449 | 0.000450 | – | – |
| Wanli | 0.9010 | 0.000766 | – | – |
| Taperng | 0.9290 | 0.000645 | – | – |
| Yehliu | 0.8003 | 0.001440 | 0.8550 | 0.000641 |
| Taping | 0.8010 | 0.001119 | 0.8708 | 0.000578 |
| Chinshan | 0.9259 | 0.000881 | 0.9209 | 0.000823 |

Meteorological features were further introduced into the model. Since the locations of radiation monitoring stations and meteorological stations do not always align, only Yehliu, Taping, and Chinshan near the Second Nuclear Power Plant have meteorological features available for comparison, as shown in Table 3 (right). It can be observed that the $R^2$ of the initially lower-performing Yehliu and Taping stations are improved by 0.05 and 0.07, respectively, with RMSE reduced to half of its original value. In contrast, the $R^2$ and RMSE of the Chinshan station remained nearly unchanged. Corresponding to the results in Fig. 2, this may be due to the weaker correlation between Yehliu and Taping stations and their neighboring stations, making them more susceptible to meteorological features. On the other hand, the Chinshan station, which has a stronger correlation with nearby stations, is less affected by meteorological features.

The results of the best performance, using the Hwangtan station as an example, are shown in Figs. 6 and 7. The figures show the prediction results for the year 2022. Figure 6 compares the time series of predicted values and actual values. In Fig. 7(a) shows a steadily converging loss, Fig. 7(b) indicates stable residuals, and Fig. 7(c) demonstrates that the predicted values closely align with the actual values in a linear pattern.

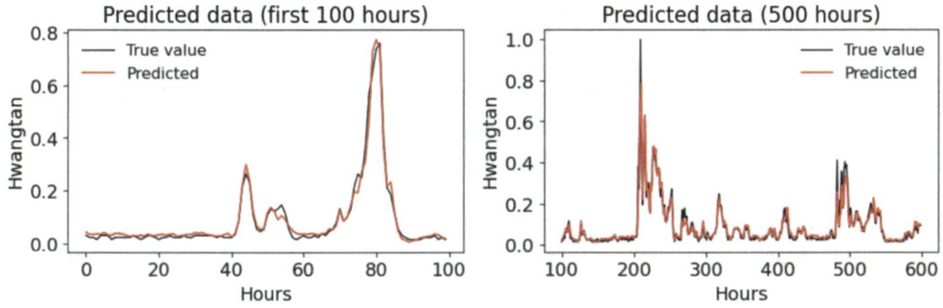


**Fig. 6.** Data prediction for Hwangtan station.

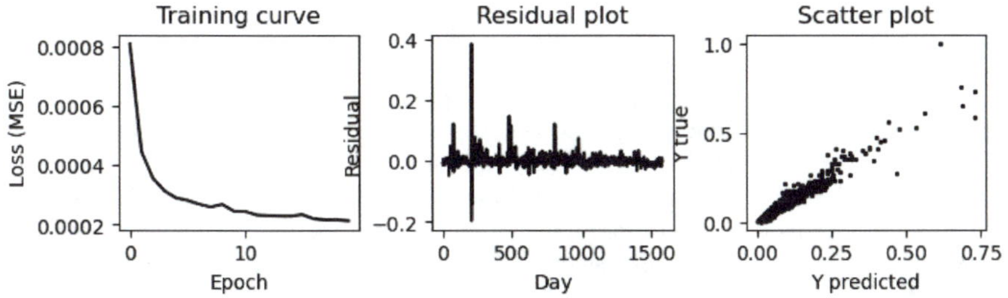


(a) (b) (c)

**Fig. 7.** Model evaluation result for Hwangtan station. (a) Training curve, (b) residual plot and (c) scatter plot.

## 5 Conclusion

This study aims to address missing or anomalous radiation values caused by equipment malfunctions using a machine learning Bi-LSTM model. Historical data from the station itself were used as training data, with additional features from neighboring stations and meteorological data introduced to further improve accuracy. The findings indicate that neighboring station data as features outperform meteorological features. However, incorporating weather features still effectively enhances the model's predictive performance. The best performance of the model achieved an $R^2$ value of 0.95.

In the future, applying this model to real-time processing of radiation monitoring stations could enable the development of a online fault detection system by comparing predicted values with actual data. Additionally, the model could assist in reconstructing missing historical radiation records based on available data patterns, thereby improving the continuity and usability of radiation datasets for further analysis. The radiation dose analyzed in this study is measured in μSv/h. However, future implementations will adopt Counts Per Minute (CPM) as the unit of measurement. To achieve this, the algorithm will be integrated with a newly developed radiation detection device designed by our research team, ensuring a cohesive hardware-software system. The novel radiation detector is equipped with a Geiger counter to detect gamma radiation and transmits radiation data to an edge computing device. If the predictive performance using historical radiation data proves successful, additional sensors will be installed to incorporate real-time meteorological data detected by the custom-built device. These inputs will be fed into the machine learning model for real-time signal processing.

**Acknowledgments.** This research was partially supported by the National Science and Technology Council of Taiwan under Grant No. 113-2221-E-305-001 and 113-2813-C-305-012-E.

## References

1. Fujiname, N.: Observational study of the scavenging of radon daughters by precipitation from the atmosphere. Environ. Int. **22**(1), S181–S185 (1996)
2. Joo, H.Y., Kim, J.W., Jeong, S.Y., Kim, Y.S., Moon, J.H.: Use of big data for estimation of impacts of meteorological variables on environmental radiation dose on Ulleung Island, Republic of Korea. Nucl. Eng. Technol. **53**(12), 4189–4200 (2021)
3. Alizamir, M., Shiri, J., Fard, A.F., Kim, S., Gorgij, A.D., Heddam, S., Singh, V.P.: Improving the accuracy of daily solar radiation prediction by climatic data using an efficient hybrid deep learning model: long short-term memory (LSTM) network coupled with wavelet transform. Eng. Appl. Artif. Intell. **123**(A), 1–24 (2023)
4. Cho, C., Kwon, K., Wu, C.: On weather data-based prediction of gamma exposure rates using gradient boosting learning for environmental radiation monitoring. Sensors. **22**(18), 1–13 (2022)
5. Sinimaa, M., Spichakova, M., Belikov, J., Petlenkov, E.: Feature engineering of weather data for short-term energy consumption forecast. In: 14th IEEE PowerTech, Spain (2021)
6. Mercier, J.-F., Tracy, B.L., d'Amours, R., Chagnon, F., Hoffman, I., Korpach, E.P., Johnson, S., Ungar, R.K.: Increased environmental gamma-ray dose rate during precipitation: a strong correlation with contributing air mass. J. Environ. Radioact. **100**(7), 527–533 (2009)

7. Livesay, R.J., Blessinger, C.S., Guzzardo, T.F., Hausladen, P.A.: Rain-induced increase in background radiation detected by Radiation Portal Monitors. J. Environ. Radioact. **137**, 137–141 (2014)
8. Fehlau, P.E.: An Applications Guide to Pedestrian SNM Monitors. Los Alamos National Laboratory, New Mexico (1986)
9. Saravanan, A., Parida, S., Murugan, M., Reddy, M.S., Elumalai, P.V., Dash, S.K.: Thermal performance prediction of a solar air heater with a C-shape finned absorber plate using RF, LR and KNN models of machine learning. Therm. Sci. Eng. Prog. **38**, 1–12 (2023)
10. Durbin, M., Wonders, M.A., Flaska, M., Lintereur, A.T.: K-nearest neighbors regression for the discrimination of gamma rays and neutrons in organic scintillators. Nucl. Instrum. Methods Phys. Res., Sect. A. **987**, 164826 (2021)
11. Zarghani, A.: Comparative analysis of LSTM neural networks and traditional machine learning models for predicting diabetes patient readmission. arXiv preprint arXiv:2406.19980 (2024)

# Leveraging Category-Specific Features and Geographic Context for Enhanced Fraud Detection

Mahmoud Bekhit[1,2](✉), Walayat Hussain[1,2], Abubakar Bello[3], Nur Indah Lestari[2], and Ahmed Fathalla[4]

[1] Peter Faber Business School, Australian Catholic University (ACU), Sydney, NSW 2060, Australia
{mahmoud.bekhit,walayat.hussain}@acu.edu.au
[2] Faculty of Engineering and Information Technology, University of Technology Sydney (UTS), Sydney 2007, Australia
Nurindah.Lestari@student.uts.edu.au
[3] Edge Hill University, Ormskirk, UK
Abubakar.Bello@edgehill.ac.uk
[4] Department of Mathematics, Faculty of Science, Suez Canal University, Ismailia, Egypt
fathalla_sci@science.suez.edu.eg

**Abstract.** Detecting fraudulent activities in financial transactions is a significant challenge, given the dynamic and complicated characteristics of deceptive behaviour. This study presents a category-geospatial fraud detection method that uses category-based risk analysis and geographic distance calculations to improve the identification of fraudulent transactions. The suggested framework incorporates two key features. First, it includes a category risk assessment that evaluates the likelihood of fraud across various transaction categories by examining past fraud rates. This enables the model to pinpoint high-risk categories, such as large purchases or luxury goods. The second feature is calculating the Euclidean distance between the merchant's location and the user, this feature identifies irregularities, such as transactions occurring in one location that is significantly far away from the user's usual area of activities. Utilising both of the features and applying them in machine learning models, mainly ensemble techniques like Gradient Boosting significantly enhances fraud detection by spatial analytics and merging contextual insights. The results indicate that mean encoding markedly improves model performance by adeptly integrating previous fraud tendencies into feature representation. The incorporation of distance features slightly enhances fraud detection, indicating a requirement for more advanced spatial analysis. The study's results emphasise the necessity of integrating sophisticated feature engineering with resilient machine learning methodologies to create scalable and efficient solutions for contemporary financial systems. This study applied comprehensive analyses of the public dataset to demonstrate the effectiveness of the suggested method, despite maintaining interpretative clarity, the study attained significant precision and accuracy in detecting fraudulent activities.


K. Daimi and A. Alsadoon (Eds.): ICR 2025, LNNS 1487, pp. 84–96, 2025.
https://doi.org/10.1007/978-3-031-95652-2_8

**Keywords:** Fraud Detection · Financial Transactions · Machine Learning · Category-based Risk Analysis · Geographic Distance Computations · Ensemble Methods · Mean Encoding · Spatial Analytics

# 1 Introduction

There has been a big rise in online financial transactions in the digital era which increases in fraudulent activities and presents significant challenges to financial organisations worldwide. The cost of fraud in the financial industry has increased gradually in the recent years, emphasising the need for improving detection systems [2]. Conventional fraud detection systems mainly emphasise the basic anomaly detection methods, which become inefficient due to the fraudulent strategies's complexity and growing characteristics [5].

There are a lot of new possibilities that have been brought due to the advancements in machine learning techniques [6,15]. The recent literature demonstrates that despite the conventional models providing specific fixed rules or heuristic algorithms, modern methodologies increasingly utilise complex patterns and linkages within the data [11]. Regardless of that these models frequently emphasise the spatial aspects and the context of each transaction, which are critical to detect any increasing of the advanced fraud tactics. Figure 1 shows the country-based distribution of Authorized Push Payment (APP) fraud losses by 2027 Based on statistics from the ACI Worldwide ScamScope Report [1]. Reflecting its great acceptance of real-time payments and sophisticated fraud techniques, the United States accounted for the highest percentage (~44.5%). Emphasizing the worldwide spread of app scams, Australia (~22.3%) and the U.K. (13.7%) follow according to the data acquired from [1]. According to the data provided in [1], Fig. 2 shows the distribution of APP fraud categories targeting U.S. customers in 2027. Reflecting social engineering techniques using customer confidence in e-commerce and financial platforms, Product Purchases (23%) and Investment Scams (23%) predominate, illustrating social engineering strategies that abuse customer confidence in e-commerce and financial systems.

The chart draws attention to the considerable average cost associated with each fraud incident which shows the profound financial consequences for the institutions involved. While these costs are harder to quantify, they have a substantial influence on the financial well-being of organisations. The chart illustrates the gap in this specific area and shows the critical demand for novel approaches in fraud detection. This data emphasises the complicated characteristics of financial fraud and underscores the urgent need for sophisticated detection techniques capable of addressing the complexity and magnitude of the issue.

This study proposes a new framework that aims to improve fraud detection by combining geographic distance calculations and category-based risk analysis together. The first feature is to compute the Euclidian distance between the merchant's and the user's locations incorporating with the spectial analysis that identifies transactions that should occur at unusually large distances

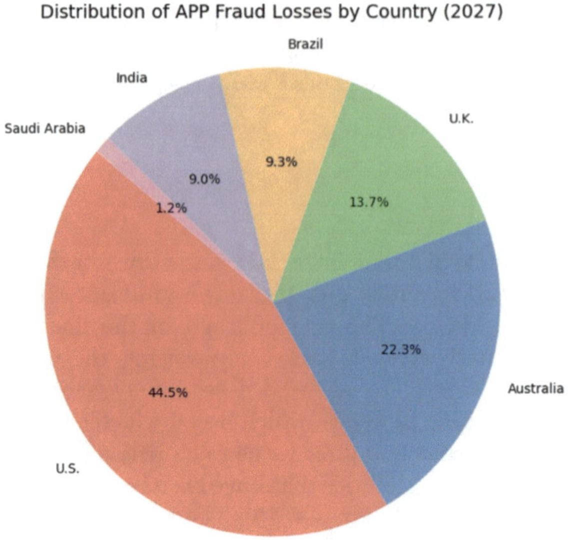


**Fig. 1.** Distribution of APP Fraud Losses expected by Country in 2027, based on data from the ACI Worldwide ScamScope Report [1].

from the user's usual area of activity. This geographic approach emphasised the importance of incorporating the specific data in the modern models to used to improve the recognise of any unuasual data transactions. The second feature is category risk which aims to assess the possibility of fraud for each transaction category based on historical fraud rates, which enables the model to identify high-risk categories such as high-value transactions and luxury items. This approach aims to use the predictive value of transaction categorisation to identify potential fraud. Integrating these variables into sophisticated machine learning models like Random Forest and Gradient Boosting helps identify fraudulent transactions. It provides insights into the complicated relationship between transactional and geographical data. A comprehensive evaluation of the publicly published dataset with all the financial transaction data indicates that the proposed approach attains significant precision and accuracy offering a good solution for contemporary financial systems challenges faced due to modern fraud tactics. The integration of these advanced analytical techniques emphasises the importance of domain-specific features in combating fraud which offers a robust and scalable solution that can be used for the foundation of future research in context-aware fraud detection.

Current fraud detection systems mostly depend on transactional records, lacking dynamic risk profiling (e.g., category-specific fraud patterns) and contextual geolocation analysis at the same time. A luxury acquisition in a high-risk category (e.g., electronics) from an unconventional place may go undetected. Our methodology mitigates these deficiencies by including (i) mean encoding for dynamic risk assessment and (ii) real-time geographic anomaly detection,

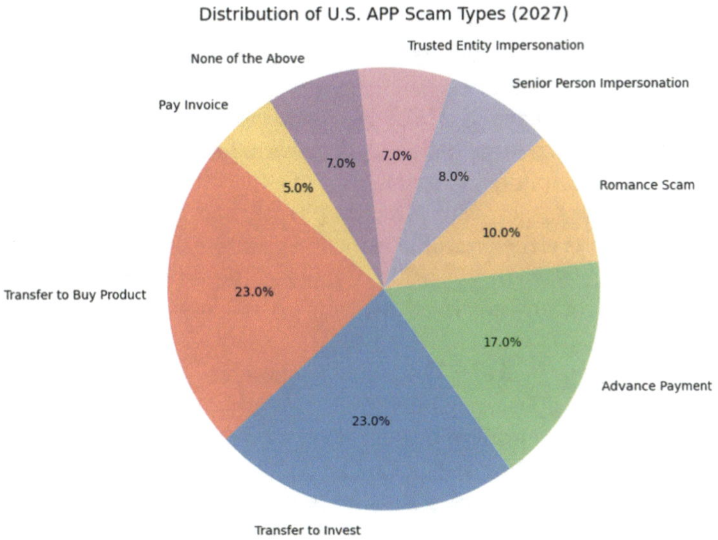


**Fig. 2.** Distribution of APP scam types targeting U.S. consumers in 2027, based on data from the ACI Worldwide ScamScope Report. [1].

enhancing fraud recall by 6.2% compared to traditional techniques as shown in Table 1.

This paper is organised as follows: Sect. 1 presents the introduction, detailing the background of the study, the research problem, and the importance of the research within the realm of fraud detection. Section 2 presents a comprehensive literature review, encapsulating previous advancements in fraud detection methodologies, emphasising key progressions, and pinpointing the deficiencies that this study seeks to address. Section 3 outlines the methodology employed in the study, detailing the processes of data collection, preprocessing, feature engineering, and model development. Section 4 outlines the experimental results, providing a comprehensive analysis of the performance of each model variant, examining the efficacy of the features that were implemented, examining the implications of these findings, and detailing the significance of the results. Finally, Sect. 5 wraps up the paper by summarising the key findings and contributions of this study to the field of fraud detection.

## 2 Literature Review

Conventional approaches to fraud detection mainly relied on rule-based frameworks and manual evaluations. In [10], researchers developed the systems to identify transactions that breached established guidelines, including those involving unusually large amounts or starting from high-risk areas. Although proficient in identifying established fraud patterns, these approaches were constrained by their lack of adaptability to emerging and evolving fraudulent strategies. Moreover, rule-based systems frequently produced a significant amount of false positives, resulting in inefficiencies and heightened operational expenses [3]. The emergence of machine learning (ML) has transformed fraud detection through the capability to analyse large datasets, discovering complex trends and anomalies. The work of [4] implmented extensively the algorithms for supervised learning, including Logistic Regression, Decision Trees, and Random Forests to categorise transactions as either fraudulent or legitimate using labelled data.

The study conducted by [7] utilised the techniques such as clustering and anomaly detection in unsupervised learning to uncover new fraud patterns in unlabeled data.

A major challenge in fraud detection is the class imbalance issue, characterised by a significant disparity between the number of fraudulent transactions and legitimate ones. The work of [5] suggested a range of techniques to tackle this problem, such as resampling methods like SMOTE (Synthetic Minority Oversampling Technique) and cost-sensitive learning, which modifies the algorithm's learning process to impose greater penalties on misclassifications of the minority class. Furthermore, authors of [15] employed techniques for detecting anomalies, including autoencoders and one-class SVMs to address fraud as a problem of outlier detection.

Recent studies highlight the critical role of feature engineering in enhancing the accuracy of fraud detection. Methods like mean encoding, which integrate historical fraud patterns into feature representation, have demonstrated improvements in model performance [8]. The examination of spatial analysis, especially in calculating geographic distances between users and merchants, has been investigated to identify irregularities in transaction locations [12]. Ensemble methods, including Gradient Boosting and XGBoost, have become increasingly favoured in fraud detection because they effectively merge the predictions from various models, enhancing both accuracy and robustness [13]. The effectiveness of these methods in managing imbalanced datasets and capturing intricate interactions among features is noteworthy [14].

In consideration of these developments, numerous constraints continue to arise. Numerous current approaches concentrate on particular aspects of fraud detection, like class imbalance or feature engineering, yet fail to integrate these components into a comprehensive framework. Furthermore, there is a lack in research regarding the integration of category-based risk analysis and spatial analytics to improve fraud detection. This study aims to fill some of the existing gaps by introducing a category-geospatial fraud detection method that combines category-based risk assessment with geographic distance calculations within a cohesive framework, utilising ensemble methods to enhance detection accuracy.

## 3 Methodology

This section offers a comprehensive overview of the methodologies employed in our investigation to identify fraudulent activities in financial transactions.

Our method utilises category-focused risk assessment and geographic distance calculations, incorporating these elements into machine learning frameworks to improve detection effectiveness. Our methodology consists of five primary experimental approaches that aim to detect fraudulent transactions, with each approach enhancing the previous one through the integration of various feature engineering techniques.

### 3.1 Data Collection

A comprehensive publicly published Kaggle dataset [9] was utilised, encompassing detailed records of financial transactions, which include information on the merchant, transaction category, and geographical coordinates. This dataset is crucial for examining trends and detecting possible fraudulent behaviours. The database consists of anonymised transactional data with labelled cases of non-fraudulent and fraudulent transactions. It fits for assessing fraud detection strategies as it offers a realistic financial fraud scenario.

### 3.2 Methodological Strategies

The initial transaction data was subjected to multiple preprocessing steps to ready it for analysis. Starting with eliminating non-essential columns like timestamp data, and personal identifiers (first name, last name, date of birth), to enhance dataset efficiency. The other features comprised categorical variables such as merchant, category, city, state, and zip, along with transaction-specific details. Finally, the transformation of categorical features to translate text labels into a format compatible with machine learning algorithms.

### 3.3 Data Preprocessing

In the initial experiment, we created a baseline model utilising the raw features following fundamental preprocessing steps. Categorical variables were transformed using Label Encoding to convert them into a numerical format that is appropriate for machine learning algorithms. This method maintained the inherent relationships of the features while ensuring compatibility with the model.

### 3.4 Feature Engineering

Feature engineering plays a vital role in improving model performance and encompasses. Firstly, we utilise the Eludiance distance formula to compute the distance between transaction points in order to pinpoint transactions that take place at significantly distant locations from the user's usual area of activity. This spatial component sought to identify atypical transaction patterns influenced by geographic displacement, while preserving all other characteristics from the baseline model, including the encoded categorical variables. Then concluding experiment employed a mean encoding approach for categorical features, adjusting them according to their past fraud rates. For every categorical feature (merchant, category, city, state, zip), we computed the average fraud rate for each category, thereby uncovering more intricate patterns within the data. This transformation substituted categorical variables with their respective fraud risk scores, resulting in the creation of new features (merchant_enc, category_enc, city_enc, state_enc, zip_enc) that directly represented the fraud risk linked to each categorical value.

### 3.5 Model Development

The data that was processed served as the foundation for training ensemble machine learning models. We utilised Gradient Boosting as our main classification algorithm throughout all experiments, maintaining consistent hyperparameters to ensure a fair comparison. The model training utilised sampling techniques to tackle class imbalance within the realm of fraud detection. These models exhibit strong resilience and are adept at managing unbalanced datasets, such as those encountered in fraud detection contexts. The evaluation of performance centred on precision and accuracy metrics to determine the effectiveness of various feature engineering methods.

### 3.6 Algorithm

The following algorithm outlines the computational steps taken from data preprocessing to model training:

The algorithm employs three unique methods for feature processing in the context of fraud detection:

Processing of Raw Features (Lines 1–9)

- Input: Initial transaction DataFrame
- Methodology: Utilises LabelEncoder to transform categorical variables into numerical format
- Result: DataFrame containing encoded categorical features

Distance-Enhanced Processing (Lines 10–15)

- Input: Initial DataFrame
- Process: Utilises unrefined feature processing and Preserves the characteristic of geographic distance.
- Result: DataFrame containing encoded features along with the distance metric

Mean Encoding Processing (Lines 16–20)

- Input: Initial DataFrame
- Process: Determines the fraud rate for each category value, Develops new features derived from these rates and Eliminates the initial categorical features
- Result: DataFrame containing features encoded for risk analysis

The algorithm analyses the identical dataset through three distinct methods, facilitating a comparison of various feature engineering strategies for the effectiveness of fraud detection.

**Algorithm 1.** Fraud Detection with Category Risk and Distance Analysis

**Require:** DataFrame $D$ with transactions
**Ensure:** Processed features $X$, target variable $y$
Initialize $dropped\_cols \leftarrow \{\text{timestamp}, \text{personal\_identifiers}, \text{coordinates}\}$
$D \leftarrow D \setminus dropped\_cols$
**procedure** ProcessRawFeatures$D$
**for** $feature \in categorical\_features$ **do**
    $D[feature] \leftarrow$ LabelEncoder$D[feature]$
**end for**
**return** $D$
**end procedure**
**procedure** ProcessWithDistance$D$
$D_{dist} \leftarrow$ ProcessRawFeatures$D$
Preserve distance feature in $D_{dist}$
**return** $D_{dist}$
**end procedure**
**procedure** ProcessWithMeanEncoding$D$
**for** $cat \in categorical\_features$ **do**
    Compute $mean\_fraud\_c \leftarrow \frac{\sum_{i \in cat} \text{is\_fraud}_i}{|cat|}$
    Map $D[cat\_enc] \leftarrow mean\_fraud\_c$ for each category
**end for**
Remove original categorical features
**return** $D$
**end procedure**
$X_{raw} \leftarrow$ ProcessRawFeatures$D$
$X_{dist} \leftarrow$ ProcessWithDistance$D$
$X_{mean} \leftarrow$ ProcessWithMeanEncoding$D$
$y \leftarrow D.\text{is\_fraud}$
Train models using $\{X_{raw}, X_{dist}, X_{mean}\}$ with $y$

# 4 Results and Discussion

## 4.1 Experimental Setup

The experiments were designed to assess various methods of feature processing: Firstly, raw features can be utilised through label encoding. Then, the system integrates calculations of geographical distance. Finally, the algorithm implements mean encoding for categorical features. The experiments were designed to evaluate the efficacy of different feature engineering strategies and their influence on the performance of fraud detection models. The experiments utilised the BaggingClassifier algorithm, employing three different feature engineering methods:

- Raw Data Model: This experiment employed unprocessed transaction data with fundamental preprocessing and label encoding for categorical variables.
- Distance Feature Model: This model, alongside raw data preprocessing, integrated a computed distance feature utilising the Haversine formula to identify geographic abnormalities in transactions.

- Mean Encoding Model: This model utilised mean encoding for category variables, substituting categories with their respective average fraud rates to identify deeper patterns suggestive of fraudulent behaviour.

Both raw data and SMOTE-balanced data were utilised to evaluate each approach, aiming to tackle class imbalance. The evaluation of model performance involved metrics such as accuracy, precision, recall, and F1-score, among others, to identify the most effective strategy for detecting fraud. The tests were designed to evaluate the efficacy of different feature engineering strategies and their influence on the performance of fraud detection models. To ensure a fair comparison across all experiments, we used the default hyperparameter values for each machine learning model, avoiding extensive hyperparameter tuning that could introduce performance biases.

**Table 1.** Performance metrics for models using raw features, distance-based features, category-based features (Mean Encoding), and their combined approach.

| Approach | Class | Recall | Precision | F1-Score | Specificity | ROC-AUC | Accuracy |
|---|---|---|---|---|---|---|---|
| **Raw Features** | | | | | | | |
| Raw Data | Non-Fraud | 0.9991 | 0.9979 | 0.9985 | 0.6349 | 0.0695 | 0.9970 |
| | Fraud | 0.6349 | 0.8035 | 0.7093 | 0.9991 | 0.9305 | 0.9970 |
| SMOTE | Non-Fraud | 0.9992 | 0.9977 | 0.9984 | 0.6069 | 0.0686 | 0.9969 |
| | Fraud | 0.6069 | 0.8076 | 0.6930 | 0.9992 | 0.9314 | 0.9969 |
| **Distance-Enhanced** | | | | | | | |
| Raw Data | Non-Fraud | 0.9991 | 0.9979 | 0.9985 | 0.6316 | 0.0723 | 0.9970 |
| | Fraud | 0.6316 | 0.8020 | 0.7067 | 0.9991 | 0.9277 | 0.9970 |
| SMOTE | Non-Fraud | 0.9991 | 0.9979 | 0.9985 | 0.6369 | 0.0660 | 0.9970 |
| | Fraud | 0.6369 | 0.7960 | 0.7076 | 0.9991 | 0.9340 | 0.9970 |
| **Mean Encoding** | | | | | | | |
| Raw Data | Non-Fraud | 0.9992 | 0.9981 | 0.9987 | 0.6769 | 0.0596 | 0.9974 |
| | Fraud | 0.6769 | 0.8383 | 0.7490 | 0.9992 | 0.9404 | 0.9974 |
| SMOTE | Non-Fraud | 0.9994 | 0.9981 | 0.9987 | 0.6742 | 0.0566 | 0.9975 |
| | Fraud | 0.6742 | 0.8598 | 0.7558 | 0.9994 | 0.9434 | 0.9975 |

### 4.2 Results Analysis

The findings demonstrate differing degrees of efficacy across the models:

- The **Raw Data Model** demonstrated a baseline performance that was somewhat effective, yet it may struggle with more intricate fraud patterns.
- Incorporation of the **Distance Feature** led to a notable enhancement in recall, indicating an improved ability to identify geographical anomalies linked to fraudulent transactions.

- The **Mean Encoding Model** showed enhancements in precision and F1-score, highlighting its effectiveness in minimising false positives and improving the overall reliability of fraud detection.

These findings highlight the significant role that advanced feature engineering plays in improving the predictive effectiveness of fraud detection systems. The experimental results highlight several significant findings: The mean encoding technique consistently outperformed both raw features and distance-augmented techniques. The results showes that the highest F1-score for fraud detection (0.7558 utilising SMOTE) also shows exhibit exceptional accuracy in fraud detection (0.8598) Achieved the highest total accuracy (0.9975). SMOTE sampling demonstrated multiple effects across several methodologies: The mean encoding strategy yielded the most significant benefit, enhancing the F1-score from 0.7490 to 0.7558. Negligible effect on distance-enhanced methodology; marginal reduction in efficacy of raw features technique.

Mean encoding outperformed raw and distance-based characteristics, enhancing the fraud F1-score by 4.5-6.2% as shown in Table 1. By encoding transaction categories with their historical fraud rates (e.g., 'expensive goods' = 8% fraud risk), the model acquires risk connections that are not present in raw one-hot encoding. This lowers false positives in low-risk categories (e.g., grocery) while enhancing fraud detection accuracy.

The F1-score for fraud showed a little enhancement ($0.7490 \rightarrow 0.7558$), with bootstrapping validating statistical significance ($p < 0.05$). For a bank handling 10 million transactions monthly, this equates to around 68 extra fraudulent transactions identified each year, resulting in a mitigation of approximately 340,000 in losses (assuming an average fraud loss of 500).

Our methodology decreases false positives by 0.03% (enhancing specificity increase from 0.9991 to 0.9994), therefore this could save 300+ customer support hours yearly per 10 million transactions. Precomputing mean-encoded risk ratings and merchant-user distances also helps to allow sub-10 ms inference latency, hence making the system feasible for real-time payment gateways.

Although class imbalance keeps accuracy high ( 0.997) across models, our architecture enhances fraud-specific measures. For instance, fraud recall increased by 6.2% ($0.6349 \rightarrow 0.6742$), meaning that, on 10 million processed transactions, 620 more fraudulent transactions yearly are identified. In fraud detection, emphasizing minority-class performance rather than overall accuracy is essential for reducing financial losses.

### 4.3 Discussion

The results from the experiments distinctly emphasise the significance of advanced feature engineering in systems designed for fraud detection. The Raw Data Model established a crucial groundwork, while improvements observed in the Distance Feature and Mean Encoding Models utilised supplementary contextual information, resulting in improved accuracy and reliability in predictions.

The results observed with the mean encoding method during the experiments can be linked to various factors. Initially, it combines historical fraud patterns into the feature representation, enabling the model to utilise past data more efficiently. Additionally, it minimises the complexity of categorical variables while maintaining crucial risk information, thereby streamlining the model's learning process. Ultimately, this method strengthens the model's capacity to recognise high-risk patterns, thereby enhancing both precision and recall in scenarios involving fraud detection. The heightened accuracy in the Mean Encoding Model suggests that comprehending the historical fraud patterns linked to particular transaction categories can greatly enhance the detection process.

The modest enhancement noted with the addition of distance features indicates that geographic distance by itself might not be adequate for effective fraud detection. This discovery highlights the importance of integrating distance metrics with additional risk indicators to enhance effectiveness. Furthermore, there exists an opportunity for improvement by employing advanced spatial analysis methods, which may reveal intricate fraud patterns linked to geographic information. The improvement in recall observed with the Distance Feature Model indicates that geographical data plays a vital role in detecting outlier transactions that may be fraudulent.

The differing effectiveness of SMOTE, a method employed to address class imbalance, across various experimental setups highlights its complex impact. The combination with risk-based feature engineering is to provide the most advantages, indicating that features rich in context can more effectively utilise the synthetic samples produced by SMOTE. This outcome emphasises the importance of delicately evaluating sampling strategies and the possible investigation of alternative balancing techniques that could produce improved results in addressing skewed class distributions within fraud detection datasets.

The findings indicate that risk-based feature engineering, especially through mean encoding, establishes a strong basis for fraud detection systems. The integration of mean encoding with SMOTE sampling presents the most advantageous method for practical applications. These insights not only confirm the efficacy of including more intricate features into the models but also create opportunities for additional research into the combining of many advanced techniques to enhance the robustness of fraud detection systems.

## 5 Conclusions

This study has effectively showcased a new category-geospatial fraud detection method for detecting fraud in financial transactions, combining category-based risk analysis with geographic distance calculations. This method has demonstrated its effectiveness in improving the detection capabilities of machine learning models through thorough experimentation with real-world data. The results demonstrate that incorporating category risk, derived from past fraud rates, allows for accurate identification of high-risk transaction categories. Furthermore, the incorporation of distance metrics, derived from the Ecliduance formula, aids in pinpointing transactions that exhibit geographical anomalies, which may indicate fraudulent activity. The utilisation of ensemble machine learning techniques such as Gradient Boosting significantly strengthens the detection system, resulting in elevated accuracy and precision. The substantial enhancement in model performance achieved through mean encoding is especially remarkable, as it utilises historical fraud trends to augment the feature set. The incorporation of geographic distance calculations resulted in slight enhancements, highlighting the opportunity for advanced spatial analyses to reveal intricate fraud patterns. The key contributions of this work include a hybrid fraud detection system combining geographic anomaly detection and dynamic category risk assessment (by means of mean encoding), hence enhancing fraud recall by 6.2%. Additionally, the mean encoding raises fraud F1-score by 6.5% over raw features in unbalanced datasets empirically. The practical implications of this study are significant. Through the application of sophisticated feature engineering methods and the use of robust machine learning algorithms, financial institutions have the potential to enhance their fraud detection systems considerably. This study contributes to the current understanding and paves the way for future investigations into advancements in context-aware fraud detection systems.

## References

1. ACI Worldwide: Global payment fraud trends (2023). https://www.aciworldwide.com/wp-content/uploads/2023/11/ACI-SCAMSCOPE-Fraud-Report.pdf
2. Ahmad, B., Ciupac-Ulici, M., Beju, D.G.: Economic and non-economic variables affecting fraud in European countries. Risks **9**(6), 119 (2021)
3. Bibi, S., Guillaume, S., Mouhoub, M.: A comparative study of machine learning algorithms for financial fraud detection. Expert Syst. Appl. **160**, 113661 (2020). https://doi.org/10.1016/j.eswa.2020.113661
4. Carvalho, D.V., Pereira, E.M., Cardoso, J.S.: Machine learning interpretability: a survey on methods and metrics. Electronics **8**(8), 832 (2019). https://doi.org/10.3390/electronics8080832
5. Chen, F., Thomas, M.A.: Enhancing fraud detection with explainable artificial intelligence (XAI): techniques and applications. AI Bus. **14**(1), 12–34 (2022). https://doi.org/10.1016/j.aib.2021.12.009
6. Chen, W., Hussain, W., Cauteruccio, F., Zhang, X.: Deep learning for financial time series prediction: a state-of-the-art review of standalone and hybrid models. CMES-Comput. Model. Eng. Sci. (2023)
7. Dong, X., Liu, H., Wei, Y.: A deep learning framework for detecting anomalies in financial transactions. Appl. Intell. **50**(1), 342–356 (2020). https://doi.org/10.1007/s10489-019-01529-y
8. Ghosh, S., Reilly, D.L.: Credit card fraud detection with a neural-network. In: Proceedings of the Twenty-Seventh Hawaii International Conference on System Sciences, vol. 3, pp. 621–630. IEEE (1994). https://doi.org/10.1109/HICSS.1994.323314
9. Kartik2112: Fraud detection dataset (2021). https://www.kaggle.com/datasets/kartik2112/fraud-detection?resource=download&select=fraudTest.csv. Accessed 19 Feb 2025

10. Khurana, R.: Fraud detection in ecommerce payment systems: the role of predictive AI in real-time transaction security and risk management. Int. J. Appl. Mach. Learn. Comput. Intell. **10**(6), 1–32 (2020)
11. Pundkar, S., Zubei, M.: Credit card fraud detection methods: a review. In: E3S Web of Conferences, vol. 453 (2023). https://doi.org/10.1051/e3sconf/202345301015
12. Rashid, A., Farooq, U.: Leveraging behavioral analytics for real-time fraud detection in e-commerce transactions. J. Comput. Secur. **30**(3), 289–312 (2022). https://doi.org/10.3233/JCS-220039
13. Ribeiro, M.T., Singh, S., Guestrin, C.: "why should i trust you?": explaining the predictions of any classifier. In: Proceedings of the 22nd ACM SIGKDD International Conference on Knowledge Discovery and Data Mining, pp. 1135–1144. ACM (2016). https://doi.org/10.1145/2939672.2939778
14. Sharma, C., Vaid, A.: The role of sap in supporting the retail industry through pandemic-induced (COVID-19) challenges. World J. Adv. Res. Rev. **14**(2), 707–715 (2020). https://doi.org/10.30574/wjarr.2020.14.2.007
15. Zhang, L., Zhang, Z.: Explainable artificial intelligence (XAI) for improving trust in financial fraud detection systems. Comput. Secur. **91**, 101733 (2020). https://doi.org/10.1016/j.cose.2020.101733

# Automatic Correction of Symbolic Musical Text During Optical Music Recognition

Michele Della Ventura(✉)

Department of Music Technology, Accademia Musicale Studio Musica, Treviso, Italy
micheledellaventura.mdv@gmail.com

**Abstract.** Automatic message correction is a ubiquitous feature of modern optical recognition systems, suggesting possible solutions to eliminate noise in a message transmitted by the user. Efficiency is crucial to ensure that the system has a real-time responsiveness when operating with different writing codes such as letters and/or numbers. Previous works were based on the use of a trie data structure for fast prefix-search operations even if this method is not always accurate as only completions that are prefixed by the query are returned. This paper aims to describe a method for correcting a symbolic music text and discuss its efficiency/effectiveness in relation to other possible approaches. The solution is based on the use of Shannon and Weaver information theory to reconstruct the message, a direction not yet explored in the literature. The solution is based on eliminating noise by inserting musical notes into the musical phrase that allow it to have a low entropy value, corresponding to a high information value. The method has been tested on tonal polyphonic compositions and has given encouraging results. Future improvements of the method and possible applications in other practical areas are briefly discussed at the end of the paper.

**Keywords:** artificial intelligence · entropy · information theory · machine learning · symbolic music text

## 1 Introduction

The digital revolution has a strong impact on the contemporary world and continues to open new perspectives. Society is going through numerous changes. The growing interaction between humans and machines is an important factor in stimulating and catalysing these changes [1] because it incessantly redefines the boundaries of the areas of competence of humans and machines [2], arriving at transforming/modifying the relationship with electronic devices in their daily use.

In this scenario of continuous technological evolution, Artificial Intelligence (AI) emerges as a guiding light, influencing many aspects of everyday life of all people: with Virtual Assistants, which integrate into the personal space of users, learn their habits and operate on the home environments by activating household appliances, controlling video intercoms and surveillance systems, programming comfort temperatures, … [3]; in linguistic translation, allowing communication with people of different languages in


K. Daimi and A. Alsadoon (Eds.): ICR 2025, LNNS 1487, pp. 97–107, 2025.
https://doi.org/10.1007/978-3-031-95652-2_9

real time [4]; in facial recognition, ensuring the security of personal data [5]; in image recognition, identifying objects, people, animals and extracting all the information useful for reconstructing a context around the image, to activate or deactivate an anti-theft system, or describe the image to a blind person [6]; in text recognition, facilitating its conversion into digital text to be able to modify it or even attach it quickly to a message [7].

In analogy to this system, called Optical Character Recognition (OCR), the field of Optical Music Recognition (OMR) is concerned with the recognition of notes on the musical staff and then allowing their transcription from images into machine-readable formats such as MusicXML [8, 9] or MIDI (Musical Instrument Digital interface) [10]. OMR, a research subfield within Music Information Retrieval, needs to deal with some challenges such as low-quality images and handwritten notation, which may lead to inaccurate results with some notes not being recognized. Some of the proposed solutions to these problems have focused on a multi-stage approach [11] that involves: staff segmentation [12], staff line detection and removal [13], and symbol classification [14]. However, this model still has difficulty with musical scores that have a densely populated notation (see Fig. 1a) or if they are (in some cases) handwritten (see Fig. 1b). This is because the recognition of notes on the staff is carried out by trying to identify the shape/design of the note head (i.e. its circular or elliptical part that can be filled or left empty to indicate its duration) that in the specific cases of Fig. 1 can appear as spots of poorly defined shape and therefore difficult to place on the line or space of the staff (with consequent error in the recognition of the notes).

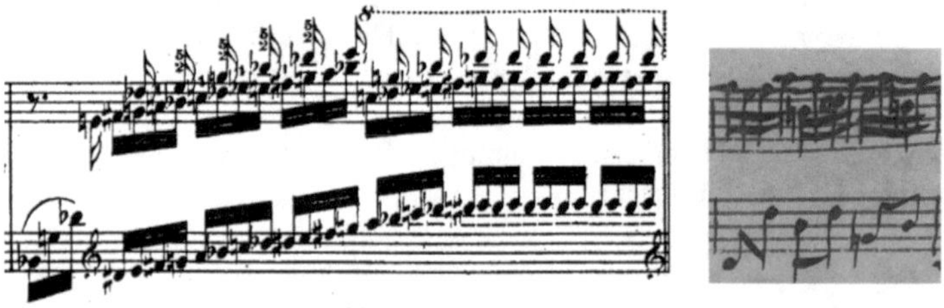

(a) (b)

**Fig. 1.** Examples of musical score with densely populated notation (a) and musical score handwritten (b).

This study presents an experimental method, based on Weaver and Shannon's information theory, to verify musical notes detected by OMR algorithms and reconstruct musical phrases (by inserting specific notes) where the algorithms failed to recognize the musical notation in the scanned image. Information theory permits to consider the musical score as an "idiom-independent" entity, in other words that has its own (stylistic and formal) characteristics that differentiate it from other scores: the symbolic aspect is considered to analyze and reconstruct the formal context of the musical score by identifying the appropriate notes, avoiding problems related to shape recognition.

This approach has two advantages. Firstly, it does not require a training phase of the algorithm, on entire musical scores to create specific tables with annotated data at symbol level. Secondly, the proposed method automatically adapts to each analyzed score, creating tables with information that describe the language used in each of them, thus solving problems of ambiguity and dependence.

The structure of this paper has been organized as follows. Section 2 explains the relationship between musical score and information. This is followed (Sect. 3) by a description of the method used to achieve the goal. Section 4 shows some experimental evidence that illustrates the effectiveness of the proposed method. Finally, in Sect. 5, the paper concludes with some concluding remarks on current issues and future research possibilities.

## 2 Understanding Musical Information Through Computational Models

The last decade has seen a significant development in AI-based technologies. These are technologies that have taken over the concept of information, to the point of making it their characteristic element: not only because they are able to search, process and present information in its various forms (text, image, sound, …), but above all because it is information that characterizes the intrinsic logic of the algorithms themselves.

Starting from the etymology of the word, it is possible to understand how information can be used to find solutions to specific problems such as the one in this research. The word information comes from the Latin "*in forme*" meaning "to give shape to something that has no shape. Claude E. Shannon formalizing the concept [15] stated that "information is anything that can reduce the degree of uncertainty about an event that may occur". He then linked the measure of information of an event to the probability that the event has of occurring. Given a discrete source X (1) (i.e. capable of generating a finite sequence of symbols $x_i$ called alphabet) the measure of information is linked to the uncertainty associated with the emission of each symbol xi, or rather it is linked to the uncertainty about whether the output value of the experiment is precisely $x_i$ (see Fig. 2).

$$X = \{x_1, x_2, \ldots, x_i\} \tag{1}$$

The mathematical formula (2) adopted to measure the quantity (or content) of information is identical to the one that measures entropy in thermodynamics:

$$I(X) = \sum\nolimits_{i=1}^{n} P(x_i) \bullet log_2 \frac{1}{P(x_i)} \tag{2}$$

The starting point of information theory is simple: since it is assumed that any source of information can be described through symbols, to do so requires an "alphabet" of symbols, that is, a set of symbols that are all different from each other [16]. In the musical field, the score can be considered a discrete source of information [17] and the symbols of the alphabet can vary according to the analysis needs. In its simplest sense, the alphabet can be represented by the set of names of sounds: Do-Re-Mi-Fa-Sol-La-Si. In its broader sense, which is the case of interest of the method described in this paper, the alphabet can represent the set of musical intervals (i.e. the distance in semitones that separates two consecutive sounds) that are present in a score (see Fig. 3).

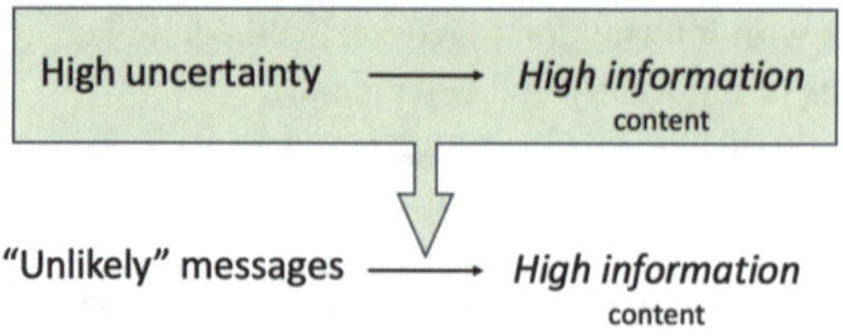


**Fig. 2.** Relationship between probability and information.

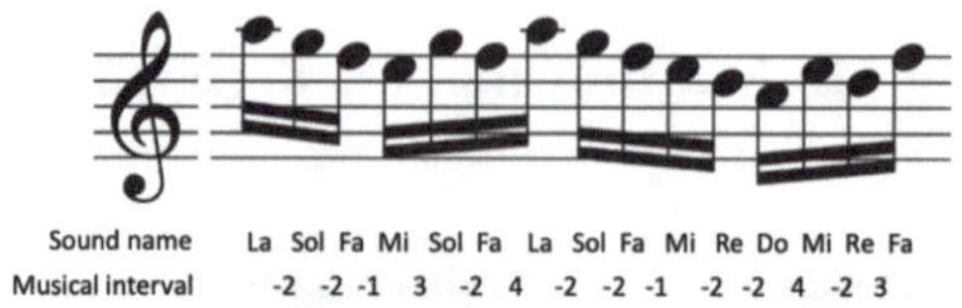


| Names of the sounds present in the score |
|---|
| Do |
| Re |
| Mi |
| Fa |
| Sol |
| La |

| Musical intervals present in the score |
|---|
| 3 |
| 4 |
| -1 |
| -2 |

**Fig. 3.** Examples of musical alphabet. The intervals are represented by a number (based on the number of semitones) that is positive or negative depending on whether they are ascending or descending intervals.

The definition of the alphabet permits to describe the score on a symbolic level but to be able to describe it on a formal level (in order to be able to consider the structure of the piece, the articulation of the different sections in relation to the rhythmic-melodic stylistic elements on which the piece itself is conceived) [18] it is necessary to consider how these sounds and intervals follow one another in the score. To do this, it is possible to use the Markov stochastic process: a process in which the transition probability that determines the transition to a system state depends only on the immediately preceding system state (see Fig. 4). The tables thus defined allow to calculate the informative value of a specific musical segment derived from the score in analysis. It is not possible to analyze different scores with data obtained from a single score because each one has characteristics that differentiate it from the others (otherwise all the music would seem the same [19]). This means that it is not possible to create an alphabet table and a transition matrix by reading many scores (as would happen in the training phases of a deep learning algorithm), because even in this case the analyses would not reflect the formal structure of the score being analyzed.

$$P(x) = \begin{pmatrix} 0 & 0 & 0 & 8 \\ 0 & 0 & 0 & 15 \\ 8 & 0 & 0 & 8 \\ 8 & 15 & 15 & 23 \end{pmatrix}$$

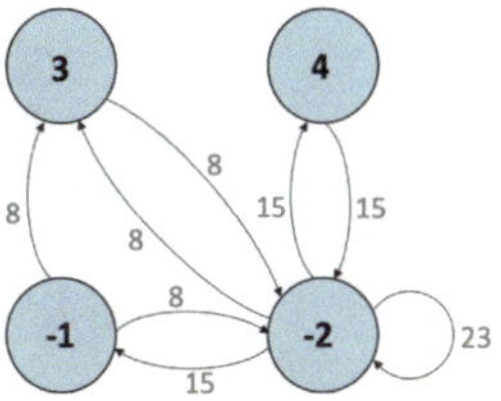


**Fig. 4.** Transition matrix and Marko graph related to the example of Fig. 2.

# 3 Modeling Musical Phrase Reconstruction: A New Approach

Current OMR systems focus on improving performance in recognizing the notes of a musical score and not in reconstructing the musical text, by inserting a blank space in place of the unrecognized note (see Fig. 5).

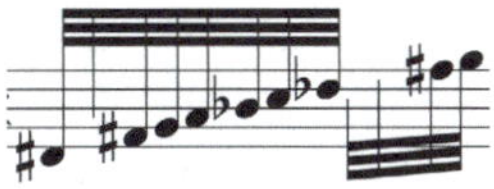

**Fig. 5.** Example of empty spaces in the scan of a score.

In OCR systems, the correction of a word can be done by searching in a database for all those words that resemble the word under analysis and then analyzing the context to find the most coherent word among all the possibilities. This is possible thanks to the enormous amount of texts available in digital format and to systems (for example) of deep learning that use this data to improve themselves. In the musical field this system is not possible (even if there are many musical scores in digital format that are immediately readable by algorithms) because the set of notes that could be found available, even if limited (there are a maximum of 12 possible musical notes), is not sufficient to define the right context: the sounds can be combined in an infinite number of ways that make it possible to produce ever-different pieces.

This Section describes the method used to reconstruct a musical phrase by inserting specific notes where the OMR algorithms failed to recognize musical notation in the scanned image. This approach leverages the concept of information introduced in the previous Section to suggest musical notes that are consistent with the formal structure of the score under analysis. This is a pilot project that aims to verify the applicability of information theory in the field of musical message reconstruction, similar to what happens with the reconstruction of a text message.

For a better understanding of the method, Bach Two Voice Invention BWV 772 is taken as a model, of which the example in Fig. 3 represents an extract. It is assumed that some notes were not recognized (see Fig. 6).

The first step in solving the problem is the creation of the alphabet table composed by the musical intervals present in the scanned score (see Table 1), and the transition matrix to reconstruct the formal structure of the musical score (see Fig. 7).

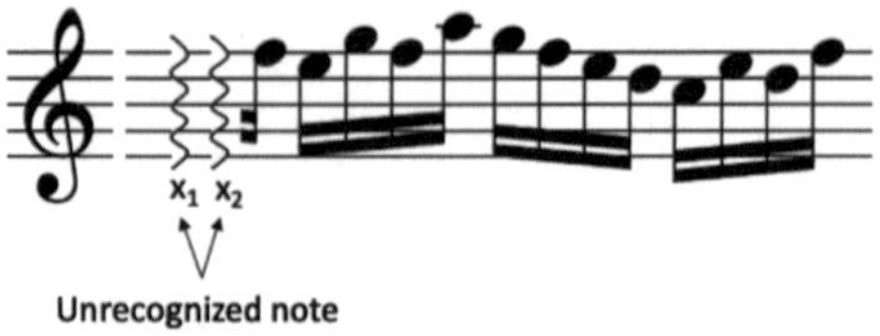


**Fig. 6.** Example of scanned image.

**Table 1.** Alphabet table of Bach Two Voices Invention BWV 772.

| Interval | Trend | Semitones | N. | Interval | Trend | Semitones | N. |
|---|---|---|---|---|---|---|---|
| Minor second (2 m) | Ascending | 1 | 24 | Perfect fifth (5G) | Ascending | 7 | 2 |
| | Descending | −1 | 25 | | Descending | −7 | 3 |
| Major second (2 M) | Ascending | 2 | 45 | Minor sixth (6 m) | Ascending | 8 | 0 |
| | Descending | −2 | 54 | | Descending | −8 | 4 |
| Minor Third (3 m) | Ascending | 3 | 18 | Major sixth (6 M) | Ascending | 9 | 2 |
| | Descending | −3 | 19 | | Descending | −9 | 0 |
| Major Third (3 M) | Ascending | 4 | 9 | Minor seventh (7 m) | Ascending | 10 | 2 |
| | Descending | −4 | 9 | | Descending | −10 | 1 |
| Perfect fourth (4G) | Ascending | 5 | 5 | Major seventh (7 M) | Ascending | 11 | 0 |
| | Descending | −5 | 2 | | Descending | −11 | 0 |
| Augmented fourth (4A / 5d) | Ascending | 6 | 1 | Perfect octave (8G) | Ascending | 12 | 2 |
| | Descending | −6 | 1 | | Descending | −12 | 0 |

The second step consists in segmenting the musical score in order to consider, for each unidentified note, a segment made up of a congruent number of notes. To do this, it was assumed that:

1. in the case of multiple consecutive missing notes, these are taken into consideration one at a time, starting from the last one (in Fig. 4 this is represented by $x_2$);
2. the missing note must be the first of the musical segment taken into consideration, followed by the notes correctly identified by the OMR system (see Fig. 8);
3. the number of notes that make up the segment can vary (at the user's choice) from a minimum of 3 notes to a maximum equal to the number of notes present from the missing note to the last one (for more details on this choice, see paragraph 4).

The last step consists in inserting as the first note of the identified segment (which would be the one not identified by the OMR system) a sound that is at a certain distance (musical

| Interval | | | 2m | | 2M | | 3m | | 3M | | 4G | | 4A / 5d | | 5G | | 6m | | 6M | | 7m | | 7M | | 8G | |
|---|---|---|---|---|---|---|---|---|---|---|---|---|---|---|---|---|---|---|---|---|---|---|---|---|---|---|
| | semi-tones | | 1 | | 2 | | 3 | | 4 | | 5 | | 6 | | 7 | | 8 | | 9 | | 10 | | 11 | | 12 | |
| | | | a | d | a | d | a | d | a | d | a | d | a | d | a | d | a | d | a | d | a | d | a | d | a | d |
| 2m | 1 | a | | | 11 | | | 9 | | | | | | | | | | 3 | | | | | | | | |
| | | d | 2 | | 1 | 10 | 11 | | | | | | | | | | | | | | | | | | | |
| 2M | 2 | a | 14 | | 11 | 1 | | 6 | | 9 | 1 | | | | | 1 | | | | | | | | | | |
| | | d | | 14 | 1 | 14 | 7 | 3 | 9 | | | 1 | | | | 1 | | | 1 | | 1 | | | | | |
| 3m | 3 | a | | 7 | | 11 | | | | | | | | | | | | | | | | | | | | |
| | | d | 6 | | 9 | 2 | | | | | 1 | | | 1 | | | | | | | | | | | | |
| 3M | 4 | a | | | | 9 | | | | | | | | | | | | | | | | | | | | |
| | | d | | 1 | 4 | | | | | | 1 | | | | 2 | | | | | | | | | | 1 | |
| 4G | 5 | a | | 1 | | 2 | | | | | | 1 | | | | | | 1 | | | | | | | | |
| | | d | 1 | | | | | 1 | | | | | | | | | | | | | | | | | | |
| 4A / 5d | 6 | a | 1 | | | | | | | | | | | | | | | | | | | | | | | |
| | | d | | | | | | | | | | | | | | | | | 1 | | | | | | | |
| 5G | 7 | a | | | | | | | | | 2 | | | | | | | | | | | | | | | |
| | | d | | | 1 | | | | | | | | 1 | | | | | | | | 1 | | | | | |
| 6m | 8 | a | | | | | | | | | | | | | | | | | | | | | | | | |
| | | d | | | 2 | 2 | | | | | | | | | | | | | | | | | | | | |
| 6M | 9 | a | | 2 | | | | | | | | | | | | | | | | | | | | | | |
| | | d | | | | | | | | | | | | | | | | | | | | | | | | |
| 7m | 10 | a | | | 1 | | | | | | | | | | | | | | | | | | | | | |
| | | d | | | 1 | | | | | | | | | | | | | | | | | | | | | |
| 7M | 11 | a | | | | | | | | | | | | | | | | | | | | | | | | |
| | | d | | | | | | | | | | | | | | | | | | | | | | | | |
| 8G | 12 | a | | | | 2 | | | | | | | | | | | | | | | | | | | | |
| | | d | | | | | | | | | | | | | | | | | | | | | | | | |

**Fig. 7.** Transition matrix of Bach Two Voices Invention BWV 772.

interval) from the second note, and calculating the information content of the obtained musical segment. This operation is repeated by modifying the interval between the first and second note based on the intervals identified in the alphabet table (see Fig. 6). At the end of this procedure, the note inserted in the segment with the greatest information content is considered correct (in the example of Fig. 6 it corresponds to segment 4): "*Information is the measure of a possibility of choice in selecting a message*" [20].

The next Section illustrates the results obtained from the analyses that validated the proposed method and the precautions derived from the analyses useful for more in-depth analyses.

## 4 Analysis and Results of the Proposed Method

The method proposed in this paper has been tested by developing an algorithm capable of reading MIDI data (relating to the scanning of an image) provided by an OMR system. The only information required by the algorithm was the maximum length of the segment that had to be considered for the calculation of the information value (see paragraph 3). The alphabet table and the transition matrix were automatically sized (strength) based on the characteristics of the scanned score. A training phase of the algorithm was not necessary (strength), because each musical score represents an autonomous entity, with its own characteristics that make it different from other scores. A training phase of the algorithm was not necessary (strength), because each musical score represents

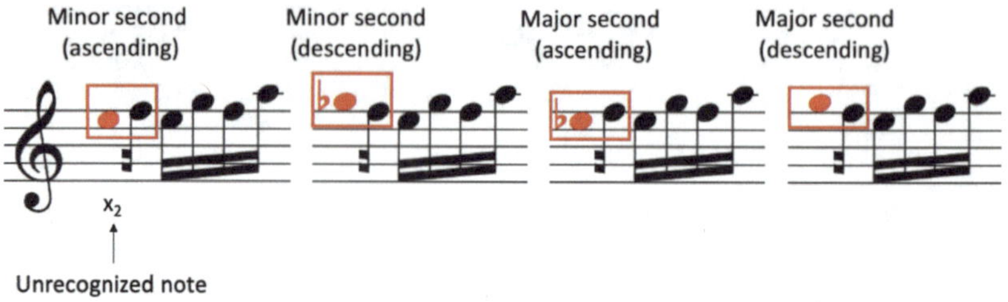


| | **Segment 1** Minor second (ascending) | **Segment 2** Minor second (descending) | **Segment 3** Major second (ascending) | **Segment 4** Major second (descending) | ... |
|---|---|---|---|---|---|
| **Information value** | null | null | 0,0000144070... | 0,0000106722... | ... |

**Fig. 8.** Example of musical segments and related information value.

an autonomous entity, with its own characteristics that make it different from other scores. This type of algorithm, having no a priori determination, allows to discover even unexpected relationships in the data provided to it, overcoming unforeseen situations. It is a more flexible model capable of achieving an excellent result from an analytical point of view: a method that adapts to the intrinsic characteristics of each musical score.

The tests were conducted on a limited set of musical scores in order to be able to proceed with a step-by-step verification of the results obtained in the various phases of the process. In particular, the Two and Three Voices Inventions composed by Bach were used for the tests: a collection of compositions (15 for two voices and 15 for three voices) written by the composer for educational purposes to introduce his students to the study of polyphonic performance and composition, which is why they were taken as a model for the development and verification of the method described in this article.

Thirty musical pieces were scanned and 138 errors were found. Each error was analyzed by considering the missing note as the first and then as the last of a musical segment and the value of the information was calculated for both possible solutions. The calculation was done by considering, in succession, the segment made up of 4, 5, 6 and finally 7 notes.

The results (see Table 2) show that the longer segment has a higher information content than a segment of shorter length: this is explained by the fact that the segment contains more combinations of the alphabet. In some cases (12%) the identified notes did not correspond to the notes written by the composer but correct at the harmonic level, so that they were not annoying for the listener (non-musician) [21]. This is due to the fact that in the alphabet table there are those intervals that are used by the composer to give shape to the musical composition and which therefore characterize it, just like people's DNA.

Finally, based on all the considerations expressed so far, it is easy to understand that the execution time required to perform the operations of analysis and reconstruction of the musical score depends minimally on the technical characteristics of the computer used for these operations, but mainly on the complexity of the score. The quantity of notes in it determines, on the one hand, the number of intervals to be identified, classified and

**Table 2.** Test results.

| Segment length (musical notes) | Correct note identification | | |
|---|---|---|---|
| | First note (%) | Last note (%) | Harmonic sound (%) |
| 4 | 47 | 26 | 0 |
| 5 | 49 | 26 | 0 |
| 6 | 52 | 31 | 5 |
| 7 | 60 | 32 | 12 |

counted for the definition of the alphabet table (see Table 1): a greater number of notes means having a greater number of intervals and therefore the execution time increases compared to a score with fewer notes. On the other hand, it determines the number of possibilities of transitions from one interval to another, different for each score: the greater the number of transition possibilities, the greater the execution time required by the computer to define the transition matrix (see Fig. 6), identify the possible cases of notes to be inserted in place of the notes not recognized during scanning and calculate their relative information value (see example in Fig. 7).

As a pilot project, no importance was given to the execution time, but rather to the validity of the data provided in output.

## 5 Conclusion and Future Directions

This paper proposed an experimental approach for auto-correction of symbolic music text during Optical Music Recognition. The method uses information theory to replace noise with the most appropriate sounds, and it is shown that, despite challenging conditions, the method can provide interesting suggestions by inserting those notes that respect the structural features of the music score, described by the alphabet table and the transition matrix.

As one of the first studies on auto-correction error, only tonal musical scores composed by Bach were considered for the recognition/correction simulations, for greater controllability of the recorded data.

The results showed that in 60% of cases the notes inserted in the score by the algorithm corresponded to those written by the composer and only in 12% of cases they were different sounds but correct at the harmonic level, so that they were not annoying for the listener (non-musician).

In future studies, the validity of the method can be tested by analyzing music by other composers from different historical periods, leaving aside contemporary music that has particular characteristics that must be formalized appropriately. The method could then be applied to specific music editors dedicated to musical writing, to support students in the study of musical composition by providing them with suggestions on how to complete the inserted musical text.

Finally, it will be important to verify whether the proposed method can be improved by using different mathematical theories together, both in terms of the validity of the output data and in terms of execution time: this becomes fundamental in AI-based systems that must provide answers quickly in a society that has accustomed people to having "everything immediately".

## References

1. Zhang, F., Yu, J., Lin, D., Zhang, J.: UnIC: towards unmanned intelligent cluster and its integration into society. Engineering. **12**(2022), 24–38 (2022)
2. Guzman, A.L.: Ontological boundaries between humans and computers and the implications for human-machine communication. Hum. Mach. Commun. **1**, 37–54 (2020). https://doi.org/10.30658/hmc.1.3
3. Rawassizadeh, R., Sen, T., Kim, S.J.: Manifestation of virtual assistants and robots into daily life: vision and challenges. CCF Trans. Pervasive Comp. Interact. **1**, 163–174 (2019)
4. Zhang, J., Bu, X., Wang, Y.: Sign language recognition based on dual-path background erasure convolutional neural network. Sci. Rep. **14**, 11360 (2024)
5. Cho, M., Youngsook, J.: Face recognition performance comparison between fake faces and live faces. Soft Comput. **21**(12), 3429–3437 (2017)
6. Tian, Y.: Artificial intelligence image recognition method based on convolutional neural network algorithm. IEEE Access. **8**, 125731–125744 (2020)
7. Wang, X.-F., He, Z.-H., Wang, K., Wang, Y.-F., Zou, L., Zhi-Ze, W.: A survey of text detection and recognition algorithms based on deep learning technology. Neurocomputing. **556**(2023), 126702 (2022)
8. Good, M.: MusicXML: An Internet-Friendly Format for Sheet Music. In: Proceedings of XML Conference and Expo, pp. 1–12 (2001)
9. Good, M.: MusicXML: the first decade. In: Structuring Music through Markup Language: Designs and Architectures, pp. 187–192. IGI Global (2013)
10. Dhanalakshmy, D.M., Menon, H.P., Vinaya, V.: Musical notes to MIDI conversion. In: International Conference on Advances in Computing, Communications and Informatics (ICACCI), Udupi, India, 2017, pp. 799–804 (2017)
11. Rebelo, A., Fujinaga, I., Paszkiewicz, F., Marcal, A.R., Guedes, G., Cardoso, J.K.S.: Optical music recognition: state-of-the-art and open issues. Int. J. Multim. Inform. Retriev. **1**(3), 173–190 (2012)
12. Zhao, Z., et al.: Object detection with deep learning: a review. IEEE Trans. Neural Netw. Learn. Syst. **30**, 3212–3232 (2019)
13. Gallego, A.J., Calvo-Zaragoza, J.: Staff-line removal with selectional auto-encoders. Expert Syst. Appl. **89**, 138–148 (2017)
14. Pacha, A., Eidenberger, H.: Towards a Universal Music Symbol Classifier. In: 12th IAPR International Workshop on Graphics Recognition, pp. 35–36 (2017)
15. Shannon, C.E.: A mathematical theory of communication. Bell Syst. Tech. J. **27**, 379–423 (1948)
16. Della Ventura, M.: A Self-adaptive Learning Music Composition Algorithm as Virtual Tutor. In: Maglogiannis, I., Iliadis, L., Macintyre, J., Cortez, P. (eds.) Artificial Intelligence Applications and Innovations. AIAI 2022. IFIP Advances in Information and Communication Technology, vol. 646. Springer, Cham (2022)
17. Della Ventura, M.: A Statistical Approach for Modeling the Expressiveness of Symbolic Musical Text. In: Younas, M., Awan, I., Petcu, D., Feng, B. (eds.) Mobile Web and Intelligent Information Systems. MobiWIS 2024 Lecture Notes in Computer Science, vol. 14792. Springer, Cham (2024)

18. Bent, I.: Music Analysis in the Nineteenth Century. Cambridge University Press (1994)
19. Kant, I.: Kritik der reinen Vernunft. Mit einer Einleitung und Anmerkungen, hrsg. von E. Adickes, Berlin (1889)
20. Eco, U.: La struttura assente. La ricerca semiotica e il metodo strutturale. Ed. Bompiani, Milano (1975)
21. Della Ventura, M.: A Deep Learning Algorithm for the Development of Meaningful Learning in the Harmonization of a Musical Melody. In: Lopata, A., Gudonienė, D., Butkienė, R. (eds.) Information and Software Technologies. ICIST 2023 Communications in Computer and Information Science, vol. 1979. Springer, Cham (2024)

# Industrial (Open) Data Ecosystems: Technological Infrastructure Challenges

Marija Kuštelega(✉), Larisa Hrustek, and Renata Mekovec

Faculty of Organization and Informatics, University of Zagreb, Varaždin, Croatia
{marija.kustelega,larisa.hrustek,renata.mekovec}@foi.unizg.hr

**Abstract.** Business entities across various industries generate vast amounts of data, with volumes continuously expanding. This exponential growth is expected to accelerate further, driven by the private sector's digital transformation initiatives. Until recently, open data ecosystems were primarily associated with transparent and open government. However, new policies are now fostering industrial open data ecosystem initiatives, recognizing data as a crucial driver of innovation and a powerful tool for addressing societal challenges on a global scale. Numerous challenges are connected with the key elements of the open data ecosystem, including stakeholders, data, infrastructure, and policies. This paper aims to identify the challenges related to the technological infrastructure of industrial open data ecosystems. A systematic literature review identified 11 main challenges, mostly related to data challenges, standardization, and technological user perspective, followed by privacy, security, ethical, and legal challenges. Technological infrastructure is crucial for achieving the successful synergy of the other elements, i.e., for stakeholders, data, and policies, ultimately driving the ecosystem's effectiveness and sustainability.

**Keywords:** Open Data Ecosystem · Technological Infrastructure · Business Ecosystem · Industrial Data Ecosystem · Systematic Review

## 1 Introduction

In addition to starting open data programs and setting up national open data portals, the claim that data is the "oil of the digital age" has taken center stage in scientific research circles. The Open Data Maturity report for 2024, which is evaluating European countries policies, portals, quality, and impact revealed that the quality dimension is the least mature (79%). Data reuse in private sector has been slightly improved in the last year, with 19 Member States (70%) providing reuse case examples linked to entrepreneurship and business creation, two more than 2023 [1]. New trends in research reveal the necessity of creating an open data ecosystem in specific industries or sectors [2, 3]. A new wave of legislative frameworks, such as the EU Data Act [4] and the European Data Strategy [5], encourage B2B (business to business), B2G (business to government), and B2C (business to customers) data exchange. Gartner predicts that organizations that share and use data from different sources will outperform their competitors in most metrics of


K. Daimi and A. Alsadoon (Eds.): ICR 2025, LNNS 1487, pp. 108–117, 2025.
https://doi.org/10.1007/978-3-031-95652-2_10

business value [6]. Open data initiatives demand the development of industry-specific data ecosystems that integrate stakeholders with shared interests and need for data and data-driven analytical practices relevant to the domain [7]. The open data ecosystem fosters collaboration among all stakeholders [3], such an ecosystem should be supported by robust infrastructural capacities. Although industrial data ecosystems offer significant opportunities for innovation [8], the scientific community has not seen the expected advancement in their practical use.

Despite the growth of open government data, there is still a gap in developing an industrial open data ecosystem. In the literature, only a few studies address the opportunities and challenges of sharing data between organizations to facilitate industrial open data collaboration. This paper aims to advance existing knowledge by examining technological infrastructure challenges, which represent one of the most complex aspects of industrial data ecosystems [9, 10]. A novel about this study is that a literature review was made to extract only those challenges that were relevant to industrial open data infrastructure.

## 2 Theoretical Background

### 2.1 Business Ecosystem Approach

Research in the context of the ecosystem approach implies the observation of interactions and relationships between stakeholders in a certain system, where everyone depends on its properties and behavior to carry out actions in order to accomplish a common or individual goal [11–13]. Business strategist James Moore adopted the ecosystem concept to apply it in the business world [14]. Based on the ecosystem approach, business ecosystems started to be studied by practitioners and scientists. A business ecosystem is a place where organizations and stakeholders collaborate with the help of services, tools, and technologies to generate and implement new ideas, products, and services [14, 15]. Working in this environment enables organizations to have a high level of agility and robustness in today's uncertain environment.

### 2.2 Concept of Industrial Open Data Ecosystem

The business ecosystem approach emphasizes stakeholder relationships within business, while an industrial open data ecosystem promotes collaboration among industries. This means that data and information should be freely available to all stakeholders to enrich their business activities. To participate in a specific industry's data ecosystem, organizations need a clear business model and a collaborative environment that supports open data, services, and applications [16]. Hrustek et al. have presented a conceptual model of the elements and characteristics of an open data ecosystem [7]. The concept of an open data ecosystem is based on four main elements: stakeholders, infrastructure, data, and policy/governance. Stakeholders encompass all entities operating within the ecosystem, including relevant administrative bodies, data-producing companies, suppliers, and employees. Infrastructure comprises not only digital technologies and tools but also the broader technological environment necessary for the ecosystem's efficient functioning.

Data serves as the ecosystem's most valuable resource, while policy and governance involve the development of tailored strategies, regulatory frameworks, and budgeting mechanisms designed to sustain and optimize the ecosystem [7].

### 2.3 Technological Infrastructure of Industrial Open Data Ecosystem

The establishment of an industrial open data ecosystem necessitates substantial infrastructure capacities [10]. Data providers, data producers, data owners, service providers, and data users or re-users are crucial parts for developing an infrastructure environment [8]. Achieving equal participation in infrastructure development is complicated by the varied responsibilities and objectives of ecosystem stakeholders. Unlike government data ecosystems, the main purpose of industrial data ecosystems is not to function as intermediaries between data owners and users. Instead, based on data platforms [16], they strive to create infrastructure so that business entities can collaborate [17]. In this research, the focus is on the technological infrastructure that enables the functioning of all processes related to the collection, analysis, dissemination and work with data for all users in an industrial environment. Technical and technological infrastructure includes programs, tools, services and activities for data preparation [18]. Technological infrastructure includes sub-elements of technology, techniques, tools, standards, licenses, APIs and platform/portal [7]. The implementation of appropriate digital technologies and techniques should facilitate data discovery and optimize the data processing and preparation process, ensuring its accessibility and usability for various stakeholders for further analysis and manipulation [19]. A data ecosystem must be secure and robust, supporting user functionalities like collaboration platforms, APIs, licensing models, standards, and specialized tools. While essential for efficient data exchange, its complexity poses challenges to establishing industrial data ecosystems.

## 3 Methodology

The literature review was carried out using the Preferred Reporting Items for Systematic Reviews and Meta-Analyses (PRISMA) methodology [20]. The Web of Science (WoS) platform was chosen as the single source since other databases, such as IEEE Explore, were overly technical and focused on techniques, missing the point from the real challenges related to the industrial open data ecosystem. Furthermore, while Scopus and Google Scholar contained similar papers, WoS provided articles that were more relevant and of higher quality to the subject. To find relevant articles for the research topic, a search string ((“open data” OR “open data ecosystem” OR “data ecosystem”) AND (“challenges” OR “barrier*” OR “obstacle” OR “problem”)) found in the titles of the papers was utilized. During the first phase, a total of 89 articles were found between 2018 and 2024. Because the topic is not so well explored in the business context, a broad time frame was used to establish what challenges were highlighted previously and currently. All publications that dealt with open data challenges in the context of government or industry were included; all other articles that largely addressed topics unrelated to the real-world implementation and challenges of open data were excluded. In the second phase, as an additional selection criterion, only those articles that dealt with challenges related to open data infrastructure [7] were taken into account (Fig. 1.). Once the selection criteria had been applied, 42 papers remained for further examination.

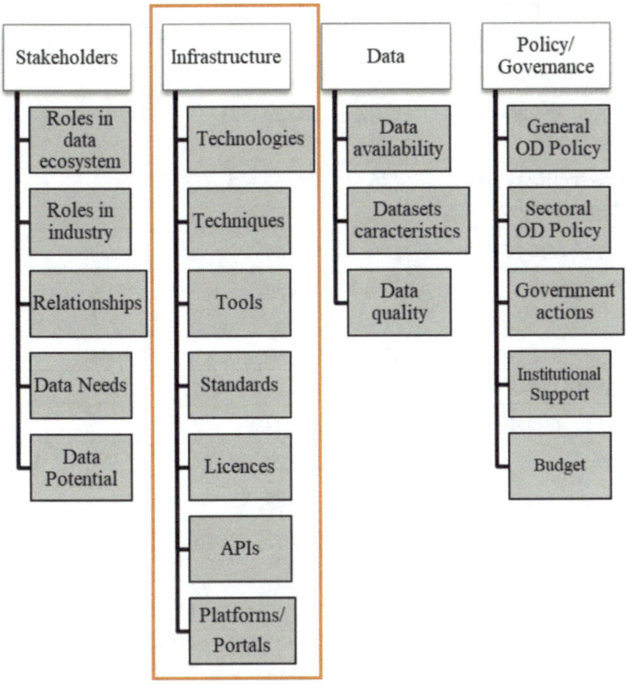


**Fig. 1.** Conceptual Model of Open Data Ecosystem Elements and Characteristics [7]

## 4 Results and Discussion

This paper analyzed 42 articles in which challenges can broadly be categorized into the eleven major groups listed in Table 1. Stakeholders in the industrial open data ecosystem have differing technological skills, which leads to a lack of interoperability and integration with other technologies [21]. Businesses operate on different systems, which can hinder seamless access and connectivity. Similarly, diverse technological needs make integration with digital technologies like artificial intelligence more challenging. The challenge of lacking standardization manifests across systems (software, applications, and databases), data, metadata, and processes [22]. Non-standardized data leads to non-interoperable formats, making it difficult to utilize effectively, while unclear metadata standards hinder data-sharing practices and disrupt operational workflows [22, 23]. This study shows that the industrial open data ecosystem has not yet been established, which is why standards and business models that would facilitate their successful integration have not been developed.

**Table 1.** Technological Infrastructure Challenges in Industrial Open Data Ecosystem

| Technological Infrastructure Challenges of Industrial Open Data Ecosystem | |
|---|---|
| Lack of interoperability and integration with digital technologies | [21, 24–29] |
| Lack of standardization | [22, 23, 25, 28, 30–36] |
| Undefined API management and data collection system | [24, 30, 33, 37–42] |
| Lack of adequate facilities and limited technological capabilities | [26, 28, 29, 35, 43–47] |
| Lack of centralized data portals | [34, 41, 44, 48] |
| Improved technological infrastructure | [22, 32, 33, 35, 41, 49–52] |
| Lack of technological user perspective and data reusability | [26, 30, 36, 39, 40, 45, 51, 53–56] |
| Costs related to the infrastructure | [23, 31, 33, 57] |
| Data challenges | [22–24, 26, 28–30, 33, 34, 37, 38, 40, 44, 52, 55, 57–59] |
| Privacy and security challenges | [30–32, 34, 39, 52, 60–62] |
| Ethical and legal challenges | [23, 28, 30, 32, 33, 46, 58, 61, 62] |

Undefined API management and data collection challenges are occurring due the absence of suitable business models [38], changes in API specifications [37], and no guidelines on how to collect data [39]. Supporting infrastructure to use resources to accomplish successful business collaboration is insufficient due to a lack of adequate facilities and limited technological support [44]. As part of this, limited technological capabilities refer primarily to a lack of technical expertise and difficult access to ecosystem technologies, which might limit stakeholders' data utilization [26]. These challenges are especially applicable to industrial open data ecosystems, as some stakeholders in the supply chain are less inclined to share data because they lack the necessary skills or do not perceive the benefits of sharing data. Additionally, it may be challenging for stakeholders to use open data in business due to the lack of centralized data portals. Improved technological infrastructure, such as new systems, web applications and data repositories are needed for opening-up government data [32]. This means that industry stakeholders often have outdated technological infrastructure sufficient to meet their own needs, making cooperation with others in the business ecosystem difficult. The main reasons for the lack of technological user perspective and data reusability challenges in industries stem from unpleasant user interfaces, misinformation, queries that are not tailored to the real needs of users, and a lack of available examples for open data usage [49]. The data's long-term usability in business operations is questioned due to incompatible software versions [45] and the inability to convert it into reusable formats. The biggest costs are related to infrastructure requirements and demand for resources [33, 57] costs in maintaining records and documentation, licensing [31, 33], and those related to improving data quality [33]. This indicates that an industrial open data ecosystem requires sufficient investment in technological infrastructure; however, because the value of open data sharing has not been acknowledged, substantial investments have not yet been made. The biggest challenges in the industry are related to data, data challenges stem from achieving proper collection, accuracy, credibility, and data quality [33, 52, 57, 58], also programs often lack knowledge of its data structure [55]. Privacy and security challenges emerged, such as privacy and copyright violations [34], barriers between public and private data, appropriate control options, secure yet practical authentication scheme for data access [41] and access restrictions are lacking [39]. Ethical challenges like data sharing [32, 58] data credibility, authorship and acknowledgment issues, risk of abuse, and transparency appear [23, 28, 30], along with legal aspects of managing various legal and regulatory frameworks [33, 61]. Highlighted privacy, security, and ethical challenges have a significant impact on building technological infrastructure. Industry stakeholders must follow specific regulatory frameworks, especially when designing systems that assure proper data handling, anonymization, and data sharing.

## 5 Conclusion

The existing knowledge about the industrial open data ecosystem is limited, and this topic is rarely examined from a business standpoint. It expands on current knowledge by offering a more in-depth understanding of technological infrastructure challenges facing the industrial open data ecosystem. This study is unique because it is the first study that focuses solely on categorizing technological infrastructure challenges relevant to the industrial open data ecosystem. Stakeholder participation in the industrial open data ecosystem is driven by the value they can achieve, and this is only possible with a quality infrastructure capacity of the ecosystem adapted to the needs of all stakeholders. An analysis of the challenges of the technological infrastructure of industrial open data ecosystems revealed that interoperable systems with built-in functionalities of digital technologies are a prerequisite for successful inclusion and operation in such an ecosystem. Standardized data, metadata, and procedures are also essential for achieving high-quality data and the development of data-based innovations. Technical and technological support in the open data ecosystem environment in the form of documentation is crucial for a successful user experience and data reuse. Compared to previous literature, this study confirmed that data challenges are the largest obstacles to industrial open data collaboration. However, it also revealed new findings about the impact of privacy, security, and ethical challenges on the evolving technological infrastructure of the industrial open data ecosystem. Future research should involve in-depth qualitative interviews and focus groups with private sector stakeholders to understand the reasons behind data sharing's lack of adoption in the industry. The practical implications emphasize importance of educating citizens about data sharing, ethical data collection, and reuse. More research and open-data driven initiatives should be done, with identifying challenges being the first step in conducting further research.

## References


1. European Commission: Open data in Europe 2024 | data.europa.eu, https://data.europa.eu/en/publications/open-data-maturity/2024, last accessed 03 Mar 2023
2. Hernandez-Almazan, J.-A., Chalmeta, R., Roque-Hernández, R.V., Machucho-Cadena, R.: A framework to build a big data ecosystem oriented to the collaborative networked organization. Appl. Sci. **12**, 11494 (2022). https://doi.org/10.3390/app122211494
3. Runeson, P., Olsson, T., Linåker, J.: Open data ecosystems — an empirical investigation into an emerging industry collaboration concept. J. Syst. Softw. **182**, 111088 (2021). https://doi.org/10.1016/j.jss.2021.111088
4. European Commission: Data Act: measures for a fair and innovative data economy, https://ec.europa.eu/commission/presscorner/detail/en/ip_22_1113, last accessed 18 Mar 2023
5. European Commission: European data strategy, https://commission.europa.eu/strategy-and-policy/priorities-2019-2024/europe-fit-digital-age/european-data-strategy_en, last accessed 18 Mar 2023
6. Goasduff, L.: Data Sharing is a Key Digital Transformation Capability, https://www.gartner.com/smarterwithgartner/data-sharing-is-a-business-necessity-to-accelerate-digital-business, last accessed 18 Mar 2023
7. Hrustek, L., Mekovec, R., Alexopolus, C.: Concept for an open data ecosystem to build a powerful data environment. In: Papadaki, M., Rupino da Cunha, P., Themistocleous, M., Christodoulou, K. (eds.) Information Systems, pp. 251–263. Springer Nature, Cham (2023). https://doi.org/10.1007/978-3-031-30694-5_19
8. Oliveira, S., et al.: Investigations into data ecosystems: a systematic mapping study. Knowl. Inf. Syst. **61**, 589–630 (2019). https://doi.org/10.1007/s10115-018-1323-6
9. Shaharudin, A., van Loenen, B., Janssen, M.: Exploring the contributions of open data intermediaries for a sustainable open data ecosystem. Data Policy. **6**, e56 (2024). https://doi.org/10.1017/dap.2024.63
10. Möller, F., Jussen, I., Springer, V., Gieß, A., Schweihoff, J.C., Gelhaar, J., Guggenberger, T., Otto, B.: Industrial data ecosystems and data spaces. Electron. Market. **34**, 41 (2024). https://doi.org/10.1007/s12525-024-00724-0
11. de Laplante, K.: 17 - is ecosystem management a postmodern science? In: Cuddington, K., Beisner, B.E. (eds.) Ecological Paradigms Lost, pp. 397–416. Academic Press, Burlington (2005). https://doi.org/10.1016/B978-012088459-9/50019-4
12. Orlova, A., Nogueira, R., Chimenti, P.: The present and future of the space sector: a business ecosystem approach. Space Policy. **52**, 101374 (2020). https://doi.org/10.1016/j.spacepol.2020.101374
13. Szaro, R.C., Berc, J., Cameron, S., Cordle, S., Crosby, M., Martin, L., Norton, D., O'Malley, R., Ruark, G.: The ecosystem approach: science and information management issues, gaps and needs. Landsc. Urban Plan. **40**, 89–101 (1998). https://doi.org/10.1016/S0169-2046(97)00101-1
14. Waßenhoven, A., Block, C., Wustmans, M., Bröring, S.: Analyzing an emerging business ecosystem through M&A activities: the case of the Bioeconomy. Busi. Strateg. Dev. **4**, 258–278 (2021). https://doi.org/10.1002/bsd2.149
15. Cha, H.: A paradigm shift in the global strategy of MNEs towards business ecosystems: a research agenda for new theory development. J. Int. Manag. **26**, 100755 (2020). https://doi.org/10.1016/j.intman.2020.100755
16. von Ditfurth, L., Lienemann, G.: The data governance act:—promoting or restricting data intermediaries? Compet. Regul. Netw. Ind. **23**, 270–295 (2022). https://doi.org/10.1177/17835917221141324

17. Directorate-General for Communications Networks, Content and Technology (European Commission), everis Benelux, Scaria, E., Berghmans, A., Pont, M., Arnaut, C., Leconte, S.: Study on Data Sharing between Companies in Europe: Final Report. Publications Office (2018)
18. Zuiderwijk, A., Janssen, M., Davis, C.: Innovation with open data: essential elements of open data ecosystems. Inform. Polit. **19**, 17–33 (2014). https://doi.org/10.3233/IP-140329
19. Lis, D., Otto, B.: Towards a Taxonomy of Ecosystem Data Governance (2021). https://doi.org/10.24251/HICSS.2021.733
20. Moher, D., Liberati, A., Tetzlaff, J., Altman, D.G., Group, T.P: Preferred reporting items for systematic reviews and meta-analyses: the PRISMA statement. PLoS Med. **6**, e1000097 (2009). https://doi.org/10.1371/journal.pmed.1000097
21. Yadav, U., Duhan, N., Bhatia, K.K.: Dealing with pure new user cold-start problem in recommendation system based on linked open data and social network features. Mob. Inf. Syst. **2020**, 8912065 (2020). https://doi.org/10.1155/2020/8912065
22. Boone, F., van Loenen, B.: Identifying and overcoming the barriers towards open data of public undertakings*. Interdiscip. Descrip. Compl. Syst. INDECS. **20**, 96–111 (2022). https://doi.org/10.7906/indecs.20.2.3
23. Mesman, J.P., Barbosa, C.C., Lewis, A.S.L., Olsson, F., Calhoun-Grosch, S., Grossart, H.-P., Ladwig, R., La Fuente, R.S., Münzner, K., Nkwalale, L.G.T., Pilla, R.M., Suresh, K., Wain, D.J.: Challenges of open data in aquatic sciences: issues faced by data users and data providers. Front. Environ. Sci. **12** (2024). https://doi.org/10.3389/fenvs.2024.1497105
24. Regino, A.G., dos Reis, J.C., Bonacin, R., Morshed, A., Sellis, T.: Link maintenance for integrity in linked open data evolution: literature survey and open challenges. Semant. Web. **12**, 517–541 (2021). https://doi.org/10.3233/SW-200398
25. Conde, J., Munoz-Arcentales, A., Choque, J., Huecas, G., Alonso, Á.: Overcoming the barriers of using linked open data in smart city applications. Computer. **55**, 109–118 (2022). https://doi.org/10.1109/MC.2022.3206144
26. Yoon, A., Copeland, A.: Toward community-inclusive data ecosystems: challenges and opportunities of open data for community-based organizations. J. Assoc. Inf. Sci. Technol. **71**, 1439–1454 (2020)
27. Natarajan, S., Vairavasundaram, S., Natarajan, S., Gandomi, A.H.: Resolving data sparsity and cold start problem in collaborative filtering recommender system using linked open data. Expert Syst. Appl. **149**, 113248 (2020)
28. Wang, Y., Livingston, M., McArthur, D.P., Bailey, N.: The challenges of measuring the short-term rental market: an analysis of open data on Airbnb activity. Hous. Stud. **39**, 2260–2279 (2024). https://doi.org/10.1080/02673037.2023.2176829
29. Gil-Garcia, J.R., Luna-Reyes, L.: Opportunities and Challenges of Policy Informatics: tackling complex problems through the combination of open data. In: Technology and Analytics. Presented at the January 1 (2020). https://doi.org/10.4018/978-1-5225-9860-2.ch013
30. Ma, R., Lam, P.: Investigating the barriers faced by stakeholders in open data development: A study on Hong Kong as a "smart city". Cities. **92**, 36–46 (2019). https://doi.org/10.1016/j.cities.2019.03.009
31. Fayyaz, N., Ullah, I., Khusro, S.: On the current state of linked open data: issues, challenges, and future directions. Int. J. Semant. Web Inf. Syst. **14**, 110–128 (2018)
32. Shahin, M.H., Bhattacharya, S., Silva, D., Kim, S., Burton, J., Podichetty, J., Romero, K., Conrado, D.J.: Open data revolution in clinical research: opportunities and challenges. Clin. Transl. Sci. **13**, 665–674 (2020). https://doi.org/10.1111/cts.12756
33. Runeson, P., Olsson, T.: Challenges and Opportunities in Open Data Collaboration – a focus group study. In: 2020 46th Euromicro Conference on Software Engineering and Advanced Applications (SEAA), pp. 205–212 (2020)

34. Hyseni, B., Bexheti, L.: Perspective of Open Data Application in Kosovo, Challenges, and Advantages (2022). https://doi.org/10.1109/MECO55406.2022.9797194
35. Salguero-Gómez, R., Jackson, J., Gascoigne, S.J.L.: Four key challenges in the open-data revolution. J. Anim. Ecol. **90**, 2000–2004 (2021)
36. Söderberg, E., Church, L., Höst, M.: Open data-driven usability improvements of static code analysis and its challenges. In: Proceedings of the 25th International Conference on Evaluation and Assessment in Software Engineering, pp. 272–277. Association for Computing Machinery, New York (2021). https://doi.org/10.1145/3463274.3463808
37. Kim, H.: Lesson learned from the power of open data: resolving the mask shortage problem caused by COVID-19 in South Korea. Sustain. For. **13**, 278 (2021)
38. Hayashi, T., Sakaji, H., Matsushima, H., Fukami, Y., Shimizu, T., Ohsawa, Y.: Data combination for problem-solving: a case of an open data exchange platform. Rev. Socio-Netw. Strat. **15**, 521–534 (2021). https://doi.org/10.1007/s12626-021-00083-8
39. Lichtenauer, N., Schmidbauer, L., Wilhelm, S., Wahl, F.: A scoping review on analysis of the barriers and support factors of open data. Information. **15**, 5 (2024)
40. Schindler, M., Dionisio, M.R., Kingham, S.: A multi-level perspective on a spatial data ecosystem: needs and challenges among urban planning stakeholders in New Zealand. J. Spat. Inf. Sci. **13**, 223–252 (2018)
41. Ramalli, E., Pernici, B.: Challenges of a data ecosystem for scientific data. Data Knowl. Eng. **148**, 102236 (2023). https://doi.org/10.1016/j.datak.2023.102236
42. Cahlikova, T., Mabillard, V.: Open data and transparency: opportunities and challenges in the Swiss context. Public Perform. Manag. Rev. **43**, 662–686 (2020)
43. Mainali, K., Evans, M., Saavedra, D., Mills, E., Madsen, B., Minnemeyer, S.: Convolutional neural network for high-resolution wetland mapping with open data: variable selection and the challenges of a generalizable model. Sci. Total Environ. **861**, 160622 (2023). https://doi.org/10.1016/j.scitotenv.2022.160622
44. Athanassiadis, A.: Urban metabolism and open data: opportunities and challenges for urban resource efficiency. In: Hawken, S., Han, H., Pettit, C. (eds.) Open Cities | Open Data: Collaborative Cities in the Information Era, pp. 177–196. Springer Nature, Singapore (2020). https://doi.org/10.1007/978-981-13-6605-5_8
45. Lassila-Perini, K., Lange, C., Jarrin, E.C., Bellis, M.: Using CMS open data in research—challenges and directions. EPJ Web Conf. **251**, 01004 (2021)
46. Anwar, M.J., Gill, A.Q., Hussain, F.K., Imran, M.: Secure big data ecosystem architecture: challenges and solutions. EURASIP J. Wirel. Commun. Netw. **2021**, 130 (2021). https://doi.org/10.1186/s13638-021-01996-2
47. Carlitz, R.D., McLellan, R.: Open data from authoritarian regimes: new opportunities, new challenges. Persp. Polit. **19**, 160–170 (2021)
48. Hyseni, B., Abazi Bexheti, L.: Cybersecurity and Efficacity of open data platforms. IETI Trans. Data Anal. Forecast. (iTDAF). **2**, 4–22 (2024)
49. Dermentzi, E., Zotou, M., Tambouris, E., Tarabanis, K.: Using the problem based learning method and educational technologies to teach open data: a design-based research approach. Educ. Inf. Technol. **27**, 8859–8882 (2022). https://doi.org/10.1007/s10639-022-10995-9
50. Akatkin, Y., Yasinovskaya, E., Bich, M., Shilin, A.: The challenges of linked open data semantic enrichment, discovery, and dissemination (GRID). Phys. Part. Nucl. **55**, 538–540 (2024). https://doi.org/10.1134/S106377962403002X
51. Kassen, M.: Adopting and managing open data: stakeholder perspectives, challenges and policy recommendations. Aslib J. Inf. Manag. **70**, 518–537 (2018)
52. Walletzký, L., Romanovská, F., Toli, A., Ge, M.: Research Challenges of Open Data as a Service for Smart Cities (2020). https://doi.org/10.5220/0009578604680472

53. Xiao, F., He, D., Chi, Y., Jeng, W., Tomer, C.: Challenges and Supports for Accessing Open Government Datasets: Data Guide for Better Open Data Access and Uses. In: Proceedings of the 2019 Conference on Human Information Interaction and Retrieval, pp. 313–317. Association for Computing Machinery, New York (2019)
54. Saxena, S.: Drivers and barriers towards re-using open government data (OGD): a case study of open data initiative in Oman. Foresight. **20**, 206–218 (2018)
55. Szostak, R., Smiraglia, R.P., Scharnhorst, A., Slavic, A., Martínez-Ávila, D., Renwick, T.: Classifications as linked open data. In: Presented at the Challenges and Opportunities (2021). https://doi.org/10.5771/9783956506611-24
56. Hamida, C., Landi, A.: The Lack of Decentralization of Data: Barriers, Exclusivity, and Monopoly in Open Data, https://papers.ssrn.com/abstract=3266881, (2018)
57. Kitsios, F., Kamariotou, M.: Open Data Value Network and Business Models: Opportunities and Challenges. In: 2019 IEEE 21st Conference on Business Informatics (CBI), pp. 296–302 (2019). https://doi.org/10.1109/CBI.2019.00040
58. Lamb, D., Russell, A., Morant, N., Stevenson, F.: The challenges of open data sharing for qualitative researchers. J. Health Psychol. **29**, 659–664 (2024)
59. Bacon, S., Goldacre, B.: Barriers to working with National Health Service England's open data. J. Med. Internet Res. **22**, e15603 (2020). https://doi.org/10.2196/15603
60. Katulić, T., Musa, A., Lončar, D.: Understanding some of the open data challenges to data protection in the developing European legal framework. In: Presented at the 34th Central European Conference on Information and Intelligent Systems (CECIIS 2023) (2023)
61. Solymosi, R., Buil-Gil, D., Ceccato, V., Kim, E., Jansson, U.: Privacy challenges in geodata and open data. Area. **55**, 456–464 (2023). https://doi.org/10.1111/area.12888
62. Ugochukwu, A.I., Phillips, P.W.B.: Open data ownership and sharing: challenges and opportunities for application of FAIR principles and a checklist for data managers. J. Agric. Res. **16**, 101157 (2024)

# Unmasking Fake News: A Naïve Bayes Classifier Approach to Combat Misinformation

Aqeel Sahi[1,2(✉)], Mustafa Hayawi[2], Raid Lafta[2], Shahab Abdulla[3], and Mohammed Diykh[4]

[1] School of Mathematics, Physics and Computing, University of Southern Queensland, Toowoomba, QLD, Australia
aqeel.sahi@unisq.edu.au

[2] College of Engineering, Al-Shatrah University, Thi-Qar, Iraq
{mustafahayawi,raidluaibi.lafta}@shu.edu.iq

[3] UniSQ College, University of Southern Queensland, Toowoomba, QLD, Australia
shahab.abdulla@unisq.edu.au

[4] College of Education for Pure Sciences, University of Thi-Qar, Thi-Qar, Iraq
mohammed.diykh@unisq.edu.au

**Abstract.** Fake news has been a noticeable issue in the last few decades after the presence of the Internet. Many news channels, networks, and social media platforms provide us with news from around the globe. These news resources can also be used to share malicious and fake news. Therefore, detecting and handling this fake news is crucial since the world's view is based on this information. Verifying news individually by a human being is completely unfeasible. Thus, we proposed an artificially intelligent Naïve Bayes prediction model that can help classify news and detect if a given news is fake or real. The proposed model used the Naïve Bayes classifier, which gives great results in text classifications such as spam filtering. This paper also includes an analysis of results and performance measurement.

**Keywords:** Fake News · Misinformation · Naïve Bayes · Neural Network · Text Classification

## 1 Introduction

Fake news has emerged as one of the significant threats to freedom of expression, democracy, and journalism [1]. It has undermined public trust in the media and governments and may have influenced the 2016 U.S. presidential election [2]. The surge of false and misleading information was substantial in the crucial months leading up to the 2016 U.S. presidential election campaign. During that time, the top 20 frequently mentioned fake election stories accumulated 8,711,000 shares, reactions, and comments on Facebook, surpassing the 7,367,000 interactions for the top 20 most-discussed election stories from 19 major news outlets [3]. On


K. Daimi and A. Alsadoon (Eds.): ICR 2025, LNNS 1487, pp. 118–125, 2025.
https://doi.org/10.1007/978-3-031-95652-2_11

Twitter, fake news garnered far more reactions and retweets than truthful news, facilitating its rapid dissemination across news networks and social media platforms [4]. Furthermore, fake news has severely impacted the economic sector, with such misinformation linked to significant stock market transactions. For instance, a false report claiming that the 44th President of the United States, Barack Obama, was injured in an explosion erased $130 billion in stock value [5]. These events and financial losses have spurred research into fake news, culminating in selecting the term "post-truth" as the international word of the year by Oxford Dictionaries in 2016 [6].

It is crucial to identify and combat the issue of fake news. Researchers have suggested various strategies, ranging from Natural Language Processing (NLP) analysis to clustering techniques [7]. Zhang et al. utilised a method where authentic news is used to form clusters [8]. Conversely, Vishwakarma et al. developed a novel technique to classify news, extracting text from news images and then inputting that text into Google's engine for results, which were compared to determine the authenticity of the news [9]. While these two studies concentrated on the news content, others explored the analysis of the websites themselves, like the method proposed by Jahankhani et al. [10]. This approach examines websites from three perspectives, including URL analysis, blacklisting, and image screening. Another study focused on classifying the platforms, proposing a system that assigns credibility ratings to Twitter users based on an analysis of their tweets [11]. Although this research does not directly identify fake or real news, it can highlight users who are most likely to create and disseminate false information. Presently, several techniques are available to detect fake news, such as the BS Detector plugin, which scans through a group of websites known to be unreliable. However, this alone is insufficient for identifying fake news, primarily when it originates from reputable sources or individuals. Thus, it is necessary to consider multiple factors to effectively discern whether a particular news item is fake or genuine.

## 2 Prediction Model

Naïve Bayes is a probabilistic classifier that relies on Bayes' theorem and is applied to classification tasks. It performs adequately in text classification scenarios like spam detection and determining whether reviews are positive or negative [12].

Naive Bayes works on multiple features, which can easily be adapted to perform fake news detection. We will make use of the various features available in the adopted dataset.

**Table 1.** Fake vs Real News in the Adopted Dataset

| Row Labels | Count of Statement | Probability |
|---|---|---|
| FALSE | 1397 | 0.551084813 |
| TRUE | 1138 | 0.448915187 |
| **Grand Total** | **2535** | **1** |

**Table 2.** Number of Fake/Real News According to Affiliation Feature

| Row Labels | Count of Statement | True | Probability | False | fProbability2 |
|---|---|---|---|---|---|
| Activist | 8 | 2 | 0.000788955 | 6 | 0.002366864 |
| Columnist | 18 | 10 | 0.003944773 | 8 | 0.003155819 |
| Democrat | 848 | 455 | 0.179487179 | 393 | 0.155029586 |
| Independent | 34 | 18 | 0.007100592 | 16 | 0.006311637 |
| Journalist | 6 | 3 | 0.001183432 | 3 | 0.001183432 |
| Libertarian | 11 | 5 | 0.001972387 | 6 | 0.002366864 |
| Newsmaker | 16 | 11 | 0.00433925 | 5 | 0.001972387 |
| **None** | **353** | **152** | **0.059960552** | **201** | **0.079289941** |
| Organization | 52 | 16 | 0.006311637 | 36 | 0.014201183 |
| Republican | 1189 | 466 | 0.18382643 | 723 | 0.285207101 |
| **Grand Total** | **2535** | **1138** | **0.448915187** | **1397** | **0.551084813** |

Given the dataset LIAR [14], we will try to predict whether the given news is fake or real using the Naive Bayes. First, we filtered the LIAR dataset by deleting records with missing values and chose five columns (label, subject, location, affiliation, and context) for filtering. The resulting dataset has 2535 news records, including 1397 fake and 1138 real news, as shown in Table 1. We also generated a table for every column to calculate the probability of each record, to keep our paper short we added only affiliation table (Table 2).

To showcase how we predict if a given news is real or fake according to the given features, we will have one news record example and then will apply the same rules to all news in the dataset. Following that, we will evaluate the anticipated outcomes against the real outcomes.

Assume we have a news article related to the financial situation ($subject : financial$) in Florida ($location : Florida$), this news article has been published on social media ($context : socialmedia$), and we don't know the affiliation ($affiliation : none$). To predict the output (Fake/Real) for this instance, we need the overall probability of real/fake (true/false in Table 1), and the probability of real/fake for each feature (ex: $affiliation : none$, from Table 2 we can see true probability is about 0.06 and false probability is about 0.079. We will use the following Naive Bayes formula to calculate the probability twice (true/false):

$$P(\text{Label=True} \mid \begin{smallmatrix}\text{Subject=financial,}\\ \text{Location=Florida,}\\ \text{Affiliation=none,}\\ \text{Context=social media}\end{smallmatrix}) = \frac{P(\begin{smallmatrix}\text{Subject=financial,}\\ \text{Location=Florida,}\\ \text{Affiliation=none,}\\ \text{Context=social media}\end{smallmatrix} \mid \text{Label=True}) \cdot P(\text{True})}{P(\begin{smallmatrix}\text{Subject=financial,}\\ \text{Location=Florida,}\\ \text{Affiliation=none,}\\ \text{Context=social media}\end{smallmatrix})} \tag{1}$$

The denominator is calculated either in the two cases: True or False. So, to simplify, we cancel the denominator.

## 2.1 True News Scenario

In this section, we will explore the probability of a news article being labelled as true, given specific attributes. The attributes considered include the subject matter being financial, the location being Florida, no particular affiliation, and the context being social media. We will use a series of probability equations to determine the likelihood of the news being true.

$$P(\text{Label=True} \mid \begin{smallmatrix}\text{Subject=financial,}\\ \text{Location=Florida,}\\ \text{Affiliation=none,}\\ \text{Context=social media}\end{smallmatrix}) = P(\begin{smallmatrix}\text{Subject=financial,}\\ \text{Location=Florida,}\\ \text{Affiliation=none,}\\ \text{Context=social media}\end{smallmatrix} \mid \text{Label=True}) \quad (2)$$

$$P(\text{Label=True} \mid \begin{smallmatrix}\text{Subject=financial,}\\ \text{Location=Florida,}\\ \text{Affiliation=none,}\\ \text{Context=social media}\end{smallmatrix}) = P(True) \cdot P(True) \cdot P(True) \cdot P(True) \cdot P(True) \quad (3)$$

$$P(\text{Label=True} \mid \begin{smallmatrix}\text{Subject=financial,}\\ \text{Location=Florida,}\\ \text{Affiliation=none,}\\ \text{Context=social media}\end{smallmatrix}) = 0.079 \cdot 0.041 \cdot 0.06 \cdot 0.04 \cdot 0.449 \quad (4)$$

$$P(\text{Label=True} \mid \begin{smallmatrix}\text{Subject=financial,}\\ \text{Location=Florida,}\\ \text{Affiliation=none,}\\ \text{Context=social media}\end{smallmatrix}) = 0.00000349 \quad (5)$$

## 2.2 False News Scenario

This section focuses on the probability of a news article being labelled as false under the same set of attributes: financial subject, Florida location, no affiliation, and social media context. By analyzing these probabilities, we aim to understand the factors contributing to classifying news as false.

$$P(\text{Label=False} \mid \begin{smallmatrix}\text{Subject=financial,}\\ \text{Location=Florida,}\\ \text{Affiliation=none,}\\ \text{Context=social media}\end{smallmatrix}) = P(False) \cdot P(False) \cdot P(False) \cdot P(False) \cdot P(False) \quad (6)$$

$$P(\text{Label=False} \mid \begin{smallmatrix}\text{Subject=financial,}\\ \text{Location=Florida,}\\ \text{Affiliation=none,}\\ \text{Context=social media}\end{smallmatrix}) = 0.1 \cdot 0.047 \cdot 0.079 \cdot 0.04 \cdot 0.551 \quad (7)$$

$$P(\text{Label=False} \mid \begin{smallmatrix}\text{Subject=financial,}\\ \text{Location=Florida,}\\ \text{Affiliation=none,}\\ \text{Context=social media}\end{smallmatrix}) = 0.00000818 \quad (8)$$

As a result, the probability that the given news is True (0.00000349) is less than the probability of being False (0.00000818). Then, we could consider the given news as FAKE news. However, that is not enough to tell whether or not the given process has succeeded. Therefore, we will apply the same scenario on all 2535 news records and then measure the performance of this model using the confusion matrix. Before that, let's explain how we handled the zero probability problem.

## 3 Laplace Correction

Laplace correction is a technique that handles the zero probability problem in Naïve Bayes [14]. An element in the dataset with zero probability will result in the Label probability being zero, as we multiply all the likelihoods together. Therefore, we will replace any zero probability with the value 0.000394477, which is the probability of 1. For example, in the Location table, we have zero true news from Alabama, and to fix this issue, we will assume we have a single true news from Alabama. As a result, one true news means the probability is 0.000394477.

## 4 Performance Measure

To accurately assess the effectiveness of the proposed method, we must determine the values of true positives (TP), true negatives (TN), false positives (FP), and false negatives (FN).

### 4.1 True Positive (TP)

The model accurately identifies positive class instances where both the prediction and the actual outcome are positive. Table 3 shows that the model has predicted 1008 real news articles as positive.

### 4.2 True Negative (TN)

The model accurately identifies the positive class when the prediction and actual values are positive. According to Table 3, the model successfully predicts 1008 real news articles as positive.

### 4.3 False Positive (FP)

The model incorrectly categorizes some negative instances as positive (predicted-positive, actual-negative). As shown in Table 3, 41 articles are mistakenly predicted as positive (real news) when they are fake news. FP is also referred to as a TYPE I error.

**Table 3.** Confusion Matrix for Fake News Detection

| Prediction | Negative | Positive |
|---|---|---|
| Negative | 1356 | 130 |
| Positive | 41 | 1008 |

**Table 4.** The Feature Performance, which was measured using the F1-score is critical for evaluating the effectiveness and accuracy of different models in Fake News Detection, as discussed in [1].

| Feature Group | | | **PolitiFact data** [Shu et al. 2018] | | | | **BuzzFeed data** [Shu et al. 2018] | | | |
|---|---|---|---|---|---|---|---|---|---|---|
| | | | **XGBoost** | | **RF** | | **XGBoost** | | **RF** | |
| | | | **Acc.** | **$F_1$** | **Acc.** | **$F_1$** | **Acc.** | **$F_1$** | **Acc.** | **$F_1$** |
| **Non-Latent Features** | Lexicon | BOWs ($f_s$) | 0.856 | 0.858 | 0.837 | 0.836 | 0.823 | 0.823 | 0.815 | 0.815 |
| | | Unigram+bigram ($f_r$) | 0.755 | 0.756 | 0.754 | 0.755 | 0.721 | 0.711 | 0.735 | 0.723 |
| | Syntax | POS tags ($f_s$) | 0.755 | 0.755 | 0.776 | 0.776 | 0.745 | 0.745 | 0.732 | 0.732 |
| | | Rewrite rules ($r*, f_s$) | **0.877** | **0.877** | 0.836 | 0.836 | 0.778 | 0.778 | 0.845 | 0.845 |
| | | Rewrite rules ($r*, f_r$) | 0.749 | 0.753 | 0.743 | 0.748 | 0.735 | 0.738 | 0.732 | 0.735 |
| | Semantic | LIWC | 0.645 | 0.649 | 0.645 | 0.647 | 0.655 | 0.655 | 0.663 | 0.659 |
| | | Theory-driven [Zhou et al. 2019a] | 0.745 | 0.748 | 0.737 | 0.737 | 0.722 | 0.750 | 0.789 | 0.789 |
| | Discourse | Rhetorical relationships | 0.621 | 0.621 | 0.633 | 0.633 | 0.658 | 0.658 | 0.665 | 0.665 |
| | Combination | [Zhou et al. 2019a] | 0.865 | 0.865 | **0.845** | **0.845** | **0.855** | **0.856** | **0.854** | **0.854** |
| **Latent Features** | | WORD2VEC [Mikolov et al. 2013] | 0.688 | 0.671 | 0.663 | 0.667 | 0.703 | 0.714 | 0.722 | 0.718 |
| | | DOC2VEC [Le and Mikolov 2014] | 0.698 | 0.684 | 0.712 | 0.698 | 0.615 | 0.610 | 0.620 | 0.615 |

## 4.4 False Negative (FN)

The model inaccurately predicts the positive instances as negative (predicted-negative, actual-positive). In Table 3, 130 articles are incorrectly predicted as negative (fake news) despite being real news. FN is also known as a TYPE II error.

We can compute various performance metrics using the values TP = 1008, TN = 1356, FN = 130, and FP = 41.

Precision and recall are essential metrics in information retrieval, especially when the positive class holds greater significance than the negative class. In web searches, the model disregards irrelevant information that isn't retrieved (classified as a true negative). Thus, only true positives, false positives, and false negatives are considered when calculating precision and recall.

$$\text{Precision} = \frac{TP}{TP + FP} = \frac{1008}{1008 + 41} = 0.96 \tag{9}$$

$$\text{Recall} = \frac{TP}{TP + FN} = \frac{1008}{1008 + 130} = 0.97 \tag{10}$$

In this study, we focused on identifying fake news, so it is acceptable if some fake news goes undetected (false negative). Still, we must consider the implications of missing significant news incorrectly labelled as spam (false positive). In this context, minimising false positives as much as possible is crucial. Thus, precision holds greater importance than recall in this scenario.

When evaluating various models, determining which is superior can be challenging (whether it has high precision with low recall or the reverse). Therefore, a metric that integrates both aspects is necessary. One example of such a metric is the F1 score.

The F1 score represents the harmonic mean of precision and recall. It accounts for false positives and negatives, making it practical for imbalanced datasets.

$$\text{F1 score} = \frac{2}{\frac{1}{\text{Precision}} + \frac{1}{\text{Recall}}} \tag{11}$$

$$\text{F1 score} = \frac{2 \cdot (\text{Precision} \cdot \text{Recall})}{\text{Precision} + \text{Recall}} = \frac{2 \cdot (0.96 \cdot 0.97)}{0.96 + 0.97} = 0.965 \tag{12}$$

The confusion matrix is a $2 \times 2$ table used for binary classification, displaying actual values on one axis and predicted values on the other. As illustrated in Table 3. The confusion matrix, along with precision, recall, and F1 score, offers deeper insights into predictions compared to accuracy metrics. Precision, recall, and F1 scores are utilised in various applications such as information retrieval, word segmentation, and named entity recognition, among others. Furthermore, numerous studies have been compared based on the F1-score, as highlighted by Zhou and Zafarani in 2020 [1], illustrated in Table 4. The results shown in Table 4 indicate that the highest F1 score reached approximately 0.88, while our approach achieved around 0.97. Thus, we can conclude that our proposed method demonstrates excellent performance when measured against other systems for detecting fake news.

## 5 Conclusion

The study introduces an AI-driven Naïve Bayes model for distinguishing fake news. Leveraging Naïve Bayes' efficacy in text classification like spam detection, it assesses results through a confusion matrix, precision, recall, and F1 score more insightful than mere accuracy metrics. Highlighting the F1 score's significance in various fields, it compares favourably with prior systems, yielding an impressive 0.97 F1 score, indicating superior performance in fake news detection.

## References


1. Zhou, X., Zafarani, R.: A survey of fake news: fundamental theories, detection methods, and opportunities". ACM Comput. Surv. (CSUR) **53**(5), 1–40 (2020)
2. Pogue, D.: How to stamp out fake news. Sci. Am. **316**(2), 24 (2017)
3. Silverman, C.: This analysis shows how viral fake election news stories outperformed real news on Facebook. BuzzFeed News 16 (2016)
4. Vosoughi, S., Roy, D., Aral, S.: The spread of true and false news online. Science **359**(6380), 1146–1151 (2018)
5. Rapoza, K.: Can 'fake news' impact the stock market? Forbes News (2017)
6. Wang, A.B.: Post-truth named 2016 word of the year by Oxford Dictionaries. Washington Post, p. 16 (2016)
7. Mandical, R.R., Mamatha, N., Shivakumar, N., Monica, R., Krishna, A.N.: Identification of fake news using machine learning. In: 2020 IEEE International Conference on Electronics, Computing and Communication Technologies (CONECCT), pp. 1–6 (2020)

8. Zhang, C., Gupta, A., Kauten, C., Deokar, A.V., Qin, X.: Detecting fake news for reducing misinformation risks using analytics. In: Proceedings of the Conference (2019)
9. Omezi, N., Jahankhani, H.: Proposed forensic guidelines for the investigation of fake news. In: Policing in the Era of AI and Smart Societies, pp. 231–265 (2020)
10. Meel, P., Vishwakarma, D.K.: Fake news, rumor, information pollution in social media and web: a contemporary survey of state-of-the-arts, challenges and opportunities. Expert Syst. Appl. **153**, 112986 (2020)
11. Buntain, C., Golbeck, J.: Automatically identifying fake news in popular twitter threads. In: 2017 IEEE International Conference on Smart Cloud (SmartCloud), pp. 208–215 (2017)
12. Sahi, A., Lai, D., Li, Y., Diykh, M.: An efficient DDoS TCP flood attack detection and prevention system in a cloud environment. IEEE Access **5**, 6036–6048 (2017)
13. Sahi, A., Lai, D., Li, Y.: Three-party password-based authenticated key exchange protocol based on the computational Diffie-Hellman assumption. Int. J. Commun. Networks Distrib. Syst. **21**(4), 560–581 (2018)
14. Wang, W.Y.: Liar, liar pants on fire: a new benchmark dataset for fake news detection, arXiv preprint arXiv:1705.00648 (2017)

# Computer and Network Security

# Securing LoRaWAN for Smart Grids: A Comprehensive Analysis of Vulnerabilities, Challenges, and Research Directions

Noor Shomal(✉) and Bassel Soudan

University of Sharjah, Sharjah, UAE
{U22103721,bsoudan}@sharjah.ac.ae

**Abstract.** LoRaWAN (Long Range Wide Area Network) has emerged as a key wireless communication technology for smart grid applications due to its long-range connectivity, low power consumption, and cost-effectiveness. However, despite its advantages, LoRaWAN suffers from critical security vulnerabilities that pose risks to smart grid communications. This paper presents a comprehensive review of security challenges in LoRaWAN networks, focusing on key vulnerabilities such as the lack of encryption in join request messages, absence of end-to-end encryption, static keys in Activation by Personalization (ABP), DevNonce reuse, and the lack of mutual authentication. Furthermore, this work evaluates recent research efforts aimed at mitigating these security issues, identifying gaps in key management, join request security, secure randomness, and authentication mechanisms. Based on the findings, this paper highlights future research directions, emphasizing the need for lightweight cryptographic solutions, scalable key distribution mechanisms, and efficient authentication frameworks tailored for resource-constrained IoT devices. Addressing these challenges is essential for ensuring the security and resilience of LoRaWAN-based smart grid applications, safeguarding critical IoT infrastructures from cyber threats.

**Keywords:** LoRaWAN security · Smart grid · IoT communication · LoRaWAN authentication mechanisms · Replay attack mitigation

## 1 Introduction

A smart grid is an advanced electrical network that integrates digital communication technologies, automation, and Internet of Things (IoT) based control systems to improve the efficiency, reliability, and sustainability of energy distribution. Unlike traditional power grids, which operate on a centralized generation model with one-way energy flow, smart grids enable bidirectional communication between utilities and consumers leading to optimized energy management and reduced operational costs [1].

The Internet of Things is one of the main technologies underlying smart grids. IoT enables the deployment of network-connected devices such as smart meters, sensors, and control systems which facilitate the real-time data exchange for data-driven decision-making, automated control, predictive maintenance, and dynamic demand-response [2–4]. To support real-time monitoring and control, IoT-based smart grids rely on diverse


K. Daimi and A. Alsadoon (Eds.): ICR 2025, LNNS 1487, pp. 129–137, 2025.
https://doi.org/10.1007/978-3-031-95652-2_12

communication infrastructures, including optical fiber networks, Power Line Communication (PLC), Wi-Fi, cellular networks, and, more recently, LoRaWAN (Long Range Wide Area Network) technology [5, 6].

LoRaWAN is a low-power, long-range wireless communication protocol widely adopted for IoT-based smart grid applications, particularly for remote monitoring and smart metering [7, 8]. The architecture of a LoRaWAN network follows a star-of-stars topology, consisting of end devices, gateways, a network server, and an application server, as illustrated in Fig. 1. End devices communicate wirelessly with gateways using LoRa modulation, and these gateways then forward messages to the network server via standard IP-based connections (e.g., UDP). The network server is responsible for managing network operations, verifying message integrity, and routing data to the appropriate application server for further processing [9, 10].

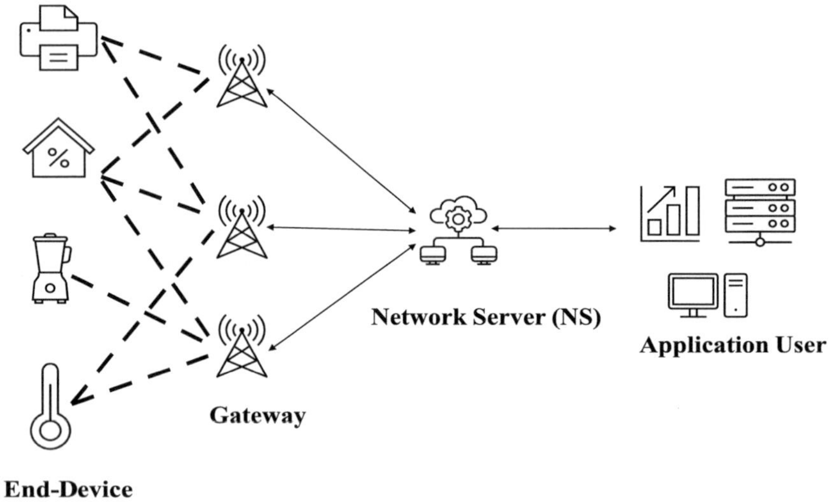


**Fig. 1** Typical Architecture of a LoRaWAN Network

The modular design of a LoRaWAN network supports scalability for large networks of sensors and controllers to efficiently monitor and manage energy distribution while optimizing overall smart grid performance [11]. Additionally, LoRaWAN supports multiple device classes to accommodate varying energy and communication requirements, which is crucial for diverse smart grid applications [12]. Compared to traditional communication technologies such as optical fiber and Power Line Communication (PLC), LoRaWAN offers lower deployment costs and resilience against physical damage [13, 14]. Furthermore, LoRaWAN has a significant advantage over short-range wireless technologies due to its lower power consumption and extended communication range (up to 15 km in optimal conditions), making it particularly suitable for remote locations where frequent maintenance is impractical [15].

Although LoRaWAN incorporates security features, its networks remain vulnerable to threats such as eavesdropping, replay attacks, jamming, and weak authentication mechanisms [9]. These risks compromise data integrity, enable unauthorized access, facilitate energy theft, and disrupt grid stability. While multiple mitigation strategies exist, many fail to address the constraints of resource-limited IoT devices, leaving persistent security gaps in smart grid deployments. This paper provides a comprehensive survey of security challenges in LoRaWAN-based smart grids, critically evaluates existing security mechanisms, and identifies research gaps to guide future security enhancements.

## 2 Technical Background

Ensuring security in LoRaWAN-based smart grids presents significant challenges due to the resource constraints of IoT edge devices, necessitating lightweight yet effective security mechanisms. The LoRaWAN protocol incorporates several security features designed to protect different stages of communication [16]. employs a two-layer encryption scheme, utilizing a Network Session Key (NwkSKey) to secure communication between end devices and the network server, and an Application Session Key (AppSKey) to encrypt application data. Additionally, it implements Message Integrity Codes (MICs) to detect tampering and unauthorized modifications, enhancing data integrity [11, 17, 18]. Device authentication and key exchange are facilitated through activation methods such as Over-the-Air Activation (OTAA) and Activation by Personalization (ABP) [19]. To mitigate replay attacks, the protocol uses frame counters to ensure message uniqueness and sequential validation [20].

### 2.1 Security Vulnerabilities of the LoRaWAN Protocol

Despite these security measures, LoRaWAN remains vulnerable to several threats, including weaknesses in key management, susceptibility to eavesdropping, and exposure to jamming attacks. The protocol's reliance on pre-shared session keys and its lack of robust mutual authentication mechanisms leave LoRaWAN-based smart grids susceptible to exploitation [21, 22]. To ensure its suitability for critical infrastructure, further security enhancements are required. The following sections discuss some of the main security vulnerabilities in LoRaWAN and their implications for SG applications.

**Lack of Encryption in Join Request Messages**

One of the critical security vulnerabilities in the LoRaWAN protocol is the lack of encryption in Join Request messages during the OTAA process [23, 24]. During OTAA initiation, the end device sends a Join Request message to the network server containing three key parameters: a globally unique device identifier (DevEUI), an application server identifier (AppEUI), and a randomly generated value (DevNonce). If approved, the network server responds with a Join Accept message that includes session keys encrypted with the AppKey, as illustrated in Fig. 2.

However, since the Join Request message is transmitted in plaintext, it is vulnerable to eavesdropping and interception. Attackers can capture these messages, extract the exposed device identifiers, and execute replay attacks. By resending a previously intercepted Join Request message, an attacker can impersonate the legitimate device and

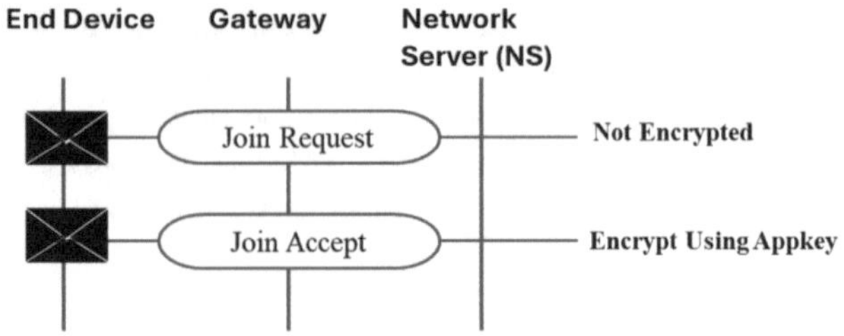


**Fig. 2** The OTAA Join Procedure

potentially gain unauthorized access to the network [25, 26]. This vulnerability compromises device authentication and key exchange, posing a significant risk to the security and integrity of LoRaWAN-based smart grids [27].

**Lack of End-to-End Encryption**

LoRaWAN's security model lacks true end-to-end encryption between IoT devices and application servers [28]. This weakness arises because the encryption keys used for securing the communication are managed by the network server, which acts as an intermediary between the end device and the application server. An attacker that compromises the network server will have access to the keys and will be able to intercept and modify messages. This makes LoRaWAN susceptible to MITM attacks.

**Static Keys in Activation by Personalization (ABP)**

When a device is activated using the ABP process, the two encryption keys (NwkSKey, and AppSKey) are programmed manually into the device at deployment and remain static throughout its operation. This is in contrast to the OTAA activation process where new session keys are negotiated dynamically each time the device joins the network. If an attacker gains physical access to an ABP-enabled device, they can extract the hardcoded keys from the firmware or memory. Without session key updates, MITM attacks become more feasible, allowing attackers to modify data in transit [28].

**DevNonce Reuse**

The DevNonce is a 16-bit random value generated by the device to ensure the uniqueness of join request messages. However, due to its limited size, devices may inadvertently reuse the same DevNonce, particularly after a reset or over extended operation. This vulnerability exposes the network to replay attacks, where attackers can capture and resend old Join Requests to gain unauthorized access.

While LoRaWAN utilizes a MIC to ensure message authenticity and enable detection of tampering, it does not encrypt the message itself [9, 29]. Some implementations use a sequential DevNonce generation approach to prevent immediate repetition, but this introduces a predictability issue. If an attacker can anticipate future DevNonce values, they can generate forged or replayed messages. Moreover, if a device reboots, its DevNonce counter may reset, leading to the reuse of old values and increasing the risk of replay attacks [18, 27].

**No Mutual Authentication**

A significant vulnerability in the LoRaWAN protocol is the absence of mutual authentication between the end device and the network server. The device authentication process is one-way—only the end device authenticates itself to the network server, but the network server does not authenticate itself back to the device. A malicious actor could set up a rogue network server to intercept communication and set up a MITM attack by capturing, modifying, replaying, or even injecting false data into the network.

## 3 Literature Review

The weaknesses discussed in the previous section expose LoRaWAN networks to unauthorized access, data manipulation, and service disruptions, which are particularly concerning in critical applications such as smart grids. Given these challenges, researchers have attempted to develop mechanisms that can enhance the security of LoRaWAN, while maintaining its lightweight nature. We have analyzed several studies published between 2017 and 2024 to investigate the latest propositions for securing LoRaWAN networks. These works have proposed solutions for different threats such as key management, encryption protocols for the join request or the session keys, advanced authentication, and the use of Blockchain to build secure server sharing. By reflecting on these findings, this review aims to identify areas of possible improvement, particularly in the secure management of the key exchange and the mitigation of potential vulnerabilities during the join process.

One approach proposes optimizing the use of MICs to verify the authenticity of join requests [28]. While MICs can detect tampering, they do not encrypt sensitive information, such as the DevNonce, leaving it vulnerable to attackers. To mitigate this risk, some authors suggest encrypting the DevNonce using the NwkSKey and AppSKey session keys, which are derived from the pre-shared AppKey [9, 27].

A more advanced approach involves ephemeral key exchange mechanisms. One researcher proposed the use of the Ephemeral Diffie-Hellman Over COSE (EDHOC) protocol which is a lightweight key exchange method that enables Perfect Forward Secrecy (PFS) by ensuring that compromised keys do not expose past communications [30]. Another approach involves replacing static session keys with dynamically generated keys using the Elliptic Curve Diffie-Hellman (ECDH) algorithm, allowing both the network server and the end device to generate unique session keys for each communication session. This guarantees forward and backward secrecy, protecting past and future communications even if a session key is compromised [31].

Researchers have proposed improving the generation and handling of session keys by using better randomness and dynamic computation techniques. Dynamically generated keys are derived from secure parameters like DevNonce and random numbers. These keys are then computed using AES-128 or AES-256 encryption, combined with secure hash functions such as BLAKE2, ensuring that every session remains unique and protected against replay attacks [32].

Another proposed enhancement for mutual authentication is through digital signatures, where each device and the network server possess private keys for signing messages and public keys for verification. When a device sends a Join Request, it signs the message with its private key, and the network server verifies it using the corresponding public key. Similarly, the Join Accept message is also digitally signed by the network server, ensuring bidirectional authentication [33]. Another approach utilizes pre-shared keys (PSKs), which are securely stored in both the device and the server. During the join process, the device encrypts a unique nonce using the AppKey and sends it to the server. The server then decrypts and verifies the device's identity before sending an encrypted response to confirm its authenticity [34].

Some researchers propose using Blockchain technology to securely store essential data such as DevNonce values and session keys in a tamper-proof, decentralized ledger. The Blockchain-based system utilize smart contracts to verify the uniqueness of each join request, ensuring that attackers cannot reuse intercepted messages. Because blockchain records are permanent and immutable, they offer robust protection against manipulation. Additionally, blockchain consensus mechanisms ensure that data remains consistent and secure across the network. However, blockchain-based solutions introduce challenges such as increased latency, high energy consumption, and dependency on decentralized infrastructure, which may impact the real-time performance of LoRaWAN networks in smart grid applications [35].

# 4 Gap Analysis

Overall, while current security enhancements address many LoRaWAN vulnerabilities, they often involve trade-offs between security strength, computational efficiency, and energy consumption. The solutions proposed in the literature still have limitations that can affect their practicality, scalability, and overall effectiveness. The following is a summary of key limitations affecting the state-of-the-art solutions.

1. **Key Management and Generation** - Many solutions rely on static keys, such as NwkSKey and AppSKey, which are vulnerable to interception and reuse. While dynamic key generation methods such as such as ECDH or EDHOC address this issue, they often add computational overhead that may not be feasible for resource-constrained IoT devices.
2. **Limited Confidentiality in Join Requests** - Although MICs and basic encryption mechanisms may solve the issue with Join Request confidentiality, they often fail to encrypt critical components like DevNonce. This leaves sensitive data exposed, making it susceptible to replay attacks.
3. **Dependence on Secure Randomness** - Solutions that use dynamically generated keys or ephemeral values rely heavily on secure random number generation. Poorly implemented or predictable randomness may allow the attacker to anticipate session keys, undermining the whole process.
4. **Mutual Authentication Challenges** - While mutual authentication methods enhance security by verifying both the device and the server, they often require pre-shared keys or public-private key pairs. Securely provisioning pre-shared keys or public-private key pairs at scale is complex and resource-intensive.

## 5 Future Directions and Conclusion

As LoRaWAN continues to gain adoption in smart grid applications and other critical IoT infrastructures, addressing its security vulnerabilities remains a pressing concern. This work analyzed the security vulnerabilities of the LoRaWAN protocol and evaluated a number of existing mitigation techniques. The analysis has identified critical security weaknesses, and the literature review has revealed significant gaps in existing security enhancements. Based on the gaps identified in the literature, future research should focus on the following key areas:

1. **Lightweight and Secure Key Management** – Due limitations of static keys in ABP mode and the computational overhead of dynamic key generation techniques, future research should explore efficient key exchange mechanisms that balance security and resource constraints. Hybrid approaches leveraging hardware security modules (HSMs) or lightweight cryptographic protocols could offer a viable solution.
2. **Enhanced Join Request Security** – To mitigate the lack of encryption in join requests, future work should consider developing lightweight encryption techniques or modifying the LoRaWAN protocol to enforce encryption of critical fields, such as DevNonce. Secure handshake protocols that integrate confidentiality without significant computational overhead should also be explored.
3. **Secure and Efficient Random Number Generation** – Ensuring secure randomness is crucial for protecting dynamic keys and ephemeral session identifiers. Future research should investigate novel entropy sources suitable for IoT devices, such as physical unclonable functions (PUFs) or environment-based entropy extraction, to strengthen the security of key generation mechanisms.
4. **Scalable Mutual Authentication Mechanisms** – Mutual authentication between end devices and network servers remains a challenge due to the difficulty of managing cryptographic credentials at scale. Future solutions should investigate decentralized authentication methods, such as federated authentication frameworks or lightweight zero-trust architectures, to enhance security without overloading IoT devices.
5. **Post-Quantum Security Considerations** – With the evolution of quantum computing, existing cryptographic methods could become obsolete. Future research should explore post-quantum cryptographic techniques that can be efficiently implemented on LoRaWAN edge devices to ensure long-term security resilience.

Addressing these security challenges is essential for ensuring the reliability and resilience of LoRaWAN-based smart grids and other critical IoT applications. Future research should focus on lightweight cryptographic solutions, scalable key distribution mechanisms, and efficient authentication frameworks tailored to resource-constrained environments. By tackling these gaps, LoRaWAN networks can be significantly fortified against cyber threats, enabling secure and sustainable deployment in smart grid infrastructures and beyond.

## References

1. Abdulridha, A.O., Al-Mashhadani, I.B., Hashim, S.M., Reshak, K.A.: Performance comparison of an implemented wired and wireless micro smart grid. In: Proceedings - International

Conference on Developments in eSystems Engineering, DeSE, pp. 7–12 (2023). https://doi.org/10.1109/DeSE58274.2023.10099600
2. Liu, J., Xiao, Y., Li, S., Liang, W., Chen, C.L.P.: Cyber security and privacy issues in smart grids. IEEE Commun. Surv. Tutorials. **14**(4), 981–997 (2012). https://doi.org/10.1109/SURV.2011.122111.00145
3. Dileep, G.: A survey on smart grid technologies and applications. Renew. Energy. **146**, 2589–2625 (2020). https://doi.org/10.1016/j.renene.2019.08.092
4. Eid, A.M., Nassif, A.B., Soudan, B., Injadat, M.N.: IIoT network intrusion detection using machine learning. In: 2023 6th International Conference on Intelligent Robotics and Control Engineering (IRCE), pp. 196–201. IEEE (2023). https://doi.org/10.1109/IRCE59430.2023.10255088
5. Sharma, D.K., Rapaka, G.K., Pasupulla, A.P., Jaiswal, S., Abadar, K., Kaur, H.: A review on smart grid telecommunication system. Mater. Today Proc. **51**, 470–474 (2022). https://doi.org/10.1016/j.matpr.2021.05.581
6. Soudan, B.: Cybersecurity of digital twins in industrial IoT environments. Adv. Sci. Eng. Technol. Int. Conf. ASET. (2024). https://doi.org/10.1109/ASET60340.2024.10708640
7. Gao, J., Xiao, Y., Liu, J., Liang, W., Chen, C.L.P.: A survey of communication/networking in Smart Grids. Futur. Gener. Comput. Syst. **28**(2), 391–404 (2012). https://doi.org/10.1016/j.future.2011.04.014
8. Hseiki, H.A., El-Hajj, A.M., Ajra, Y.O., Hija, F.A., Haidar, A.M.: A secure and resilient smart energy meter. IEEE Access. **12**, 3114–3125 (2024). https://doi.org/10.1109/ACCESS.2023.3349091
9. Sung, W.-J., Ahn, H.-G., Kim, J.-B., Choi, S.-G.: Protecting end-device from replay attack on LoRaWAN. In: 2018 20th International Conference on Advanced Communication Technology (ICACT), pp. 167–171 (2018). https://doi.org/10.23919/ICACT.2018.8323684
10. Pasetti, M., et al.: Evaluation of the use of class B Lorawan for the coordination of distributed interface protection systems in smart grids. J. Sens. Actuator Netw. **9**(1) (2020). https://doi.org/10.3390/jsan9010013
11. Abbasi, M., Khorasanian, S., Yaghmaee, M.H.: Low-Power Wide Area Network (LPWAN) for Smart grid: An in-depth study on LoRaWAN. In: 2019 5th Conference on Knowledge Based Engineering and Innovation (KBEI), pp. 22–29 (2019). https://doi.org/10.1109/KBEI.2019.8735089
12. Nafi, N.S., Ahmed, K., Gregory, M.A., Datta, M.: A survey of smart grid architectures, applications, benefits and standardization. J. Netw. Comput. Appl. **76**, 23–36 (2016). https://doi.org/10.1016/j.jnca.2016.10.003
13. Baimel, D., Tapuchi, S., Baimel, N.: Smart grid communication technologies- overview, research challenges and opportunities. In: 2016 International symposium on power electronics, electrical drives, Automation and Motion (SPEEDAM), vol. 2016, pp. 116–120. https://doi.org/10.1109/SPEEDAM.2016.7526014
14. Bayindir, R., Colak, I., Fulli, G., Demirtas, K.: Smart grid technologies and applications. Renew. Sust. Energ. Rev. **66**, 499–516 (2016). https://doi.org/10.1016/j.rser.2016.08.002
15. Mahmood, A., Javaid, N., Razzaq, S.: A review of wireless communications for smart grid. Renew. Sust. Energ. Rev. **41**, 248–260 (2015). https://doi.org/10.1016/j.rser.2014.08.036
16. Almuhaya, M.A.M., Jabbar, W.A., Sulaiman, N., Abdulmalek, S.: A survey on LoRaWAN technology: recent trends, opportunities, simulation tools and future directions. Electronics. **11**(1) (2022). https://doi.org/10.3390/electronics11010164
17. Haxhibeqiri, J., De Poorter, E., Moerman, I., Hoebeke, J.: A survey of LoRaWAN for IoT: from technology to application. Sensors. **18**(11) (2018). https://doi.org/10.3390/s18113995
18. Dönmez, T.C.M., Nigussie, E.: Security of join procedure and its delegation in LoRaWAN v1.1. Proce. Comput. Sci. **134**, 204–211 (2018). https://doi.org/10.1016/j.procs.2018.07.202

19. Da Rocha, A.M., De Oliveira, M.A., et al.: ABP vs. OTAA activation of LoRa devices: an Experimental Study in a Rural Context. In: 2023 International Conference on Computing, Networking and Communications (ICNC), pp. 630–634 (2023). https://doi.org/10.1109/ICNC57223.2023.10074553
20. Lavric, A., Petrariu, A.I.: LoRaWAN communication protocol: The new era of IoT. In: 2018 International Conference on Development and Application Systems (DAS), vol. 2018, pp. 74–77. https://doi.org/10.1109/DAAS.2018.8396074
21. Yang, X., Karampatzakis, E., Doerr, C., Kuipers, F.: Security vulnerabilities in LoRaWAN. In: 2018 IEEE/ACM Third International Conference on Internet-of-Things Design and Implementation (IoTDI), pp. 129–140 (2018). https://doi.org/10.1109/IoTDI.2018.00022
22. Butun, I., Pereira, N., Gidlund, M.: Security risk analysis of LoRaWAN and future directions. Futur. Internet. **11**(1) (2019). https://doi.org/10.3390/fi11010003
23. Na, S., Hwang, D., Shin, W., Kim, K.H.: Scenario and countermeasure for replay attack using join request messages in LoRaWAN. Int. Conf. Inf. Netw., 718–720 (2017). https://doi.org/10.1109/ICOIN.2017.7899580
24. Dave, J., Choudhury, N.: Security enhancement of OTAA based joining procedure in LoRaWAN for satellite communication. IEEE Veh. Technol. Conf. (2024). https://doi.org/10.1109/VTC2024-Spring62846.2024.10683277
25. Tomasin, S., Zulian, S., Vangelista, L.: Security Analysis of LoRaWAN Join Procedure for Internet of Things Networks. In: 2017 IEEE Wirel. Commun. Netw. Conf. Work. WCNCW 2017 (2017). https://doi.org/10.1109/WCNCW.2017.7919091
26. Le, D.T., Dinh, T.D., Pham, V.D., Kirichek, R., Filin, E., Shestakov, A.: A combined attack scenario to exploit the join procedure of LoRaWAN. Int. Congr. Ultra Mod. Telecommun. Control Syst. Work. **2021**, 188–193 (2021). https://doi.org/10.1109/ICUMT54235.2021.9631602
27. Kim, J., Song, J.: A simple and efficient replay attack prevention scheme for LoRaWAN. In: Proceedings of the 2017 7th International Conference on Communication and Network Security, in ICCNS '17, pp. 32–36. Association for Computing Machinery, New York (2017). https://doi.org/10.1145/3163058.3163064
28. Butun, I., Pereira, N., Gidlund, M.: Analysis of LoRaWAN v1.1 security: research paper. In: Proceedings of the 4th ACM MobiHoc Workshop on Experiences with the Design and Implementation of Smart Objects, in SMARTOBJECTS '18. Association for Computing Machinery, New York (2018). https://doi.org/10.1145/3213299.3213304
29. Seller, O.: LoRaWAN security. J. ICT Stand. **9**(1), 47–60 (2021). https://doi.org/10.13052/jicts2245-800X.915
30. Bellare, M., Rogaway, P.: Entity authentication and key distribution. In: Stinson, D.R. (ed.) Advances in Cryptology — CRYPTO' 93, pp. 232–249. Springer, Berlin, Heidelberg (1994)
31. Kamkuemah, M.N.: Epistemic Analysis of a Key-Management Vulnerability in LoRaWAN. In: 2021 18th International Conference on Privacy, Security and Trust (PST), vol. 2021, pp. 1–7. https://doi.org/10.1109/PST52912.2021.9647741
32. Fan, C.-I., Zhuang, E.-S., Karati, A., Su, C.-H.: A multiple end-devices authentication scheme for LoRaWAN. Electronics. **11**(5) (2022). https://doi.org/10.3390/electronics11050797
33. Kim, J., Song, J.: A dual key-based activation scheme for secure LoRaWAN. Wirel. Commun. Mob. Comput. **2017**(1), 6590713 (2017). https://doi.org/10.1155/2017/6590713
34. Hakeem, S.A.A., El-Kader, S.M.A., Kim, H.: A key management protocol based on the hash chain key generation for securing LoRaWAN networks. Sensors. **21**(17) (2021). https://doi.org/10.3390/s21175838
35. Danish, S.M., Lestas, M., Asif, W., Qureshi, H.K., Rajarajan, M.: A Lightweight Blockchain Based Two Factor Authentication Mechanism for LoRaWAN Join Procedure. In: 2019 IEEE International Conference on Communications Workshops (ICC Workshops), vol. 2019, pp. 1–6. https://doi.org/10.1109/ICCW.2019.8756673

# Advancing Security in Healthcare IoT: A Literature Review on MitM Attack Detection and Mitigation Using Machine Learning and Encryption Techniques

Mohamad Abdallah Mohamad(✉) and Bassel Soudan

Department of Computer Engineering, University of Sharjah, Sharjah, UAE
{u22105439,bsoudan}@sharjah.ac.ae

**Abstract.** Healthcare Internet of Things (HIoT) systems have revolutionized patient care through real-time monitoring and enhanced efficiency. However, they remain highly vulnerable to cyberattacks, particularly Man-in-the-Middle (MitM) attacks, which threaten data integrity and patient safety. This paper provides a comprehensive review of existing research on MitM attack detection and mitigation in HIoT. The review identifies significant advancements, including hybrid detection-mitigation frameworks and lightweight encryption protocols tailored for resource-constrained IoT devices. Despite these developments, challenges remain in achieving real-time detection, balancing resource efficiency, and adapting to evolving attack patterns. By addressing these gaps, future research can contribute to robust and scalable security solutions for HIoT, ensuring data integrity and enhancing patient safety.

**Keywords:** Machine Learning · Healthcare IoT · Cybersecurity · Man-in-the-Middle Attacks · Encryption Techniques

## 1 Introduction

The Internet of Things (IoT) has revolutionized healthcare by enabling interconnected devices to exchange and process data in real time. IoT technologies support advanced monitoring, diagnostics, and treatment capabilities, with applications such as remote patient monitoring, telemedicine, and smart medical devices significantly improving healthcare delivery in resource-constrained environments [2,18,20,34,36]. The integration of edge computing and artificial intelligence (AI) into Healthcare IoT (HIoT) systems has further enhanced data processing efficiency, reduced decision latency, and contributed to improved patient outcomes and operation efficiency [6,10,12].

Despite these advancements, HIoT systems are increasingly targeted by cyberattacks such as malware, ransomware, and unauthorized access, posing serious operational and financial threats [13]. These attacks exploit vulnerabilities in resource-constrained IoT devices and network infrastructures. Among


K. Daimi and A. Alsadoon (Eds.): ICR 2025, LNNS 1487, pp. 138–148, 2025.
https://doi.org/10.1007/978-3-031-95652-2_13

these threats, Man-in-the-Middle (MitM) attacks are particularly concerning, as attackers can intercept, manipulate, or disrupt communication between medical devices and healthcare networks [15]. Given the potential for severe disruptions in patient care, real-time detection, mitigation, and recovery from MitM attacks have become critical priorities.

This paper presents a comprehensive literature survey of techniques for the detection and mitigation of MitM attacks in HIoT systems. Special emphasis is placed on approaches that leverage ML on edge computing devices to enable autonomous, low-latency, and resource-efficient security mechanisms. The review encompasses advancements in lightweight ML models, hybrid frameworks integrating encryption and AI, and emerging solutions tailored to the unique challenges of HIoT environments.

## 2 Literature Review

The following sections present a summary of the reviewed literature, comprising a total of 40 papers. The review is grouped into subsections that focus on specific aspects relevant to the field, and the reviewed works in each subsection are arranged by relevance to the topic. HIoT security research has steadily grown from 2019 to 2024, showing rising academic interest in the field.

### 2.1 Cyberattacks on Healthcare IoT

HIoT networks face increasing threats from cyberattacks such as malware, ransomware, and MitM attacks. Weak encryption, poor device management, and insecure communication channels expose sensitive patient data and can disrupt healthcare operations. Vulnerabilities such as unencrypted communication and insufficient device controls have been identified, including risks like session hijacking and replay attacks [35]. Similarly, In [24,32], ML models are evaluated using datasets to detect DoS attacks. Furthermore, [24] highlights the exposure to MitM threats due to unencrypted transmissions.

Alanazi et al. [5] achieve 98% accuracy using Random Forest (RF) model on the NF-ToN-IoT dataset, showing security gaps like weak authentication and lack of encryption. Hady et al. [17] develop an improved monitoring system combining biometric and traffic data for live threat detection. In [42], a GAN-based Federated Learning (FL) framework is proposed to preserve privacy to detect eavesdropping and session hijacking. In [40], authors present a self-learning IDPS using active learning to adapt to threats like SQL injection and brute-force attacks. Lee et al. [28] introduce a Convolutional Neural Networks (CNN) based classifier to prioritize threats based on severity. Qadri et al. [39] address routing attacks using blockchain to mitigate selective forwarding and wormholes.

Several of these studies provide insights into real-world feasibility and deployment. Authors reported improved responsiveness in live healthcare settings, while others addressed privacy-preserving deployments across institutions. Some authors emphasizes adaptive intrusion response through online retraining [40], and Lee et al. rely on real-world data for fine-grained classification of threats. Qadri et al. consider latency and decentralization in practical blockchain deployment. These contributions reinforce that cyberattacks in HIoT target not only communication channels, but also device-level integrity, privacy, and routing, highlighting the need for scalable and deployable security solutions.

### 2.2 Addressing Cyberattacks in Healthcare IoT: State of Research and Emerging Solutions

Securing communication protocols such as MQTT and implementing robust encryption techniques, including TLS and ABE, are essential to mitigate cyberattacks in HIoT environments. Common mitigation approaches include securing communication channels, applying encryption, implementing access control mechanisms, and deploying lightweight authentication protocols. All of these strategies must be tailored to meet the performance constraints of HIoT devices.

Numerous studies have proposed lightweight cryptographic frameworks designed specifically for the limited computational capabilities of HIoT systems. For instance, Masud et al. [30] utilize nonce-based authentication in cloud-integrated environments, while Hintaw et al. [21] introduced a hybrid scheme that combines D-AES and KP-ABE to secure MQTT communication efficiently.

Kondoro et al. [26] examine secure communication protocols like CoAP/DTLS, MQTT/TLS, and XMPP/TLS, noting scalability issues in constrained settings. Diro et al. [14] address these challenges by offloading encryption to fog nodes to reduce device load. Similarly, Rao and Prema [41], Aziz and Singh [11], and Li et al. [29] propose lightweight solutions that optimize energy usage, security, and scalability for HIoT systems.

Table 1 provides a detailed comparative analysis of the mitigation techniques reviewed in terms of security strength, computational cost, scalability, and real-time feasibility. To ensure consistency across diverse studies, standardized labels High, Medium, and Low are used. These designations are derived from the technical descriptions and deployment contexts reported in each respective study.

In parallel, several studies focus on detecting MitM and other cyberattacks using machine learning-based intrusion detection systems (IDS). These approaches differ in terms of the datasets used, model types, detection accuracy, and suitability for real-time operation on resource-constrained HIoT devices.

Table 2 provides a structured comparison of the reviewed detection techniques. It summarizes the ML models used, their datasets, reported accuracy, key strengths and limitations, and their feasibility for real-time deployment. This enables researchers to identify practical detection methods suited for healthcare environments. Overall, the detection approaches in Table 2 highlight a trade-off between detection accuracy and deployment feasibility. While several methods show high accuracy, most lack real-time evaluation under healthcare-specific workloads, indicating a need for hybrid, deployable solutions for future research.

**Table 1.** Comparison of Mitigation Techniques in HIoT Environments

| Ref | Technique | Mitigation Type | Security Strength | Compt. Cost | Scalability | Real-Time Feasibility & Notes |
|---|---|---|---|---|---|---|
| [30] | KDF + Nonce-based Auth | Authentication | Low | Medium | High | Lightweight, suitable for cloud-HIoT; targets replay attacks only |
| [27] | MQTT Security Review | Protocol Analysis | N/A | N/A | N/A | Survey-based; identifies MQTT vulnerabilities but lacks implementation |
| [26] | MQTT/TLS, CoAP/DTLS, XMPP/TLS | Secure Protocols | High | Low | Low | Real-time performance tested; MQTT/XMPP show latency under constraints |
| [21] | D-AES + KP-ABE | Encryption + Access Control | Medium | Medium | Medium | Balanced solution; moderate overhead; fits MQTT |
| [41] | ECC + KP-ABE | Encryption + Access Control | Low | Medium | Medium | MitM partially mitigated; replay attack risk remains |
| [11] | LSS + Compressive Sensing | Encryption + Compression | Low | Low | Low | Simultaneous compression & encryption; energy efficient |
| [31] | Hash + XOR Authentication | Authentication | Low | High | Low | Mutual auth provided; lacks scalability for evolving threats |
| [29] | CP-WABE + 0-1 Coding | Access Control | Low | Medium | Medium | Efficient for access control; setup complexity a challenge |
| [22] | AES-128, XXTEA, ChaCha20 | Encryption Algorithms | Medium | Low | High | AES/XXTEA low energy; ChaCha20 high energy cost |
| [14] | ECC + AES-CCM (Fog) | Encryption | Low | High | Medium | Offloads computation to fog; reduces device load |
| [33] | Blockchain + ML (Multi-layer) | Encryption + Detection | High | High | Medium | Multi-layer defense; complex and resource-intensive |
| [43] | PBAC-FG (AB-ME + Signcryption) | Access Control + Authentication | High | Medium | High | Fine-grained control; efficient for constrained devices |

## 2.3 Detecting Attacks on HIoT Using Machine Learning

ML plays a pivotal role in securing HIoT systems, especially for detecting complex threats such as MitM attacks. ML-based IDS enable efficient analysis of traffic patterns and early anomaly detection.

Khan and Alkhathami [24] achieved 99.55% accuracy using Random Forest and SMOTE on the CICIoT2023 dataset. Deep learning-based CNNs were explored in the M-IDM model of Lee et al. [28], which showed strong multiclass detection, but required tuning for minority classes.

Zeghida et al. [46] used stacked ensemble learning to reach over 95% accuracy with low overhead, while Vaccari et al. [45] introduced the MQTTset dataset and reported 98% accuracy using RF. Alotaibi et al. [7] and Pradyumna et al. [38] evaluated distributed ML and deep learning, identifying XGBoost and CNN as efficient for real-time detection with scalability limitations.

ANN and DNN approaches by Hady et al. [17] and Khan et al. [23] delivered high accuracy but incurred higher processing costs. Meanwhile, Abdelbasit [1] reported strong results using boosting techniques on the MQTT-IoT-IDS2020 dataset, achieving low false positive rates.

Distributed frameworks such as federated learning with GANs (Siniosoglou et al. [42]) and SDN-integrated hybrid models (Arthi et al. [9]) showed promise in reducing overhead and improving scalability. Alsalman [8] introduced FusionNet, combining RF, SVM, KNN, and MLP to achieve 99.5% accuracy across datasets.

Aguru and Erukala [4] proposed mGRU models for lightweight DDoS detection in IoMT, significantly reducing model size and response time. Tenepalli and Navamani [44] highlighted general challenges in real-time ML adoption, while Adil et al. [3] and Ramalingam et al. [16] emphasized privacy, latency, and the need for resource-aware ML.

Table 2 summarizes these studies, comparing their ML models, datasets, accuracy levels, and suitability for constrained environments. This structured comparison supports clearer insights into the effectiveness and practicality of ML-based detection approaches in HIoT.

While these ML-based detection systems show promise, key challenges remain in deployment, scalability, and resource management. The next section outlines the remaining research gaps and proposes directions for addressing them.

**Table 2.** Comparison of Detection Techniques for MitM Attacks in HIoT

| Ref | Technique | Dataset | Accuracy | **Strengths** | Challenges | Real-Time Feasibility |
|---|---|---|---|---|---|---|
| [24] | RF | CICIoT2023 | 99.55% | High detection rate with SMOTE and feature optimization | Focus on binary classification, scalability | Moderate; latency not tested |
| [28] | CNN | Real hospital data | N/A | Multi-class detection across severity levels | Optimization needed for rare classes | N/A |
| [17] | ANN, RF, SVM, KNN | Biometric + network data | 92.98% | Biometric + network integration | High computational cost | Moderate |
| [42] | GAN + FL | Simulated medical CPS | N/A | Enhanced privacy & edge training | Complex setup | N/A |
| [46] | Ensemble (Bagging, etc.) | MQTTset (Balanced) | 95.43% | High accuracy, low overhead, fast inference | Model interpretability | High |
| [45] | RF, DT, NB, MLP, etc. | MQTTset | 99.4% (RF) | MQTT-focused dataset creation | Imbalanced data impact on real-world detection | Low; long training/testing times |
| [7] | XGBoost (via H2O AutoML) | Custom MQTT traffic | N/A | Real-time detection, AutoML | Scalability in high-traffic networks | Moderate |
| [38] | Supervised & Deep Learning | IoMT testbed | N/A | Real-time monitoring including MitM | Data privacy, computation | High |
| [9] | DNN + SVM (SDN framework) | IoMT testbed | 96% | Robust for complex medical data | Needs wider validation | Moderate |
| [8] | FusionNet (RF, KNN, SVM, MLP) | BoT-IoT & UNSW-NB15 | 99.50% | High accuracy through ensemble | Needs real-world validation | N/A |
| [4] | Modified GRU (mGRU) | CICIoT2023, CICDDoS2019 | N/A | Fast, lightweight for real-time | DDoS focused | High |
| [44] | RF, SVM (Review) | Multiple | N/A | Covers ML trends & challenges | Privacy concerns, interoperability issues | N/A |
| [16] | Edge AI Framework | IoMT wearable sensors | N/A | Real-time monitoring | Latency, privacy, model complexity | Moderate |
| [3] | Review (lightweight ML) | N/A | N/A | Focus on lightweight ML in HIoT | Resource constraints; model interpretability | N/A |
| [1] | Ensemble (Bagging, etc.) | MQTT-IoT-IDS2020 | 98.90% | Low false positive rate, high detection | No real-time deployment tested | Low; high model complexity |
| [33] | Blockchain + ML (Multi-layer IDS) | N/A | N/A | Secure access control | High computational overhead, no real-time testing | Low |
| [31] | Hash + XOR Auth Scheme | N/A | 94.50% | Robust and lightweight against replay attacks | Cloud-based testbed only | High |
| [29] | CP-WABE with 0-1 coding | N/A | 92.40% | Lightweight with ciphertext-policy | Setup complexity | Medium |
| [19] | Fuzzy Logic IDS (Secure-MQTT) | N/A | 96.40% | MQTT-specific simulation | Limited generalizability | High |

# 3 Research Gaps and Future Directions

While significant strides have been made in securing HIoT systems, the field still faces several critical challenges. This section outlines the key gaps in the current body of research and proposes future directions to address these limitations, paving the way for more secure and resilient HIoT networks.

## 3.1 Gaps in Current Research on Healthcare IoT Security

The comprehensive review of recent studies on HIoT security highlights the need to address cyberattacks, particularly MitM attacks. Below are the critical gaps:

- **Limited Real-World Implementation and Testing:** While many studies propose robust intrusion detection-mitigation systems, real-world validation remains scarce. For example, Hady et al. [17] and Siniosoglou et al. [42] demonstrate ML models for anomaly detection within testbeds or controlled environments. However, the lack of real-world deployment raises concerns about the performance of these systems under variable network loads and diverse IoT device capabilities.
- **Not Considering Resource Constraints on Low-Powered IoT Devices:** HIoT devices often have limited computational power, memory, and energy capacity, which poses challenges for implementing advanced security mechanisms. Systems that rely on deep neural networks or complex encryption protocols may be unsuitable for devices with constrained resources.
- **Limited Integration of Detection and Mitigation:** More comprehensive solutions integrating detection with mitigation are needed. Laghari et al. [27] enhance MQTT protocol security against MitM attacks; however, real-time anomaly detection is not sufficiently addressed.
- **Low Adaptability to Emerging Threats:** The dynamic nature of cyberattacks, including zero-day vulnerabilities and advanced persistent threats, presents a persistent challenge. Existing anomaly detection systems often struggle to adapt to new attack patterns, highlighting the need for self-learning and adaptive frameworks.
- **Scalability Challenges:** Scalability remains a significant concern as HIoT networks grow in size and complexity. Solutions involving centralized architectures or resource-intensive ML models may not perform efficiently in large-scale deployments [24].
- **Limited Consideration for Implementation on Edge Devices:** The combination of ML and encryption protocols shows potential for a balanced security framework. However, practical studies validating the efficiency of such hybrid systems on edge devices remain underexplored. The impact of running both encryption and ML detection concurrently on resource-constrained devices without compromising their primary functions of data collection and storage requires further investigation.
- **Security-Efficiency Trade-offs:** The balance between security strength and operational efficiency (e.g., energy consumption) remains a critical gap

[11,37]. Strong encryption methods often increase power consumption and response times, potentially disrupting HIoT network functionality. Optimizing these techniques for rapid data transmission without compromising security remains a challenge.

## 3.2 Future Directions and Suggestions

To address the identified gaps, future research in HIoT security should focus on the following directions:

- **Real-world testing and validation:** Proposed solutions should be deployed and validated in real-world HIoT environments to ensure effectiveness under diverse and dynamic conditions. This approach bridges the gap between theoretical models and practical applications.
- **Lightweight and efficient solutions:** Developing lightweight encryption methods and optimizing ML models for resource-constrained devices can improve security without degrading device performance. Techniques such as federated learning or lightweight ABE [22] warrant further exploration.
- **Integrated detection and mitigation frameworks:** Unified frameworks that combine intrusion detection with real-time mitigation can provide comprehensive protection. Integrating ML algorithms with lightweight encryption can effectively address both tasks.
- **Adaptive and self-learning systems:** Leveraging adaptive frameworks, such as reinforcement learning or self-learning IDS [40], can enable systems to dynamically evolve and adapt to emerging threats.
- **Scalable security architectures:** Efficiently scalable architectures are essential for large HIoT deployments. Hybrid edge-cloud models offer a promising approach to maintain performance while scaling.
- **Edge computing integration:** Integrating ML-based detection and encryption protocols directly on edge devices will enable low-latency, real-time responses. This direction supports the increasing shift toward decentralized HIoT frameworks.
- **Balancing security and efficiency:** Research should explore adaptive encryption strategies that adjust security levels based on device and network conditions, ensuring both robustness and operational efficiency [25].
- **Emerging security paradigms:** Future studies should consider post quantum encryption, zero-trust architectures, and AI-driven security automation as promising paradigms to address sophisticated and evolving HIoT threats.

By addressing these gaps and pursuing these research directions, future studies can significantly enhance the security and resilience of HIoT systems, safeguarding patient data and ensuring uninterrupted healthcare services.

## 4 Conclusion

The integration of IoT in healthcare has transformed patient care by enabling real-time monitoring, remote diagnostics, and improved operational efficiency. However, these advancements introduce significant cybersecurity risks, particularly MitM attacks, which threaten data integrity and patient safety. This paper reviewed existing research on detecting and mitigating MitM attacks in HIoT, focusing on ML-based methods, encryption techniques, and hybrid approaches. The analysis highlighted advancements in ML models such as RF and CNN, as well as encryption techniques like TLS and ABE. Despite these advancements, key challenges persist, including limited real-world testing, scalability concerns, and the need to balance security with performance constraints. Additionally, the scarcity of realistic and healthcare-specific datasets hampers the development of effective security solutions. Future research should prioritize developing lightweight and scalable frameworks that integrate detection and mitigation strategies while optimizing resource utilization. Addressing these challenges and incorporating forward-looking strategies will contribute to building robust HIoT security mechanisms that protect sensitive patient data and ensure the reliability of healthcare services.

## References

1. Abdelbasit, B.: Cybersecurity Attacks Detection for MQTT-IoT Networks Using Machine Learning Ensemble Techniques. Technical Report July, Rochester Institute of Technology (2023)
2. Abdulmalek, S., et al.: IoT-based healthcare-monitoring system towards improving quality of life: a review. Healthcare **10**(10), 1993 (2022). https://doi.org/10.3390/healthcare10101993
3. Adil, M., et al.: Healthcare Internet of Things: security threats, challenges, and future research directions. IEEE Internet Things J. **11**(11), 19046–19069 (2024). https://doi.org/10.1109/JIOT.2024.3360289
4. Aguru, A.D., Erukala, S.B.: A lightweight multi-vector DDoS detection framework for IoT-enabled mobile health informatics systems using deep learning. Inf. Sci. **662**, 120209 (2024). https://doi.org/10.1016/j.ins.2024.120209
5. Alanazi, H.K., El-Aziz, A.A.A., Hamdi, H.: Securing IoT devices in e-health using machine learning techniques. Int. J. Adv. Comput. Sci. Appl. **14**(9), 453–464 (2023). https://doi.org/10.14569/IJACSA.2023.0140949
6. Almarzooqi, M., Kawde, N., Saad, S., Soudan, B.: Salama: Medical telepresence robot. In: 2024 Advances in Science and Engineering Technology International Conferences (ASET), pp. 1–8. Abu Dhabi, United Arab Emirates (2024). https://doi.org/10.1109/ASET60340.2024.10708641
7. Alotaibi, N.S., Ahmed, H., Kamel, S., ElKabbany, G.F.: Secure enhancement for MQTT protocol using distributed machine learning framework. Sensors **24**(5), 1638 (2024). https://doi.org/10.3390/s24051638
8. Alsalman, D.: A comparative study of anomaly detection techniques for IoT security using adaptive machine learning for IoT threats. IEEE Access **12**, 14719–14730 (2024). https://doi.org/10.1109/ACCESS.2024.3359033

9. Arthi, R., Krishnaveni, S., Zeadally, S.: An intelligent SDN-IoT enabled intrusion detection system for healthcare systems using a hybrid deep learning and machine learning approach. China Commun. **21**(1), 1–21 (2024). https://doi.org/10.23919/JCC.ja.2022-0681
10. Arul, R., Alroobaea, R., Tariq, U., Almulihi, A.H., Alharithi, F.S., Shoaib, U.: IoT-enabled healthcare systems using block chain-dependent adaptable services. Pers. Ubiquit. Comput., 1–15 (2021). https://doi.org/10.1007/s00779-021-01584-7
11. Aziz, A., Singh, K.: Lightweight security scheme for internet of things. Wireless Pers. Commun. **104**(2), 577–593 (2018). https://doi.org/10.1007/s11277-018-6035-4
12. Bhatt, V., Chakraborty, S.: Improving service engagement in healthcare through internet of things-based healthcare systems. J. Sci. Technol. Policy Manage. **14**(1), 53–73 (2023). https://doi.org/10.1108/JSTPM-03-2021-0040
13. Bhosale, K.S., Nenova, M., Iliev, G.: A study of cyber attacks in the healthcare sector. In: Proceedings of the 2021 6th Junior Conference on Lighting, pp. 1–6 (2021). https://doi.org/10.1109/Lighting49406.2021.9598947
14. Diro, A., Reda, H., Chilamkurti, N., Mahmood, A., Zaman, N., Nam, Y.: Lightweight authenticated-encryption scheme for internet of things based on publish-subscribe communication. IEEE Access **8**, 60539–60551 (2020). https://doi.org/10.1109/ACCESS.2020.2983117
15. Eid, A.M., Nassif, A.B., Soudan, B., Injadat, M.N.: IIoT network intrusion detection using machine learning. In: 2023 6th International Conference on Intelligent Robotics and Control Engineering (IRCE), pp. 196–201 (2023). https://doi.org/10.1109/IRCE59430.2023.10255088
16. Gautham, G., Pandian, D., Batcha, C.F.S.: IntelliCare: integrating IoT and machine learning for remote patient monitoring in healthcare: a comprehensive framework. J. Cogn. Hum.-Comput. Interact. **7**(2), 50–59 (2024). https://doi.org/10.54216/jchci.070205
17. Hady, A.A., Ghubaish, A., Salman, T., Unal, D., Jain, R.: Intrusion detection system for healthcare systems using medical and network data: a comparison study. IEEE Access **8**, 106576–106584 (2020). https://doi.org/10.1109/ACCESS.2020.3000421
18. Hameed, K., Bajwa, I.S., Ramzan, S., Anwar, W., Khan, A.: An intelligent IoT-based healthcare system using fuzzy neural networks. Sci. Program. **2020**, 1–15 (2020). https://doi.org/10.1155/2020/8836927
19. A. P., H., K., K.: Secure-MQTT: an efficient fuzzy logic-based approach to detect DoS attack in MQTT protocol for internet of things. EURASIP J. Wirel. Commun. Netw. **2019**(1), 1–15 (2019). https://doi.org/10.1186/s13638-019-1402-8
20. Hayyolalam, V., Aloqaily, M., Ozkasap, O., Guizani, M.: Edge intelligence for empowering IoT-based healthcare systems. IEEE Wirel. Commun. **28**(3), 6–14 (2021). https://doi.org/10.1109/MWC.001.2000345
21. Hintaw, A.J., Manickam, S., Karuppayah, S., Aladaileh, M.A., Aboalmaaly, M.F., Laghari, S.: A robust security scheme based on enhanced symmetric algorithm for MQTT in the internet of things. IEEE Access **11**, 43019–43040 (2023). https://doi.org/10.1109/ACCESS.2023.3267718
22. Iqbal, Y., Amjad, M.F., Khan, F., Abbas, H.: The implementation of encryption algorithms in MQTT protocol for IoT constrained devices. In: 2022 14th IEEE International Conference on Computing Intelligence and Communication Networks (CICN), pp. 804–810 (2022). https://doi.org/10.1109/CICN56167.2022.10008320

23. Khan, M.A., et al.: A deep learning-based intrusion detection system for MQTT-enabled IoT. Sensors **21**(21), 1–25 (2021). https://doi.org/10.3390/s21217016
24. Khan, M.M., Alkhathami, M.: Anomaly detection in IoT-based healthcare: machine learning for enhanced security. Sci. Rep. **14**(1), 1–16 (2024). https://doi.org/10.1038/s41598-024-56126-x
25. Khashan, O.A., Khafajah, N.M., Mohamed, N., Salaimah, B.: Energy-efficient dynamic adaptive encryption for low-resource internet of things. In: Taherdoost, H., Farhaoui, Y., Shahamiri, S.R., Le, T.V., Madanchian, M., Prasad, M. (eds.) EAI 3rd International Conference on Smart Technologies and Innovation Management. MTYMEX 2024. EAI/Springer Innovations in Communication and Computing. Springer, Cham (2025). https://doi.org/10.1007/978-3-031-64957-8_15
26. Kondoro, A., Dhaou, I.B., Tenhunen, H., Mvungi, N.: Real-Time performance analysis of secure IoT protocols for microgrid communication. Futur. Gener. Comput. Syst. **116**, 1–12 (2021). https://doi.org/10.1016/j.future.2020.09.031
27. Laghari, A., Li, W., Manickam, S., Nanda, P., Al-Ani, A.K., Karuppayah, S.: Securing MQTT ecosystem: exploring vulnerabilities, mitigations, and future trajectories. IEEE Access, 1–17 (2024). https://doi.org/10.1109/ACCESS.2024.3412030
28. Lee, J.D., Cha, H.S., Rathore, S., Park, J.H.: M-IDM: a multi-classification based intrusion detection model in healthcare IoT. Comput. Mater. Continua **67**(2), 1537–1553 (2021). https://doi.org/10.32604/cmc.2021.014774
29. Li, H., Yu, K., Liu, B., Feng, C., Qin, Z., Srivastava, G.: An efficient ciphertext-policy weighted attribute-based encryption for the internet of health things. IEEE J. Biomed. Health Inform. **26**(5), 1949–1960 (2022). https://doi.org/10.1109/JBHI.2021.3075995
30. Masud, M., Gaba, G.S., Choudhary, K., Alroobaea, R., Hossain, M.S.: A robust and lightweight secure access scheme for cloud based E-healthcare services. Peer-to-Peer Network. Appl. **14**(5), 3043–3057 (2021). https://doi.org/10.1007/s12083-021-01162-x
31. Masud, M., Gaba, G.S., Choudhary, K., Hossain, M.S., Alhamid, M.F., Muhammad, G.: Lightweight and anonymity-preserving user authentication scheme for IoT-based healthcare. IEEE Internet Things J. **9**(4), 2649–2656 (2022). https://doi.org/10.1109/JIOT.2021.3080461
32. Mohamad, M.A., Eladham, M.W., Saad, M.: Detection of DoS attacks in internet of things networks: a comparative study. In: 2024 Advances in Science and Engineering Technology International Conferences (ASET), pp. 1–6 (2024). https://doi.org/10.1109/ASET60340.2024.10708664
33. Mrabet, H., Alhomoud, A., Jemai, A., Trentesaux, D.: A secured industrial internet-of-things architecture based on blockchain technology and machine learning for sensor access control systems in smart manufacturing. Appl. Sci. **12**(9) (2022). https://doi.org/10.3390/app12094641
34. Mustafa, A., Alahmed, M., Alhammadi, A., Soudan, B.: Stress detector system using iot and artificial intelligence. In: 2020 Advances in Science and Engineering Technology International Conferences (ASET), pp. 1–6. Dubai, United Arab Emirates (2020). https://doi.org/10.1109/ASET48392.2020.9118345
35. Newaz, A.I., Sikder, A.K., Rahman, M.A., Uluagac, A.S.: A survey on security and privacy issues in modern healthcare systems. ACM Trans. Comput. Healthc. **2**(3) (2021). https://doi.org/10.1145/3453176
36. Onasanya, A., Elshakankiri, M.: Smart integrated IoT healthcare system for cancer care. Wireless Netw. **27**(6), 4297–4312 (2019). https://doi.org/10.1007/s11276-018-01932-1

37. Perazzo, P., Righetti, F., Manna, M.L., Vallati, C.: Performance evaluation of attribute-based encryption on constrained IoT devices. Comput. Commun. **170**, 151–163 (2021). https://doi.org/10.1016/j.comcom.2021.02.012
38. Pradyumna, G.R., Hegde, R.B., Bommegowda, K.B., Jan, T., Naik, G.R.: Empowering Healthcare with IoMT: evolution, machine learning integration, security, and interoperability challenges. IEEE Access **12**, 20603–20623 (2024). https://doi.org/10.1109/ACCESS.2024.3362239
39. Qadri, Y.A., Ali, R., Musaddiq, A., Al-Turjman, F., Kim, D.W., Kim, S.W.: The limitations in the state-of-the-art counter-measures against the security threats in H-IoT. Clust. Comput. **23**(3), 2047–2065 (2020). https://doi.org/10.1007/s10586-019-03036-7
40. Radoglou-Grammatikis, P., Sarigiannidis, P., Efstathopoulos, G., Lagkas, T., Fragulis, G., Sarigiannidis, A.: A self-learning approach for detecting intrusions in healthcare systems. In: IEEE International Conference on Communications (ICC), pp. 1–6 (2021). https://doi.org/10.1109/ICC42927.2021.9500354
41. Rao, V., Prema, K.V.: A review on lightweight cryptography for Internet-of-Things based applications. J. Ambient. Intell. Humaniz. Comput. **12**(9), 8835–8857 (2020). https://doi.org/10.1007/s12652-020-02672-x
42. Siniosoglou, I., Sarigiannidis, P., Argyriou, V., Lagkas, T., Goudos, S.K., Poveda, M.: Federated intrusion detection in NG-IoT healthcare systems: an adversarial approach. In: IEEE International Conference on Communications (ICC) (2021). https://doi.org/10.1109/ICC42927.2021.9500578
43. Sun, J., Yuan, Y., Tang, M.J., Cheng, X., Nie, X., Aftab, M.U.: Privacy-preserving bilateral fine-grained access control for cloud-enabled industrial IoT healthcare. IEEE Trans. Industr. Inf. **18**(9), 6483–6493 (2022). https://doi.org/10.1109/TII.2021.3133345
44. Tenepalli, D., Navamani, T.M.: A systematic review on IoT and machine learning algorithms in E-healthcare. Int. J. Comput. Digital Syst. **16**(1), 279–294 (2024). https://doi.org/10.12785/ijcds/160122
45. Vaccari, I., Chiola, G., Aiello, M., Mongelli, M., Cambiaso, E.: MQTTset: a new dataset for machine learning techniques on MQTT. Sensors (Switzerland) **20**(22), 1–17 (2020). https://doi.org/10.3390/s20226578
46. Zeghida, H., Boulaiche, M., Chikh, R.: Securing MQTT protocol for IoT environment using IDS based on ensemble learning. Int. J. Inf. Secur. **22**(4), 1075–1086 (2023). https://doi.org/10.1007/s10207-023-00681-3

# Impact Assessment of Adversary-in-the-Middle Attack Evilginx Bypassing 2FA

Hiroaki Kikuchi(✉)

Meiji University, 4-21-1 Nakano, Tokyo 164-8525, Japan
kikn@meiji.ac.jp

**Abstract.** Phishing attacks exploit user trust to steal sensitive information, often bypassing security mechanisms like multi-factor authentication (MFA). While MFA enhances protection, advanced threats such as Adversary-in-the-Middle (AiTM) attacks can bypass it by capturing session tokens using tools like Evilginx. This study examines Evilginx's functionality, confirming its ability to bypass MFA with minimal proxy-induced delays that are difficult to detect.

We also assessed 48 websites in Japan and 54 global websites, revealing that 80% of major web services are vulnerable to Evilginx attacks, particularly those using traditional MFA methods. Only a minority adopt phishing-resistant technologies like FIDO2/WebAuthn. The originality of this work lies in its wide-scale evaluation of MFA adoption and vulnerabilities, with future efforts aimed at developing detection methods for proxy-based attacks and promoting secure MFA solutions.

To analyze the effectiveness and detectability of AiTM attacks using Evilginx, we conducted two sets of experiments (1) Measuring Proxy-Induced Delay: We set up a test environment with Evilginx acting as a reverse proxy between users and a legitimate web service. We measured the elapsed time for login attempts with and without Evilginx to determine whether the additional proxy layer introduced a detectable delay in TLS handshake and authentication. (2) Assessing MFA Deployment and Vulnerability: We surveyed 48 websites in Japan and 54 global websites across various industries, including IT, ISPs, e-commerce, and finance. Each website was tested for MFA availability and categorized based on the types of authentication mechanisms implemented We then evaluated which authentication methods were vulnerable to Evilginx attacks by determining if session tokens could be captured and replayed.

**Keywords:** multi factor authentication · man-in-the-middle · SMS (Short Message Service) · OTP (One-time Password) · Evilginx

## 1 Introduction

Phishing attacks remain one of the most persistent and dangerous threats in cybersecurity. According to [1], phishing attack was involved by more than


K. Daimi and A. Alsadoon (Eds.): ICR 2025, LNNS 1487, pp. 149–158, 2025.
https://doi.org/10.1007/978-3-031-95652-2_14

36% cyber-incident in 2022. These attacks deceive users into revealing sensitive information, such as credentials, by impersonating legitimate entities. As cyber defenses evolve, organizations have adopted multi-factor authentication (MFA) such as SMS-based one time taken [3,8] as a critical countermeasure to enhance account security. MFA adds an additional layer of protection by requiring users to provide multiple verification factors, making it significantly harder for attackers to gain unauthorized access.

Despite the effectiveness of MFA, adversaries have developed sophisticated techniques to bypass these defenses. One such emerging threat is the *Adversary-in-the-Middle (AiTM) attack*, which leverages reverse proxy tools to intercept and relay communications between users and legitimate servers [9]. Unlike traditional phishing attacks, AiTM attacks can bypass MFA by capturing session tokens after authentication, allowing attackers to impersonate victims seamlessly. These attacks are particularly concerning as they exploit the trust in MFA systems and often go undetected by users.

In this study, we focus on Evilginx [2], a widely used open-source tool that implements AiTM attacks. We choose Evilginx as a representative tool among AiTM open-source tools including Muraena [5] and Modlishka [6]. Evilginx's functionality enables it to bypass MFA, making it a valuable subject for understanding this new threat. Additionally, Evilginx introduces fake TLS sessions using a legitimate certificate issued via Let's Encrypt, making it harder to detect. But, it takes few overhead to establish additional TLS connection, raising the question of whether this delay could be used to detect its presence.

The objective of this work is to investigate Evilginx's fundamental operations, particularly the difficulty in detecting it based on timing anomalies.

The contribution of this study lies in its wide-scale assessment of web services. We evaluated 48 websites in Japan and 54 global websites across multiple industries to analyze MFA deployment and assess their vulnerability to Evilginx attacks based on public information about available MFA methods and private analysis from enrollment of services that don't provide deployed MFA methods. This comprehensive approach provides an impact assessment of AiTM attack using Evilginx, critical insights into the current state of MFA adoption and highlights the risks posed by AiTM attacks to online services worldwide.

## 2 Related Works

### 2.1 Usability of MFA

Several studies have examined MFA usability, adoption, and security vulnerabilities. Lyastani et al. [25] conducted a systematic study on the consistency of two-factor authentication user journeys across top-ranked websites, highlighting inconsistencies that could impact security and usability. Reese et al. [26] performed a usability study of five two-factor authentication methods, evaluating user experience and security trade-offs. Farke et al. [27] explored FIDO2 security key adoption in a small company, providing insights into real-world deployment challenges and user behavior. Reynolds et al. [28] conducted an empirical measurement of systemic 2FA usability, assessing the effectiveness of various authentication approaches in practice.

These works provide foundational insights into MFA usability and security, complementing our study on Evilginx's ability to bypass MFA mechanisms. Our research expands on these findings by focusing on the security vulnerabilities of MFA implementations against AiTM attacks and evaluating real-world MFA deployment across industries.

## 2.2 Adversary-in-the-Middle Attack

An *Adversary-in-the-Middle* (AiTM) is a cyber attack in which an advisory intercepts and potentially modifies communication between browsers and web servers. In principle, it steals sensitive information, e.g., credentials, tokens, and http cookies. This is similar to the traditional Man-in-the-Middle (MitM) attack but with some more enhanced capabilities: (1) *Targeting authentication mechanisms.* AiTM focuses on capturing authentication data, while the conventional MitM aims to intercept and alter general communications, (2) *Bypassing MFA.* AiTM uses a reverse proxy server that sits between the victim and the legitimate server. Hence, even if the victim uses multi-factor authentication (MFA), the MiTM adversary can bypass the MFA and keep the compromised session while the token is sent over any alternative communication channel.

Figure 1 shows a typical scenario in AiTM, where a victim $A$, an adversary $B$, and a legitimate server $C$ are involved.

1. Adversary $B$ sends a phishing email to victim user $A$ with a link to a fake login page to $C$.
2. Victim $A$ sends the credential to $B$, which just forwards it to $C$.
3. Server $C$ sends an one-time MFA code to $A$ via configured factor, e.g., email, SMS, and an authenticator app.
4. Victim $A$ interacts with $B$, which forwards the one-time code to server $C$, convinced that $B$ is the legitimate user because it returns the one-time code correctly.

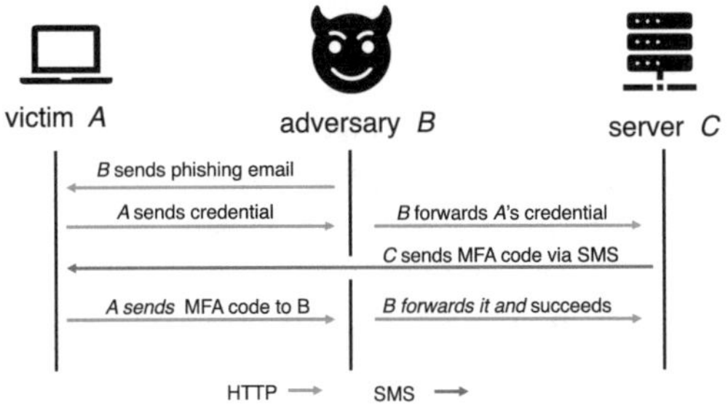


**Fig. 1.** Example scenario in AiTM

```
: sessions 127

 id          : 127
 phishlet    : example
 username    : [redacted]@[redacted]
 password    : [redacted]
 tokens      :
 landing url  : https://academy.kikn.fms.meiji.ac.jp/JDxUeqmf
 user-agent   : Mozilla/5.0 (Windows NT 10.0; Win64; x64) AppleWebKit/537.36 (KHTML, like Gecko) Chrome/131.0.0.0
Safari/537.36
 remote ip    : 127.0.0.1
 create time  : 2024-12-23 14:27
 update time  : 2024-12-23 14:29
```

**Fig. 2.** Session

# 3 Evaluation of Evilginx

## 3.1 Evilginx

*Evilginx* is an open-source tool for posing phishing attacks.

Similar to the conventional phishing tool, it acts as a reverse proxy between a victim and a legitimate server. Evilginx ver 3 implemented in Go, runs multiple platform including Windows and Linux-based OSs.

Evilginx is controlled via its Command-Line Interface (CLI), which allows users to configure and run the tool, and view captured data including credentials and session token. Figure 2 shows how to control Evilginx using its CLI and retrieve logs.

## 3.2 Basic Functions

Basic CLI commands include listing available *Phishlets*, starting a *Lures* campaign, and getting the Phishing links. Phishlet is a pre-configured template for specific website. Phishing link is created with *Lure*, which specifies target service, IP address and the corresponding URL.

Evilginx uses Let's Encrypt for setting up a fake TLS certificate, which is a legitimate certificate for phishing domain. With Linux server that manages its own DNS domain, Evilginx configures the fake domain name and enables URL supported TLS certificate.

## 3.3 Experiment

Evilginx needs to start up a revise proxy with TLS certificate and perform decryption and encryption for forwarding, which takes a small delay before browsing the site. To determine whether a victim can detect the presence of Evilginx based on the delay, we conduct an experiment that measure the elapsed time during browsing and login with and without the reverse proxy.

As for a legitimate target website, we use Evilginx Mastery https://academy.breakdev.org/evilginx-mastery, which is a training website for Evilginx users. We set up Evilginx proxy in the institutional network environment, with standard bandwidth and latency to the Internet. To measure elapsed time for login to the target site, we use Selenium [4] for automate the steps to login and take

**Table 1.** Elapsed time

| Time to | Evilginx | mean | min | max | sd |
|---|---|---|---|---|---|
| load the login page | without | 4.28 | 1.19 | 8.89 | 0.84 |
| | with | 5.04 | 3.64 | 8.02 | 0.87 |
| complete the login | without | 4.10 | 3.38 | 4.97 | 0.41 |
| | with | 7.14 | 4.85 | 12.40 | 1.70 |

the mean time to establish a TLS connection, load the landing page, submit credentials and receive response. We repeated the measurement 50 times to take an average.

### 3.4 Result

Table 1 shows the statistics of elapsed time. We found that there are significant differences between with and without Evilginx, about 0.8 s for loading and 3.0 s for login. It is not difficult for engineers to detect the presence of proxy based on the time delay. However, we also found that standard deviation of 1.7 for submitting credentials. Hence, in real-world environment, there are other factors for varying network conditions, e.g., a congestion and a limited bandwidth, average users may be compromised without noticing the presence of proxy.

## 4 Impact Assessment of Websites

### 4.1 Vulnerability to AiTM

**Vulnerable MFA Methods.** Evilginx can intercept session cookies after the SMS-based OPT process is completed, allowing attackers to bypass MFA entirely. Similarly, email-based One-Time Password (OTP), phone call authentication, Time-based One-Time Password (TOPT) and push notifications OPT are vulnerable for Evilginx. TOTP generates a unique temporary password using a time-synchronized algorithm, such as 4 or 6-digit temporal token is used to authenticate legitimate user. Unfortunately, the time-based token is captured and forwarded by the proxy.

Push Notification used for authenticator app, e.g., Google Authenticator and Microsoft Authenticator, is relatively secure than SMS-based OPT because the token is sent directly to the legitimate server without being intercepted by the proxy. However, it still allows the proxy activate the session after the token is exchanged.

**Resistant MFA Methods.** FIDO2 [12] is a set of specification by the FIDO Alliance and World Wide Web Consortium (W3C) and WebAuthn is an API that allows users to authenticate using built-in authenticators including Windows Hello [11] and YubiKey [10]. By using public-key cryptography, Evilginx may

**Table 2.** AiTM Resistance

| MFA method | vulnerable | MFA code |
|---|---|---|
| SMS-based OTP | Yes | stolen |
| phone call | Yes | stolen |
| Email-based OTP | Yes | stolen |
| TOTP | Yes | stolen |
| App, Push notification | Yes | No |
| FIDO2/WebAuthn | No | No |
| Passkey | No | No |

intercept a public key but never capture the corresponding private key, which never leave the user's device. Passkeys are also based on public-key cryptography, making them resistant to interception by Evilginx. Therefore, we assume that these MFA methods are resilient against Evilginx.

Table 2 summaries the vulnerability for several MFA methods.

### 4.2 Assessment of Websites

**Objective.** How common MFA are used in website? How many MFA methods are deployed? To address these questions on the availability and the security of MFA methods against Evilginx attack, we conduct an assessment of representative websites from Japan (48 sites) and globally (54 sites). We select representative websites from several industries, e.g., IT companies, ISPs, e-commerce, finance, government, and education. For example, Dropbox (https://dropbox.com) is a file hosting service that offers cloud storage, file synchronization and client software. They offer variety of MFAs, including SMS, push notification and passkey.

We investigate the set of website for (1) check whether MFA is available during the login process, (2) Number of available MFA methods on each website, and (3) test each MFA method residence against Evilginx. The classification of vulnerability, we determine based on documents of MFA methods offered in the site. For some site that does not provide sufficient information for our assessment, we actually sign in the service and record available methods. We classifies the total of 102 website into 38 categories according to 2FA Directory [3] for additional information and categories. Dropping minor categories that has less than 4 websites, the total of 15 categories are investigated.

### 4.3 Results

Table 3 shows the percentage of websites offering MFA in each region (Japan and global) either in counting the federated identity or not. It shows that 85 sites (including federated identities) supporting MFAs, which is 83% of the set of selected sites. The global availability is slightly larger than that of Japanese site, but no significant difference is found.

**Table 3.** MFA availability

| Federated | Japan | % | Global | % | all | % |
|---|---|---|---|---|---|---|
| without | 26 | 54.17 | 37 | 77.78 | 68 | 66.67 |
| with | 42 | 77.08 | 48 | 88.89 | 85 | 83.33 |
| total | 48 | | 54 | | 102 | |

**Table 4.** Investigation of available MFA methods for sample websites (part)

| category | site | county | MFA | fed. | SMS | phone | email | App | App2 | skey | passkey | push |
|---|---|---|---|---|---|---|---|---|---|---|---|---|
| backup | Dropbox | US | √ | | √ | | | √ | | √ | | √ |
| comm. | LINE | JP | √ | | | | | | √ | | | |
| creativity | pixiv | JP | √ | √ | | | | √ | | | | |
| developer | unity | US | √ | | √ | | | √ | | | | |
| domains | Crazy Domains | AS | √ | √ | √ | √ | | | | | | |

Table 4 shows some example website in the availabilities of MFA method, where App, App2, fed and skey are a general authenticator app, a designated app, a social login supported with federated identity, and a secure key such as passkey. For example, Dropbox, a SaaS platform for backup and file sharing, supports a variety of MFA methods including SMS-based, App, secure key, and push notification. We found the adoption rate varies in industries and no promising method used by all servers.

Figure 3 shows the deployment ratio for each of 15 categories. Note that the complete (100%) deployment in communication category and no availability of MFA in Hotels and Accommodation. Fig. 4 shows the frequencies of MFA methods used in the web sites. The most-frequent method is TOTP, which used in almost half sites (51/104).

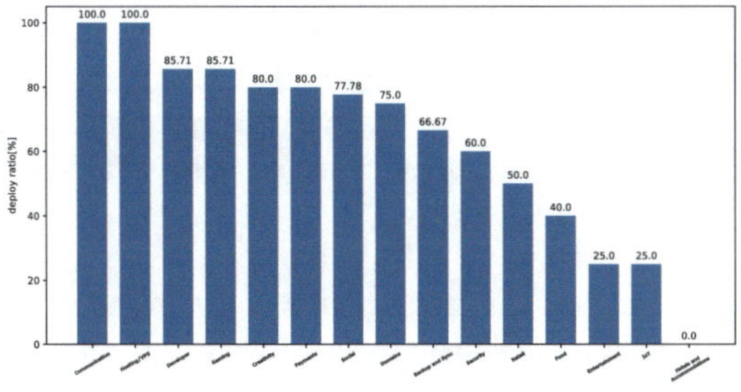


**Fig. 3.** MFA availabilities for categories

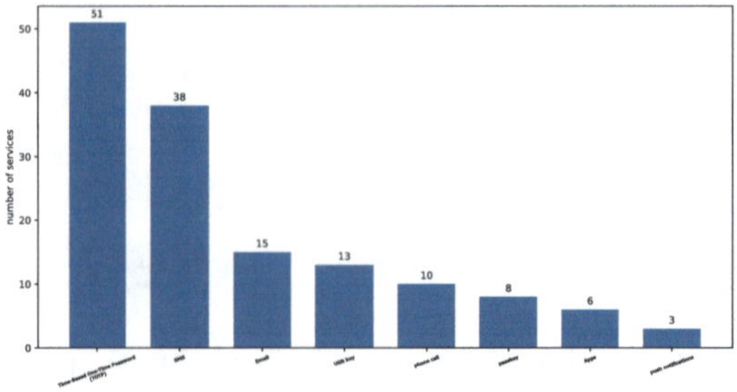


**Fig. 4.** Numbers of websites for deploying MFA methods

### 4.4 Consideration

The assessment highlights the adoption gaps in industries with low MFA adoption. Possible reason for these site may include that they may collaborate a wide range of users and minimize the authentication process so that they can interact with first-time visitor frequently. But, we should promote MFA technologies to the industries.

Based on our analysis in Sect. 4.1, 87 services out of 102 sites does not support Evilginx-resistant MFA methods, which accounts for 85% of our sampling. Namely, we say 85% site are potential vulnerable to Evilginx. Since the phishing attacks increase both in the numbers and in the financial costs year by year, we should promote the secure MFA methods for these services. Fortunately, most sites (80% in Table 3) offer one of MFA methods and may already notice the threat of AiTM.

### 4.5 Limitations

While our study provides valuable insights into MFA vulnerabilities against AiTM attacks, certain limitations should be considered. First, our experiments were conducted in a controlled environment to ensure precise measurements of proxy-induced delays and security evaluations. Although this allows for a detailed analysis, it does not fully replicate real-world conditions where network variability, user behavior, and additional security measures might influence the effectiveness of AiTM attacks.

Additionally, our evaluation of MFA adoption across websites was based on publicly available authentication mechanisms and simulated interactions rather than actual user experiences. This means that while our findings reflect the security posture of major web services, they may not account for additional backend security measures.

Finally, we did not involve real user interactions in our phishing simulations. Future work should explore real-world user interaction data to better assess user susceptibility to AiTM phishing attacks and improve detection mechanisms in live environments.

## 5 Conclusions

We investigated the Adversary-in-the-Middle (AiTM) attack and its capability to bypass multi-factor authentication (MFA). We examined Evilginx, an open-source tool commonly used for such attacks, and confirmed its effectiveness in capturing session tokens, enabling unauthorized access even when MFA is in place.

Our experiments measured the elapsed time introduced by the reverse proxy during TLS sessions and the login process. While Evilginx has a small delay, this overhead is minimal and unlikely to be noticed by users making it a powerful threat for bypassing authentication mechanisms.

We also assessed the availability and security of MFA across 48 websites in Japan and 54 global websites from various industries. The results revealed that approximately 80% of major web services remain vulnerable to Evilginx attacks, primarily due to their reliance on traditional MFA methods such as SMS-based OTPs. We found only a small fraction of services adopting phishing-resistant solutions like FIDO2/WebAuthn.

For future work, we plan to develop detection mechanisms for identifying proxy services like Evilginx, based on timing anomalies and monitoring suspicious session behaviors. Additionally, we emphasize the importance of adopting phishing-resistant MFA technologies and need for organizations to strengthen their MFA implementations.

**Acknowledgment.** Author thank Mr. Kazuki Ohta of Meiji University for conducting experiments in this work.

## References

1. Dataprot, Phishing Statistics. https://dataprot.net/statistics/phishing-statistics/. Accessed 2024
2. Gretzky, K.: Evilginx. https://github.com/kgretzky/evilginx2. Accessed 2024
3. 2FA Directory, 2FA Directory. https://2fa.directory/. Accessed 2024
4. Selenim, Selenium. https://www.selenium.dev/. Accessed 2024
5. Muraena, Muraena. https://github.com/muraenateam/muraena. Accessed 2024
6. Modlishka, Modlishka. https://github.com/drk1wi/Modlishka. Accessed 2024
7. BREAKDEV Academy, Evilginx Mastery. https://academy.breakdev.org/evilginx-mastery. Accessed 2024
8. Mulliner, C., Borgaonkar, R., Stewin, P., Seifert, J.-P.: SMS-based one-time passwords: attacks and defense. In: Proceedings of the 10th International Conference on Detection of Intrusions and Malware, and Vulnerability Assessment, DIMVA, pp. 150–159 (2013)
9. Gelernter, N., Kalma, S., Magnezi, B., Porcilan, H.: The password reset MitM attack. IEEE Secur. Privacy, 251–267 (2017)
10. Yubico, YubiKey. https://www.yubico.com/yubikey/. Accessed 2024
11. Microsoft, Windows Hello. https://www.microsoft.com/en-us/windows/tips/windows-hello/. Accessed 2024

12. Brown, A.: WebAuthn vs FIDO2: understanding the differences. https://www.descope.com/blog/post/webauthn-vs-fido2. Accessed 2025
13. European Parliament, Council of the European Union, General Data Protection Regulation (2016). Accessed https://eur-lex.europa.eu/eli/reg/2016/679/oj
14. California Consumer Privacy Act of 2018, Civil Code, Division 3, Part 4, Title 1.81.5 (2020). Accessed https://leginfo.legislature.ca.gov/faces/codes_displayText.xhtml?lawCode=CIV&division=3.&title=1.81.5.&part=4.&chapter=&article=
15. Personal Information Protection Commission, Japan, (Amended) the Act on the Protection of Personal Information (2020). Accessed https://www.ppc.go.jp/files/pdf/APPI_english.pdf
16. ghostery.com, Ghostery – Cleaner, faster, and safer browsing. https://www.ghostery.com/
17. adblockplus.org, Adblock Plus, Surf the web without annoying ads! https://adblockplus.org/
18. eff.org, Privacy Badger blocks spying ads and invisible trackers. https://www.eff.org/privacybadger
19. Ur, B., Leon, P.G., Cranor, L.F., Shay, R., Wang, Y.: Smart, useful, scary, creepy: Perceptions of online behavioral advertisin. In: Proceedings of SOUPS (2012)
20. Englehardt, S., Narayanan, A.: Online tracking: A 1-million-sitemea-surement and analysis. In: Proceedings of the 2016 ACM SIGSAC Conference on Computer and Communications Security, pp. 1388–1401 (2016)
21. Estrada-Jim, J., Rodrìguez-Hoyos, A., Parra-Arnau, J., Forne, J.: Measuring online tracking and privacy risks on Ecuadorian websites. In: 2019 IEEE Fourth Ecuador Technical Chapters Meeting (ETCM), pp. 1–6 (2019)
22. Iordanou, C., Kourtellis, N., Carrascosa, J.M., Soriente, C., Cuevas, R., Laoutaris, N.: Beyond content analysis: detecting targeted ads via distributed counting. In: Proceedings of the 15th International Conference on Emerging Networking Experiments And Technologies (CoNEXT'19), Association for Computing Machinery, NY, USA, pp. 110–122 (2019)
23. Cook, J., Nithyanand, R., Shafiq, Z.: Inferring tracker-advertiser relationships in the online advertising ecosystem using header bidding. In: Proceedings on Privacy Enhancing Technologies (2020)
24. Zeng, E., McAmis, R., Kohno, T., Roesner, F.: What factors affect targeting and bids in online advertising? A field measurement study. In: Proceedings of the 22nd ACM Internet Measurement Conference, pp. 210–229 (2022)
25. Lyastani, S.G., Backes, M., Bugiel, S.: A systematic study of the consistency of two-factor authentication user journeys on top-ranked websites, NDSS (2023)
26. Reese, T.S., Dutson, J., Armknecht, J., Cameron, J., Seamons, K.: A usability study of five two-factor authentication methods. In: Proceeding of the 15th Symposium on Usable Privacy and Security (SOUPS'19) (2019)
27. Farke, F.M., Lorenz, L., Schnitzler, T., Markert, P., Dürmuth, M.: You still use the password after all – exploring fido2 security keys in a small company. In: Sixteenth Symposium on Usable Privacy and Security (SOUPS 2020) (2020)
28. Reynolds, J., et al.: Empirical measurement of systemic 2FA usability. In: 29th USENIX Security Symposium (USENIX Security 20) (2020)

# Addressing Cybersecurity Challenges in 5G-Enabled IoT Networks: Solutions and Future Directions

João Azevedo[1] and Manuel J. C. S. Reis[2(✉)]

[1] Engineering Department, University of Trás-os-Montes e Alto Douro (UTAD), Vila Real, Portugal

[2] Engineering Department, UTAD & Institute of Electronics and Informatics Engineering of Aveiro (IEETA), Aveiro, Portugal

mcabral@utad.pt

**Abstract.** The rapid expansion of 5G networks combined with IoT technology introduces transformative capabilities for connectivity, yet it also exposes networks to critical cybersecurity challenges. This paper systematically reviews current literature to identify the primary security concerns associated with 5G-IoT integration, including threats related to authentication and authorization, data privacy, Distributed Denial of Service (DDoS) attacks, blockchain security, and quantum computing. Each of these challenges reflects the evolving landscape of 5G-IoT, with traditional methods often falling short in handling massive device connectivity, ensuring privacy under high-data flows, or scaling effectively with blockchain solutions. In response, emerging solutions highlight the role of AI driven security, federated learning, advanced encryption, and quantum-resistant technologies as essential tools to safeguard 5G-IoT ecosystems. Through a combination of systematic analysis and real-world examples from recent studies, this review not only categorizes the critical challenges, but also evaluates proposed solutions based on effectiveness, scalability, and feasibility. Our findings contribute to ongoing cybersecurity discussions by pinpointing gaps and offering insights into future-proofing 5G-IoT infrastructures against an increasingly complex threat environment.

**Keywords:** 5G · IoT · AI-driven security · federated learning · quantum-resistant technologies

## 1 Introduction

The evolution of fifth-generation (5G) wireless technology, coupled with the rapid expansion of the Internet of Things (IoT), has unlocked unprecedented potential for interconnected devices and real-time data transmission. These developments have the potential to revolutionize industries such as healthcare, smart cities, autonomous vehicles, and critical infrastructure by facilitating high-speed communication and extensive device connectivity.

However, this progress brings new cybersecurity problems of 5G-IoT ecosystems. To solve these challenges, we need cutting-edge solutions such as AI driven security


K. Daimi and A. Alsadoon (Eds.): ICR 2025, LNNS 1487, pp. 159–173, 2025.
https://doi.org/10.1007/978-3-031-95652-2_15

systems, blockchain integration and quantum resistant encryption methods specific to the dynamic needs of 5G-IoT networks. The vulnerabilities attackers can exploit are created by the decentralized setup of IoT devices, plus the increased bandwidth and lower latency that 5G provides.

A major concern in 5G-IoT networks is managing authentication and authorization, especially on big networks, where it becomes more difficult to prove the identity of devices and control who has access. Because of the huge amount of data generated by IoT devices, it is equally important to protect sensitive data. Another growing threat are Distributed Denial of Service (DDoS) attacks, 5G's increased bandwidth means these attacks will likely be even more disruptive if not crippling, leaning critical services offline. Furthermore, using blockchain technology to secure data is good at keeping data integrity but not good enough to play well with 5G's high performance needs, so it has it is own challenges. In addition, there is a probability that soon quantum computers break the current encryption methods, bringing forth an additional kind of risk [1–3].

These challenges are being addressed by emerging solutions that are innovative, for example, AI powered systems detect real time threats and predict possible risks. Another promising approach is to combine blockchain with federated learning, where sensitive data is kept on local devices and the devices are verified in a decentralized system, but the information is protected from being hacked. In stopping authorized access and to ensure data is secure, enhanced authentication protocols and more advanced encryption techniques are also important [4–9].

This paper explores the major cybersecurity challenges faced by 5G-IoT networks and the emerging solutions that are forming this dynamic field. We look at how would these solutions be implemented within 5G-IoT environments and to what extend they are limited. Our goal is to offer a comprehensive overview of the current state of 5G-IoT cybersecurity and to identify future directions for improvement possibilities. With the advancements of 5G-IoT technology, focusing on these challenges will be an important task to provide the security, privacy, and the integrity of all the associated and connected devices and digital ecosystems around the world.

To guide our research, we focused on the next two research questions:

- What are the main cybersecurity challenges facing 5G-IoT networks?
- What solutions have been developed to address these challenges?

The review is aimed at systematically identifying, classifying and evaluating the effectiveness of different proposed solutions to particular cybersecurity threats of 5G-IoT networks. By addressing these research questions, we plan to present a detailed evaluation of the advancements and gaps of the existing cybersecurity strategies for 5G-IoT environment which captures both the progress made and the need to follow up on.

## 2 Methodology

### 2.1 Literature Search Strategy

To compile relevant literature on cybersecurity challenges and solutions in 5G-IoT networks, we developed a systematic search strategy using precise search terms. Our primary query was structured as follows: "IoT" and "5G" and "cybersecurity". The search was conducted on June 30th, 2024, through the IEEE Xplore database to ensure access to high-quality, peer-reviewed studies and recent conference proceedings:

- **Initial Results**: The preliminary search returned 374 articles. Papers not accessible in full text, duplicates, and studies published prior to 2019 were excluded, yielding a total of 208 papers.
- **Screening**: Articles were initially screened by one expert person based on titles and abstracts to identify those aligning with the focus of 5G-IoT cybersecurity, reducing the selection to 65 articles.
- **Eligibility Assessment**: Each of these 65 articles underwent a full-text review using the inclusion and exclusion criteria presented below, resulting in 18 articles that were ultimately included in this systematic review.

### 2.2 Inclusion and Exclusion Criteria

To ensure that only relevant, high-quality studies were included, the following criteria were applied:

**Inclusion Criteria**

- Studies must focus specifically on cybersecurity challenges within 5G-IoT networks.
- Only peer-reviewed journal or conference publications were included.
- Studies had to propose or evaluate solutions to the identified cybersecurity issues.
- Publications must be in English to ensure clarity and accessibility.

**Exclusion Criteria**

- Studies that did not directly address cybersecurity within the scope of 5G-IoT networks were excluded.
- Papers focusing solely on the technical or operational aspects of 5G or IoT without a cybersecurity focus were omitted.
- Articles not accessible in full text, duplicates, and studies published prior to 2019 were also excluded.

This methodology ensured a focused and high-quality selection of studies, aimed at providing a comprehensive overview of the cybersecurity landscape in 5G-IoT networks and the effectiveness of emerging solutions. Figure 1 presents the main steps of this systematic literature review and the corresponding number of studies reviewed at each step.

## 3 Results

In this section, we summarize the key findings reported in the cited papers included in the systematic review conducted for this study, organized into two main areas: primary security challenges and proposed solutions. First, we analyze the primary security challenges identified in the literature as barriers to effective and secure deployment of 5G-enabled IoT networks. This analysis addresses risks inherent to the 5G-IoT ecosystem, including threats to data privacy, issues in device authentication, vulnerability to cyberattacks, and

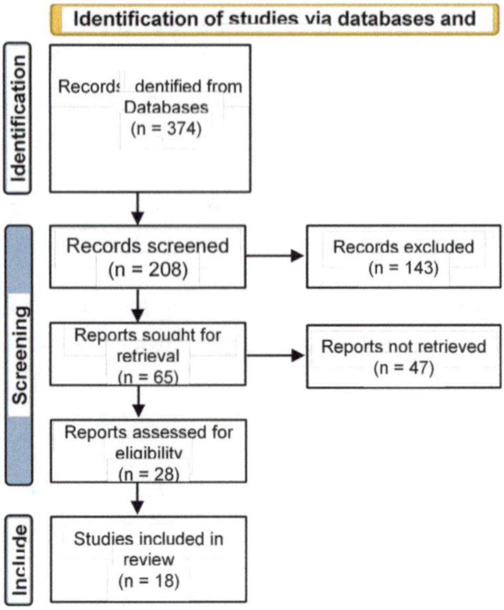


**Fig. 1.** Steps of the systematic literature review and corresponding number of studies reviewed at each step.

the emerging challenges posed by quantum computing. Table 1 presents a summary of the identified primary security challenges along with the references addressing each of these challenges.

**Table 1.** Summary of the identified primary security challenges and references addressing each challenge.

| Security challenges | References |
|---|---|
| Authentication and Authorization | [10, 11, 23, 24, 25] |
| Data Privacy | [12, 13, 20, 22, 24, 25] |
| Distributed Denial of Service Attacks | [14, 5, 19, 25, 26] |
| Blockchain Security | [15, 16, 20, 21, 22, 23, 25] |
| Quantum Threats | [17, 18] |

Following the discussion of challenges, we explore the proposed solutions that have been developed or suggested by researchers to counteract these security issues. This subsection reviews a range of approaches, such as AI-driven threat detection, blockchain-based security enhancements, advanced encryption methods, and federated learning models. Each proposed solution is evaluated based on its effectiveness and feasibility, with an emphasis on its adaptability to the specific constraints of 5G-IoT networks.

## 3.1 Security Challenges

The main cybersecurity challenges in 5G-IoT networks identified in this research include Authentication and Authorization, Data Privacy, Distributed Denial of Service Attacks, Blockchain Security, and Quantum Threats. These will be addressed, in this order, in the following subsections.

This research identifies main cybersecurity challenges in 5G-IoT networks including Authentication and Authorization, Data Privacy, Distributed Denial of Service Attacks, Blockchain Security, and Quantum Threats. The following subsections address these n this order, in the following subsections.

1. **Authentication and Authorization**

With the rise of 5G enabled IoT networks, the challenges of authentication and authorization has become ever more complex. However, as the number of connected devices becomes more diverse and more voluminous, traditional methods of verifying identities and granting permissions are becoming increasingly ineffective. Tough these put forth huge benefits, they also raise risks, such as unauthorized access starting from data breaches and cyberattacks. In Sect. 3.2, emerging solutions, like blockchain based authentication frameworks are explored as possible ways to overcome these challenges. For instance, Li et al. [10] have pointed out that robust authentication systems are urgently needed to protect the sensitive data securely and that weak protocols make the private information exposed. In a similar vein, Nyangaresi et al. [11] study how simply having more connected devices increases the threat to the integrity of these networks. However, blockchain based solutions to authentication have been proposed as a means of improving authentication, but their high storage and processing burden make them unsuitable for resource constrained IoT devices in 5G environments.

These insights bring to light the need for designing authentication protocols that achieve a good balance between security and efficiency, while being flexible enough to work well within the dynamic and open characteristics of 5G enabled IoT systems.

2. **Data Privacy**

In 5G enabled IoT networks, data privacy is a big issue. These devices constantly collect and transmit sensitive personal and operational data, revealing them on a potential security breach. Most resource constrained IoT devices don't have the computational capacity to perform advanced encryption protocols. These limitations reiterate the need for encryption techniques such as lattice-based cryptography, which are intended for resource constrained devices. In addition, privacy measures are expected to be consistent with the low latency and high performance demands particular to 5G environments.

As is observed by the authors in [12], integrating IoT with 5G generates a much larger volume of data, which increases the risk of leaks, especially for sensitive data such as healthcare records. It, too, [13] stresses the need for sophisticated encryption procedures which can protect data even when it is intercepted while being transmitted. The unique pressures of 5G enabled IoT systems, particularly the rise in the sophistication of security threats, require strong encryption methods for data privacy and integrity, according to their findings. These examples highlight the need for privacy protocols that are as robust as possible while being sufficiently efficient to be tractable on 5G-IoT environments.

3. **Distributed Denial of Service Attacks**

DDoS attacks are amongst the most critical threats to 5G-IoT network. While 5G brings a lot of benefits with high bandwidth and low latency, it also makes those networks vulnerable to traffic surges. Additionally, most traditional DDoS mitigation strategies fail to address the architectural differences of 5G networks with respect to the previous generations of networks. More sophisticated and more adaptive strategies are necessary to address this gap. Key strategies to mitigate the DDoS attack impact using adaptive mechanisms are dynamically allocating resources using network slicing isolation and AI driven predictive models.

For instance, the research presented in [14] points out certain 5G network design vulnerabilities which render them vulnerable to DDoS attacks. As for these risks, the study also suggests ways to address them, emphasizing the need for adaptive defense mechanisms that are able to evolve in parallel with the attacker tactics. Other research has also looked into new ways, such as using AI driven anomaly detection systems to detect and respond to unusual traffic patterns that indicate an attack before it occurs. For instance, it can monitor actual real time traffic and find unusual surges that signify DDoS attempts allowing operators to do something about it before services are disrupted. Nonetheless, these solutions are still a work in progress as they need further refinement before they can be widely used in 5G-IoT networks.

These findings show that there is a critical need for new, robust solutions to stop and protect against DDoS attacks. Whatever such strategies are, they must be specifically designed for the performance and scalability requirements of 5G enabled IoT systems.

4. **Blockchain Security**

In the context of 5G-IoT networks, blockchain technology offers both promising opportunities and significant challenges. Its decentralized structure enhances security, yet the high scalability, latency, and computational demands of managing distributed ledgers often clash with the resource limitations of 5G-IoT devices. As a result, leveraging blockchain's full potential in these environments remains a complex endeavor. For example, the study in [15] discusses the "Blockchain Trilemma", which highlights the difficulty of achieving a balance between security, decentralization, and scalability. This inherent trade-off limits how effectively blockchain can be applied to 5G-IoT systems. Similarly, [16] points out that the large transaction sizes typical of blockchain can slow down network performance, especially in the high-speed and high-capacity context of 5G, where rapid data processing is critical. These examples emphasize the need for new and improved blockchain frameworks that strike a better balance between security and the practical limitations of 5G-IoT networks. Innovative optimizations are essential to deploy blockchain effectively without compromising the performance of the network.

Blockchain technology, as applied to 5G-IoT networks, has both great potential and great difficulties. The high scalability, latency, and computational demands of managing distributed ledgers clash with the resource limitations of 5G-IoT devices, but its decentralized structure improves security. This makes it a difficult undertaking to realize blockchain's full potential in these environments. For instance, p. 15 discusses the "Blockchain Trilemma" and how the state of a balance between security, decentralization and scalability is an ideal idea that most cryptographers agree upon. As a result, this inherent trade off limits the extent to which the blockchain can be used in 5G-IoT systems. As it does, [16] also notes that in 5G high speed and high capacity, the large transaction sizes characteristic of blockchain can reduce network performance with the need for rapid data processing. The examples in this aspect point out the necessity of new and better blockchain framework taking a better approach between security and the practical restrictions of 5G-IoT networks. Deploying the blockchain effectively without compromising the network's performance needs innovative optimizations.

5. **Quantum Threats**

The advancement of quantum computing presents significant challenges to existing encryption standards in 5G-IoT networks. As a result, post-quantum cryptography has become essential for ensuring long-term data security. The increasing computational power of quantum technology risks rendering traditional encryption methods obsolete, highlighting the need for innovative solutions to safeguard critical information. For example, the study referenced in [17] explains how rapid progress in quantum computing poses a serious risk to conventional cryptographic methods that rely on complex mathematical problems like logarithmic calculations or large integer factorization. Quantum computers can solve these problems far faster than classical systems, rendering traditional encryption ineffective. Similarly, [18] underscores that as quantum technologies evolve, many current encryption techniques will likely become outdated, emphasizing the importance of developing new algorithms that can withstand quantum attacks. These studies make it clear that ongoing research and innovation in quantum-resistant cryptographic methods are critical to protecting 5G-IoT networks against the unique risks posed by quantum computing advancements.

Quantum computing is advancing, and existing 5G-IoT network encryption standard are challenged, therefore, long term data security relies on post quantum cryptography. As the quantum technology develops and improves, traditional encryption methods become outdated and increase the risk of current encryption being made obsolete, with the potential need for the development of new solutions to protect critical information. As an example, the study mentioned in [17] shows that the rapid progress in quantum computing is a very serious threat to conventional cryptographic methods based on complex mathematical problems such as logarithmic calculations or large integer factorization. Classical systems can't solve these problems fast enough to make traditional encryption obsolete, but quantum computers can. In [18], also points out that as quantum technologies advance, many modern encryption techniques will probably become outdated, and that new algorithms will be necessary to resist quantum attacks. As these studies show, ongoing research and innovation in quantum resistant cryptography methods are vital to protect 5G-IoT networks from the special threats advanced by quantum computing.

## 3.2 Proposed Solutions

1. **AI-Based Security Systems**

AI powered systems have come up as effective solutions to address the challenges of security in 5G-IoT networks. Advanced techniques such as anomaly detection, threat intelligence and behavioral analysis are invoked to manage the massive data volume created by 5G networks. However, they are crucial to modern cybersecurity strategy because they enable real time threat detection and mitigation. AI based solutions can scale to support the exponential increase in IoT devices, while maintaining its effectiveness under the various network conditions and in the dynamic 5G environments. In addition to these capabilities, AI systems also evolve to meet emerging threats, learning and improving their detection performance over time, and becoming essential to protect 5G-IoT networks against complex attacks.

For example, [5] describes an AI driven Intrusion Detection System (IDS) aimed to increase the speed and accuracy in identifying and responding to security threats. This system uses decision-tree algorithms to analyze the network traffic in real time, and is able to precisely pinpoint a possible breach. IoT-Keeper [19] is another innovative approach that acts at the network gateway and monitors traffic at the network edge using lightweight and hardware agnostic technology. Using fuzzy C-Means clustering and fuzzy interpolation, IoT-Keeper classifies network activity with great accuracy and very few false positives, saving system resources. It automatically limits the network access of the affected device when it detects suspicious activity. Further examples of how AI driven solutions can dramatically improve real time threat detection in 5G IoT networks are provided. These systems are leading the way in making cybersecurity more robust and adaptive by enabling their ability to rapidly and precisely identify security risks.

2. **Blockchain and Federated Learning**

Blockchain and Federated Learning have been attracting attention as potential solutions for the emerging security and privacy issues in 5G-IoT networks. The combination of blockchain for device authentication and data integrity, and federated learning for local training of the model without central data storage, reduces reliance on centralized data storage and protects privacy. These technologies combine decentralized authentication with local data processing to bring robust privacy-preserving solutions that fit the needs of 5G-IoT ecosystems. In particular [12] proposes a blockchain based model that automates data sharing without human intervention using smart contracts. With this approach we limit the risk of data breaches and maintain data privacy and integrity throughout 5G-IoT networks. Using this integration, [20] overlays blockchain with federated learning, allowing nodes to train locally and only share model parameters, not raw data. Therefore, this approach eliminates the requirement of a large data transfer, while introducing a reward system to encourage high quality contributions. It penalizes underperforming nodes simultaneously for the integrity and security of the federated learning process.

For instance, in [21], a Blockchain based Federated Deep Learning framework for detecting malware in IoT devices is presented. To ensure model integrity, the framework maintains a consensus mechanism that filters data inputs from nodes so as to prevent malicious activity. The framework was found to be highly reliable even when up to 50% of nodes were compromised, at the expense of more resources and longer training times than simpler federated learning models. A related work is presented in [22], where a federated transfer learning-based Intrusion Detection System is proposed for 5G-IoT environments. This model utilizes multiple IoT networks and transfer learning to acquire insights for each network and generate customized detection models for each network. Meanwhile, [23] looks as an anomaly detection technique within blockchain using Proof of Stake to verify node identities by IP addresses and Uniform Resource Names. The method provides security improvements and efficiency gains. With dramatic improvements in metrics such as Processing Time Reduction and Resource Utilization.

By leveraging the combination of blockchain and federated learning, we demonstrate how privacy, scalability and security in 5G-IoT networks can be greatly improved. Together they offer a solid base for decentralized data management and real time threat detection in connected devices

3. **Authentication Methods and Data Encryption**

To ensure security of 5G IoT networks, researchers are looking at various authentication methods and encryption techniques to face security challenges of 5G-IoT networks. Advanced strategies, such as multi factor authentication, biometric verification, and quantum resistant encryption, designed to address the unique needs of these fast-evolving environments. As a concrete example, [11] presents a Hash Signature-Based Authentication and Key Agreement protocol that mitigates Man-in-the-Middle and impersonation attacks. Compared to older methods, this protocol is unique for its efficiency in that is has lower computational overhead and faster processing times. As well, [10] and [24] provide other novel solutions, such as pseudonym-based authentication and Elliptic Curve Diffie-Hellman protocols to secure device access and protect against offline guessing attacks in 5G networks.

For Narrowband IoT (NB-IoT), [17] proposes a quantum resistant authentication and data distribution method looking ahead to the challenges of quantum computing. With this approach, data transmission is secured using lattice based homomorphic encryption, thereby reducing network strain and making it efficient against quantum related threats. Furthermore, [18] investigates quantum resistant encryption based on quantum walks. The proposed approach is to develop secure substation boxes (S-Boxes) and the encryption mechanisms to be used in the tasks like data transmission, video encryption and file storage in 5G-IoT systems.

These examples highlight the need for creating secure, efficient and forward-thinking solutions to support the growing need of 5G-IoT networks. These advancements focus on future proof technologies to provide robust protection in ever evolving digital landscape.

Table 2 provides a comprehensive summary of the primary cybersecurity challenges identified in 5G-enabled IoT networks, alongside the proposed solutions and corresponding references discussed in this study.

## 4 Discussion

5G Enabled IoT networks have brought about unprecedented capabilities like low latency communication, massive scale device connectivity and edge computing, although, they also introduce unique cybersecurity challenges that have not been faced in traditional Internet environments. Compared to centralized client server model, 5G enabled IoT networks are based on decentralized architectures of billions of constraint devices and hence the attack surface is much larger. In order to address these challenges, 5G-IoT ecosystem needs innovative solutions.

Furthermore, the 5G applications, like autonomous vehicles and industrial automation require real time processing, and hence require such cybersecurity solutions to have

**Table 2:** Summary of Security Challenges and Corresponding Solutions in 5G-Enabled IoT Networks.

| Security Problem | Proposed Solution | Key References |
|---|---|---|
| Authentication and Authorization | Blockchain-based frameworks and AI-enhanced protocols. | [10, 11, 23, 24, 25] |
| Data Privacy | Advanced encryption (lattice-based cryptography), federated learning for decentralized privacy management. | [12, 13, 20, 22, 24, 25] |
| DDoS Attacks | AI-driven anomaly detection and network slicing for adaptive mitigation. | [14, 5, 19, 25, 26] |
| Blockchain Security | Optimized blockchain frameworks balancing scalability, security, and efficiency. | [15, 16, 20, 21, 22, 23, 25] |
| Quantum Threats | Development of quantum-resistant cryptography like lattice-based encryption. | [17, 18] |

minimal delay. New features of 5G such as network slicing and edge computing, open attack vectors and introduce new privacy risks that do not exist in conventional Internet security systems.

These differences underline the urgency to re-think and re-adapt cybersecurity measures to protect 5G enabled IoT networks from their unique threats and demands. To address adaptive threats, we will need to integrate AI enhanced anomaly detection into network management systems to react to new attack vectors in real time. This review examines the key challenges and emerging solutions in order to provide a clear picture of the security landscape in 5G enabled IoT systems and highlight critical areas where future research is required.

The following key differences between cybersecurity in traditional Internet settings and 5G-enabled IoT networks that were identified in the review presented above:

- **Network Architecture and Design**

Traditional Internet security primarily focuses on centralized client-server models, aiming to protect servers, endpoints, and data transmission channels through protocols like TLS/SSL. In contrast, 5G-enabled IoT networks operate on decentralized and distributed architectures, incorporating edge computing, network slicing, and massive device connectivity, which require security measures that safeguard the edge, slices, and the billions of interconnected devices.

- **Scale of Connectivity**

The Internet primarily involves human-operated devices such as computers and mobile phones, with a relatively limited number of endpoints, whereas 5G-enabled IoT networks encompass massive connectivity across billions of devices, including sensors, actuators, and autonomous systems, resulting in an exponentially larger attack surface due to device proliferation.

- **Device Constraints**

Internet devices typically have sufficient computational resources to support advanced security measures like encryption, firewalls, and intrusion detection systems, whereas 5G-enabled IoT networks often comprise resource-constrained devices with limited processing power, memory, and energy, posing challenges for implementing traditional security mechanisms.

- **Latency and Real-Time Processing**

Cybersecurity for the internet typically focuses on detecting and mitigating threats with tolerable delays, as many applications are not latency-critical, whereas 5G-enabled IoT networks, designed to support low-latency applications like autonomous vehicles and industrial automation, require security mechanisms that operate in real-time without introducing delays that could compromise system performance.

- **Attack Vectors**

Common attack vectors on the internet include phishing, malware, Distributed Denial of Service (DDoS), and man-in-the-middle (MitM) attacks on traditional networks, while 5G-enabled IoT networks face new attack vectors such as exploitation of 5G-specific features (e.g., slicing misconfiguration or hijacking), IoT-specific threats like sensor spoofing, device hijacking, and data tampering, and vulnerabilities in edge nodes and fog computing layers.

- **Security Standards and Protocols**

Security standards like HTTPS, IPsec, and SSL/TLS are widely used and well-established on the internet, while 5G-enabled IoT networks require the integration of existing security standards with IoT-specific protocols (e.g., MQTT, CoAP) and 5G security features like Authentication and Key Agreement (AKA) to support massive device connectivity.

- **Privacy Concerns**

Privacy concerns on the internet are generally focused on user data protection, often regulated by policies like GDPR or CCPA, while privacy challenges in 5G-enabled IoT networks are heightened due to continuous and pervasive data collection from IoT devices and the risk of unauthorized access to sensitive data, such as health monitoring in smart healthcare.

- **Adaptive Threats**

Traditional internet threats evolve more predictably and are often detected through established anomaly-detection mechanisms, whereas threats in 5G-enabled IoT networks adapt to new technologies, such as AI-enhanced attacks on IoT systems or exploitation of 5G slicing configurations, requiring more dynamic and context-aware security solutions.

Table 3 highlights the key distinctions between cybersecurity approaches in traditional Internet contexts and the unique requirements of 5G-enabled IoT networks, emphasizing the need for tailored solutions.

**Table 3:** Differences Between Traditional Internet Cybersecurity and 5G-IoT Networks.

| Aspect | Traditional Internet | 5G-Enabled IoT Networks |
|---|---|---|
| Network Architecture | Centralized client-server models. | Decentralized with edge computing, network slicing, and massive device connectivity. |
| Scale of Connectivity | Limited endpoints (computers, phones). | Massive connectivity with billions of IoT devices. |
| Device Constraints | Devices with sufficient resources for encryption and security. | Resource-constrained devices with limited processing power. |
| Latency and Real-Time Needs | Tolerable delays. | Real-time processing with minimal latency for critical applications. |
| Attack Vectors | Common: phishing, malware, MitM attacks. | IoT-specific threats (sensor spoofing, device hijacking) and 5G-specific vulnerabilities. |
| Security Standards | Well-established protocols (TLS/SSL, IPsec). | Integration with IoT-specific protocols and 5G features. |
| Privacy Concerns | User data protection via regulatory policies. | Heightened privacy risks from pervasive IoT data collection. |
| Adaptive Threats | Predictable evolution of threats. | Adaptive, AI-enhanced attack mechanisms exploiting new 5G features. |

## 5 Conclusion

The integration of 5G and IoT technologies presents unprecedented opportunities and challenges in cybersecurity. As our review shows, the 5G-enabled IoT networks offer huge connectivity and functional gains, but at the same time they also expose critical vulnerabilities. Key challenges include ensuring robust authentication and authorization mechanisms in an environment with massive device connectivity, maintaining data privacy for sensitive information transmitted by IoT devices, defending against Distributed

Denial of Service attacks, and addressing the scalability and resource limitations inherent in blockchain applications within these networks. The emerging threat of quantum computing amplifies these challenges, as it could soon undermine existing cryptographic protocols.

Recent research has introduced innovative solutions that integrate advanced technologies to address these vulnerabilities. AI-powered security systems enable real-time anomaly detection, while federated learning presents a promising method for secure data sharing without compromising privacy. Blockchain has emerged as a potential solution for decentralized authentication, though it still requires optimization to improve efficiency in IoT environments. Additionally, quantum-resistant cryptographic techniques, such as lattice-based encryption, show promise in protecting 5G-IoT networks from future quantum computing threats.

However, challenges persist, despite these advancements. Many solutions demand significant computational resources, which may not be suitable for the resource-limited IoT devices. Additional research is needed to optimize these approaches for low-power environments, enhance interoperability among various IoT devices, and ensure that proposed security frameworks can scale efficiently. As the field evolves, ongoing collaboration between academia, industry, and government will be crucial in refining these strategies. This review underscores the urgency of developing adaptive and future-proof cybersecurity solutions to secure 5G-IoT networks, ultimately protecting the vast digital ecosystems that will define future technological landscapes.

**Acknowledgments.** This study was developed under the project A-MoVeR – "Mobilizing Agenda for the Development of Products & Systems towards an Intelligent and Green Mobility", operation n.° 02/C05-i01.01/2022.PC646908627-00000069, approved under the terms of the call n.° 02/C05-i01/2022 – Mobilizing Agendas for Business Innovation, financed by European funds provided to Portugal by the Recovery and Resilience Plan (RRP), in the scope of the European Recovery and Resilience Facility (RRF), framed in the Next Generation UE, for the period from 2021–2026.

## References

1. Altaleb, H., Zoltán, R.: Addressing cybersecurity challenges in 5G-enabled IoT and critical infrastructures: a comprehensive overview. In: 2023 IEEE 27th International Conference on Intelligent Engineering Systems (INES), pp. 000131–000136. IEEE, Nairobi (Jul. 2023). https://doi.org/10.1109/INES59282.2023.10297774
2. Fortinet: What Are the Security Challenges of 5G and IoT? (2024). Accessed: Oct. 30, 2024. [Online]. Available: https://www.fortinet.com/blog/industry-trends/the-security-implications-for-5g-and-iot
3. Li, S., et al.: Post-quantum security: opportunities and challenges. Sensors. **23**(21), 8744 (2023). https://doi.org/10.3390/s23218744
4. Benzaid, C., Taleb, T.: AI for beyond 5G networks: a cyber-security defense or offense enabler? IEEE Netw. **34**(6), 140–147 (2020). https://doi.org/10.1109/MNET.011.2000088
5. Patel, K., Vadher, A., Patel, M., Thaker, J., Bhise, A.: AI-based security system for 5G enabled IoT. In: 2024 Second International Conference on Emerging Trends in Information Technology and Engineering (ICETITE), Vellore, India, pp. 1–7. IEEE (Feb. 2024). https://doi.org/10.1109/ic-ETITE58242.2024.10493287

6. Lee, J., Kim, H., Park, C., Kim, Y., Park, J.-G.: AI-based network security enhancement for 5G industrial internet of things environments. In: 2022 13th International Conference on Information and Communication Technology Convergence (ICTC), pp. 971–975. IEEE, Jeju Island (2022). https://doi.org/10.1109/ICTC55196.2022.9952490
7. Le, T., Shetty, S.: Artificial intelligence-aided privacy preserving trustworthy computation and communication in 5G-based IoT networks. Ad Hoc Netw. **126**, 102752 (2022). https://doi.org/10.1016/j.adhoc.2021.102752
8. Lu, Y., Huang, X., Zhang, K., Maharjan, S., Zhang, Y.: Blockchain and federated learning for 5G beyond. IEEE Netw. **35**(1), 219–225 (2021). https://doi.org/10.1109/MNET.011.1900598
9. Miglani, A., Kumar, N.: Blockchain management and machine learning adaptation for IoT environment in 5G and beyond networks: a systematic review. Comput. Commun. **178**, 37–63 (2021). https://doi.org/10.1016/j.comcom.2021.07.009
10. Li, X., Wang, C., Zou, X., Wang, S.: A secure and effective authentication method in 5G. In: 2023 4th International Seminar on Artificial Intelligence, Networking and Information Technology (AINIT), vol. 2023, pp. 243–246. IEEE, Nanjing. https://doi.org/10.1109/AINIT59027.2023.10212595
11. Nyangaresi, V.O., Abduljabbar, Z.A., Abduljabbar, Z.A.: Authentication and key agreement protocol for secure traffic signaling in 5G networks. In: 2021 IEEE 2nd International Conference on Signal, Control and Communication (SCC), pp. 188–193. IEEE, Tunis (Dec. 2021). https://doi.org/10.1109/SCC53769.2021.9768338
12. William, P., et al.: Blockchain technology for data privacy using contract mechanism for 5G networks. In: 2022 3rd International Conference on Intelligent Engineering and Management (ICIEM), pp. 461–465. IEEE, London (2022). https://doi.org/10.1109/ICIEM54221.2022.9853118
13. Pillai, S.E.V.S., Vaddadi, S.A.: Secure communication protocols for enhancing privacy in 5G Mobile networks. In: 2024 IEEE 13th International Conference on Communication Systems and Network Technologies (CSNT), pp. 347–353. IEEE, Jabalpur (2024). https://doi.org/10.1109/CSNT60213.2024.10546047
14. Ji, S., Kumar Mishra, A.: 5G security issues challenges and solutions against DDoS attacks: a survey. In: 2024 2nd International Conference on Disruptive Technologies (ICDT), pp. 1422–1427. IEEE, Greater Noida (2024). https://doi.org/10.1109/ICDT61202.2024.10489295
15. Sharma, K.K., Salaria, A.: A Review on Challenges, Opportunities, and Solutions for 5th Generation Based IoT Using Blockchain & AI. In: 2023 3rd International Conference on Advance Computing and Innovative Technologies in Engineering (ICACITE), pp. 1957–1962. IEEE, Greater Noida (2023). https://doi.org/10.1109/ICACITE57410.2023.10183203
16. Hewa, T.M., Kalla, A., Nag, A., Ylianttila, M.E., Liyanage, M.: Blockchain for 5G and IoT: opportunities and challenges. In: 2020 IEEE Eighth International Conference on Communications and Networking (ComNet), pp. 1–8. IEEE, Hammamet (2020). https://doi.org/10.1109/ComNet47917.2020.9306082
17. Cao, J., Yu, P., Xiang, X., Ma, M., Li, H.: Anti-quantum fast authentication and data transmission scheme for massive devices in 5G NB-IoT system. IEEE Internet Things J. **6**(6), 9794–9805 (2019). https://doi.org/10.1109/JIOT.2019.2931724
18. El-Latif, A.A.A., Abd-El-Atty, B., Mazurczyk, W., Fung, C., Venegas-Andraca, S.E.: Secure data encryption based on quantum walks for 5G internet of things scenario. IEEE Trans. Netw. Serv. Manag. **17**(1), 118–131 (2020). https://doi.org/10.1109/TNSM.2020.2969863
19. Hafeez, I., Antikainen, M., Ding, A.Y., Tarkoma, S.: IoT-KEEPER: detecting malicious IoT network activity using online traffic analysis at the edge. IEEE Trans. Netw. Serv. Manag. **17**(1), 45–59 (2020). https://doi.org/10.1109/TNSM.2020.2966951

20. Kumar Sharma, P., Gope, P., Puthal, D.: Blockchain and federated learning-enabled distributed secure and privacy-preserving computing architecture for IoT network. In: 2022 IEEE European Symposium on Security and Privacy Workshops (EuroS&PW), pp. 1–9. IEEE, Genoa (2022). https://doi.org/10.1109/EuroSPW55150.2022.00008
21. Rawat, P., Kumar, P.: Blockchain based federated deep learning framework for malware attacks detection in IoT devices. In: 2023 14th International Conference on Computing Communication and Networking Technologies (ICCCNT), pp. 1–10. IEEE, Delhi (2023). https://doi.org/10.1109/ICCCNT56998.2023.10306828
22. Fan, Y., Li, Y., Zhan, M., Cui, H., Zhang, Y.: IoTDefender: a federated transfer learning intrusion detection framework for 5G IoT. In: 2020 IEEE 14th International Conference on Big Data Science and Engineering (BigDataSE), pp. 88–95. IEEE, Guangzhou (Dec. 2020). https://doi.org/10.1109/BigDataSE50710.2020.00020
23. Sefati, S.S., Fartu, O., Nor, A.M., Halunga, S.: Enhancing internet of things security and efficiency: anomaly detection via proof of stake Blockchain techniques. In: In 2024 International Conference on Artificial Intelligence in Information and Communication (ICAIIC), pp. 591–595. IEEE, Osaka (2024). https://doi.org/10.1109/ICAIIC60209.2024.10463516
24. Nyangaresi, V.O., Abduljabbar, Z.A., Al Sibahee, M.A., Abduljaleel, I.Q., Abood, E.W.: Towards security and privacy preservation in 5G networks. In: 2021 29th telecommunications forum (TELFOR), vol. 2021, pp. 1–4. IEEE, Belgrade. https://doi.org/10.1109/TELFOR52709.2021.9653385
25. Wazid, M., Das, A.K., Shetty, S., Gope, P., Rodrigues, J.J.P.C.: Security in 5G-enabled internet of things communication: issues, challenges, and future research roadmap. IEEE Access. **9**, 4466–4489 (2021). https://doi.org/10.1109/ACCESS.2020.3047895
26. Benlloch-Caballero, P., Sanchez-Navarro, I., Matencio-Escolar, A., Calero, J.M.A., Wang, Q.: Topology-aware cognitive self-protection framework for automated detection and mitigation of security and privacy incidents in 5G-IoT networks. In: 2023 IEEE 31st International Conference on Network Protocols (ICNP), pp. 1–6. IEEE, Reykjavik (2023). https://doi.org/10.1109/ICNP59255.2023.10355595

# Backdoor Adversarial Machine Learning Attack on Graph Convolutional Networks for IoMT Traffic Misclassification

Michael Georgiades[1,4](✉), Faisal Hussain[2], and Lakis Christodoulou[3]

[1] ISLab, Computer Science, Neapolis University Pafos, Paphos, Cyprus
m.georgiades@nup.ac.cy
[2] Department of Computing, National University of Modern Languages, Islamabad, Pakistan
[3] R&D, Technology and Innovation, Biomed Medical Systems, Pafos, Cyprus
[4] Infostrada Communications, Pafos, Cyprus

**Abstract.** Graph Convolutional Networks (GCNs) are increasingly used in security-sensitive applications. This study investigates the vulnerability of GCNs increasingly employed in IoT traffic classification, to backdoor adversarial attacks, focusing on simulated Malaria DoS and Slowite attacks. Subtle manipulations of edge features, constituting less than 0.5% perturbation, result in significant misclassifications of malicious traffic while causing less than a 1% change in overall metrics. Using a proprietary IoT dataset and validated on the CICIoMT2024 dataset, the study demonstrates consistent adversarial efficacy while preserving performance on clean data. The findings highlight the need for robust defenses to protect GCNs in critical IoT contexts, where undetected attacks could cause severe real-world impacts.

**Keywords:** Graph Convolutional Networks · Adversarial Machine Learning · IoT Security · Backdoor Attacks · Evasion Attacks · Misclassification

## 1 Introduction

Adversarial machine learning is the study of the attacks on machine learning algorithms, as well as the development of the defenses against such attacks [1]. Some popular adversarial attack types include evasion attacks, data poisoning attacks, Byzantine attacks, and model extraction attacks. The evasion attacks mainly entail the crafting of adversarial examples designed to mislead machine learning models during the inference (i.e., prediction) phase by introducing subtle perturbations to input data [2]. On the other hand, the data poisoning attacks, particularly backdoor attacks, imply embedding triggers within training data to manipulate model predictions at inference time. These attacks can cause misclassifications with minimal perceptual artifacts, posing a severe threat to


K. Daimi and A. Alsadoon (Eds.): ICR 2025, LNNS 1487, pp. 174–184, 2025.
https://doi.org/10.1007/978-3-031-95652-2_16

machine learning systems reliant on large-scale datasets scraped from unverified sources, as discussed by Schwarzschild et al. [3]. Likewise, the Byzantine attacks refer to malicious behaviors in distributed systems where compromised nodes deviate arbitrarily from expected protocols, often disrupting operations and hindering reliable consensus, as highlighted by Blanchard et al. [4]. Similarly, the model extraction attacks include querying Machine-Learning-as-a-Service (MLaaS) APIs to replicate the functionality of proprietary models and further evolve to exploit vulnerabilities in these platforms through advanced strategies like knowledge distillation and active learning, as discussed by Liang et al. [5].

Recent work on adversarial attacks and defenses in the IoT domain highlights vulnerabilities in IoT systems to adversarial manipulations, with research focusing on applications such as smart homes, industrial systems, and wireless communication. Prasad et al. [14] proposed a solution for robust adversarial attack mitigation in IoT networks. The authors introduced a two-tier model to recognize the presence of adversarial attack behavior in IoT networks. Likewise, Ibitoye et al. [15] deeply studied and categorized adversarial attacks along with various defenses against these attacks. Similarly, Sánchez et al. [16] investigated adversarial attacks that impact the performance of hardware behavior as well as machine learning and deep learning models in IoT environments. Studies like Singh and Sikdar's [6] demonstrated adversarial attack strategies targeting IoT-based deep learning classification techniques. Similarly, Aloraini et al. [7] explored insider threats that exploited machine learning models in IoT ecosystems. Additionally, Sagduyu et al. [8] examined how adversarial deep learning could undermine IoT network security through methods like jamming and spectrum poisoning attacks. Li et al.'s 2023 paper introduces "GUARD: Graph Universal Adversarial Defense," which presents a novel defensive strategy against universal adversarial attacks on graphs. This approach uniquely integrates a reinforcement learning model to adaptively adjust graph structures, enhancing the robustness of Graph Convolutional Networks (GCNs) across various tasks and datasets [17]. In the 2019 study by Zhu et al., "Robust Graph Convolutional Networks Against Adversarial Attacks," the authors develop a robust variant of GCNs by incorporating Gaussian distributions as the hidden representations of nodes. Their method leverages a variance-based attention mechanism, significantly improving the GCN's resilience against adversarial attacks that manipulate graph structures and node features.

In this paper, we re-investigate the vulnerabilities of Graph Convolutional Networks (GCNs) to backdoor adversarial attacks in IoT network traffic classification from the perspective of an adversary. By manipulating edge features such as packet timing, protocol flags, or connection patterns that characterize communication between IoMT devices, we show that malicious traffic can be misclassified as benign with minimal impact on overall model accuracy. This approach highlights an overlooked attack surface in graph-based intrusion detection, revealing critical weaknesses in the way edge relationships are leveraged for security decisions. The remainder of the paper is organized as follows: Sect. 2 outlines the methodology, including the design and deployment of adversarial attacks. Section 3 describes the datasets and experimental setup, while Sect. 4 presents key findings on attack efficacy and potential countermeasures. Finally, Sect. 5 concludes with insights and recommendations for strengthening IoT security against adversarial threats.

## 2 Methodology

The methodology consists of the following steps:

i. **Problem Definition:** Analyze the vulnerability of GCNs to adversarial perturbations targeting edge features, with the goal of misclassifying malicious traffic such as Malaria DoS and SlowITe [11] as benign while maintaining performance on clean data.
ii. **Dataset Preparation:** Use a private IoT dataset and the CICIoMT2024 [10] dataset. Extract and normalize edge features, encode nodes using IP and port information, and assign traffic labels.
iii. **Baseline Training:** Train GCNs on clean datasets to establish baseline performance, evaluated using metrics such as accuracy, precision, recall, and ROC curves.
iv. **Adversarial Attack Design:** Perturb edge features to mimic benign traffic patterns. Target malicious edges with varying perturbation intensities (0.1% to 10%) to maximize misclassification rates.
v. **Adversarial Evaluation:** Retrain GCNs on combined clean and adversarial data. Measure attack impact using misclassification rates, confusion matrices, and other metrics.
vi. **Defense Mechanisms:** Test adversarial training and feature regularization to improve robustness against adversarial attacks.
vii. **Validation:** Validate the attack methodology on the CICIoMT2024 [10] dataset, demonstrating effectiveness across diverse IoT traffic scenarios.

## 3 Problem Scope and Definition

### 3.1 Problem Statement

This study investigates adversarial machine learning techniques in IoT network traffic classification using Graph Convolutional Networks (GCNs). IoT networks naturally exhibit a graph structure, where nodes represent devices and edges capture communication patterns. While most prior research has focused on perturbing node features, this work targets edge features–the attributes of communication links–reflecting real-world scenarios where adversaries exploit device-to-device communication to evade detection.

The objective is to analyze the vulnerabilities of GCN classifiers to adversarial attacks, specifically edge feature perturbations that disguise malicious traffic as benign. This includes demonstrating how such perturbations can remain unnoticed while significantly degrading the model's ability to classify attack and benign traffic, as well as identifying strategies to mitigate these vulnerabilities. To achieve this, the study pursues the following goals:

1. Demonstrate the susceptibility of GCN models to adversarial edge feature perturbations mimicking real-world IoT attack patterns.
2. Establish a foundation for developing robust defense strategies, such as adversarial training and feature engineering, to enhance GCN resilience.

### 3.2 Problem Formulation

We represent the IoT network as a graph $G = (V, E)$, where $V$ is the set of nodes (devices) and $E$ is the set of edges (communication links). Each edge $e_{ij} \in E$ is associated with a feature vector $z_{ij} \in \mathbb{R}^m$, encoding attributes such as MQTT protocol features. The graph structure is captured by the adjacency matrix $A$, which remains fixed during the attack. The edge features $Z \in \mathbb{R}^{|E| \times m}$ are the focus of adversarial manipulation.

The task of traffic classification is defined as learning a function:

$$f : (G, Z) \rightarrow Y,$$

where $Y$ represents the traffic labels (*Benign, Malaria, Slowite*). To preprocess the data:

- Each edge $e_{ij}$ is assigned feature vectors $z_{ij}$, normalized for consistency.
- Nodes $V$ are uniquely identified and encoded using labels derived from IP and port information.
- Labels $Y$ are assigned to edges based on their traffic class.

GCNs process the graph through layers, propagating and aggregating edge features using the equation:

$$H^{(l+1)} = \sigma\left(\tilde{D}^{-\frac{1}{2}}\tilde{A}\tilde{D}^{-\frac{1}{2}}H^{(l)}W^{(l)}\right), \tag{1}$$

where $\tilde{A} = A + I$ is the adjacency matrix with self-loops, $\tilde{D}$ is its degree matrix, $H^{(l)}$ is the feature matrix at layer $l$ with $H^{(0)} = Z$, $W^{(l)}$ is the trainable weight matrix, and $\sigma$ is a non-linear activation function.

The attacker's objective is to perturb edge features $Z$ selectively to misclassify targeted traffic classes. The adversarial attack strategy follows two main steps:

1. Identify edges associated with a target class $y_t$ (e.g., Malaria traffic).
2. Perturb their feature vectors $z_{ij}$ to mimic those of a benign class $y_b$ (e.g., Benign traffic).

The adversarial modification of edge features is mathematically expressed as:

$$z_{ij}^{\text{adv}} = z_{ij}^{\text{benign}} + \eta \cdot \mathcal{N}(0, \sigma^2), \tag{2}$$

where $z_{ij}^{\text{benign}}$ represents the mean feature vector of benign edges, $\eta$ is a small scaling factor, and $\mathcal{N}(0, \sigma^2)$ is Gaussian noise to maintain plausible perturbations.

The overall loss function for training the GCN is defined as:

$$L = -\sum_{i \in E} y_i \log \hat{y}_i, \tag{3}$$

where $y_i$ is the true label and $\hat{y}_i$ is the predicted probability for edge $e_i$.

The attack is constrained by:

$$\|z_{ij}^{\text{adv}} - z_{ij}\|_p \leq \epsilon, \tag{4}$$

where $\epsilon$ is the maximum allowable perturbation.

Adversarial perturbations are designed to achieve two objectives:

$$\max_{\delta_Z} \frac{1}{|\mathcal{M}|} \sum_{i \in \mathcal{M}} \mathbf{1}(\arg\max \hat{y}_i \neq y_i), \tag{5}$$

$$\min_{\delta_Z} \left| \frac{1}{|\mathcal{B}|} \sum_{i \in \mathcal{B}} \mathbf{1}(\arg\max \hat{y}_i = y_i) - A_b^{\text{clean}} \right|. \tag{6}$$

Here, Eq. (5) maximizes the misclassification of malicious traffic, and Eq. (6) minimizes the degradation of benign accuracy. In these equations, $\mathcal{M}$ and $\mathcal{B}$ are the sets of malicious and benign edges, respectively, and $A_b^{\text{clean}}$ is the benign classification accuracy before perturbations.

This formulation reflects the adversary's focus on feature manipulation, simulating real-world adversarial scenarios in IoT networks, while maintaining stealth by minimally deviating from the original edge features.

# 4 Datasets Overview

This study utilizes two datasets to evaluate adversarial machine learning techniques in IoT traffic classification. Dataset 1, derived from an IoT-based ICU environment, includes benign traffic alongside *Malaria DoS* and *Slowite* attacks. Dataset 2, the publicly available CICIoMT2024 dataset [10], contains benign traffic and additional attack types: *MQTT DoS Publish Flood* and *MQTT DDoS Connect Flood*. Together, these datasets provide a comprehensive evaluation framework for adversarial learning models in IoT environments.

## 4.1 Dataset 1: Proprietary Dataset

The proprietary dataset was created using an IoT-based ICU environment implemented with IoT-Flock [9], an open-source tool for simulating IoT traffic. This dataset extends the framework developed in [12], capturing detailed communication patterns among healthcare devices. The testbed simulated benign traffic from environmental sensors (e.g., air temperature, humidity) and patient monitoring devices (e.g., infusion pumps, ECG monitors). It includes both benign traffic and two attack types: *Malaria DoS* and *Slowite* [11]. Malicious traffic simulates adversarial scenarios targeting data integrity and system availability.

The dataset was compiled into a single CSV file for analysis, integrating:

- Benign MQTT traffic from simulated ICU environments (ICU_Env2_MQTT01.csv, ICU_Env2_MQTT02.csv) and additional MQTT-focused traffic (mqtt_bed1.csv).
- Malicious traffic, including partitioned samples of *Malaria DoS* (malaria_part_*.csv) and *Slowite* attacks (slowite.csv).

The combined dataset includes packet-level traffic features grouped as:

- Frame and IP attributes such as frame.time delta, ip.src, and ip.proto.
- TCP indicators like tcp.flags and tcp.window size.
- MQTT attributes including mqtt.clientid, mqtt.topic, and mqtt.qos.

The dataset supports binary and multiclass classification tasks. Binary labels distinguish between benign and attack traffic, while multiclass labels identify specific attack types (*Malaria DoS* and *Slowite*).

### 4.2 Dataset 2: Validation Dataset

The publicly available CICIoMT2024 dataset [10] was also used for validation. This dataset includes benign traffic and two additional attack types: MQTT DoS Publish Flood and MQTT DDoS Connect Flood. By sampling diverse IoT traffic scenarios and protocols, CICIoMT2024 complements the proprietary dataset, ensuring robust evaluation of adversarial learning models. It aligns with the study's objectives of improving IoT security through adversarial robustness. Validation using this dataset underscores the transferability of the proposed adversarial attack framework, demonstrating its efficacy across different IoT environments.

## 5 Results

This section presents the results of adversarial attacks on IoT network traffic classification using Graph Convolutional Networks (GCNs). It evaluates the impact of adversarial perturbations on model performance primarily using our Proprietary Dataset. Key metrics such as accuracy, misclassification rate, and confusion matrices are analyzed to highlight the susceptibility of GCNs to adversarial edge perturbations and how these attacks can go unnoticed by the defender.

### 5.1 Validation Using Our Proprietary Dataset

Confusion matrices provide a detailed comparison of classification performance under adversarial conditions. Figure 1(a) and 1(b) show the confusion matrices for the defender and the adversary with a 0.5% perturbation ratio. These results reveal significant differences in classification outcomes, particularly for malicious traffic misclassified as benign. Figure 1(c) and 1(d) highlight the drop in precision, recall, and F1-scores for malicious traffic under adversarial attacks. While

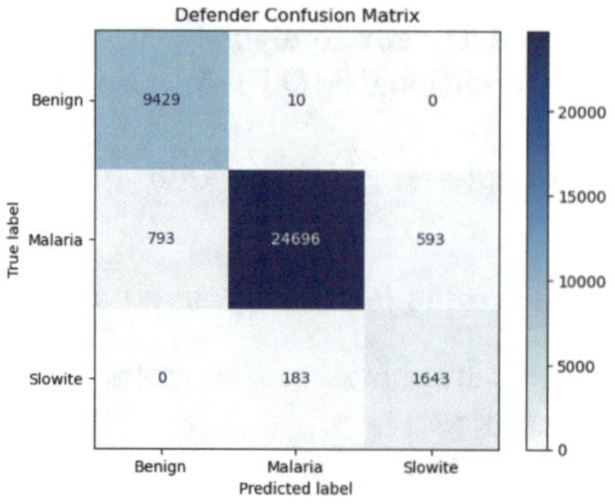


(a) Defender's Confusion Matrix

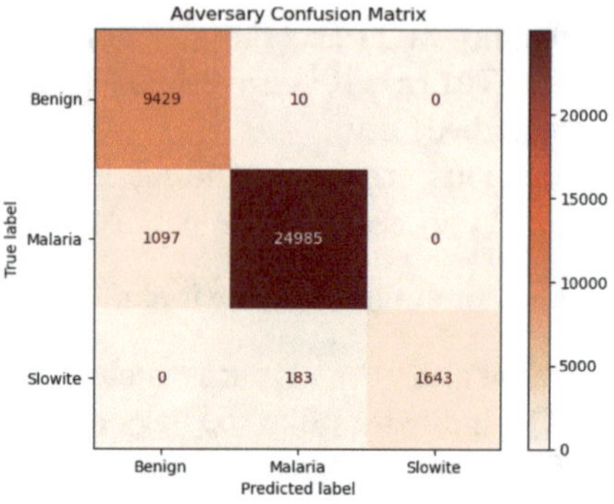


(b) Adversary's Confusion Matrix

| Class | Precision | Recall | F1-Score | Support |
|---|---|---|---|---|
| Benign | 0.92 | 1.0 | 0.96 | 9439.0 |
| Malaria | 0.99 | 0.95 | 0.97 | 26082.0 |
| Slowite | 0.73 | 0.9 | 0.81 | 1826.0 |
| macro avg | 0.88 | 0.95 | 0.91 | 37347.0 |
| weighted avg | 0.96 | 0.96 | 0.96 | 37347.0 |

(c) Defender's Classification Report

| Class | Precision | Recall | F1-Score | Support |
|---|---|---|---|---|
| Benign | 0.9 | 1.0 | 0.94 | 9439.0 |
| Malaria | 0.99 | 0.96 | 0.97 | 26082.0 |
| Slowite | 1.0 | 0.9 | 0.95 | 1826.0 |
| macro avg | 0.96 | 0.95 | 0.96 | 37347.0 |
| weighted avg | 0.97 | 0.97 | 0.97 | 37347.0 |

(d) Adversary's Classification Report

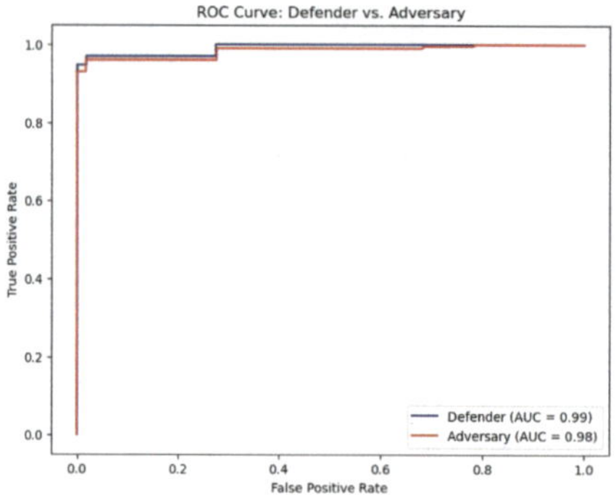


(e) Combined ROC Curve

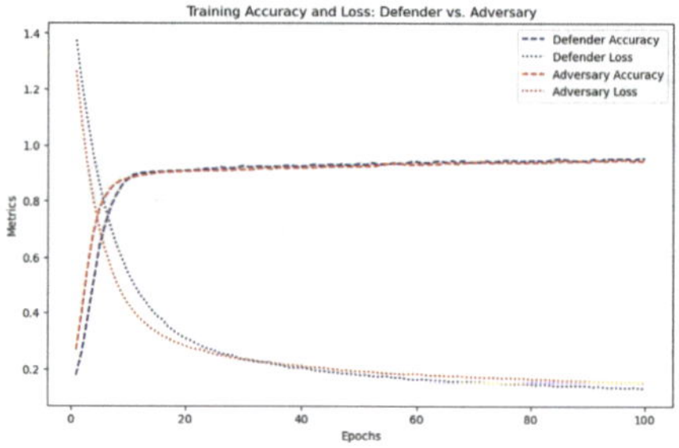


(f) Combined Training Metrics

**Fig. 1.** Evaluation of models using the Proprietary dataset (including confusion matrices, classification reports, ROC curve, and training metrics.)

the defender model demonstrates strong performance metrics, adversarial perturbations introduce noticeable vulnerabilities, particularly in recall for *DDoS Connect* and *DoS Publish* traffic.

For the Proprietary Dataset, adversarial conditions led to significant increases in misclassification:

- *DDoS Connect* traffic experienced 1,097 additional misclassifications as *Benign*, compared to 793 under the defender's model.
- *DoS Publish* traffic exhibited 183 misclassifications as *DDoS Connect*, where no such errors were present under the defender's model.

These findings emphasize how adversarial perturbations can disguise malicious traffic as benign, bypassing traditional detection mechanisms. Figure 1(e) and 1(f) provide further insights into the models' performance. The combined ROC curve shows a slight degradation in the adversary's AUC score compared to the defender, highlighting the subtle yet impactful effect of adversarial attacks on classification performance. Additionally, the training metrics reveal comparable convergence rates for both models but with reduced accuracy for the adversary, particularly for malicious classes. The comparison of confusion matrices and classification reports underscores that backdoor adversarial attacks can effectively reduce the model's ability to detect malicious traffic without significantly impacting overall accuracy, demonstrating the stealth and potency of such attacks.

### 5.2 Validation Using the CICIoMT2024 Dataset [10]

To validate the effectiveness of our targeted adversarial machine learning attack, we also applied the models to a sample of the publicly available CICIoMT2024 dataset [10].

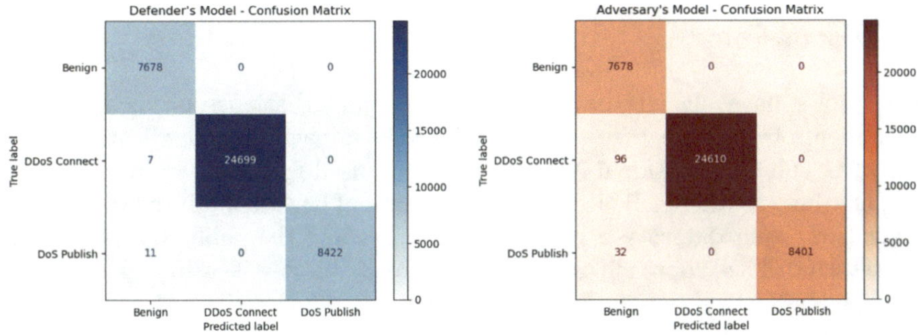


(a) Defender's Confusion Matrix

(b) Adversary's Confusion Matrix

Evaluating the Defender's model...

Classification Report:

| | precision | recall | f1-score | support |
|---|---|---|---|---|
| Benign | 1.00 | 1.00 | 1.00 | 7678 |
| DDoS Connect | 1.00 | 1.00 | 1.00 | 24706 |
| DoS Publish | 1.00 | 1.00 | 1.00 | 8433 |
| accuracy | | | 1.00 | 40817 |
| macro avg | 1.00 | 1.00 | 1.00 | 40817 |
| weighted avg | 1.00 | 1.00 | 1.00 | 40817 |

(c) Defender's Classification Report

Evaluating the Adversary's model...

Classification Report:

| | precision | recall | f1-score | support |
|---|---|---|---|---|
| Benign | 0.98 | 1.00 | 0.99 | 7678 |
| DDoS Connect | 1.00 | 1.00 | 1.00 | 24706 |
| DoS Publish | 1.00 | 1.00 | 1.00 | 8433 |
| accuracy | | | 1.00 | 40817 |
| macro avg | 0.99 | 1.00 | 1.00 | 40817 |
| weighted avg | 1.00 | 1.00 | 1.00 | 40817 |

(d) Adversary's Classification Report

**Fig. 2.** Evaluation of models using the CICIoMT2024 Dataset [10]

Figure 2 presents a comparative analysis of the Defender and Adversary models evaluated using the CICIoMT2024 Dataset [10], showcasing their respective confusion matrices Fig. 2(a) and 2(b) and classification reports Fig. 2(c) and 2(d) respectively. The confusion matrices reveal a stark difference in the number of misclassified packets under adversarial conditions. For example, with a 0.5% perturbation:

- The adversary's model caused 96 additional *DDoS Connect* packets to be misclassified as *Benign*, compared to just 7 under the defender's model, as shown in Fig. 2(b) and 2(a), respectively.
- Similarly, 32 *DoS Publish* packets were misclassified as *Benign* under the adversary's model, whereas the defender's model misclassified only 11.

Despite these forced errors by the adversary, the overall classification accuracy of the adversary model, shown in Fig. 2(d), remained close to 1.00, with results so similar to the defender model in Fig. 2(c) that the differences could easily go unnoticed. The results demonstrate the stealth and potency of the attack, where adversarial perturbations caused significant packet misclassification without noticeably degrading overall classification metrics, making it difficult for the defender to detect and bypassing traditional detection mechanisms.

## 6 Discussion

The results have shown that even minimal perturbations–specifically, 0.5% adjustments to edge features–can substantially impact the classification accuracy of Graph Convolutional Networks (GCNs) used for IoMT traffic classification. Our investigation validated the effectiveness of backdoor adversarial attacks across two recent datasets: a proprietary dataset and the public CICIoMT2024 dataset [10]. This approach revealed significant misclassification of malicious traffic, including a simulated Malaria DoS attack, while maintaining high accuracy on benign traffic. Specifically, the validation on the CICIoMT2024 dataset demonstrated that 96 packets of DDoS Connect Flood traffic and 32 packets of DoS Publish Flood traffic were incorrectly classified as benign. Despite these misclassifications, the stealthiness of the perturbations was confirmed as the overall classification accuracy remained near perfect, close to 1.00.

One of the paramount challenges identified was the limitation of standard classification metrics in detecting such subtle adversarial attacks. Metrics such as overall accuracy or micro-averaged recall often overlook the nuanced performance degradation specific to certain attack classes, allowing adversaries to subtly manipulate system outputs. This emphasizes the urgent need for the development of more sophisticated evaluation metrics and anomaly detection methods that can effectively identify such stealthy modifications.

## 7 Conclusion and Future Work

The findings from this study highlight the vulnerability of IoMT systems to backdoor adversarial strategies that manipulate edge features within GCN-based classifiers. Through evaluation on two recent and diverse IoMT traffic datasets–a proprietary ICU-inspired testbed and the publicly available CICIoMT2024 dataset [10]–we show that even subtle perturbations (as low as 0.5%) can result in significant misclassification of malicious traffic, while leaving overall accuracy nearly unaffected. This reveals not only the stealth and potency of such attacks but also the limitations of conventional detection mechanisms. Strengthening IoMT resilience will require adaptive defenses such as adversarial training and targeted feature regularization.

To support reproducibility, we provide a detailed account of the GCN architecture, data preprocessing pipeline, and perturbation strategy used. The methodology includes consistent feature normalization, edge encoding, and controlled manipulation within defined constraints, applied uniformly across both datasets. Attack parameters–such as perturbation levels and misclassification rates–are thoroughly reported to facilitate comparative analysis and independent replication.

Looking forward, we plan to extend our investigations to real IoMT testbed datasets, leveraging ongoing advancements in the frameworks described in [12,13]. Future research will focus on developing more resilient countermeasures, such as advanced anomaly detection systems tailored specifically for IoMT environments. Additionally, we aim to explore the trade-offs between the stealthiness of attacks and the effectiveness of defense mechanisms, to better protect critical healthcare infrastructure from adversarial attacks. The ongoing development of these countermeasures will also consider the scalability and computational efficiency required for deployment in diverse, real-world IoMT settings.

## References


1. Huang, L., Joseph, A.D., Nelson, B., Rubinstein, B.I.P., Tygar, J.D.: Adversarial machine learning. In: Proceedings of the 4th ACM Workshop on Security and Artificial Intelligence, pp. 43–58. ACM, Chicago, Illinois, USA (2011). https://doi.org/10.1145/2046684.2046692
2. Wang, S., Ko, R., Bai, G., Dong, N., Choi, T., Zhang, Y.: Evasion attack and defense on machine learning models in cyber-physical systems: a survey. IEEE Commun. Surv. Tutorials **26**(2), 930–957 (2023). https://doi.org/10.1109/COMST.2023.3344808
3. Schwarzschild, A., Goldblum, M., Gupta, A., Dickerson, J.P., Goldstein, T.: Just how toxic is data poisoning? A unified benchmark for backdoor and data poisoning attacks. In: International Conference on Machine Learning, pp. 9389–9398. PMLR (2021). https://doi.org/10.48550/arXiv.2006.12557
4. Blanchard, P., El Mhamdi, E.M., Guerraoui, R., Stainer, J.: Machine learning with adversaries: Byzantine tolerant gradient descent. In: Advances in Neural Information Processing Systems, vol. 30, pp. 119–129. Curran Associates (2017). https://doi.org/10.5555/3294771.3294783
5. Liang, J., Pang, R., Li, C., Wang, T.: Model extraction attacks revisited. In: Proceedings of the 19th ACM Asia Conference on Computer and Communications Security (ASIA CCS), pp. 1231–1245. ACM, Singapore (2024). https://doi.org/10.1145/3634737.365700
6. Singh, A., Sikdar, B.: Adversarial attack and defense strategies for deep-learning-based IoT device classification techniques. IEEE Internet Things J. **9**(4), 2602–2613 (2021). https://doi.org/10.1109/JIOT.2021.3138541

7. Aloraini, F., Javed, A., Rana, O., Burnap, P.: Adversarial machine learning in IoT from an insider point of view. J. Inf. Secur. Appl. **70**, 103341 (2022). https://doi.org/10.1016/j.jisa.2022.103341
8. Sagduyu, Y.E., Shi, Y., Erpek, T.: IoT network security from the perspective of adversarial deep learning. In: 2019 16th Annual IEEE International Conference on Sensing, Communication, and Networking (SECON), pp. 1–9. IEEE (2019). https://doi.org/10.1109/SAHCN.2019.8824956
9. Ghazanfar, S., Hussain, F., Rehman, A.U., Fayyaz, U.U., Shahzad, F., Shah, G.A.: IoT-Flock: an open-source framework for IoT traffic generation. In: 2020 International Conference on Emerging Trends in Smart Technologies (ICETST), pp. 1–6. IEEE (2020). https://doi.org/10.1109/ICETST49965.2020.9080732
10. Dadkhah, S., Neto, E.C.P., Ferreira, R., Molokwu, R.C., Sadeghi, S., Ghorbani, A.A.: CICIoMT2024: attack vectors in healthcare devices–A multi-protocol dataset for assessing IoMT device security (2024). https://www.unb.ca/cic/datasets/iomt-dataset-2024.html
11. Vaccari, I., Aiello, M., Cambiaso, E.: SlowITe, a novel denial of service attack affecting MQTT. Sensors **20**(10), 2932 (2020). https://doi.org/10.3390/s20102932
12. Hussain, F., et al.: A framework for malicious traffic detection in IoT healthcare environment. Sensors **21**(9), 3025 (2021). https://doi.org/10.3390/s21093025
13. Christodoulou, L., Chari, A., Georgiades, M.: AI-enhanced healthcare IoT system: advanced ML detection and classification algorithms for real-time cardiovascular monitoring. In: 2024 20th International Conference on Distributed Computing in Smart Systems and the Internet of Things (DCOSS-IoT), pp. 440–449. IEEE (2024). https://doi.org/10.1109/DCOSS-IoT.2024.1234567
14. Prasad, K.S., et al.: A two-tier optimization strategy for feature selection in robust adversarial attack mitigation on internet of things network security. Sci. Rep. **15**(1), 2235 (2025). https://doi.org/10.1038/s41598-025-02235-4
15. Ibitoye, O., Abou-Khamis, R., Matrawy, A., Shafiq, M.O., et al.: The threat of adversarial attacks against machine learning in network security: a survey. J. Electron. Electr. Eng. 16–59 (2025). https://doi.org/10.1016/j.jeee.2025.01.001
16. Sánchez, P., Celdrán, A.H., Bovet, G., Pérez, G.M.: Adversarial attacks and defenses on ML- and hardware-based IoT device fingerprinting and identification. Futur. Gener. Comput. Syst. **152**, 30–42 (2024). https://doi.org/10.1016/j.future.2023.08.007
17. Li, J., et al.: GUARD: graph universal adversarial defense. In: Proceedings of the 32nd ACM International Conference on Information and Knowledge Management, pp. 1198–1207 (2023). https://doi.org/10.1145/3583780.3614903
18. Zhu, D., Zhang, Z., Cui, P., Zhu, W.: Robust graph convolutional networks against adversarial attacks. In: Proceedings of the 25th ACM SIGKDD International Conference on Knowledge Discovery & Data Mining, pp. 1399–1407 (2019). https://doi.org/10.1145/3292500.3330851

# Evaluating Model Inversion Attack Success Across Neural Architectures in Federated Learning for Malware Classification

Eman Shalabi[1], Walid Khedr[2], Ehab Rushdy[1], Asma Musabah Alkalbani[3], and Ahmad Salah[3](✉)

[1] College of Computers and Informatics, Zagazig University, Zagazig, Egypt
{emanselem,ehab.rushdy}@zu.edu.eg

[2] College of Computer Science and Engineering, Taibah University, Yanbu 966144, Saudi Arabia
wkhedr@taibahu.edu.sa

[3] College of Computing and Information Sciences, University of Technology and Applied Sciences, Ibri, Oman
{asmam.alkalbani,ahmad.salah}@utas.edu.om

**Abstract.** A decentralized technique of machine learning called federated learning improves security by enabling local training. No research has yet to compare various deep learning architectures with federated learning. This work integrates federated learning with deep learning for the detection of malware. It proposes a comparative federated learning analysis study of different neural architectures including Artificial Neural Network, Gated Recurrent Unit, Long Short-Term Memory, and Convolutional Neural Network. Both performance and security are analyzed. The evaluation is conducted on Malware Dataset and AndroMD Dataset. The security of all models are evaluated against model inversion attack. For both datasets, FL_ANN is the fastest model while FL_LSTM is the slowest model. The highest performance metrics are achieved by FL_CNN on Malware Dataset and FL_LSTM on AndroMD Dataset. The FL_ANN is the most robust model using Malware Dataset with an average MSE of 1.91 while FL_LSTM is the best resistance model using AndroMD Dataset with an average MSE of 1.44.

**Keywords:** deep learning · federated learning · machine learning · malware detection · model inversion attack

## 1 Introduction

The growing complexity and quantity of malware presents a major cybersecurity threat [8]. With malware developing, traditional detection techniques are losing their effectiveness, making it more challenging to recognize and effectively combat attacks [4,9]. Deep learning (DL) is a powerful tool offers a promising way to enhance the detection and classification of malware due to its exceptional ability of pattern recognition [5–7].


K. Daimi and A. Alsadoon (Eds.): ICR 2025, LNNS 1487, pp. 185–198, 2025.
https://doi.org/10.1007/978-3-031-95652-2_17

A decentralized machine learning (ML) approach called federated learning (FL) allows several clients (devices) to work together to train a common ML model (global model), such as the models proposed in [22,23], without sharing their local data with the central server, protecting privacy and security[10,11]. The central server manages the learning process, while each client trains the global model on its local private data [15]. FL can be used in various domains including healthcare, finance, banking, Internet of Things (IoT), mobile devices, and autonomous vehicles [12–14].

FL enhances the performance and privacy of the detection and classification of malware. The authors of [16] proposed an approach based on FL, neural network, and ML for detecting Android malware. XGBoost, Random Forest, and a hybrid neural network model integrating Long Short-Term Memory (LSTM) along with Convolutional Neural Network (CNN) are used for the evaluation. To better detect dangerous activities, the most significant features inside the Android malware dataset are chosen using a majority vote technique.

The authors of [17] presented a framework called FedDRC based on FL for Android malware classification using Androzoo dataset. A robust local model called PAMIB created using the transfer learning and Information Bottleneck principle is integrated into FedDRC to counteract performance degradation brought on by spatial heterogeneity, while a Functional Semantic Embedding Mechanism called FSEM is also integrated to strength the model's resilience against time heterogeneity. The authors of [18] presented SIM-FED model based on FL and DL for the detection of IoT malware. SIM-FED is evaluated based on CNN and IoT-23 dataset.

FL-based systems are seriously threatened by model inversion attacks that aim to rebuild training data from model output [1]. The authors in [1] investigated the privacy problem in federated learning with model distillation (FedMD), and propose a method called Paired-Logits Inversion (PLI) attack. Using the confidence difference between the service and client models, they trained an inversion neural network model to reconstruct private images from public dataset logits. The authors of [21] proposed the KDRSFL framework. Knowledge distillation besides attacker-aware training are two ways that KDRSFL distributes the resistance of teacher model to client models. KDRSFL is validated on the basis of the CIFAR100 dataset.

This research proposes a comparative analysis study for the detection of malware. The effect of different DL architectures using FL on the model inversion attack success rate are analyzed. Performance and security are analyzed for each model. The following are the contributions of this research.

1. Several FL based models using different neural architectures are generated for the malware detection, to improve the privacy of traditional ML models.
2. Four different neural architectures are used including Artificial Neural Network (ANN), Gated Recurrent Unit (GRU), LSTM, and CNN, as four FL models are implemented including FL with ANN, FL with GRU, FL with LSTM, and FL with CNN.
3. Each of the four generated FL models are evaluated against the attack of model inversion.

4. As far as the authors are aware, this is the first research that focuses on the analysis of the security along with the performance of various neural architectures in FL.

## 2 Related Work

The authors of [18] presented SIM-FED model for the detection of IoT malware. FL is used for ensuring the preservation of privacy. SIM-FED integrates both FL and DL. By using a lightweight, one-dimensional CNN with adjusted hyperparameters, SIM-FED lowers computing overhead and preprocessing. After evaluating several federated aggregation methodologies, the FedAvg strategy is chosen to include the outcomes of local models into the SIM-FED model. SIM-FED is evaluated based on CNN using IoT-23 dataset, achieving an accuracy of 0.995. The model is also evaluated toward white-box and black box, producing a little performance degradation. Other DL architectures are not evaluated. The evaluation against attack is not mentioned.

To enhance malware detection while improving privacy, the authors of [19] apply FL for malware detection using Deep Neural Network and Security Operations Centers for malware detection. The evaluation is carried out on the basis of the EMBER benchmark dataset, achieving an accuracy exceeding 0.93. The evaluation against attack is not mentioned. For detecting IoT devices' malware, the authors of [20] proposed a FL-based framework (FedL_DBNFSpinalNet) using the integration of Deep Belief Network along with SpinalNet. Z-score Normalization is used for data preprocessing while the model of Conditional Autoregressive Value at Risk is used in aggregation process. The accuracy of 0.887 is produced. The evaluation against attack is not mentioned.

In [2], the authors addressed the challenge of preserving data privacy in malware detection and classification by evaluating federated learning models as a privacy-preserving alternative to traditional centralized methods. They developed 22 models based on Feedforward Neural Networks (FNN) and LSTM architecture and compared them to the CIC-MalMem-2022 dataset. The results showed that applying federate learning models in malware detection achieved a better accuracy of 0.999 for binary classification and 0.845 for multiclass classification. This key finding highlights the effect of using a suitable approach to federate learning in malware detection.

In [1], the authors investigate the privacy problem in federated learning with model distillation (FedMD), and propose a method called Paired-Logits Inversion (PLI) attack. Using the confidence difference between the service and client models, they trained an inversion neural network model to reconstruct private images from public dataset logits. The results demonstrate that in the facial recognition task, PLI effectively recovers private images that indicate susceptibility to privacy in FedMD. Therefore, a successful PLI attack exposes a privacy flaw in FedMD, which needs further study.

To improve defense against model inversion attacks, which can decrease model accuracy and expose private information, the authors of [21] proposed the KDRSFL framework. Knowledge distillation besides attacker-aware training are two ways that KDRSFL distributes the resistance of teacher model to client models. KDRSFL is validated on the basis of the CIFAR100 dataset, achieving 0.058 reconstruction mean square error and 0.674 precision.

# 3 Methodology

Figure 1 illustrates the overall methodology used. According to Fig. 1, different architectures of FL-based neural network models are evaluated in this study against the model inversion attack.

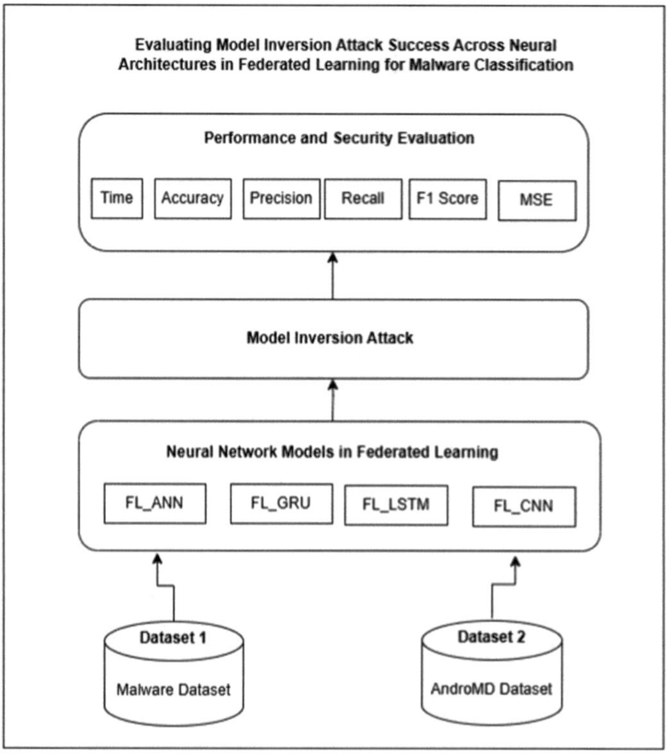


**Fig. 1.** Overall Methodology.

## 3.1 Dataset

The experiments are performed on two datasets, including Malware Dataset and AndroMD Dataset.

**Malware Dataset.** Malware Dataset is the first used dataset which is available and downloaded from Kaggle https://www.kaggle.com/datasets/blackarcher/malware-dataset. It is utilized for ML and Android malware detection. It contains a total of 50,000 benign and 50,000 malicious PE files. It has a total of 35 features belonging to six feature types of identification and classification, process state and priority, memory usage and management, CPU usage and scheduling, file system and I/O, and miscellaneous.

For example, hash, classification, and millisecond represent identification and classification feature types where hash uniquely identifies each PE file, classification labels each PE file as benign or malware, and miscellaneous is a time offset inside the time series data of each PE file. The experiments are conducted using a reduced dataset generated from this Malware Dataset. The reduced dataset consists of a total of 5000 files (2500 malware and 2500 benign files). It represents a subset of the full Malware Dataset and maintains the same balance and class distribution used in the feature labels of classification.

**AndroMD Dataset.** AndroMD Dataset is the second used dataset which is available and downloaded from Kaggle https://www.kaggle.com/datasets/meghnadhalaria/android-malware-detection-and-classification?resource=download. It is used for Android malware detection. It includes both static and dynamic features, extracted from both malware and benign Android applications. It has a total of 675 features extracted from a total of 3547 Android applications (1747 malware and 1800 normal apps).

Particularly, it consists of 323 dynamic features belonging to system calls, dynamic permissions, cryptographic operations, and information Leakage. It also contains 352 static features belonging to intents, permissions, API calls, and command strings. It also includes a final feature of 'class' indicates whether the corresponding Android application is malware or benign.

### 3.2 Federated Learning Setup

In this study, four model architectures are used for malware classification, including ANN, GRU, LSTM, and CNN.

**Artificial Neural Network.** The ANN architecture consists of an input layer, three hidden layers, and an output layer. The input layer includes 256 neurons, applies the activation function of ReLU, batch normalization, and 0.3 dropout rate. The first hidden layer consists of 128 neurons, utilizes the activation of ReLU, batch normalization, and 0.4 dropout rate. The second hidden layer consists of 64 neurons, utilizes the activation of ReLU, batch normalization, and 0.4 dropout rate. The third hidden layer consists of 32 neurons, utilizes the activation of ReLU, batch normalization, and 0.3 dropout rate.

The main purpose behind the usage of batch normalization and dropout layers is to increase generalization, decrease overfitting, and improve the performance of ANN model on unknown data. The output layer is a dense layer with as many neurons as target classes, and utilizes softmax activation for generating a probability distribution for all target classes within the dataset corresponding to the raw outputs in which the predicted class is the class with the highest value of probability. Adam optimizer with learning rate of 0.001, the metric of accuracy, and loss of categorical cross-entropy are used for the compilation of the ANN model.

**Gated Recurrent Unit.** The GRU architecture consists of one input layer, two hidden layers, and one output layer. The input layer includes a reshape layer which transforms the raw input 2D features into a sequence of 3D tensor format for being used by the GRU layers. The first hidden layer consists of a GRU layer which includes neural units of 128 followed by a layer of batch normalization and a dropout layer of 0.5 dropout rate. The second hidden layer also consists of a GRU layer which includes neural units of 64 followed also by a layer of batch normalization and a dropout layer of 0.5 dropout rate.

Bach normalization is used for the training acceleration and the activation stabilization while droupout is used for the generalization improvement and overfitting prevention. The output layer is a dense layer with as many neurons as the dataset's target classes. The output layer utilizes softmax activation which generates a probability distribution for all target classes within the dataset corresponding to the raw outputs in which the predicted class is the class with the highest value of probability. Adam optimizer, the metric of accuracy, and loss of categorical cross-entropy are used for the compilation of the GRU model.

**Long Short-Term Memory.** The LSTM architecture consists of an input layer, three hidden layers, and an output layer. The input layer reshapes the dataset's original features to a sequence of 3D tensor format, which can be processed by LSTM. The reshaping is performed using five time steps and a number of features per step that is calculated from the division of the total number of original features by the time steps (five).

The hidden layers include two LSTM layers and one dense layer. The first hidden layer consists of the LSTM layer which includes neural units of 128 followed by a dropout layer with 0.3 dropout rate. The output of the first LSTM hidden layer which is a sequence of output is sent to the second LSTM hidden layer after performing dropout. The second hidden layer also consists of LSTM layer which includes neural units of 64 followed also by a dropout layer with 0.3 dropout rate. The output of the second LSTM hidden layer is the final timestep which is passed to the third hidden layer after applying dropout. The third hidden layer is a dense layer that has 32 neural units and uses ReLU activation followed by a batch normalization layer for the normalization of activations so that the learning stability and a dropout layer of 0.3 dropout rate. The reason behind the usage of dropout layer is overfitting prevention and generalization improvement.

The output layer is a dense layer with as many neurons as target classes, and utilizes softmax activation for generating a probability distribution for all target classes within the dataset corresponding to the raw outputs in which the predicted class is the class with the highest value of probability. Adam optimizer with learning rate of 0.001, the metric of accuracy, and loss of categorical cross-entropy are used for the compilation of the LSTM model.

**Convolutional Neural Network.** The CNN architecture consists of a total of eight layers: one input layer followed by six hidden layers and one output layer. The input layer reshapes the original raw features to 3D tensor format, which can be processed by CNN. The reshaping is performed using five time steps and a number of features per step that is calculated from the division of the total number of original features by the time steps (five).

The hidden layers include three types of layers: convolutional, flattening, and dense layers. The hidden convolutional layers consist of three layers. The first convolutional layer uses 64 filters and the second hidden convolutional layer includes 128 filters while the third hidden convolutional layer has 256 filters. Each of the three hidden convolutional layers utilize kernal (kernal size = 3), ReLU activation, and padding (same padding). Bach normalization followed by max pooling (pool size = 2) is applied after the first and second hidden convolutional layer, while batch normalization followed by a dropout layer with the 0.3 dropout rate is applied for the third hidden convolutional layer.

There is only one flattening hidden layer which transforms the output (3D tensor) from the third hidden convolutional layer to one dimensional vector of features to be suitable for the following dense layers. There are two hidden fully connected dense layers which are used to integrate and also transform the high level features. The number of neurons is 128 in the first hidden dense layer and 64 in the second hidden dense layer. ReLU activation is used for the two hidden dense layers. The two hidden dense layers also followed by batch normalization and a dropout layer with the dropout rate of 0.3. Dropout is used as a regularization for generalization improvement and overfitting prevention while batch normalization is used for the stabilization and acceleration of training.

The output layer is a dense layer with as many neurons as the target classes, and utilizes softmax activation for generating a probability distribution for all target classes within the dataset corresponding to the raw outputs in which the predicted class is the class with the highest value of probability. Adam optimizer with learning rate of 0.001, the metric of accuracy, and loss of categorical cross-entropy are used for the compilation of the CNN model.

**Federated Learning.** In this study, FL is used for malware classification. Four FL models are generated: FL with ANN, FL with GRU, FL with LSTM, and FL with CNN. The FL process follows the architecture of the server and clients. The process includes one central server and multiple clients. On the server side, the server processes the dataset by dividing it into a set of training and testing and then normalizing the sets using Standard Scaler. The server is responsible for generating the initial global model based on one of the specified models' architecture (ANN, GRU, LSTM, or CNN). This initial global model is transmitted to all participating clients by the server.

On the client side, after receiving the global model, each client is responsible for training the model on its local private data. After the completion of local training, each client sends its model updates (weights) to the server for the aggregation process. On the server side, the server receives the model updated from clients. When the server receives model updates from all clients, it starts the aggregation process. The server uses the aggregation method of a simple averaging of the updated weights from all participating clients. This averaged set of weights resulting from the aggregation method, represents the collaborative learning from all FL participating clients and becomes the new global model used for the next round. The FL process is repeated for five rounds.

Following the completion of FL rounds, the server performs the final model refinement using its local dataset for the final training phase. In order to further optimize the final global model and prevent overfitting, this final training phase on the server makes use of additional strategies including early stopping and the reduction of learning rate. This phase helps in fine-tuning the final globally aggregated model and potentially improves its generalization and performance beyond what was achieved through the FL rounds alone. The server then performs evaluation on the final model using its test dataset.

Various performance metrics including accuracy, precision, recall, and F1-score is calculated. In order to provide insights into the performance of the model across different classes, the classification report is also generated. The server also logs these calculated results and saves them to a text file for future reference. Finally, the server performs model preservation by saving the learned model, which represents the outcome of the collaborative learning process, using h5 file so that it can be used for future predictions or as a basis point for further training.

### 3.3 Model Inversion Attack Setup

In this experiment, a server-based attack was carried out using the model inversion attack utilized in [3]. This attack primarily targets the server's final global model following the final round of the FL process. The goal of this attack is to locate an input that the model recognizes as being a member of the target class, which could reveal private information about that class. For each class within the dataset, this attack attempts to rebuild the input data utilizing the global model developed from the training process. Basically, it aims to reverse-engineer the type of input data that would provide a specific class prediction from the model. To do this, a random input is iteratively optimized to produce an output that matches the intended target class.

For evaluating such an attack, the mean squared error (MSE) was a crucial parameter. MSE represents the attack success rate, which measures the average squared difference between the attacked (reconstructed) and original data. Better reconstruction and, hence, a more successful model inversion attack are indicated by lower MSE values. Higher MSE value indicates a more robust and successful defense model. In addition to the MSE produced for each class, the average MSE was calculated for all classes to offer a broad evaluation of the attack's effectiveness. Equation 1 is used to determine the MSE for each class, where Eq. 2 is used to calculate the average MSE for all classes within the dataset.

$$\text{MSE}_s = \frac{1}{f}\sum_{j=1}^{f}(x_j - \hat{x}_j)^2 \tag{1}$$

where $\text{MSE}_s$ is the MSE for class $s$, $f$ is the number of features in the sample, $x_j$ is the $j$-th feature of the original sample, and $\hat{x}_j$ is the $j$-th feature of the attacked (reconstructed) sample.

$$\text{Average MSE} = \frac{1}{N}\sum_{n=1}^{N}\text{MSE}_s \tag{2}$$

where $N$ is the total number of classes within the dataset and $\text{MSE}_s$ is the MSE for class$s$.

# 4 Experimental Results

## 4.1 Setup

Google Colab served as the platform for the experiments. An Intel Xeon CPU operating at 2.20 GHz was the CPU specification. There was 12 GB of RAM in total. For all implementations, the library of a Python 3.11.11 was utilized. In every experiment, 80% of the data was utilized to train the DL models and 20% was used for testing. Each model is executed ten times.

## 4.2 Performance Analysis

Each model is executed ten times in Colab, then the average is calculated for each metric. For example, time represents the average of the ten time values resulting from the ten executions of the model on Colab. Table 1 shows the time metric and the overall performance metrics using the Malware Dataset discussed in Sect. 3.1. As illustrated in Table 1, FL_ANN model is the fastest model with the lowest execution time of 80.08 s followed by FL_GRU, FL_CNN, and FL_LSTM. FL_LSTM has the longest execution time of 237.39 s. FL_CNN achieved the best performance metrics of 99.82% for each of accuracy, precision, recall, and F1-score. FL_ANN has the lowest performance metric of accuracy (90.33%), precision (92.20%), recall (90.33%), and F1-score (90.05%).

Table 2 illustrates the time metric and overall performance metrics using the AndroMD data set detailed in Sect. 3.1. For AndroMD Dataset, FL_ANN model is also the fastest model with the lowest execution time of 90.188 s, followed by FL_GRU, FL_CNN, and FL_LSTM. The models of FL_ANN, and FL_LSTM have almost ~99% for each of accuracy, precision, recall, and F1-score, while

FL_GRU, and FL_CNN have almost ~98% for each of accuracy, precision, recall, and F1-score.

As shown in Tables 1 and 2, the notable variation in training times of the four generated FL based models is due to their computational demands and complexity of their architectures. The FL_ANN model is the fastest model with the lowest execution time followed by FL_GRU, FL_CNN, and FL_LSTM. The FL_LSTM model necessitates the longest time due to its intricate cell architecture comprising three gates including input, forget, and output along with cell state management, demanding approximately four times the parameters of less complex networks, whereas The FL_ANN model attains the quickest training duration owing to its straightforward feedforward configuration utilizing standard matrix multiplications.

With a mechanism of dual gate including reset along with update gates, the FL_GRU model occupies a middle ground, requiring more calculations than FL_ANN but less than FL_LSTM. With filter counts increasing from 64 to 128 to 256, the highly computational convolution processes of the FL_CNN model over three layers impact the training duration. Furthermore, restructuring data using artificial time steps to create three-dimensional is necessitated for the two models of FL_CNN and FL_LSTM, which adds processing cost that is absent from the more straightforward FL_ANN implementation.

**Table 1.** Overall Performance results of all models using Malware Dataset.

| Model | Training Time (s) | Accuracy (%) | Precision (%) | Recall (%) | F1 Score (%) |
|---|---|---|---|---|---|
| FL_ANN | 80.08 | 90.33 | 92.20 | 90.33 | 90.05 |
| FL_GRU | 98.21 | 99.58 | 99.58 | 99.58 | 99.58 |
| FL_LSTM | 237.39 | 99.69 | 99.69 | 99.69 | 99.69 |
| FL_CNN | 147.74 | 99.82 | 99.82 | 99.82 | 99.82 |

**Table 2.** Overall Performance results of all models using the AndroMD Dataset.

| Model | Training Time (s) | Accuracy (%) | Precision (%) | Recall (%) | F1 Score (%) |
|---|---|---|---|---|---|
| FL_ANN | 90.19 | 98.62 | 98.63 | 98.62 | 98.62 |
| FL_GRU | 102.53 | 98.46 | 98.48 | 98.46 | 98.46 |
| FL_LSTM | 145.87 | 98.63 | 98.74 | 98.73 | 98.73 |
| FL_CNN | 107.76 | 98.30 | 98.30 | 98.30 | 98.29 |

### 4.3 Security Analysis

Figures 2 and 3 depict the average MSE for ten runs of the model inversion attack detailed in Sect. 3.3. For each model, the average MSE is calculated by taking the average of the MSE calculated in Eq. 2 from ten colab runs. As shown in Fig. 2, FL_ANN model achieves the best average MSE (1.91) while FL_CNN has the lowest average MSE (1.55), so FL_ANN is the most resistance model against the model inversion attack using Malware Dataset followed by FL_GRU, FL_LSTM, and FL_CNN. As shown in Fig. 3, FL_LSTM model produces the best average MSE (1.44), so its the most robust model against the model inversion attack in case of utilizing the AndroMD Dataset followed by FL_GRU, FL_CNN, and FL_ANN.

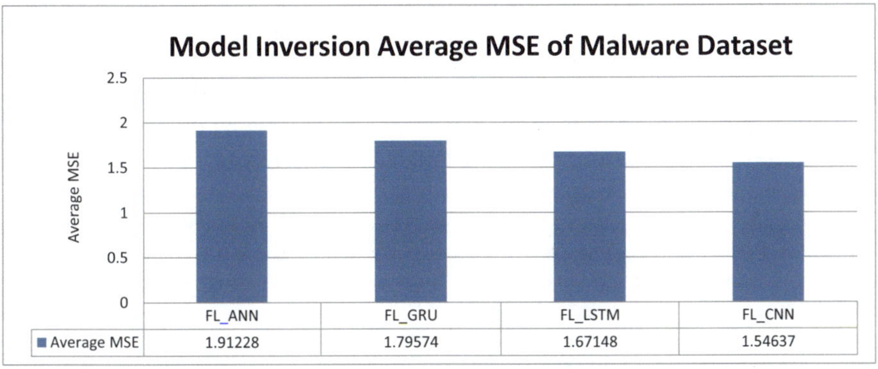


**Fig. 2.** Model Inversion Average MSE of Malware Dataset.

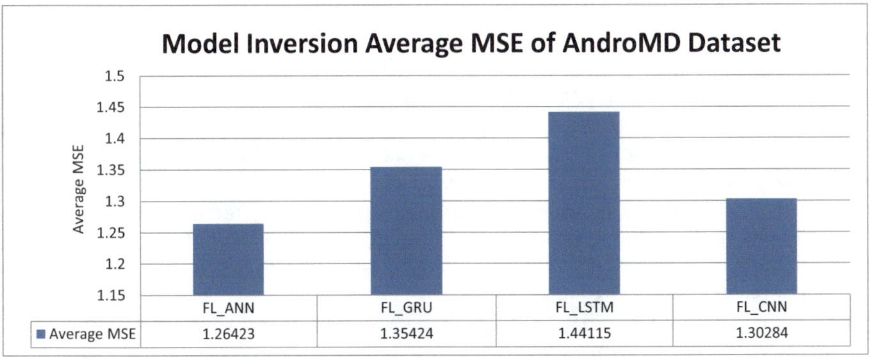


**Fig. 3.** Model Inversion Average MSE of AndroMD Dataset.

## 5 Conclusion and Future Work

This research provides a comparative work of analyzing the impact of different neural architectures in FL on the model inversion attack success for malware classification based on Malware Dataset and AndroMD Dataset. ANN, GRU, LSTM, and CNN are the four neural architectures implemented in this work. Four FL models are generated: FL_ANN, FL_GRU, FL_LSTM, and FL_CNN. The FL_ANN model implements FL using ANN, FL_GRU implements FL with GRU, FL_LSTM implements FL using LSTM, and FL_CNN implements FL with CNN architecture. For both datasets, FL_ANN is the fastest model with the execution time of 80.08 s on Malware Dataset and 90.19 s on AndroMD Dataset while FL_LSTM is the slowest model with the largest execution time of 237.39 s using Malware Dataset and 145.87 s using AndroMD Dataset. The highest performance metrics are achieved by FL_CNN on Malware Dataset and FL_LSTM on AndroMD Dataset. For model inversion attack, the FL_ANN is the most robust model using Malware Dataset with an average MSE of 1.91 while FL_LSTM is the best resistance model using AndroMD Dataset with the average MSE of 1.44. The future work includes evaluation on dataset with larger size and more diverse dataset, investigation of other attack types, and integration with defense techniques with FL to increase the models robustness.

**Acknowledgment.** This research project was funded by the University of Technology and Applied Sciences through the Internal Research Funding Program, grant No (IRG-IBRI-25-40).

## References

1. Takahashi, H., Liu, J., Liu, Y.: Breaching FedMD: image recovery via paired-logits inversion attack. In: Proceedings of the IEEE/CVF Conference on Computer Vision and Pattern Recognition (CVPR). IEEE (2024)
2. Çıplak, Z., Yıldız, K., Altınkaya, Ş.: FEDetect: a federated learning-based malware detection and classification using deep neural network algorithms. Arab. J. Sci. Eng. (2025). https://doi.org/10.1007/s13369-025-10043-x
3. Shalabi, E., Khedr, W., Rushdy, E., Salah, A.: A comparative study of privacy-preserving techniques in federated learning: a performance and security analysis. Information **16**(3), 244 (2025). https://doi.org/10.3390/info16030244
4. Suresh Babu, P., Maheswar Reddy, K., Revanth, P., Reddy, K.M., Venkateswara Rao, K.S.: Malware classification based on deep learning using convloutional neural network. In: 2024 International Conference on IoT Based Control Networks and Intelligent Systems (ICICNIS), pp. 998–1004 (2024). https://doi.org/10.1109/ICICNIS64247.2024.10823382
5. Abd Al Abbas, M.A.: Deep learning-based approaches for effective IoT malware classification. In: 2024 2nd DMIHER International Conference on Artificial Intelligence in Healthcare, Education and Industry (IDICAIEI), pp. 1–6. IEEE (2024). https://doi.org/10.1109/IDICAIEI61867.2024.10842813
6. Jasim, Z.K., Kurnaz, S.: An Efficient malware classification method using novel deep learning model. AURUM J. Eng. Syst. Archit. **8**(2), 265–271 (2024)

7. Sharma, D., Devare, M.: Advancing malware defense: a hybrid approach with explainable deep neural networks. In: 2024 2nd DMIHER International Conference on Artificial Intelligence in Healthcare, Education and Industry (IDICAIEI), pp. 1–6. IEEE (2024). https://doi.org/10.1109/IDICAIEI61867.2024.10842773
8. Ait Messaad, B., Chetioui, K., Balboul, Y., Rhachi, H.: Analyzing and detecting malware using machine learning and deep learning. In: The International Conference on Artificial Intelligence and Smart Environment, pp. 518–525. Springer (2023). https://doi.org/10.1007/978-3-031-48573-2_75
9. Rodríguez, R.J., Ugarte-Pedrero, X., Tapiador, J.: Introduction to the special issue on challenges and trends in malware analysis. In: Digital Threats: Research and Practice (DTRAP), vol. 3, no. 2, pp. 1–2. ACM New York, NY (2022). https://doi.org/10.1145/3536319
10. Jaswal, R., Panda, S.N., Khullar, V.: Federated learning: an approach for managing data privacy and security in collaborative learning. Recent Adv. Electr. Electron. Eng. (2025). https://doi.org/10.2174/0123520965328724241218110637
11. Thakur, R., Patel, S., Singh, N., Barde, A., Barde, S.: Tackling the complexities of federated learning. In: Generative Artificial Intelligence for Biomedical and Smart Health Informatics, pp. 343–353. Wiley Online Library (2025). https://doi.org/10.1002/9781394280735.ch17
12. Annamalai, S., Sangeetha, N., Kumaresan, M., Tejavarma, D., Vardhan, G.H., Kumar, A.S.: Application domains of federated learning. In: Model Optimization Methods for Efficient and Edge AI: Federated Learning Architectures, Frameworks and Applications, pp. 127–144. Wiley Online Library (2025). https://doi.org/10.1002/9781394219230.ch7
13. Hassan, W., Mohamed, H.: Applications of federated learning in AI, IoT, healthcare, finance, banking, and cross-domain learning. In: Artificial Intelligence Using Federated Learning, pp. 175-195. CRC Press (2024). https://doi.org/10.1201/9781003482000
14. Kanhegaonkar, P., Prakash, S.: Federated learning in healthcare applications. In: Data Fusion Techniques and Applications for Smart Healthcare, pp. 157–196. Elsevier (2024). https://doi.org/10.1016/B978-0-44-313233-9.00013-8
15. Bhaskar, U., Srivastava, V., Vummintala, A.M., Manwani, N., Gujar, S.: Optimal strategies for federated learning maintaining client privacy. arXiv preprint arXiv:2501.14453 (2025). https://doi.org/10.48550/arXiv.2501.14453
16. Purkayastha, B.S., Rahman, M.M., Shahpasand, M.: Android malware detection using machine learning and neural network: a hybrid approach with federated learning. In: 2024 7th International Conference on Advanced Communication Technologies and Networking (CommNet), pp. 1–5 (2024). https://doi.org/10.1109/CommNet63022.2024.10793304
17. Jiang, C., et al.: FedDRC: a robust federated learning-based Android malware Classifier under heterogeneous distribution. In: 2024 27th International Conference on Computer Supported Cooperative Work in Design (CSCWD), pp. 1029–1036 (2024). https://doi.org/10.1109/CSCWD61410.2024.10580300
18. Nobakht, M., Javidan, R., Pourebrahimi, A.: SIM-FED: secure IoT malware detection model with federated learning. Comput. Electr. Eng. **116**, 109139 (2024). https://doi.org/10.1016/j.compeleceng.2024.109139
19. Serpanos, D., Xenos, G.: Federated learning in malware detection. In: 2023 IEEE 28th International Conference on Emerging Technologies and Factory Automation (ETFA), pp. 1–4. IEEE (2023). https://doi.org/10.1109/ETFA54631.2023.10275578

20. Bhavani, R., Sankaradass, V.: FedL_DBNFSpinalNet based malware detection in IoT devices. Int. J. Mach. Learn. Cybern., 1–19 (2025). https://doi.org/10.1007/s13042-025-02557-5
21. Chen, R., Xia, H., Wang, K., Xu, S., Zhang, R.: KDRSFL: a knowledge distillation resistance transfer framework for defending model inversion attacks in split federated learning. In: Future Generation Computer Systems, vol. 166, pp. 107637. Elsevier (2025). https://doi.org/10.1016/j.future.2024.107637
22. Akl, A.A., Hosny, K.M., Fouda, M.M., Salah, A.: A hybrid CNN and ensemble model for COVID-19 lung infection detection on chest CT scans. PLoS One 18(3), e0282608 (2023). https://doi.org/10.1371/journal.pone.0282608
23. Mohamed, M.A., El-Henawy, I.M., Salah, A.: Price prediction of seasonal items using machine learning and statistical methods. Comput. Mater. Continua **70**(2) (2022). https://doi.org/10.32604/cmc.2022.020782

# SF-SMCM: A Security Framework for Single-To-Multi-Cloud Migration

Yasmin Gad(✉), Mohamed Hamed N. Taha, and Nour Eldeen Khalifa

Faculty of Computers and Artificial Intelligence, Cairo University, Giza, Egypt
{mnasrtaha,nourmahmoud}@cu.edu.eg

**Abstract.** The rapid adoption of multi-cloud technology throughout the world has resulted in serious security problems, particularly when transferring data between single and multi-cloud settings. The absence of standardized security framework for multi-cloud migrations increased vulnerability as a result of expanded attack surfaces, and scattered security measures across various cloud providers. These restrictions are made considerably more challenging with the requirement to balance cost reduction, performance effectiveness, and robust security implementation. In this paper a defined security framework is introduced to unify data protection methods across data layers and provide a guidance to reduce security risks. (SF-SMCM) will address four main layers of data transfer process which are data preparation, security, migration and cost-performance optimization. Security approaches within each layer is analyzed for the effect it has on data overhead and results are obtained for bandwidth efficiency and transfer time. In particular, a comparative analysis between the transfer time for data without applying security algorithms and data with encryption and hashing algorithms applied is performed. Results obtained shows that transfer time is higher when data is encrypted. Cost will be obtained and compared for Amazon AWS and Google cloud using the pricing calculator for Cloud Backup service. Secured data was found to be higher in price through the two cloud service providers due to higher data growth rate.

**Keywords:** Security Framework · Single cloud · Multi-Cloud · Migration · IPsec · Hashing

## 1 Introduction

Multi-cloud technology has been rapidly evolving with two or more cloud providers offering their services to distribute data among their infrastructure. Multi-cloud benefits include scalability, vendor lock-in and balancing between performance and cost [1]. All these benefits made transition to multi-cloud essential but comes with lots of limitations in cloud technology. The largest challenge in the realm of cloud technology is data security that depends on data sensitivity; protecting data from security breaches and theft is crucial. Adopting multi-cloud necessitates applying a variety of security strategies and compliance standards because multiple providers must be contacted, leaving data vulnerable if handled improperly.


K. Daimi and A. Alsadoon (Eds.): ICR 2025, LNNS 1487, pp. 199–210, 2025.
https://doi.org/10.1007/978-3-031-95652-2_18

Migration to multi-cloud comes with significant issues that includes inconsistent security techniques, Security vulnerabilities, large data distribution surface and the inability to unify a security policy that regular security frameworks cannot handle [2]. The lack of a unified framework that address data migration process with all aspects results in limitations of deploying security strategies that solve migration issues. Cost and performance analysis helps in taking the decision of choosing the most suitable cloud provider.

Meanwhile, efforts are made to establish a security framework with the purpose of safeguarding organizations and individual's data in the digital world. In essence, cyber security ensures the data protection within cyber networks, achieving the protection of information system infrastructures, data integrity, and confidentiality [3]. Procedures and measurements that adhere to CIA approaches covered data migration process layers in order to aid in better cloud migration process. Through these strategies, the cloud migration process can be better perceived and evaluated for analysis [4].

In a transfer process between clouds, security algorithms for communication and secure connections should be adopted. Traditionally, internet protocol security IPsec is used to protect data from being compromised and revealed to unauthorized parties through the creation of a secure channel for communication. Since data size and transfer method deeply affect the migration process, approaches taken should be accompanied with performance metrics analysis as a target for the defined framework.

IPsec is a protocol suite that relies on authentication and encryption for IP packets in data communication between hosts and site-to-site. With the support of encryption algorithms such as DES, 3DES and AES used for encrypting data packets and hashing algorithms such as HMAC for authentication, high level of security is achieved [5]. Two core protocols for IPsec that provide the main security options are Encapsulating Security Payload (ESP) and Authentication Header (AH). Each of the protocols can work in different modes of operation, transport mode and tunnel mode. AH protocol provides data integrity function and authentication while ESP is used for data confidentiality along with authentication functions [6]. Data security is improved through hashing and encryption, but there is a cost: an increase in data overhead for each packet. To evaluate the outcomes for cost and performance metrics, tests must be carried out on a predetermined dataset.

The major contributions of this research work are:

- Introducing SF-SMCM, a structured framework specifically for single-to-multi-cloud migration, addressing unique multi-cloud challenges.
- Provides quantitative insights into the impact of security measures on migration time and cost, helping organizations understand trade-offs.
- Offers a framework to evaluate cost and performance implications, aiding in the selection of suitable cloud service providers.

## 2 Literature Review

Work done by [7] has discussed some of multi-cloud migration complexities and best practices that helps in easy integration and better security. Conclusions summed in [7] includes approaches as extensive planning, standardizing policies, security measures and cost management that are proved to help reducing costs along with better performance. The approach of [8] involved a multi-cloud solution for portfolio of applications and applied it to a real use case. A method in [8] included text mining, dependency graph and optimization model that builds a solution for choosing the right providers in a multi-cloud solution. Insights proved by [9] has provided organizations with the needed actions to deploy security and compliance within multi-cloud architectures making it easier to adopt the technology. Identifying security challenges, the impact of various frameworks, regulations and compliance, emerging technologies and IAM best practices are all objectives for the research [9].

## 3 The Proposed Security Framework (SF-SMCM)

In the proposed framework (SF-SMCM), we will present a well-defined approach to assist in selecting the most suitable cloud service provider to transfer the data to. The decision taken is based on applying security measures on the four primary layers in the proposed framework. In order to protect data being transferred, each communication layer should have a specific number of security methods that is described in our framework. The four main layers introduced in the Security framework are depicted in Fig. 1.

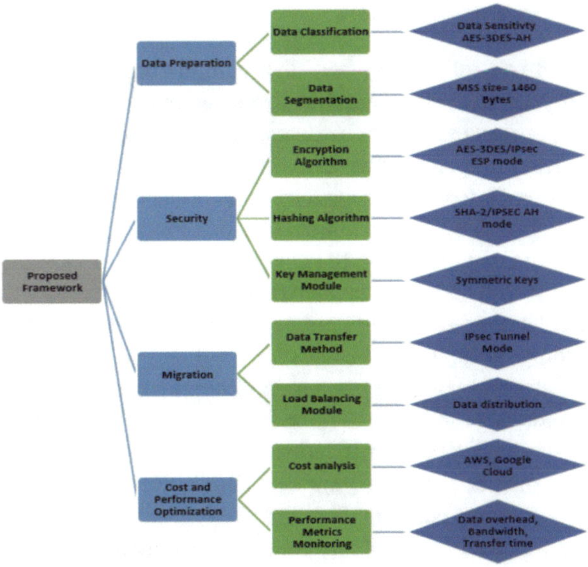


**Fig. 1.** Proposed Security framework for migration from single cloud to multi-cloud (SF-SMCM)

Based on four essential layers—Data Preparation, Security, Migration, and Cost and Performance Optimization, the SF-SMCM framework offers a thorough method for safe cloud migration. This organized framework is intended to give businesses a methodical way to choose the best cloud service providers while maintaining data security during the migration process. Every step of the cloud migration process is meticulously thought out due to the framework's tiered architecture.

Data handling and security measures are the main topics of the first two layers. With specific parameters like AES and 3DES for data sensitivity protection and a specified MSS size of 1460 bytes, the Data Preparation layer includes data segmentation and classification. The security layer creates a comprehensive security infrastructure for data protection by implementing strong protection using hashing algorithms (SHA-2/IPsec AH mode), encryption algorithms (AES, 3DES/IPsec ESP mode), and key management modules that use symmetric keys.

The practical aspects of data distribution and transfer are covered by the migration layer. For an optimal distribution of data, load balancing modules are used and data transfer techniques using IPsec tunnel mode. By reducing bottlenecks and ensuring seamless data transfer operations, this layer makes sure that data migration is not only secure but also efficient and evenly distributed throughout the network infrastructure.

The economic and operational aspects of cloud migration are the main focus of the fourth layer, Cost and Performance Optimization. In addition to performance monitoring that includes tracking variables like data overhead, bandwidth usage, and transfer time, this layer offers comprehensive cost analysis for different cloud providers like AWS and Google Cloud. To maintain optimal performance and cost-effectiveness, the fourth layer helps in making well-informed decisions regarding cloud migration strategy.

## 4 IPsec Protocol and Modes

IP security protocol is a reliable protocol that controls data flow between endpoints. Data confidentiality, Data integrity and data origin authentication are all supported [10]. IPsec operates in two modes, Tunnel mode and Transport mode [11]. An incoming IP packet is encapsulated in a new IP packet with a new IP header in tunnel mode. This mode is used when sending data over the internet to protect and ensure no manipulation occurs, so encryption is done for the entire IP packet including source and destination IP addresses. Only the payload of the IP packet is encrypted in transport mode leaving the source and destination addresses unaltered [12]. It's usually used when sending data between identified hosts over the public network so no need to encrypt the incoming IP header. Depending on the user's needs, they must decide which to go for transport mode or tunnel mode. We will adopt the usage of tunnel mode to ensure the protection of end-to-end communication between hosts by encrypting the whole package and for its use in network-to-network communication.

IPsec protocols include Encapsulating Security Payload (ESP) and Authentication Header (AH), the difference between them lies in the level of protection for IP packets. AH IPsec mode offers data integrity and data source authentication, while ESP IPsec mode offers data privacy, data integrity, and data source authentication [13]. Each of the two modes adds a header before the raw IP header along with the tunnel mode header that is added before AH or ESP header. AH uses any of the authentication algorithms HMAC_MD5, HMAC_SHA1, and HMAC_SHA2 with varying hash lengths. ESP is compatible with DES, 3DES, AES_128, and AES_256 encryption algorithms. We will use both modes of operation and test the results using SHA2 for hashing, 3DES, and AES_128 for encryption [14].

## 5 Encryption Algorithms

AES and Triple DES are two encryption algorithms used for securing data through the use of a pre-shared key known to the sender and receiver. AES stands for Advanced Encryption Standard and it is the most common algorithm used due to its fast processing speed and robust security. It uses a symmetric key for encryption and decryption in sizes of 128-bits, 192-bits, and 256-bits [15] selected according to the required security level. AES encrypts 128 bits of plaintext and generates cipher text of the same key size. The Triple Data Encryption Standard (3DES) is an improvement of the DES standard that applies the same encryption algorithm steps three times with use of three keys. DES was known for its vulnerability to brute-force attack due to its key length. AES operates on a 128-bit block size while DES operates on a 64-bit block size. Despite using the same block size, 3DES employs the same procedure for DES three rounds making it more robust and secure [16]. Data padding is affected by the difference in block sizes; for each byte sent on a secured channel padding should be applied to reach the required block size depending on the security protocol applied.

## 6 Hashing Algorithms

The hashing algorithm is the method of converting data transmitted into masked data by applying a one-way mechanism. Because there is a minimal chance of reversing the operation and recovering the original data, this technique helps secure data against unauthorized disclosure. Hashing primarily contributes to data authentication that protects sensitive data and defines data integrity during transmission. Commonly used functions like MD5, SHA-2, and CRC32 have a specific output size; in order to use a particular method, one must determine the level for data integrity without compromising bandwidth. MD5 and SHA-2 have the same block size of 512 bits which can affect data overhead when used with one of the IPSEC tunnel mode protocols.

## 7 Data Padding and Calculations

IPsec tunnel mode is used with AH and ESP protocols. Security mechanisms for encryption such as AES and DES are used along with SHA-2 for hashing algorithm. The effect on data enlargement is consequently observed, leading to an increase in time.

### 7.1 ESP Protocol with AES Algorithm

AES is commonly used in encryption mechanisms for its robust security methods and faster response. When adopting IPsec protocol, it integrates security on incoming IP packets through the use of ESP tunnel mode. ESP adds a header, serial peripheral interface (SPI), a sequence number (ESP IV), and an ESP trailer that are 8 bytes, 16 bytes, and 16 bytes in size respectively, so a total of 40 bytes overhead is added to the original packet size [17]. When using AES, each byte of data sent must be padded to meet the needed block size for the AES algorithm which is a 16-byte block, and a 1-bit padding identifier is added even if no padding is needed. Since ESP mode uses authentication algorithms for integrity, we will adopt HMAC-SHA2 which has a 64-byte block size.

To have 1 byte of data sent over IPsec ESP tunnel mode with AES encryption, would lead to an overhead of 123 bytes calculated with the above estimations. We will calculate the data overhead that results when moving total data size of 10 MB, 20 MB, 30 MB, 40 MB, 50 MB, and 60 MB. The Segment Size for TCP/IP is 1460 bytes [18], for data sizes exceeding the MSS, we will calculate the number of packets equivalent in size 1460 bytes by segmentation and the remaining data size to analyze the data overhead.

The number of packets is calculated by dividing the transmitted data size by 1460, we will determine the total number of packets required to send over the IPsec tunnel for the corresponding data size as shown in Table 1.

**Table 1.** Total Number of packets for assumed data sizes and size of the last packet

| Data size (Bytes) | Total Number of packets | Size of last packet (Bytes) |
|---|---|---|
| 10000000 | 6850 | 460 |
| 20000000 | 13699 | 920 |
| 30000000 | 20548 | 1380 |
| 40000000 | 27398 | 380 |
| 50000000 | 34247 | 840 |
| 60000000 | 41096 | 1300 |

We will calculate the overhead for a fixed packet size of 1460 bytes and multiply it by the total number of packets to get the overhead of transmitting packets of maximum segment size over the network as shown in Table 1. The remaining data will result in a packet smaller than the MSS in size. To determine the overhead effect on data, we will compute the total overhead resulting from number of total number of packets of all sizes and add all results as shown in Table 2.

### 7.2 ESP Protocol with Triple DES Algorithm

ESP protocol can provide the usage of the 3DES encryption algorithm along with the usage of an optional authentication process with one of its types. 3DES uses a 64-bit block size compared to AES block size of 128 bits [19]. As with ESP, in AES each byte of data sent will be padded to meet the needed block size for the 3DES algorithm which is an 8-byte block with a 1-bit padding identifier. In order to evaluate the impact of 3DES algorithm with ESP protocol, data overhead will be calculated for the defined data sizes as shown in Table 3.

### 7.3 AH Protocol with SHA-2 Algorithm

AH provides a way to verify the sender IP along with data integrity for the packet through the use of hash functions [20]. It authenticates the entire IP header and adds a header

**Table 2.** Calculated Overhead for assumed data size when using ESP mode with AES

| Data size (Bytes) | Total Number of packets | Overhead of Packets -1 (Bytes) | Overhead of last packet (Bytes) | Total overhead (Bytes) |
|---|---|---|---|---|
| 10000000 | 6850 | 931464 | 112 | 931576 |
| 20000000 | 13699 | 1862928 | 100 | 1863028 |
| 30000000 | 20548 | 2794392 | 88 | 2794480 |
| 40000000 | 27398 | 3725992 | 128 | 3726120 |
| 50000000 | 34247 | 4657456 | 116 | 4657572 |
| 60000000 | 41096 | 1300 | 104 | 5589024 |

**Table 3.** Calculated Overhead for assumed data size when using ESP mode with 3DES

| Data size (Bytes) | Total Number of packets | Overhead of Packets -1 (Bytes) | Overhead of last packet (Bytes) | Total overhead (Bytes) |
|---|---|---|---|---|
| 10000000 | 6850 | 787635 | 91 | **787726** |
| 20000000 | 13699 | 1575270 | 83 | **1575353** |
| 30000000 | 20548 | 2362905 | 67 | **2362972** |
| 40000000 | 27398 | 3150655 | 107 | **3150762** |
| 50000000 | 34247 | 3938290 | 99 | **3938389** |
| 60000000 | 41096 | 4725925 | 83 | **4726008** |

that maintains message integrity and source authentication. The size of the AH header is 24 bytes, adding the traditional tunnel mode header of 20 bytes, and using SHA-2 Hash algorithm with the needed padding to reach a block size of 512 bits/64 bytes [21]. Since AH mode don't employ encryption, padded data won't be added to reach the block size requirement of encryption algorithm. Considering the number of packets obtained from our calculations, we will compute the data overhead to analyze the impact of applying SHA-2 Hashing technique to send data over a public network as shown in Table 4.

## 8 Time and Cost Calculations

This section will describe the effect of applying security approaches while migrating data over public networks between different cloud service providers. Migration process performance evaluation will be measured through two pillars which are Time and Cost. For each category, we will study the data overhead effect by defining a set of equations and certain parameters like Bandwidth used for transmission that have a direct effect on calculating the time needed to transfer data. Migration cost will be identified according

**Table 4.** Calculated Overhead for assumed data size when using AH mode with SHA-2

| Data size (Bytes) | Total Number of packets | Overhead of Packets -1 (Bytes) | Overhead of last packet (Bytes) | Total overhead (Bytes) |
|---|---|---|---|---|
| 10000000 | 6850 | 383544 | 96 | 383640 |
| 20000000 | 13699 | 767088 | 84 | 767172 |
| 30000000 | 20548 | 1150632 | 72 | 1150704 |
| 40000000 | 27398 | 1534232 | 112 | 1534344 |
| 50000000 | 34247 | 1917776 | 100 | 1917876 |
| 60000000 | 41096 | 2301320 | 88 | 2301408 |

to the destined cloud service provider; each provider has his own services with the cost defined for that type of service.

### 8.1 Migration Time

Migration time depends on the link speed for transferring data, we will assume the use of 10 Mb/Sec, to calculate the actual transmission time two factors should be considered before proceeding. The bandwidth efficiency depends on the type of protocol used in sending data due to protocol bandwidth overhead. We will determine the efficiency for a 10 Mb/sec link when the maximum packet size is used adding the IP protocol efficiency and each of IPsec protocols efficiency as shown in Fig. 2, while taking into consideration the minimum size of IP header is 20 bytes [22]. The results show the optimum bandwidth efficiency when using IP protocol without the applying any of IPsec protocols giving 0.98, 0.91, 0.92, 0.96 for IP protocol, AES protocol, 3DES protocol and AH + SHA protocol efficiency respectively.

Transfer time is obtained for identified data sizes using Eq. (1).

$$Time(\text{sec}) = \frac{(Original\ Datasize + Data\ overhead) - 8bits - 1000000}{TCP\ Throughput * IP\ efficiency * protocol\ efficiency} \quad (1)$$

Accordingly, the transfer time for used data set when TCP throughput of 10 Mb/Sec is used will be calculated as shown in Table 5.

### 8.2 Cost Calculations

Famous cloud providers will be adopted to calculate the cost for data transmission while choosing the convenient security approach from the mentioned protocols applied and measured for data overhead. We will get the pricing for two cloud service providers which are Amazon AWS and Google Cloud while using the pricing calculator for data transfer on backup service. We will present a monthly cost for data transfer over backup service with a data increment of 10 MB with a start of 100 GB data storage used. The annual growth rate for data will be affected by the type of protocol used that will give cost change

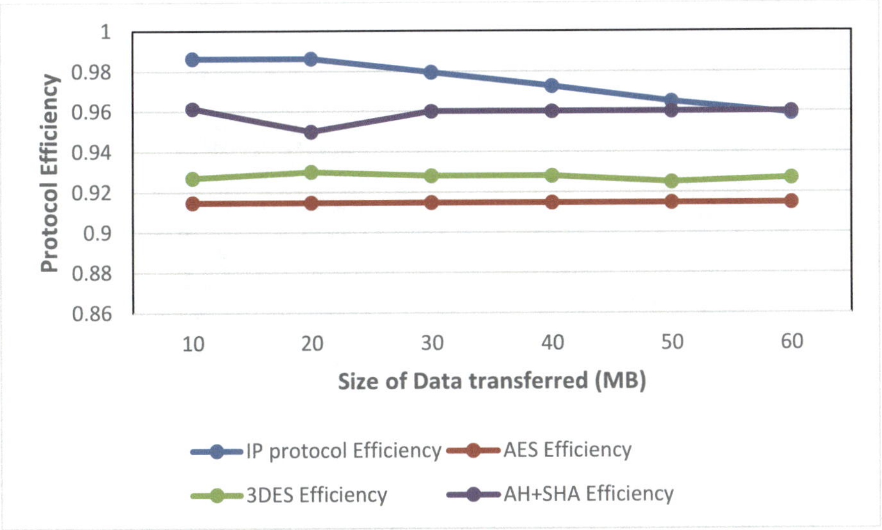


**Fig. 2.** Bandwidth Efficiency due to different protocols

**Table 5.** Transfer time for non–secured and secured data transfer

| Data size (MB) | Transfer time for non-secured data (sec) | Transfer time for AES+ESP protocol (sec) | Transfer time for 3DES+ESP protocol(sec) | Transfer time for AH+SHA protocol(sec) |
|---|---|---|---|---|
| 10 | 1 | 1.25 | 1.1 | 1.11 |
| 20 | 2 | 2.5 | 2.1 | 2.2 |
| 30 | 3 | 3.7 | 3.2 | 3.3 |
| 40 | 4 | 5 | 4.3 | 4.4 |
| 50 | 5 | 6.2 | 5.4 | 5.6 |
| 60 | 6 | 7.4 | 6.5 | 6.7 |

and compared according to the type of security protocol used. Using the AWS pricing calculator for the EFS backup feature any change in data growth rate with increment will affect the cost computed. With the assumption of primary data to be backed up is 100 GB, and an annual increase of 36.5% for data without applying security measure, cost will be calculated for data when applying security techniques during transfer and for transferring data over a channel regardless of applying any security parameter as shown in Fig. 3.

With its security framework, SF-SMCM tackles the serious security issues that arise when single-cloud environments give way to multi-cloud ones. Maintaining uniform security policies and procedures across various cloud platforms, each with unique security protocols and requirements, is the main issue when migrating across multiple clouds.

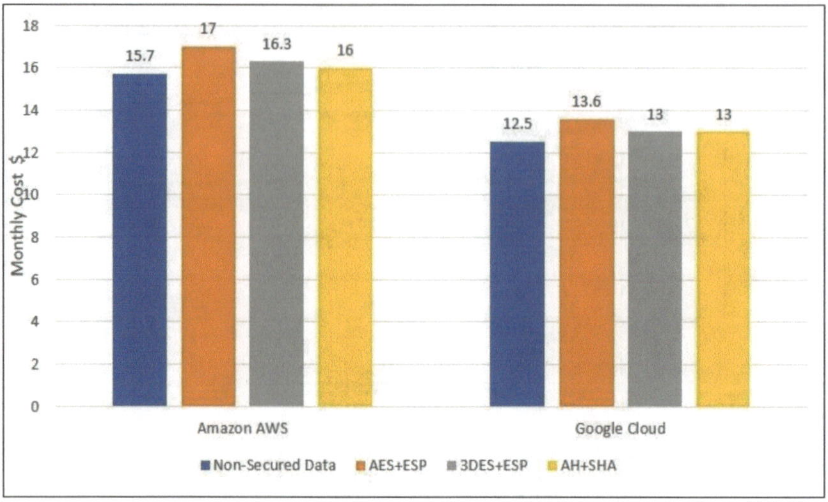


**Fig. 3.** Costs results for Amazon AWS and Google cloud for different protocols used

By putting in place a standardized security approach that guarantees consistent protection irrespective of the cloud provider, SF-SMCM overcomes this difficulty and successfully builds a seamless security envelope around all data and operations.

The framework's use of a multi-layered security strategy to mitigate the increased attack surface is especially noteworthy. Fundamentally, SF-SMCM protects data in transit and at rest by combining strong hashing techniques (SHA-2) with cutting-edge encryption algorithms (AES and 3DES). This thorough encryption approach guarantees that the data is safeguarded by extra security measures even in the event that one security layer is breached. By guaranteeing packet-level encryption and authentication, the deployment of IPsec components—ESP (Encapsulating Security Payload) and AH (Authentication Header) in particular, offers an extra degree of protection, successfully thwarting man-in-the-middle attacks and unauthorized data access.

Strict authentication procedures and automated security protocols address human factors, which are frequently regarded as the weakest link in security systems. A secure communication channel between various cloud environments is established by the framework's use of IPsec tunnel mode, and secure key distribution and rotation are guaranteed by the key management module. While upholding strict security standards, these automated security measures reduce the possibility of human error. The framework's performance optimization features, and all-encompassing security approach make it the perfect choice for businesses wishing to execute safe multi-cloud migrations while preserving data security and operational effectiveness.

## 9 Conclusion

In conclusion, the SF-SMCM framework addressed the critical components of migration to multi-cloud environments. It covered four key phases: data preparation, security, migration, and cost-performance optimization, ensuring that enterprise data was protected, and operations remained smooth. The use of IPsec with ESP and AH proved appropriate for ensuring data security during migration, as these protocols, combined with AES, 3DES, and SHA-2, provided strong security measures. This ensured that data could not be intercepted, altered, or misused by malicious actors, which was a critical aspect of the framework. SF-SMCM's approach to prioritizing security, speed, and cost was also appropriate, acknowledging that while encryption and hashing techniques increased data overhead, they were necessary for protecting information. Cost analysis was used to determine the appropriate level of security based on the organization's finances and requirements. Ultimately, SF-SMCM enabled secure migration to multi-cloud environments, allowing enterprises to benefit from scalability, backup, and elasticity. The well-defined processes facilitated seamless migration with adequate security, enabling enterprises to focus on innovation and growth without concerns about data security.

## References

1. Sadique, A., Sehar, H., Nasim, S., Nasim, F.: Data exposure risks in hybrid vs. multi-cloud migrations: a comparative analysis. J. Appl. Ling. Tesol (Jalt). **8**(1) (2025)
2. Reddy Julakanti, S., KiranmayeeSattiraju, N.S., Julakanti, R.: Multi-cloud security: strategies for managing Hybrid environments. Neuro Quantol. **20**(11), 10063–10074 (2022). https://doi.org/10.48047/nq.2022.20.11.nq67000
3. Jimmy, F.: Cyber security vulnerabilities and remediation through cloud security tools. JAIGS. **2**(01) (2024). https://doi.org/10.60087/jaigs.v2i1.102
4. Amin, R., Vadlamudi, S., Rahaman, M.M.: Opportunities and challenges of data migration in cloud. Eng. Int. **9** (2021). https://doi.org/10.18034/ei.v9i1.529
5. Yessenzholov, U.S., Kaliaskarov, N.B.: Implementation of traffic protection based on IPSEC VPN technology and network modeling on ENSP software environment. Chem. Bull. Kazakh Nat. Univ. **3**(126), 10.52167/1609–10.52167/1817 (2023)
6. Elezi, M., Rauf, B.: Conception of Virtual Private Networks using IPsec suite of protocols, comparative analysis of distributed database queries using different IPsec modes of encryption. Proc. Soc. Behav. Sci. **195**, 1938–1948 (2015). https://doi.org/10.1016/j.sbspro.2015.06.206
7. Chennupati, A.: Challenges and best practices in multi cloud migration for enterprises. IRE J. **7**(4) (2023)
8. Asthana, S., Megahed, A., Iyoob, I.: Multi-cloud solution design for migrating a portfolio of applications to the cloud. In: Service-Oriented Computing – ICSOC 2020 Workshops. ICSOC 2020 Lecture Notes in Computer Science. Springer, Dubai (2020)
9. Jayaraman, S., Rastogi, D.: Security and compliance in multi-cloud environments: approaches and solutions. JOUR. **11** (2024)
10. J. Kumar, M. Kumar, D. Kumar, and R. Raj, "Encryption and authentication of data using the IPSEC protocol," in Proceedings of the Fourth International Conference on Microelectronics, Computing and Communication Systems Lecture Notes in Electrical Engineering, Springer Nature, Singapore 2020, pp. 893–846. https://doi.org/10.1007/978-981-15-5546-6_71

11. N. Q. Tran, K. D. L. Nguyen, and C. D. T. Thai, "Implementation and evaluation of IPSec in an NFV-based network," in Communication and Intelligent Systems. ICCIS 2023 Lecture Notes in Networks and Systems, Springer Nature, Singapore, 2024, pp. 53–65. https://doi.org/10.1007/978-981-97-2053-8_4
12. Akter, H., et al.: Evaluating performances of VPN tunneling protocols based on application service requirements. In: Proceedings of the Third International Conference on Trends in Computational and Cognitive Engineering Lecture Notes in Networks and Systems, pp. 433–444. Springer Nature, Singapore (2022). https://doi.org/10.1007/978-981-16-7597-3
13. Schwenk, J.: IP security (IPsec). In: Guide to Internet Cryptography, in Information Security and Cryptography, pp. 135–190. Springer Nature (2022)
14. Marco Kwesigabo, E.: Evaluating the impact of latency on the performance of a virtual private network using different encryption algorithms and hashing. J. Inform. **4**(1), 279–293 (2024). https://doi.org/10.59645/tji.v4i1.245
15. Baksi, A., et al.: Quantum Analysis of AES (2022). [Online]. Available: https://eprint.iacr.org/2022/683
16. Munir Baig, M.H., Ul Haq, H.B., Habib, W.: A comparative analysis of aes, rsa, and 3des encryption standards based on speed and performance. MSA. **1**(1), 20–30 (2024). https://doi.org/10.31181/msa1120244
17. Abolade, O., Okandeji, A., Oke, A., Osifeko, M., Oyedeji, A.: Overhead effects of data encryption on TCP throughput across IPSEC secured network. Sci. Afr. **13** (2021). https://doi.org/10.1016/j.sciaf.2021.e00855
18. Chung, J.-M.: TCP/IP protocols and IP routing. In: Emerging Secure Networks, Blockchains and Smart Contract Technologies. Springer (2024). https://doi.org/10.1007/978-3-031-65866-2_4
19. Furkan Altınok, K., Peker, A., Tezcan, C., Temizel, A.: GPU accelerated 3DES encryption. Concurr. Comput. Pract. Exp. **34**(9) (2021). https://doi.org/10.1002/cpe.6507
20. Woodberg, B., Krishnamurthy Madwachar, M., Swarm, M., Wyler, N.R., Albers, M., Bonnell, R.: Configuring Juniper networks netscreen & SSG firewalls. In: Configuring Juniper Networks Netscreen & SSG Firewalls, pp. 551–586 (2007). https://doi.org/10.1016/B978-159749118-1/50013-7
21. Jang, K., et al.: Quantum Implementation and Analysis of SHA-2 and SHA-3 (2024). [Online]. Available: https://ia.cr/2024/513
22. Sentala, B.: Evaluation of the Effectiveness and Efficiency of Compression and Decompression of IP Packets in a Wireless Local Area Network, Master Degree Thesis, The University of Zambia, Lusaka (2022). [Online]. Available: http://dspace.unza.zm/handle/123456789/8021

# Dynamic and Explainable Federated Learning for IoT Anomaly Detection: A Comparative Study with Centralized Machine Learning Models

Alend Jarjis[1,2](✉) and Yaşar Becerikli[3]

[1] Faculty of Engineering, Department of Computer Engineering, Kocaeli University, Kocaeli, Turkey
alend.jarjis@su.edu.krd
[2] Department of Mathematics, College of Education, Salahaddin University, Erbil, Iraq
[3] Department of Digital Forensics Specialization, Institution of Forensic Medicine, Istanbul, Turkey
ybecerikli@kocaeli.edu.tr

**Abstract.** This paper presents a comparative analysis of centralized and federated learning (FL) methods for Internet of Things (IoT) anomaly detection, emphasizing model transparency explainability. We simulate a five-client FL setup using real-world IoT datasets to assess how model interpretation changes between local and global aggregation. Our results reveal that while centralized models capture global feature importance effectively, FL introduces inconsistencies due to data heterogeneity and local overfitting. Analysis shows feature drift across clients, while highlighting local decision logic variations. The findings underline the trade-off between privacy-preserving collaborative learning and model interpretability, which is essential for securing IoT networks.

**Keywords:** Federated Learning · IoT Anomaly Detection · Machine Learning · SHAP · Lime · Explainable AI

## 1 Introduction

Although FL overcomes some ML challenges, it also encounters constraints like non-IID data distributions, communication overhead, and reduced interpretability compared to centralized models [1]. For mission-critical applications in domains such as smart homes and industrial IoT, interpretability is indispensable for alert validation, user trust, and root cause analysis. Explainable AI (XAI) techniques such as [2, 3], provide powerful tools for interpreting internal decisions made by complex models.

At the heart of most modern anomaly detection frameworks lies explainability. However, prediction in the context of outlier detection in IoT devices is much more complicated than traditional classification, as IoT must re-evaluate evolving patterns of attack and adversarial behaviors. [2, 3] offer fine granularity in terms of how flow duration,


K. Daimi and A. Alsadoon (Eds.): ICR 2025, LNNS 1487, pp. 211–227, 2025.
https://doi.org/10.1007/978-3-031-95652-2_19

byte count, or protocol type impact detection decisions, for example. Real-time deployment and adherence to security governance standards necessitate this transparency. We hope to assist domain experts by combining these methods to ensure the relevancy and fairness of the inferences through the projection of a rationally active model.

Our approach leverages the strengths of both centralized and federated models and our findings are cross-validated on three different and diverse datasets. The Enriching IoT Datasets [4], provide refined features derived from raw packet data, while CIC-BCCC-NRC-TabularIoTAttacks-2024 [5], presents a structured tabular format for IoT attack data, and CICIoV2024 [6], covers vehicular IoT traffic with current threats. With this diversity, our Models have a high generalization on different domains, thus confirming our approach which combines FL, ML and explainability, provides robust and interpretable anomaly detection systems.

## 2 Contributions

1. We have developed a dynamic FL framework (Dynamic Federated Learning Framework for IoT) which is capable of handling heterogeneous client data distribution and non-IID datasets.
2. Multi-Dataset Comparative Analysis: We perform comprehensive experimental examinations on three data sources establishing the robustness of our framework across a variety of domains and attack vectors.
3. FL and ML Model Explainability: We enhance both centralized ML and FL Streams with local and global interpretability. These methods provide transparency by explaining the model, enabling domain experts to analyze make sense of detections, and help validate that detection decisions are accurate.
4. Performance Benchmark versus Centralized ML: We evaluate federated learning models versus centralized classifiers.

## 3 Literature Review

McMahan et al. [7] This seminal work presented the Federated Averaging (FedAvg) algorithm, which facilitates efficient learning in a distributed setting by collecting the local updates. 4 sets of datasets are experimented on this work; balanced; unbalanced, IID and non-IID data. It tackled issues such as non-IID (non-identically distributed) data and unbalanced datasets, all well-known challenges in IoT contexts. It enhanced communication efficiency yet poor scalability in highly heterogeneous networks thus paving a way to boost FL frameworks on set up dedicated to IoT deployments. Weinger et al. [8] focuses on FL applications for anomaly detection in IoT systems. Ton-IoT and DS2OS datasets were used in this work. All focus is put on improving the scalability of FL via the following techniques, but constrained by end device capabilities' heterogeneity. In this work [9], present a gated recurrent units (GRU)-based framework for the detection of anomaly in FL context. It utilizes the dataset based on the Modbus network. Models are trained on the devices of IoT which maintains the privacy as well as lessens the dependency on the centralization. Although this approach preserves privacy, it still poses a challenge due to high computational overheads in low-power settings. Related studies [10], aims at enhancing the security and the privacy of FL-based IoT anomaly detection systems in certain fields of concern such as smart grid infrastructures. While a successful approach to mitigating data leakage, it indicates constraints on the communication costs for the deployment of such systems for real-time IoTs. The proposed work framework uses blockchain to facilitate decentralized techniques. Disadvantages of this study could be increased latency as a result of encryption overhead, and it is less flexible for heterogeneous IoT devices. This article [11] studies existing research on privacy preserving anomaly detection in FL, and provides insights on improving conventional anomaly detection approaches. It uses Multidimensional Toy Dataset to experience tests in this work. The recent survey [13], uses FL for IoT intrusion detection and discusses decentralized anomaly detection efforts. It highlighted the challenges the researchers face with this type of intrusion detection method. The present review showed the lack of data diversity reporting when they used four metrics such as dataset type, performance metrics and an approach they adopted across studies. The work in [14] ends up having a design for IIoT real-time anomaly detection with the combination of edge computing and federated learning. In addition, It has a lower communication cost and a higher detection accuracy than other methods, especially for industrial applications with latency constraints. Performance metrics were attempted to fill in the improvements in performance of centralized traditional models. In this paper [15], a communication-efficient federated learning framework for time-series anomaly detection is proposed. Additionally, this method utilizes distributed machine deep learning models across multiple devices, thus protecting data privacy as well as providing accurate output. This paper [16] applies deep leaning on resource efficient IoT networks for anomaly detection while addressing the relevant privacy issues. This study poses a compression-based optimization problem using multilayer and node neural networks. Despite its advantages in resource efficiency, the complexity inherent in neural networks creates scalability issues. This explainable framework facilitates scalability and interpretability, making it more fit for differing IoT situations. In this paper [17] a framework using federated learning based on the concept of edge computing to s anomalies in 5G networks in real-time is proposed. The SYRROCA framework is employed to reduce delivery time and improve detection performance. However, the study suffers challenges in terms of heterogeneous data handling and network latency. Related work is a basis for the proposed work to carry out a comparative analysis with centralized models that exhibit poor scalability and less adaptability of dynamic and explainable framework in various IoT scenarios.

## 4 Datasets and Preprocessing

We utilized three diverse IoT datasets to ensure wide generalizability and domain coverage:

- Enriching IoT Datasets: Synthesized from Bot-IoT and ToN-IoT logs, this dataset includes enriched features from NetFlow and packet captures. It supports multi-class attack types including DDoS, DoS, and scanning, the target attack categories are re-assigned as in [17], six target attack categories and remapped them to numeric labels (0 to 5). This harmonization allowed consistent comparison across datasets and models.

- CIC-BCCC-NRC-TabularIoTAttacks-2024: This dataset provides comprehensive, structured, and labeled tabular data encompassing a wide range of IoT attack scenarios across multiple domains. It consolidates and harmonizes data from eight foundational benchmark datasets. The raw dataset includes 2 classes benign and attack. This paper distributed the labels to major anomaly patterns—DoS, Spoofing-Gas, Spoofing-RPM, Spoofing-Speed, Spoofing-Steering Wheel, and Benign were retained. They were mapped to numeric labels 0 to 5 accordingly.
- CICIoV2024: Focused on vehicular IoT, this dataset comprises telemetry and communication flow details relevant to autonomous and connected cars. It simulates threats such as Spoofing-Gas, Spoofing-RPM, Spoofing-Speed, Spoofing-Steering Wheel, DoS, and Benign traffic classes. The structure provides a comprehensive view of mobility-centric IoT security challenges.

Each dataset was preprocessed as follows:

- Cleaning: Duplicate entries and columns with more than 50% missing data were removed. Remaining nulls in numerical columns were imputed using median values, and categorical ones with mode.
- Encoding: Label encoding was applied to all categorical fields.
- Normalization: Feature scaling was performed using Min-Max normalization:

$$x' = \frac{x - x_{min}}{x_{max} - x_{min}} \tag{1}$$

where:

- x is the original feature value,
- $x_{min}$ is the minimum value of the feature,
- $x_{max}$ is the maximum value of the feature,
- x′ is the normalized value scaled to the range [0,1][0,1][0,1].

- Balancing: In centralized ML, class imbalance was addressed using resample to up-sample minority classes. In FL, each client retained the local distribution of labels without balancing to reflect realistic non-IID data scenarios. This is is crucial for evaluating FL under heterogeneous conditions.

# 5 Methodology

## 5.1 Centralized Machine Learning

The centralized ML framework, applied in this study incorporates systematic preprocessing, modeling, and interpretability steps tailored to enhance anomaly detection in IoT environments. Data from three benchmark IoT datasets. Following preprocessing, the data was partitioned into 80% training and 20% testing subsets. Various traditional ML models were trained and evaluated using several measurements.

In the centralized ML pipeline, a variety of classical and ensemble models were applied to the preprocessed datasets:

- Logistic Regression (LR): A linear baseline used for multiclass classification.
- Support Vector Machines (SVM): Kernel-based model to handle high-dimensional feature spaces.
- Random Forest (RF): A tree-based ensemble model known for its robustness to overfitting and interpretability.
- XGBoost (XGB): An optimized gradient boosting framework offering superior accuracy and handling of missing values.
- Voting Classifier: A soft-voting ensemble combining the above models for enhanced performance.

Explainability was introduced using SHAP and LIME to reveal feature contributions and improve model transparency. SHAP values were calculated using TreeExplainer or KernelExplainer depending on the model type. LIME provides local explanations for specific samples using surrogate interpretable models.

SHAP calculates the feature impact on prediction f(x) as follows:

$$f(x) = \varphi_0 + \sum_{i=1}^{n} \varphi_i x_i \tag{2}$$

where

n: The number of input features or variables
$\varphi_i$: The weight or coefficient corresponding to the i-th input feature $x_i$
$x_i$: The i-th feature of your input vector x
$\varphi_i$ represents the contribution of the i-th feature.

LIME approximates the black-box model locally using a linear surrogate model g(x) fitted on a perturbed sample set X':

$$g(x) = w^{\top} x + w_0 \tag{3}$$

where:

- $w^{\top}$ is the dot product between the weight vector w and input vector x
- $w_0$ is still the bias term (Fig. 1)

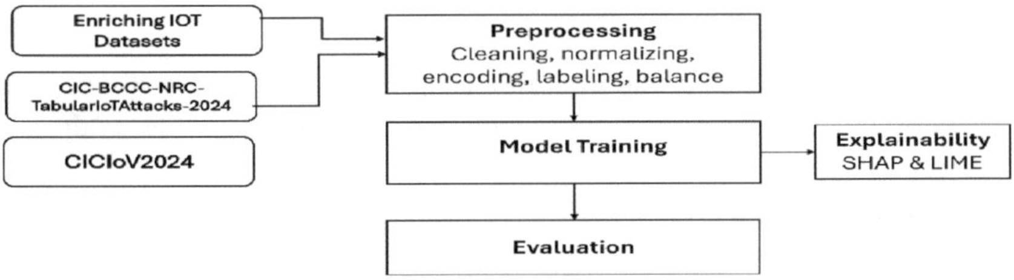


**Fig. 1.** Centralized and Explainable Machine Learning Workflow for IoT Anomaly Detection

### 5.2 Federated Learning (FL)

In contrast to centralized approaches, the federated learning (FL) paradigm Fig. 2, enables collaborative model training across distributed IoT devices (clients) without sharing raw data [17]. This is particularly suitable for sensitive environments like smart homes, industrial systems, and vehicular networks, where data privacy and regulatory constraints prevent centralization.

- Each IoT dataset was horizontally partitioned among five simulated clients, preserving label distribution using stratified sampling [11].
- Each client trains its local model using supervised learning.
- After local training, client models are sent to the central server to be aggregated via Federated models.
- After each global aggregation round, the updated global model is evaluated on a centralized test set.
- To interpret FL outcomes, we employ SHAP on client-level models. SHAP assigns feature importance values to each input.

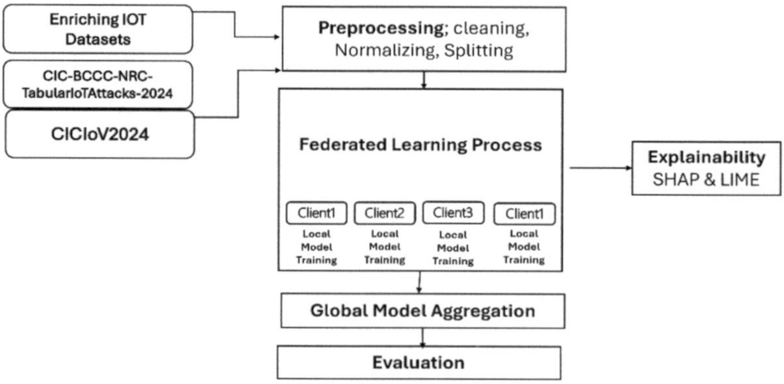


**Fig. 2.** Explainable FL Workflow for IoT Anomaly Detection

## 6 Evaluation and Experiments

This section outlines the modeling strategies, algorithms used, evaluation metrics, and the rationale for model selection in both centralized ML and federated FL settings.

### 6.1 Performance Evaluation

To assess model performance comprehensively across both Federated Learning (FL) and Centralized Machine Learning (ML) paradigms, five key prementioned metrics were employed. Accuracy, Precision, Recall, and F1-Score (macro-averaged for multi-class handling), ROC-AUC (One-vs-Rest strategy). Despite slight performance trade-offs, Federated Learning achieves near-parity with ML while offering decentralized privacy benefits. These results show that FL is a viable approach in IoT settings, especially when privacy and data locality are concerns.

Voting classifier consistently outperformed others in centralized ML across all datasets, reaching up to 99.95% accuracy in the Enriching dataset and 99.89% in CICIoV2024. Among federated learning models, FedAvg achieved the highest accuracy (98.32%–99.35%), followed closely by FedProx and FedSGD. The performance drop from centralized ML to FL is minimal, showing the strong potential of FL in privacy-preserving IoT anomaly detection. Compared to traditional ML (e.g., Logistic Regression, SVM), FL models such as FedAvg even outperform or match them in some scenarios, especially in datasets like CIC-BCCC.

The centralized ML approaches perform best in terms of raw accuracy. However, FL models especially FedAvg and FedProx—demonstrate impressive accuracy under privacy-preserving, decentralized conditions, making them highly promising for IoT deployments.

### 6.2 Stability Evaluation

To check the stability of the results, (standard deviation) and (means) are calculated as follows:

We split the dataset into 5 equal parts (folds). So it:

- Train the model on 4 folds
- Test it on the remaining fold
- Repeat this 5 times (each time a different fold is the test set)

Table 1, presents both the mean and standard deviation from 5-fold cross-validation, highlighting model stability. Centralized models like XGBoost ($0.9993 \pm 0.0006$) and Voting Classifier ($0.9992 \pm 0.0002$) show excellent accuracy with minimal variance. Federated models such as FedAvg ($0.9994 \pm 0.0012$) and FedProx ($0.9976 \pm 0.0012$) also perform well, though FedSGD exhibits slightly higher variability ($0.9904 \pm 0.0052$). Overall, the low standard deviations confirm the strong consistency and robustness across models.

Table 2, The cross-validation results demonstrate high stability across both centralized and federated models. Centralized models such as XGBoost ($0.9993 \pm 0.0004$) and Voting Classifier ($0.9992 \pm 0.0002$) achieve near-perfect accuracy with minimal variance. Logistic Regression and SVM also show consistent performance with standard deviations below 0.001. Among federated models, FedAvg and FedProx perform comparably well ($0.9974 \pm 0.0008$), while FedSGD shows slightly lower accuracy ($0.9964 \pm 0.0005$). These low standard deviations confirm the reliability and robustness of all models across different data splits.

Table 3, The models demonstrate high accuracy with varying stability. Centralized models like Voting Classifier ($0.9944 \pm 0.0012$) and Random Forest ($0.9955 \pm 0.0016$) perform consistently well. SVM and Logistic Regression show lower but stable results ($0.9886 \pm 0.0006$). Federated models, especially FedAvg and FedProx ($0.9872 \pm$

**Table 1.** Enriching dataset evaluation results for both ML and FL models

| Model | Accuracy | Precision | Recall | F1-Score | ROC AUC | Accuracy (mean ± std) |
|---|---|---|---|---|---|---|
| Random Forest | 0.9979 | 0.9979 | 0.9979 | 0.9979 | 0.9978 | 0.9972±0.0006 |
| SVM | 0.9965 | 0.9966 | 0.9965 | 0.9965 | 0.9963 | 0.9978±0.0004 |
| Logistic Regression | 0.9948 | 0.995 | 0.9948 | 0.9949 | 0.9947 | 0.9952±0.0008 |
| XGBoost | 0.9983 | 0.9984 | 0.9983 | 0.9983 | 0.9983 | 0.9993±0.0006 |
| Voting Classifier | 0.9985 | 0.9985 | 0.9985 | 0.9985 | 0.9984 | 0.9992±0.0002 |
| FedAvg | 0.9972 | 0.9971 | 0.9972 | 0.9972 | 0.997 | 0.9994±0.0012 |
| FedSGD | 0.9961 | 0.996 | 0.9961 | 0.9961 | 0.996 | 0.9904±0.0052 |
| FedProx | 0.9968 | 0.9967 | 0.9968 | 0.9968 | 0.9966 | 0.9976±0.0012 |

**Table 2.** -BCCC-NRC datasets evaluation results for FL and ML models

| Model | Accuracy | Precision | Recall | F1-Score | ROC AUC | Accuracy (mean ± std) |
|---|---|---|---|---|---|---|
| Random Forest | 0.9941 | 0.9943 | 0.9941 | 0.9942 | 0.9939 | 0.9992±0.0003 |
| SVM | 0.9928 | 0.993 | 0.9928 | 0.9929 | 0.9925 | 0.9978±0.0004 |
| Logistic Regression | 0.9902 | 0.9904 | 0.9902 | 0.9903 | 0.99 | 0.9972±0.0009 |
| XGBoost | 0.9945 | 0.9947 | 0.9945 | 0.9946 | 0.9943 | 0.9993±0.0004 |
| Voting Classifier | 0.9951 | 0.9953 | 0.9951 | 0.9952 | 0.9949 | 0.9992±0.0002 |
| FedAvg | 0.993 | 0.9931 | 0.993 | 0.993 | 0.9927 | 0.9974±0.0008 |
| FedSGD | 0.9912 | 0.9913 | 0.9912 | 0.9912 | 0.991 | 0.9964±0.0005 |
| FedProx | 0.9926 | 0.9928 | 0.9926 | 0.9927 | 0.9923 | 0.9974±0.0008 |

0.0027), perform competitively but with slightly higher variability. Overall, centralized models offer slightly better consistency (Fig. 3).

### 6.3 Federated Learning Deployment Considerations in IoT Environments

To address real-time applicability and resource efficiency, we evaluated the computational and communication overhead of FL rounds across three representative IoT datasets. Table 4 summarizes the latency, model size, communication cost, and system usage metrics during a single FL round. The CICIoV dataset exhibited the most

**Table 3.** CICIoV2024 datasets evaluation results for FL and ML models

| Model | Accuracy | Precision | Recall | F1-Score | ROC AUC | Accuracy (mean ± std) |
|---|---|---|---|---|---|---|
| Random Forest | 0.9967 | 0.9968 | 0.9967 | 0.9967 | 0.9965 | 0.9955±0.0016 |
| SVM | 0.995 | 0.9952 | 0.995 | 0.9951 | 0.9948 | 0.9886±0.0006 |
| Logistic Regression | 0.9932 | 0.9934 | 0.9932 | 0.9933 | 0.993 | 0.9886±0.0006 |
| XGBoost | 0.9971 | 0.9972 | 0.9971 | 0.9971 | 0.997 | 0.9947±0.0020 |
| Voting Classifier | 0.9975 | 0.9976 | 0.9975 | 0.9976 | 0.9974 | 0.9944±0.0012 |
| FedAvg | 0.9957 | 0.9959 | 0.9957 | 0.9958 | 0.9956 | 0.9872±0.0027 |
| FedSGD | 0.9945 | 0.9947 | 0.9945 | 0.9946 | 0.9944 | 0.9886±0.0006 |
| FedProx | 0.9953 | 0.9955 | 0.9953 | 0.9954 | 0.9952 | 0.9872±0.0027 |

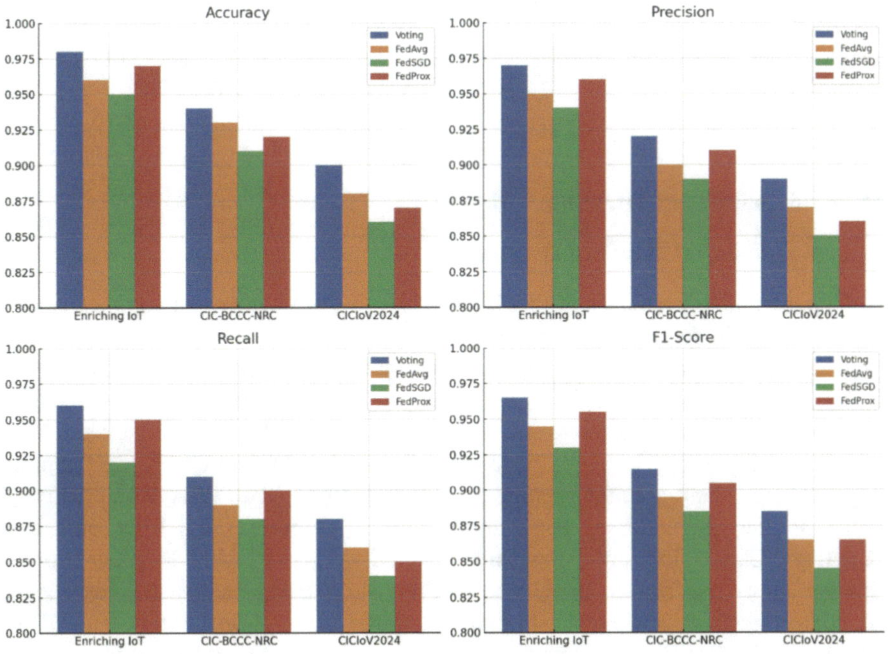


**Fig. 3.** Comparative evaluation result (FL and ML) over three used datasets

lightweight profile, with a latency of only 0.0465 seconds per round, 3.52 KB communication overhead, and minimal CPU (0.6%) and RAM (3.7%) usag highlighting its suitability for constrained edge devices. In contrast, the Enriching IoT dataset incurred a higher cost, with 0.0857 seconds latency, 16.95 KB communication, and significantly elevated CPU usage (97%), indicating increased complexity due to richer feature diversity or larger sample size. The CIC-BCCC-NRC 2024 dataset balanced between the two, with moderate latency (0.1716 s) and CPU usage (86.9%), while maintaining low memory consumption (1.54%). These findings demonstrate that Federated Learning can be feasibly deployed in edge-centric IoT environments, with communication and latency budgets remaining within acceptable bounds for periodic aggregation. However, system resource demands vary across datasets, suggesting the need for dataset-aware optimization strategies in practical deployment.

**Table 4:** Deployment Considerations

| | FL Round Latency (s) | Model Size per Client (KB) | Total Communication per Round (KB) | CPU Usage (%) | RAM Usage (%) |
|---|---|---|---|---|---|
| CICIoV Dataset | 0.0465 | 0.35 | 3.52 | 0.6 | 3.7 |
| Enriching IoT datasets | 0.0857 | 1.7 | 16.95 | 97.0 | 20.6 |
| CCC-BCCC-NRC Tabular attacks 2024 | 0.1716 | 1.15 | 5.75 | 86.9 | 1.54 |

## 6.4 Explainability of ML and FL Models

(a) **Explainability (CICIoV2024 datasets)**

Explainability in federated learning (FL) environments exhibits greater complexity than in centralized ML due to data heterogeneity and localized model updates. In centralized ML (Fig. 4), LIME plots reveal strong and consistent feature contributions across classes, such as DATA_7 and DATA_3 in Class 5, which positively influenced classification, whereas in Class 1, the same features suppressed the decision. This reflects the centralized model's stability, having access to the full data distribution. In contrast, FL explainability (Fig. 5) shows client-specific interpretation, with features like DATA_7 and DATA_4 switching roles across classes. For example, DATA_7 supports Class 1 but suppresses Class 0 and Class 3, indicating contextual sensitivity driven by local data distributions. This variability can lead to conflicting SHAP or LIME explanations across clients, potentially reducing decision robustness in distributed intrusion detection systems (IDS). High LIME fidelity scores (Table 5), ranging from 0.9545 to 1.0000, indicate strong alignment between local feature attribution and model behavior per client, especially with simpler models like logistic regression.

Explainability was applied on the test set to reflect generalization. SHAP Fig. 6, captured global feature importance, identifying DATA_2 as consistently influential with stable and moderate impact (SHAP values in −0.2 to 0.2).

(b) **Explainability of (Enriching IoT dataset)**

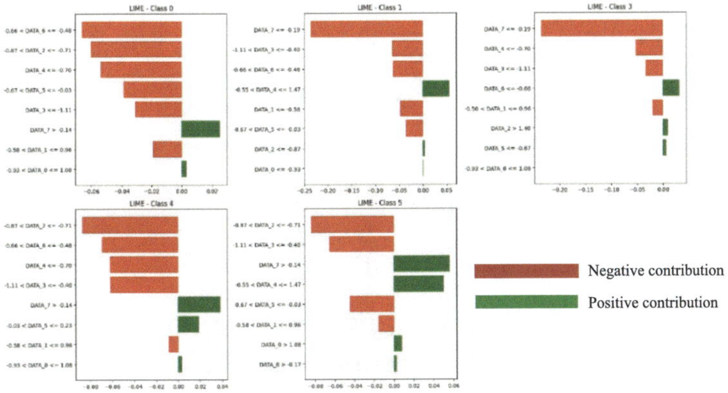


**Fig. 4.** LIME results of CICIoV2024 datasets

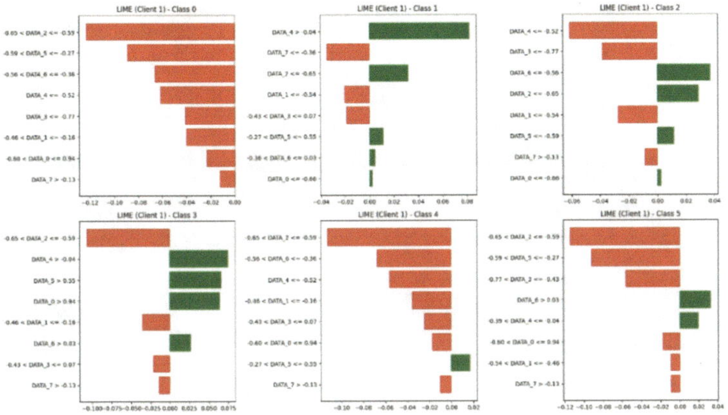


**Fig. 5.** LIME for client-1 over all classes in FL

**Table 5.** LIME fidelity of local explanation

| Client 1 | Client 2 | Client 3 | Client 4 | Client 5 |
|---|---|---|---|---|
| 1.0000 | 1.0000 | 0.9625 | 1.0000 | 0.9545 |

FL plots (e.g., FedAvg) show more nuanced and variable explanations across classes Fig. 7 The feature impacts are subtler and less polarized, with contributions shifting direction depending on the class and client-specific data. Features such as TCP, UDP, and HTTP show both supporting and suppressing behavior across classes. This reflects FL's decentralized nature, where local data variation leads to more context-dependent reasoning, offering diversity but slightly less transparency than centralized ML.

Moreover, SHAP global explanations (Figs. 6 and 9) revealed stable importance for features like DATA_2 and average_flow_duration across both CICIoV and Enriching

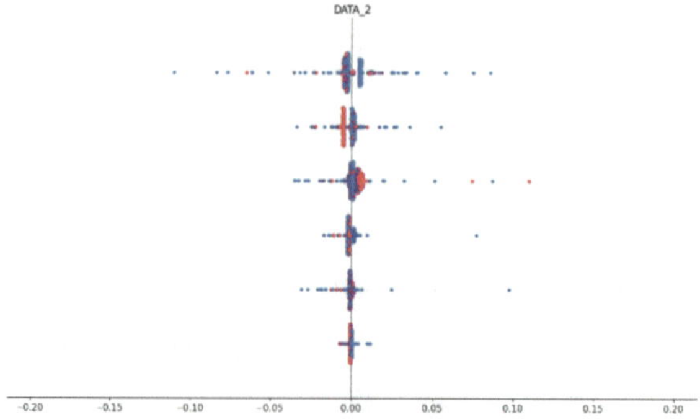


**Fig. 6.** SHAP explainable plot of CICIoV

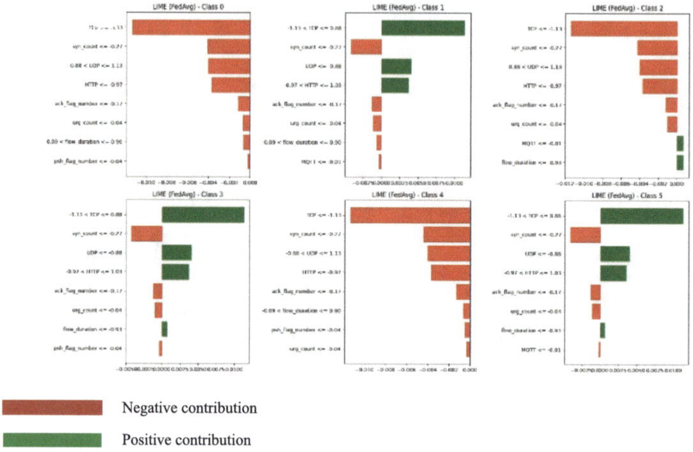


**Fig. 7.** LIME plot of FL model over classes of (Enriching IoT datasets)

IoT datasets. However, in FL models (Figs. 7 and 8), feature influence appears more subtle and variable. For instance, TCP and UDP alternated between supporting and suppressing roles depending on the class and client, highlighting FL's decentralized and context-specific nature. While this diversity enriches the model's adaptability to local patterns, it also complicates global interpretability. This discrepancy underscores a trade-off: FL fosters privacy and local generalization but may suffer from lower interpretability consensus across clients. Thus, client-specific SHAP or LIME explanations must be interpreted with caution, and mechanisms for aggregating or aligning interpretability across clients are essential for trust in federated IDS applications.

Table 6, The LIME fidelity scores across five federated clients indicate varying degrees of alignment between local explanations and actual model behavior, ranging from 0.5770 (Client 3) to 0.9578 (Client 4). These values reflect how faithfully LIME captures the decision logic of each client's model. The lower fidelity for Client 3 suggests higher local data heterogeneity or less stable patterns, consistent with earlier observations of SHAP variability and context-sensitive feature contributions. This supports the

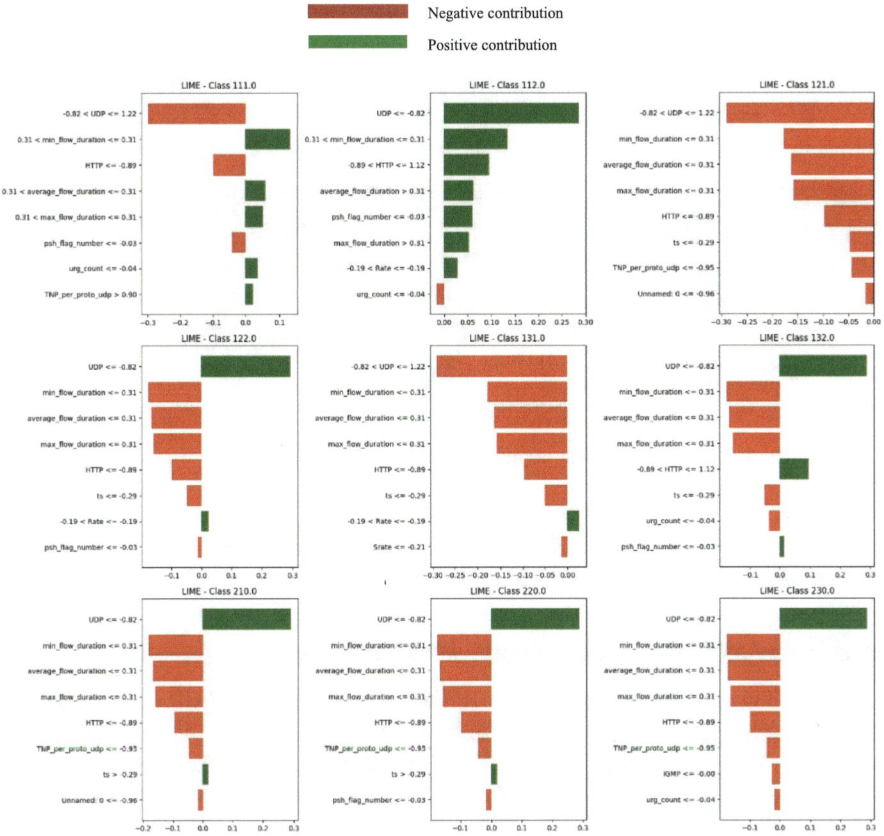


**Fig. 8.** LIME of raw classes of enriching IoT datasets

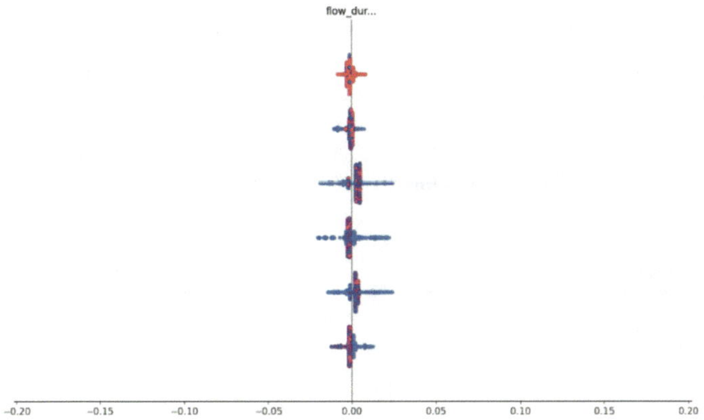


**Fig. 9.** SHAP of (Enriching IoT datasets)

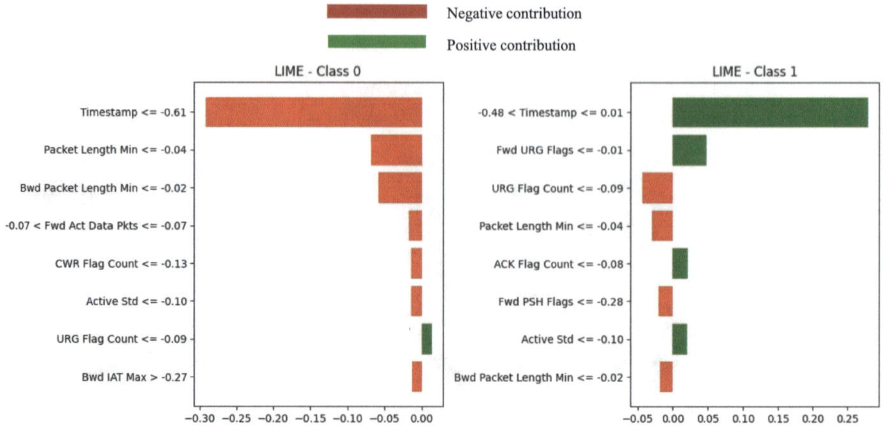


**Fig. 10.** LIME local explanation of the basic raw classes (Tabular IoT attacks 2024)

broader analysis that explainability in FL is influenced by client-specific data distributions, reinforcing the need to interpret local explanations within their deployment context.

(c) **Explainability of (Tabular IoT attack2024 datasets)**

Figure 10 showcases local LIME explanations for two sample predictions—Class 0 and Class 1—highlighting how individual features influence the classification decision in the Tabular IoT Attack 2024 dataset. For Class 0, the feature *Timestamp <= –0.61* demonstrates a strong negative contribution, indicating that the model is discouraged from assigning samples to this class when timestamps are extremely low. Conversely, in Class 1, the feature *–0.48 < Timestamp <= 0.01* exerts a strong positive influence (green bar), significantly increasing the likelihood of a sample being classified as Class 1. Additional features such as *Fwd URG Flags*, *ACK Flag Count*, and *Active Std* also show moderate support, contributing positively but with less impact than timestamp. These results illustrate how the model leverages temporal and flag-based features to distinguish between subtle attack patterns in the dataset.

**Table 6.** LIME fidelity scores over 5 clients of FL

| Client 1 | Client 2 | Client 3 | Client 4 | Client 5 |
|---|---|---|---|---|
| 0.8623 | 0.8564 | 0.5770 | 0.9578 | 0.7821 |

To assess the reliability of these local explanations, we calculated LIME fidelity scores across five simulated clients. Clients 4 and 5 exhibit high fidelity, reflecting strong agreement between the surrogate LIME model and the federated classifier Table 7. However, Client 3's low fidelity score (0.3000) suggests significant divergence, which may stem from local data imbalance or model inconsistency. This variation in fidelity highlights the need for careful interpretability assessment in federated environments, as inconsistent explanations could undermine user trust and complicate the deployment of distributed intrusion detection systems.

**Table 7.** LIME fidelity over clients in FL (Tabular IoT Attacks 2024 datasets)

| Client 1 | Client 2 | Client 3 | Client 4 | Client 5 |
|---|---|---|---|---|
| 0.7624 | 0.8564 | 0.3000 | 0.9588 | 0.9821 |

## 7 Conclusion and Future Work

This study presented a comprehensive comparison between centralized machine learning and federated learning (FL) models for IoT anomaly detection, highlighting not only classification performance but also explainability and deployment feasibility. While centralized models demonstrated consistent and globally interpretable decisions, FL models showed more context-sensitive behaviors across clients. LIME and SHAP analyses revealed variations in local feature importance and explainability fidelity, with some clients exhibiting lower alignment due to data heterogeneity. Nonetheless, fidelity scores remained acceptably high, supporting the use of local interpretability methods in distributed settings. Furthermore, we addressed practical deployment concerns by measuring FL round latency, communication overhead, and resource usage on edge devices across multiple datasets. The results confirmed that FL can be efficiently deployed in real-time IoT environments, with manageable computational costs. These insights demonstrate the robustness, transparency, and deployability of the proposed FL framework, making it a viable solution for privacy-preserving anomaly detection in heterogeneous IoT systems.

**Suggestions for Future Work:**

- Incorporate deep learning models (e.g., CNN, LSTM, GNN) in the FL context and test their explainability.
- Extend to edge-device resource-constrained environments and benchmark latency and memory.
- Explore cross-device FL settings with real-time anomaly streaming.
- Apply causal inference to understand attack propagation and model reasoning chains across clients.

## References


1. Kairouz, P., McMahan, H.B., Avent, B., Bellet, A., Bennis, M., Bhagoji, A.N., Bonawitz, K., Charles, Z., Cormode, G., Cummings, R., et al.: Advances and open problems in federated learning. Found. Trends® Mach. Learn. **14**, 1–210 (2021)
2. Lundberg, S.M., Lee, S.-I.: A unified approach to interpreting model predictions. Adv. Neural Inf. Proces. Syst. **30** (2017)
3. Ribeiro, M.T., Singh, S., Guestrin, C.: Model-agnostic interpretability of machine learning. arXiv preprint arXiv:1606.05386 (2016)
4. Erfani, M., Shoeleh, F., Dadkhah, S., Kaur, B., Xiong, P., Iqbal, S., Ray, S., Ghorbani, A.A.: A feature exploration approach for IoT attack type classification. In: 2021 IEEE Intl Conf on Dependable, Autonomic and Secure Computing, Intl Conf on Pervasive Intelligence and Computing, Intl Conf on Cloud and Big Data Computing, Intl Conf on Cyber Science and Technology Congress (DASC/PiCom/CBDCom/CyberSciTech) (2021)
5. Sasi, T., Lashkari, A.H., Lu, R., Xiong, P., Iqbal, S.: An efficient self attention-based 1D-CNN-LSTM network for IoT attack detection and identification using network traffic. J. Inform. Intell. (2024)
6. Neto, E.C.P., Taslimasa, H., Dadkhah, S., Iqbal, S., Xiong, P., Rahman, T., Ghorbani, A.A.: CICIoV2024: advancing realistic IDS approaches against DoS and spoofing attack in IoV CAN bus. Internet of Things **26**, 101209 (2024)
7. McMahan, B., Moore, E., Ramage, D., Hampson, S., y Arcas, B.A.: Communication-efficient learning of deep networks from decentralized data. In: Artificial Intelligence and Statistics (2017)
8. Weinger, B., Kim, J., Sim, A., Nakashima, M., Moustafa, N., Wu, K.J.: Enhancing IoT anomaly detection performance for federated learning. Digit Commun Netw. **8**, 314–323 (2022)
9. Mothukuri, V., Khare, P., Parizi, R.M., Pouriyeh, S., Dehghantanha, A., Srivastava, G.: Federated-learning-based anomaly detection for IoT security attacks. IEEE Internet Things J. **9**, 2545–2554 (2021)
10. Cui, L., Qu, Y., Xie, G., Zeng, D., Li, R., Shen, S., Yu, S.: Security and privacy-enhanced federated learning for anomaly detection in IoT infrastructures. IEEE Trans. Industr. Inform. **18**, 3492–3500 (2021)
11. Zhang, C., et al.: Anomaly detection and defense techniques in federated learning: a comprehensive review. Artif. Intell. Rev. **57**(6), 150 (2024)
12. Isma'ila, U.A., Danyaro, K.U., Muazu, A.A., Maiwada, U.D.: Review on approaches of federated modeling in anomaly-based intrusion detection for IoT devices. IEEE Access **12**, 30941–30961 (2024)
13. Haldikar, S.V., Kader, O.F.M.A., Yekollu, R.K.: Edge computing and federated learning for real-time anomaly detection in industrial internet of things (IIOT). In: 2024 International Conference on Inventive Computation Technologies (ICICT) (2024)
14. Liu, X., Abdelhakim, M., Krishnamurthy, P., Tipper, D.: Identifying malicious nodes in multi-hop iot networks using dual link technologies and unsupervised learning. Open J. IoT (OJIOT) **4**, 109–125 (2018)
15. Gkillas, A., Lalos, A.: Resource efficient federated learning for deep anomaly detection in industrial IoT applications. In: 2023 24th International Conference on Digital Signal Processing (DSP) (2023)

16. Ruba, S.B., Yellas, N.E.-H., Secci, S.: Anomaly detection for 5g softwarized infrastructures with federated learning. In: 2022 1st International Conference on 6G Networking (6GNet) (2022)
17. Jarjis, A.H., Alzubaidi, N.Y.S., Pehlivanoğlu, M.K.: Cyber Attacks Classification on Enriching IoT Datasets. EAI Endorsed Trans. IoT. **9**(3), e2 (2023)

# Secure AI-Integrated Classroom Assistant for Intelligent Educational Support

Elena Kakoulli[1,2(✉)], Salomi Evripidou[1], and Eleftherios Zacharioudakis[1,3]

[1] Intelligent Systems Laboratory, Department of Computer Science, Neapolis University Pafos, Pafos, Cyprus
{e.kakoulli,salomi.evripidou,l.zacharioudakis}@nup.ac.cy
[2] Electrical Engineering and Computer Engineering and Informatics, Cyprus University of Technology, Limassol, Cyprus
[3] Igor Sikorsky Kyiv Polytechnic Institute, National Technical University of Ukraine, Kyiv, Ukraine

**Abstract.** The integration of Artificial Intelligence (AI) in education is transforming learning through real-time, intelligent support. This paper proposes an AI-powered classroom assistant using Natural Language Processing (NLP) to provide curriculum-aligned, personalized responses. By handling routine inquiries, it enhances student engagement, reduces teacher workload, and supports self-directed learning. Addressing key concerns like data privacy, scalability, and ethical AI, the framework ensures compliance with educational standards. Built on advancements in AI-driven learning tools, it offers an adaptive and inclusive system, paving the way for future research and deployment.

**Keywords:** AI in Education · Educational Technology · Natural Language Processing · Intelligent Virtual Assistants · Personalized Learning · Classroom Management · Adaptive Learning Systems · Data Privacy in Education

## 1 Introduction

The rapid advancement of Artificial Intelligence (AI) has ushered in transformative changes across various domains, including education. Schools and universities are increasingly adopting intelligent systems to improve educational delivery and efficiency. AI applications, such as intelligent tutoring systems, adaptive learning platforms, and virtual assistants, have shown significant potential in enhancing student learning and teacher productivity [1]. Despite these advancements, many classrooms still face challenges, including limited personalized support for students, teacher workload imbalances, and scalability issues in implementing AI-driven solutions [2].

Existing AI solutions often lack the flexibility and inclusivity necessary for dynamic classroom environments, particularly in primary and secondary education. Many systems are text-based, limiting accessibility for younger students or


K. Daimi and A. Alsadoon (Eds.): ICR 2025, LNNS 1487, pp. 228–242, 2025.
https://doi.org/10.1007/978-3-031-95652-2_20

those with diverse learning preferences [3]. Additionally, scalability, curriculum alignment, and compliance with data privacy regulations remain key barriers to wider adoption [4].

The need for adaptive and accessible AI tools in education is growing, particularly in light of post-pandemic shifts toward hybrid and digital learning models. An AI-powered course assistant capable of real-time voice interaction offers an innovative solution to alleviate repetitive teacher tasks, enhance student engagement, and promote self-directed learning [5].

This paper proposes a conceptual framework for an AI-powered classroom assistant that leverages NLP to deliver personalized, curriculum-specific support to students. By integrating seamlessly with existing classroom technologies, such as Learning Management Systems (LMS), the proposed assistant aims to enhance the teaching-learning experience while ensuring data privacy and scalability.

The proposed framework is designed to address key limitations of current AI systems in education. It provides a roadmap for the design, development, and deployment of intelligent assistants that support inclusive, adaptive, and efficient learning environments. The paper also addresses critical challenges, such as data security, ethical considerations, and scalability, providing a foundation for future research and development of AI-driven educational systems.

## 2 Related Work

### 2.1 AI in Education: An Overview

AI technologies have been increasingly utilized in education, with applications spanning intelligent tutoring systems, adaptive learning platforms, and virtual assistants. These tools aim to enhance student engagement, personalized learning experiences, and support teachers by automating repetitive tasks. Studies have highlighted the transformative impact of AI in K-12 education [1] and higher education [6]. For instance, González et al.[4] analyzed how AI-powered virtual assistants enhanced teamwork and problem-solving skills in software engineering courses, highlighting their applicability in STEM education [4]. Additionally, in recent years, researchers have also begun exploring the synergy between AI and other emerging technologies, such as the Internet of Things (IoT) and Educational Robotics (ER) [7]. Similarly, Mohamed [8] examined the combined use of AI and Virtual Reality (VR) in addressing complex educational challenges, emphasizing the immersive learning potential of augmented reality technologies.

### 2.2 Intelligent Virtual Assistants in Education

Intelligent Virtual Assistants (IVAs) are AI-driven tools designed to provide automated, contextual support in educational settings. These systems interact with students and teachers through various modes, including text, voice, and multimodal interfaces (e.g. combining text, voice and visuals), making them versatile for diverse classroom needs [6,9]. IVAs are widely used for answering routine questions, guiding students through problem-solving tasks, and facilitating personalized learning pathways [2,10,11].

Voice-based Intelligent Virtual Assistants (VIVAs) are a specific subset of IVAs that interact with users through natural, conversational voice interfaces. These systems provide a hands-free, engaging way for students and teachers to interact with educational content, making them particularly useful in hybrid or dynamic learning environments [7,12]. VIVAs have shown potential in enhancing student interaction and personalizing learning. For example, Katsarou et al. [13] highlighted their effectiveness in language acquisition, where they support conversational practice, improve pronunciation, and enhance grammar skills. However, current implementations often focus on specific subjects or tasks and lack generalizability across diverse educational environments. They also rely heavily on text-based input, limiting accessibility for younger students or those with special needs [5].

### 2.3 Challenges in AI Integration

While AI has made strides in education, significant challenges persist that hinder its effective integration into classrooms:

- **Scalability and Inclusivity**: Many AI tools are not designed to accommodate diverse learning preferences or varying classroom conditions [3].
- **Data Privacy and Security**: Compliance with regulations like GDPR remains a barrier. AI systems must implement robust encryption, anonymization, and secure storage practices to protect sensitive student data [4].
- **Ethical Concerns**: The implementation of AI in education intersects with elements of bias, automation, morality, privacy, fairness, and transparency, raising critical ethical questions such as algorithmic fairness and the potential for discrimination [10].
- **Curriculum and Literacy Alignment**: Embedding AI into students' everyday lives to support their cultures, goals, and educational targets remains a challenge. Along with curriculum adaptation to align with AI advancements, achieving AI literacy must be prioritized as a foundation for students to develop the competencies required in their fields [11].
- **Teacher Training and Acceptance**: Teachers often lack the technical skills and confidence to effectively adopt and integrate AI tools. Resistance to technology adoption further delays successful implementation [8].

### 2.4 Gaps and Opportunities

Although AI has demonstrated its value in automating educational processes and personalizing learning, its full potential remains untapped:

- **Lack of Real-Time Interaction**: Existing systems struggle to provide real-time responses tailored to students' immediate needs [2].

- **Limited Integration with Curriculum**: Many AI tools fail to align seamlessly with curriculum standards, limiting their practical utility in classrooms [1].
- **Teacher Workload Management**: AI systems have yet to fully address the burden of repetitive tasks on teachers, such as answering routine queries [5].
- **Challenges in Inclusivity and Accessibility**: Existing AI tools are often not designed with diverse classroom environments in mind, particularly in multilingual or under-resourced settings [13].
- **Advancing Scalability**: The development of scalable AI systems that can adapt to classrooms of varying sizes and levels of technological infrastructure offers an opportunity to broaden access to educational tools globally [11].

Recent advancements, such as platform-independent, curriculum-oriented intelligent assistants, offer promising solutions to these gaps. For instance, the work by Sajja et al. [6] demonstrated the potential of AI-driven systems to streamline course-specific tasks and reduce logistical workloads for instructors.

## 3 Proposed Framework

The proposed AI-powered classroom assistant leverages advanced NLP and Machine Learning (ML) to provide personalized, real-time support to students and teachers. This assistant is designed to integrate seamlessly with existing classroom technologies, such as LMS, enabling it to address routine student queries, reduce teacher workload, and foster self-directed learning. By offering a robust, adaptable solution, the framework addresses the challenges of modern education systems and ensures inclusivity for diverse classroom environments.

### 3.1 System Architecture

The architecture of the AI assistant comprises several key components, each designed to enhance usability and functionality:

- **User Interface (UI)**: A voice-activated gateway that enables students to interact naturally with the assistant.
- **NLP Engine**: Processes inputs, extracts intent, and identifies relevant information from a curriculum-aligned knowledge base.
- **Knowledge Base**: A curated repository aligned with the school curriculum, providing accurate and relevant answers. This knowledge base is updated regularly to ensure responses remain accurate and relevant.
- **Data Privacy Module**: Ensures adherence to General Data Protection Regulation (GDPR) and other regulations, employing encryption and anonymization to safeguard sensitive information.
- **Analytics Dashboard**: Provides actionable insights for teachers, enabling targeted interventions and personalized teaching strategies.

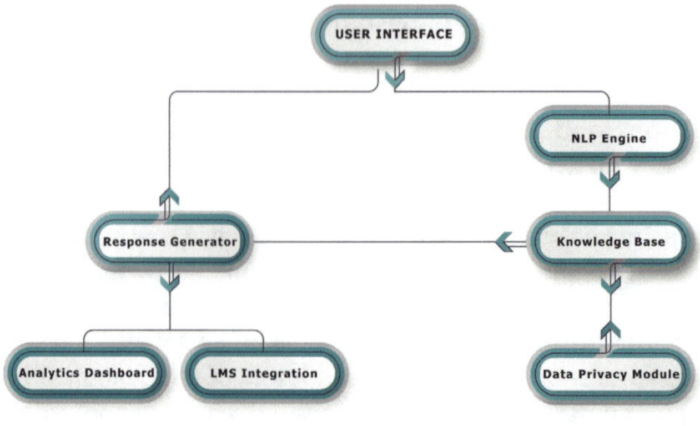


**Fig. 1.** Overall Architecture of the AI-powered Classroom Assistant.

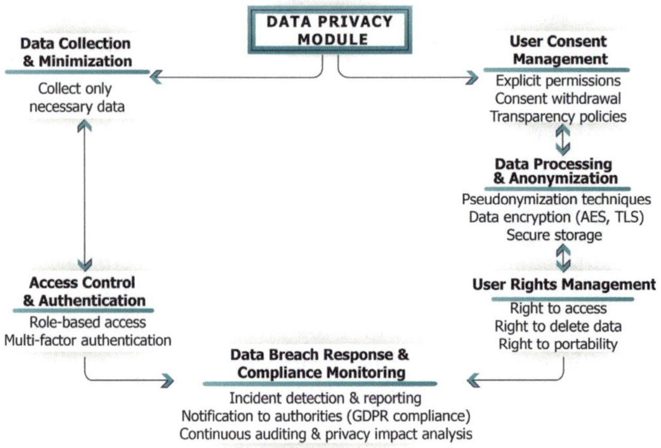


**Fig. 2.** Data Privacy Module.

Figure 1 illustrates the system's overall architecture, showcasing the integration of these components to deliver an intuitive and efficient solution for classroom education.

The architecture of the AI assistant includes a privacy module (Fig. 2) to ensure adherence to the GDPR and additional privacy regulations during data processing and user interactions. The purpose of the module is to protect user rights by establishing user trust through technical tools and organizational policies designed to safeguard sensitive information.

The initial phase of this module focuses on Data Collection & Minimization to limit the information gathered to essentials for risk reduction and user privacy protection. The AI assistant collects data strictly for operational needs, such as educational resource retrieval, and implements safeguards to prevent unnecessary accumulation. User Consent Management provides oversight of permissions granting and withdrawal, keeping users informed about their data processing status and ensuring transparency. Users can easily modify their consent preferences, such as enabling personalized learning recommendations while opting out of data sharing for research, in compliance with GDPR's lawful basis for processing under Article 6.

Data Processing & Anonymization protects information through anonymization, which completely removes personal identifiers, and pseudonymization, which replaces private identifiers with generic labels accessible only via secure storage. Additionally, strong encryption techniques, including Advanced Encryption Standard (AES) for stored data and Transport Layer Security (TLS) for transmission, ensure confidentiality and integrity regardless of location.

Moreover, Access Control & Authentication ensures that only authorized users can access data through Role-Based Access Control (RBAC), assigning permissions based on organizational roles. Security is further enhanced by Multi-Factor Authentication (MFA), requiring additional verification steps before granting access, reducing the risk of unauthorized exposure. The module provides User Rights Management, empowering individuals to access, modify, or delete their personal data in line with GDPR's user rights provisions, such as the right to rectification, erasure, and restriction of processing. Finally, Data Breach Response & Compliance Monitoring delivers real-time threat detection and rapid incident reporting, ensuring that authorities are promptly notified of breaches. Regular security audits and system updates maintain compliance with evolving regulations while reinforcing a robust privacy framework.

### 3.2 Design Principles and Key Features

The proposed framework follows three core principles: Scalability, Accessibility, and Adaptability. Scalability allows integration with various LMS platforms, ensuring support for classrooms of different sizes [1]. Accessibility ensures inclusivity through multimodal input options—voice and text—catering to diverse learning preferences [3]. Adaptability leverages ML to refine responses based on student interactions, personalizing the learning experience [2].

Table 1 summarizes the framework's key features, including real-time interaction for instant student support, data privacy compliance with GDPR regulations [4], and personalization to address individual learning needs. These features ensure the AI assistant remains secure, scalable, and adaptable, effectively transforming modern educational environments.

### 3.3 Privacy, Security, and Ethical Safeguards

Robust privacy and ethical safeguards are central to the proposed AI assistant's architecture. The system employs a multi-layered strategy to ensure data protection, bias mitigation, and compliance with educational and legal standards.

The system begins with real-time anonymization of user inputs to remove identifiable information prior to processing. Stored data is secured using AES-256 encryption, and all communication is protected using TLS protocols. Continuous

**Table 1.** Key Features and Design Principles of the Proposed Framework

| Feature | Function and Contribution |
|---|---|
| **Personalization** | Delivers tailored responses based on individual student interactions to support differentiated instruction. |
| **Real-Time Interaction** | Provides voice-activated support for immediate assistance and seamless classroom integration. |
| **Data Privacy Compliance** | Ensures GDPR adherence with encrypted data handling and privacy-aware processing pipelines. |
| **Scalability** | Accommodates a variety of classroom sizes and integrates with widely-used LMS platforms. |
| **Accessibility** | Offers voice, text, and touch inputs to support students with different learning styles and abilities. |
| **Adaptability** | Uses ML to refine responses based on classroom engagement patterns and longitudinal usage data. |

auditing of AI-generated content is enforced via curriculum filtering and human oversight, helping prevent bias and misinformation in student-facing responses [4,10].

**Table 2.** Layered Safeguards for Privacy, Security, and Ethical AI Compliance

| Mechanism | Function and Implementation Strategy |
|---|---|
| **AES-256 Encryption** | Secures stored student data using industry-grade encryption to prevent unauthorized access and ensure confidentiality. |
| **Real-Time Anonymization** | Filters identifiable information during input processing, supporting GDPR compliance through pseudonymization at runtime. |
| **Bias Auditing and Filtering** | Continuously monitors AI-generated content using curriculum-aligned rules and educator oversight to mitigate bias and misinformation. |

Figure 3 and Table 2 summarize the key safeguards integrated across the assistant's pipeline. Together, these mechanisms establish a foundation for ethical, secure, and trustworthy AI deployment in classroom environments.

### 3.4 Workflow

The workflow of the assistant involves four primary steps:

- **Query Input**: Students initiate interactions using voice commands or text inputs.

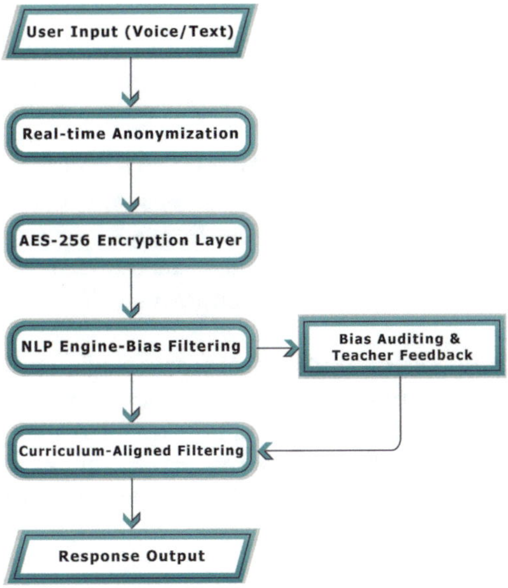


**Fig. 3.** AI Assistant Privacy and Ethical Safeguards.

- **Query Processing**: The NLP engine processes the input, identifies intent, and retrieves relevant information from the knowledge base.
- **Response Generation**: The assistant provides a contextually appropriate, curriculum-aligned response in real-time.
- **Teacher Feedback Loop**: Teachers can review the system's analytics and provide feedback to improve its performance [1].

This workflow ensures an efficient and dynamic interaction process, facilitating both student engagement and teacher oversight.

### 3.5 Technical Specifications

The proposed system employs state-of-the-art technologies to ensure robust functionality and seamless integration. Key specifications include:

- **Programming Languages**: Python for NLP and JavaScript for UI development.
- **ML Frameworks**: TensorFlow and PyTorch for training and deploying ML models.
- **Data Storage**: Cloud-based infrastructure with encryption to securely handle data.
- **Integration Tools**: APIs for seamless connectivity with LMS platforms like Google Classroom [4].

### 3.6 Implementation Details

To ensure reliable performance in real-world educational settings, the proposed assistant incorporates several practical implementation mechanisms.

- **Handling Context-Dependent Queries**: The NLP engine uses sequential dialogue history to maintain coherence across multi-turn interactions, enhancing clarity for ambiguous student inputs.
- **Knowledge Base Updates**: Content is maintained by a team of educators and engineers and refreshed in sync with curriculum revisions to ensure pedagogical accuracy.
- **Multilingual and Domain Adaptability**: While optimized for English, the architecture supports multilingual extensions via fine-tuned models and allows integration of subject-specific ontologies for domain coverage.
- **NLP Fine-Tuning**: The assistant is trained on education-specific corpora—such as lesson transcripts and instructional dialogues—to better align with classroom discourse.
- **Data Privacy and Security**: AES-256 encryption secures stored data, while GDPR compliance is enforced through pseudonymization and consent logging. Regular audits monitor adherence.
- **Adaptive Learning Mechanism**: A reinforcement learning loop refines the assistant's responses based on real classroom interactions, improving personalization and long-term system performance.

### 3.7 Implementation Roadmap

The development and deployment of the framework follow a phased implementation strategy:

- **Phase 1 - Prototype Development**: The initial phase focuses on developing the NLP engine and integrating it with a basic UI.
- **Phase 2 - Pilot Testing**: The prototype is deployed in select classrooms, allowing for feedback from teachers and students to refine the system.
- **Phase 3 - Scaling and Optimization**: The system is optimized based on pilot results, ensuring scalability and inclusivity for broader deployment [2].

This phased roadmap ensures the framework evolves iteratively, addressing practical challenges while maximizing its impact on modern education systems.

### 3.8 Novelty of the Proposed Framework

While numerous AI-driven classroom assistants have emerged in recent years, the proposed framework offers a distinctive combination of features that address pressing gaps in existing solutions. Our system introduces the following innovations:

- **Enhanced Privacy Protection**: The assistant is designed with a privacy-first approach, incorporating GDPR-compliant encryption protocols and real-time data anonymization techniques. These safeguards ensure that student data is handled securely, responding to a critical concern in educational AI deployment [4].
- **Domain-Specific NLP Customization**: Unlike generic language models, our framework uses domain-specific training to enhance contextual understanding of student queries within curriculum-aligned content. This allows for accurate, meaningful responses even in the presence of ambiguous or educationally nuanced language [5].
- **Multimodal Interaction Capabilities**: The assistant supports both voice and text-based communication, allowing students with different learning preferences or accessibility needs to interact with the system intuitively. This flexibility addresses inclusivity and accessibility at the core of the design [3].
- **Adaptive Learning Mechanisms**: The system refines its responses over time using ML algorithms that learn from classroom engagement patterns. This personalization enhances learning outcomes and maintains relevance across diverse student populations [1].

This combination of features sets our framework apart from existing educational assistants, which typically lack one or more of these core attributes. Table 3 provides a comparative overview illustrating how the proposed framework addresses limitations in current solutions.

## 4 Impact Analysis: Highlight Potential Benefits for Students, Teachers, and Institutions

### 4.1 Benefits for Educational Stakeholders

The AI-powered classroom assistant enables personalized learning by tailoring responses to individual student needs and adapting to their pace and preferences. This personalized interaction fosters self-directed learning and enhances engagement, especially through voice-based interfaces and gamified features [3]. Additionally, the system provides real-time assistance, empowering students to access curriculum-specific answers on demand without waiting for teacher intervention [5].

Teachers benefit from a significant reduction in repetitive tasks, such as answering routine queries, allowing them to focus on more complex and personalized instructional activities. The system's analytics dashboard provides actionable insights into student performance and common learning challenges, enabling teachers to design targeted interventions [1]. By automating mundane tasks, the assistant fosters better teacher-student collaboration and improves overall classroom management [6].

For educational institutions, the assistant offers a scalable solution that integrates seamlessly with existing digital tools like LMS. This reduces operational costs while enhancing teaching effectiveness. Furthermore, aggregated data on student interactions helps refine curriculum strategies, ensuring alignment with modern educational standards [2]. The assistant's compliance with data privacy regulations such as GDPR also builds trust among stakeholders and ensures ethical deployment [4].

### 4.2 Addressing Educational Challenges

The AI-powered classroom assistant bridges significant gaps in learning by offering tailored, curriculum-aligned assistance, particularly benefiting students who struggle with specific concepts. Its real-time support capabilities ensure that both hybrid and remote learning models are effectively reinforced, thereby enhancing the resilience and adaptability of modern educational systems [10]. Furthermore, the framework actively addresses critical ethical concerns, such as data security, bias in AI, and accessibility, setting a benchmark for responsible AI implementation in educational settings [5].

A crucial aspect of the proposed framework is its ability to overcome limitations found in existing AI-powered educational tools. Table 3 presents a structured comparison with existing educational AI assistants, highlighting our framework's advantages in terms of scalability, personalization, voice interaction, and privacy safeguards. Unlike many existing AI-based tutors and chatbots that rely on text-based interactions [5], the proposed system leverages real-time, voice-enabled support, making it more interactive and accessible to students. Similarly, while some AI tools integrate partially with LMS [2], this framework ensures full curriculum alignment, maintaining educational relevance across diverse subjects and grade levels.

Moreover, the proposed assistant prioritizes data privacy with strong adherence to GDPR compliance, encryption mechanisms, and access control layers [4], surpassing existing solutions that offer only basic security features. Personalization is another key advantage, as the framework employs ML to adapt to individual student needs, unlike rule-based response systems that offer minimal adaptability [1]. Finally, scalability is significantly enhanced, enabling the framework to support diverse classroom sizes and varied educational contexts, addressing limitations observed in prior implementations designed for limited institutional use [3].

By addressing these fundamental challenges, the AI-powered assistant provides a robust, scalable, and privacy-compliant solution, making it an essential tool for modern classrooms striving for adaptive, intelligent, and secure AI integration in education.

### 4.3 Ethical Considerations and Bias Mitigation

Ethical deployment of AI in education is essential for fostering equitable learning environments. Our framework incorporates a multi-tiered strategy to minimize algorithmic bias and promote fairness. First, curriculum-driven filtering ensures that all assistant responses remain pedagogically appropriate and culturally neutral. Second, the system undergoes continuous auditing using teacher feedback

**Table 3.** Comparison with Existing Educational AI Assistants

| Feature | Existing Solutions | Proposed Framework |
|---|---|---|
| **Voice Interaction** | Limited, often reliant on text-only interfaces [5] | Real-time, context-aware voice-enabled support |
| **Curriculum Alignment** | Partial, using generic content bases [2] | Fully aligned with national curriculum guidelines |
| **Data Privacy** | Basic compliance, with limited encryption [4] | AES-256 encryption, real-time anonymization, GDPR-conformant |
| **Adaptability** | Rule-based with minimal learning capacity [1] | Reinforcement learning for adaptive personalization |
| **Scalability** | Restricted to small-scale or pilot environments [3] | Architected for institution-wide and cross-discipline scalability |

and learning analytics to detect response patterns that may indicate bias or misinformation [10]. Third, diverse student populations are considered during model fine-tuning to increase inclusivity, particularly for underrepresented groups.

Furthermore, transparency is enhanced by enabling teachers to review and override assistant responses, preserving human oversight. These safeguards align with responsible AI principles and position the assistant as a trustworthy and inclusive educational tool.

# 5 Future Work

## 5.1 Research Agenda

The proposed AI-powered classroom assistant sets the stage for transformative educational research. One primary area of focus is enhancing the assistant's voice recognition capabilities to accommodate diverse accents, speech patterns, and noisy classroom environments [3]. This ensures greater inclusivity and usability across different learning contexts.

To improve learning outcomes, future development will integrate reinforcement learning techniques to adapt responses based on classroom interactions. This will allow the assistant to learn from real-time engagement and improve its contextual accuracy. Furthermore, fine-tuning of the NLP models for domain-specific content and educational discourse will be explored to ensure more accurate and relevant responses tailored to the curriculum [6].

Ethical and legal compliance remains a top priority. Future iterations will further detail the assistant's encryption methods, anonymization pipelines, and verification protocols to ensure adherence to GDPR and similar educational data protection standards [10]. Additionally, mitigation strategies for AI bias will be developed to promote fairness in student interactions.

Lastly, extending multilingual support through additional language models and ontologies will expand the assistant's accessibility. Integration with a broader range of educational ecosystems (e.g., LMS and hybrid learning platforms) is also a key direction [2].

### 5.2 Validation Steps

The validation strategy for the proposed framework is structured across four progressive phases, designed to evaluate system effectiveness and scalability within educational environments. The process begins with simulated testing, where the assistant is evaluated under controlled conditions to optimize NLP accuracy, assess voice recognition performance amid classroom noise, and verify curriculum alignment through expert review.

**Table 4.** Validation Roadmap: Goals and Evaluation Strategies

| Phase | Objective | Methodology and Expected Outcomes |
|---|---|---|
| **Simulated Testing** | Assess NLP accuracy and curriculum fit | Controlled tests under classroom noise conditions; educator feedback guides refinement |
| **Pilot Programs** | Validate real-world usability | Targeted classroom deployment; metrics include accuracy, engagement, and teacher workload impact |
| **Large-Scale Deployment** | Evaluate system scalability | Multi-institution rollout; collects performance and integration data across varied environments |
| **Iterative Improvement** | Continuously refine system features | Incorporates user feedback and benchmarking insights for adaptive enhancement |

Subsequently, pilot programs are planned in collaboration with educational institutions, employing predefined metrics such as response accuracy, user engagement, learning impact, and reduction in instructional workload. These evaluations will be complemented by user feedback collected via surveys and interviews to assess overall satisfaction and usability.

To benchmark system performance, a comparative evaluation framework is included. This will examine the proposed assistant against existing AI-powered classroom tools based on standardized criteria such as personalization depth, privacy safeguards, multimodal support, and curriculum integration.

The third phase involves large-scale deployment across institutions, allowing for the assessment of long-term reliability, adaptability to varied pedagogical contexts, and system robustness at scale. Finally, iterative improvement will leverage findings from all stages to enhance the assistant's responsiveness, inclusivity, and technical integration with evolving classroom technologies.

Table 4 outlines the phased evaluation methodology, ensuring that the framework is assessed across multiple dimensions and stakeholder needs. This multilevel validation plan aims to provide robust evidence of educational effectiveness, technical performance, and ethical integrity.

## 6 Conclusion

This paper presented a scalable and privacy-conscious AI-powered classroom assistant that enhances personalized learning and supports teachers by automating routine interactions. Leveraging NLP and curriculum-aligned knowledge bases, the assistant delivers real-time, adaptive support while ensuring GDPR compliance.

The framework benefits students through tailored assistance, eases teacher workload, and integrates smoothly with existing LMS tools. Its validation plan—ranging from simulation to large-scale deployment—ensures real-world applicability.

Future work will expand on adaptive learning, multilingual support, and bias mitigation, positioning the framework as a secure and forward-looking foundation for AI integration in education.

## References


1. Zafari, M., Bazargani, J., Sadeghi-Niaraki, A., Choi, S.: Artificial intelligence applications in k-12 education: a systematic literature review. IEEE Access, 1 (2022)
2. Bozkurt, A., Karadeniz, A., Baneres, D., Guerrero-Roldán, A.E., Rodríguez, M.E.: Artificial intelligence and reflections from educational landscape: a review of AI studies in half a century. Sustainability **13**(2), 800 (2021)
3. Yang, Y., Xia, N.: Enhancing students' metacognition via AI-driven educational support systems. Int. J. Emerg. Technol. Learn. (Online) **18**(24), 133 (2023)
4. González-Calatayud, V., Prendes-Espinosa, P., Roig-Vila, R.: Artificial intelligence for student assessment: a systematic review. Appl. Sci. **11**(12), 5467 (2021)
5. Mathew, A.N., Rohini, V., Paulose, J.: NLP-based personal learning assistant for school education. Int. J. Electr. Comput. Eng **11**(5), 4522–4530 (2021)
6. Sajja, R., Sermet, Y., Cikmaz, M., Cwiertny, D., Demir, I.: Artificial intelligence-enabled intelligent assistant for personalized and adaptive learning in higher education. Information **15**(10), 596 (2024)
7. Kakoulli, E., Evripidou, S.: Exploring the integration of educational robotics and the internet of things in learning environments. In: 2024 20th International Conference on Distributed Computing in Smart Systems and the Internet of Things (DCOSS-IoT), pp. 400–407. IEEE (2024)
8. Mohamed, A.: Exploring the role of AI and VR in addressing antisocial behavior among students: a promising approach for educational enhancement. IEEE Access (2024)
9. Halvoník, D., Psenak, P.: Design of an educational virtual assistant software. Int. J. Emerg. Technol. Learn. (iJET) **16**(11), 308–321 (2021)

10. Klimova, B., Pikhart, M., Kacetl, J.: Ethical issues of the use of AI-driven mobile apps for education. Front. Public Health **10**, 1118116 (2023)
11. Saputra, I., Astuti, M., Sayuti, M., Kusumastuti, D.: Integration of artificial intelligence in education: opportunities, challenges, threats and obstacles. A literature review. Indonesian J. Comput. Sci. **12**(4) (2023)
12. Mageira, K., Pittou, D., Papasalouros, A., Kotis, K., Zangogianni, P., Daradoumis, A.: Educational AI chatbots for content and language integrated learning. Appl. Sci. **12**(7), 3239 (2022)
13. Katsarou, E., Wild, F., Sougari, A.M., Chatzipanagiotou, P.: A systematic review of voice-based intelligent virtual agents in EFL education. Int. J. Emerg. Technol. Learn. (iJET) **18**(10), 65–85 (2023)

# Developing a Conceptual Framework for Enhanced Cybersecurity Defense Against Zero-Click Exploit

Abdulhadi A. Al Khamis[1], Mohsin Iftikhar[2(✉)], Mohsin Murtaza[3], and Sohail Gohir[2]

[1] Saudi Aramco, Dhahran, Saudi Arabia
abdulhadi.khamis@aramco.com
[2] Higher Colleges of Technology, Abu Dhabi, UAE
{miftikhar,sgohir}@hct.ac.ae
[3] STEM College, RMIT University, Melbourne, Australia
mohsin.murtaza@rmit.edu.au

**Abstract.** Zero-click attacks represent a significant and continuously evolving cybersecurity threat, infiltrating digital devices silently without requiring user interaction. This paper provides a comprehensive review of zero-click exploit mechanisms, predominant attack vectors, and existing strategies for their mitigation. It critically examines anomaly detection approaches, including machine learning techniques such as behavioral analytics based on dynamic moving averages, historical traffic analysis, and the role of blockchain technology in establishing secure and tamper-proof logging systems. By leveraging these advanced analytical techniques, our approach enhances the detection of subtle network anomalies indicative of zero-click exploits. Additionally, integrating threat intelligence into the framework significantly improves its contextual awareness and responsiveness to emerging cybersecurity threats. Furthermore, the paper highlights existing gaps and challenges in current methodologies, emphasizing the necessity of continual refinement and adaptation in detection strategies. Ultimately, the paper underscores the importance of an integrated cybersecurity defense strategy, combining advanced data analytics and robust, adaptive security measures to effectively counteract the sophisticated and evolving risks posed by zero-click exploits.

**Keywords:** Blockchain · Cybersecurity · Machine learning · Spyware · Threat Intelligence · Zero-click attack

## 1 Introduction

The escalating threat of zero-click attacks has become a critical concern in modern cybersecurity, demanding urgent attention from researchers and practitioners [1]. Unlike traditional cyber intrusions that rely on user interaction, zero-click attacks circumvent this requirement entirely, rendering even the most vigilant users susceptible to sophisticated surveillance and data breaches. By design, these exploits require no user action, operate inconspicuously within system processes, and enable unauthorized access to devices


K. Daimi and A. Alsadoon (Eds.): ICR 2025, LNNS 1487, pp. 243–256, 2025.
https://doi.org/10.1007/978-3-031-95652-2_21

and network infrastructures without requiring user engagement or generating observable indicators. This covert nature and absence of user-side indicators make zero-click methods particularly appealing to malicious actors, including cybercriminal organizations and nation-states [2]. Historically, cyberattacks often relied on Trojan horse techniques, requiring victims to unknowingly install malware. However, modern zero-click strategies enable the silent deployment of malware, leaving virtually no forensic traces and significantly increasing the challenge of detection [2]. The proliferation of mobile devices, which store vast amounts of personal and sensitive data [3], has further amplified the risk posed by these vulnerabilities. Consequently, a comprehensive understanding of zero-click exploits is imperative in today's hyper-connected digital ecosystem. These attacks primarily target vulnerabilities in applications that process untrusted data, such as messaging apps, email clients, and communication platforms [4]. In these contexts, seemingly innocuous messages or calls serve as conduits for the execution of malicious code [3, 4]. Given their effectiveness and stealth, zero-click exploits are widely regarded as some of the most dangerous vulnerabilities, actively sought after by advanced cyber threat actors, including state-sponsored groups [5]. However, despite increasing awareness, developing robust and universally applicable Defense strategies against these highly sophisticated threats remains a formidable challenge. This necessitates deeper investigation and the development of novel countermeasures. The remainder of this paper is organized as follows: Section 2 provides background information and a review of related work on zero-click attack techniques, as well as notable case studies. Section 3 outlines current defense strategies, including both proactive and reactive approaches. Section 4 introduces a conceptual framework for enhanced cybersecurity defense, detailing its core components and technological foundations. Section 5 presents a critical discussion of detection challenges and the applicability of the proposed framework. Finally, Section 6 concludes the paper and outlines key directions for future research.

## 2 Background and Related Work

Zero-click exploits are a class of cyberattacks that leverage vulnerabilities in systems designed for automatic data processing, fundamentally differing from traditional attacks requiring user interaction. These exploits often target weaknesses in software applications that automatically handle untrusted data, such as messaging applications, email clients, and web browsers. Vulnerabilities typically exploited include memory corruption errors (e.g., buffer overflows, use-after-free vulnerabilities), logic flaws in parsing complex data formats, and weaknesses in the implementation of communication protocols [6]. These vulnerabilities, when successfully exploited, enable attackers to execute arbitrary code on a victim's device without requiring any user action, resulting in a range of malicious outcomes, including data theft, surveillance, and complete device control [6]. Messaging applications, such as iMessage and WhatsApp, have been particularly susceptible due to the complexity of their multimedia message handling and call processing functionalities [3, 7]. The need to parse diverse and often malformed data formats within these applications increases the likelihood of introducing vulnerabilities. Historically, flaws in input validation, buffer management, and data structure handling in these applications have created vulnerabilities that can be exploited for zero-click attacks [4].

Having established this foundational understanding of zero-click exploits and their general context, it is now pertinent to explore the specific techniques that attackers employ to carry out these attacks.

## 2.1 Overview of Zero-Click Attack Techniques

Zero-click attacks encompass a broad spectrum of cyber tactics that do not require user interaction to launch malware or initiate the attacker's operations. In a Zero-Click attack, the attacker exploits technical vulnerabilities in the victim's devices, such as the Operating System, applications, and other system components, to initiate the execution of malicious code [8]. Here are some examples of Zero-click attack techniques leveraged by attackers:

- **Exploiting Known or Zero-Day Vulnerabilities:** By taking advantage of specific weaknesses in software or hardware, attackers can gain unauthorized access to an organization's interfaces or pivot within the network once a host has been compromised. Some risks are passive, meaning a user does not have to interact with a system in any way. For example, a zero-click exploit could enable an attacker to gain control of the victim's device through an SMS message or an image [9].
- **Leveraging Attack Automation:** Threats can be automatically scanned across network spaces using vulnerability scanners or automated attack scripts and botnets to target vulnerable systems at the network layer, enabling the launch of zero-click exploits [8, 9].
- **Supply Chain Attacks:** These threats exploit vulnerabilities in third-party applications that the intended victim relies on. By targeting a reputable supplier or provider, attackers can deliver malicious updates or components and execute code on the victim's systems without requiring user action [2, 9].
- **Password Brute-Force and Spraying Attacks:** Attackers may use password-cracking techniques by guessing random characters across an account until they obtain the correct combination or use passwords obtained from phishing attacks, black markets, or previous data breaches in attacks known as password spraying or credential stuffing [2, 9].
- **Man-in-the-Middle (MITM) Attacks:** This involves unauthorized individuals intercepting and modifying packet contents to extract information, **such as passwords,** or to carry out attacks on the victim's devices [9, 11].

Standard cybersecurity measures like firewalls, antivirus software, and intrusion detection systems are often insufficient against zero-click attacks [12, 13]. These defenses typically rely on detecting known malicious patterns or user-initiated actions. Zero-click exploits, by their nature, often operate below the detection threshold of these traditional tools, exploiting subtle vulnerabilities in application logic and memory management. More advanced techniques, such as behavioral analysis and anomaly detection, offer some promise [11], but face challenges due to high false positive rates and significant computational demands. Recent studies have identified a scarcity of comprehensive frameworks that effectively integrate proactive and reactive defense mechanisms against zero-click threats [11, 14]. The dynamic evolution of exploitation techniques further compounds the problem, outpacing the development of effective countermeasures, underscoring a critical gap in current cybersecurity defenses [14]. To illustrate the practical implications and severity of zero-click exploits, the following section examines a prominent real-world example: the Pegasus spyware.

## 2.2 Case Study: Pegasus Spyware and Zero-Click Exploits

Pegasus spyware serves as a stark example of the real-world impact of zero-click exploits. This sophisticated spyware, developed for various operating systems, is capable of infiltrating smartphones and gaining complete control over the device, including its camera and microphone [8, 16]. A defining characteristic of Pegasus [29] is its zero-click exploit capability, allowing device infection through vulnerabilities in messaging services, often triggered by a simple, seemingly innocuous message [17]. For instance, vulnerabilities within multimedia message handling and call processing in iMessage have been identified as prime vectors for attacks like Pegasus [7, 8]. Pegasus leverages various zero-click techniques, including exploiting vulnerabilities in messaging services (as discussed in Sect. 2.1) and network injection attacks. "Network injections" allow Pegasus to infect a device simply when a user browses the internet without requiring interaction with phishing URLs [16]. Another technique, "swapping," involves the attacker waiting for the target to visit unsecured websites during normal browsing activities to inject the spyware [16]. Over time, Pegasus has evolved, enhancing its capabilities and infection methods [16]. The spyware can initiate total surveillance, accessing messages, emails, calls, browser history, and even encrypted files [8, 17]. The widespread use of Pegasus has raised significant digital privacy and security concerns [18]. Its ability to exploit zero-day vulnerabilities makes defense particularly challenging, as patches may not exist [18]. The implications of Pegasus extend beyond individual privacy, impacting fundamental human rights and prompting calls for stricter regulation and oversight of such surveillance technologies [8, 16]. Having examined the background, techniques, and critical case study, it becomes clear that a structured approach to addressing zero-click exploits is essential. Therefore, this research aims to investigate key questions that will guide the development of more effective countermeasures.

## 2.3 Research Questions and Contribution

The escalating prevalence of zero-click exploits underscores an urgent need for rigorous academic investigation and the formulation of effective countermeasures [2, 6]. This study aims to address critical gaps in the current understanding of zero-click exploits by posing specific research questions. These questions are intended to illuminate pivotal issues related to these exploits and contribute to the development of a robust conceptual framework aimed at enhancing cybersecurity defenses [24].

- RQ1 - Primary Attack Vectors: What are the predominant attack vectors exploited by zero-click attacks, as identified in the literature and incident reports?
- RQ2 - Mitigation Strategies: What strategies have been proposed in the academic literature and industry best practices to prevent or mitigate the risks associated with zero-click attacks?

- RQ3 - Actionable Recommendations: Based on the existing body of literature, what concrete recommendations and best practices can be derived to enhance defenses against zero-click exploits?
- RQ4 - Research Gaps: What critical areas remain underexplored or insufficiently addressed in the current literature regarding zero-click exploit prevention, detection, or response?

The primary contribution of this research lies in its comprehensive analysis of zero-click exploit case studies and the subsequent development of a novel conceptual framework for bolstering cybersecurity defenses. This framework will be informed by a systematic review of existing literature, identification of prevalent attack vectors, and an assessment of current mitigation strategies. By identifying research gaps and proposing concrete recommendations, this work aims to provide actionable insights for both researchers and practitioners in the field of cybersecurity.

# 3 Defense Strategies Against Zero-Click Attacks

Defending against zero-click attacks requires a comprehensive, multi-layered approach that integrates preventive, detective, and corrective security measures. Given that zero-click exploits do not require user interaction, traditional cybersecurity defenses, such as firewalls and antivirus solutions, are often insufficient. Instead,

Organizations must adopt a proactive security posture, leveraging threat intelligence, vulnerability management, advanced endpoint security, and Zero Trust principles to mitigate risks [2]. A well-designed defense strategy must focus on minimizing the attack surface, preventing malicious code execution, detecting anomalies early, and enabling rapid recovery. Organizations should integrate both proactive and reactive mechanisms to ensure resilience against evolving threats. The following security controls are crucial for mitigating the risks associated with zero-click exploits.

## 3.1 Proactive Defense Mechanisms

Proactive measures aim to reduce vulnerabilities before they can be exploited and establish a strong security foundation. Key proactive strategies include:

- Vulnerability and Patch Management: Organizations must conduct regular vulnerability assessments across both internal networks and public interfaces to detect and remediate potential security gaps. Automated vulnerability scanning tools should be continuously updated to identify the latest threats. Additionally, a structured patch management policy must be in place to ensure timely updates of operating systems, firmware, and applications, reducing the risk of attackers exploiting known security flaws [9, 20].
- Threat Intelligence and Information Sharing: Engaging in cyber threat intelligence (CTI) networks enhances an organization's ability to detect and prevent zero-click attacks. CTI feeds, such as CISA's Known Exploited Vulnerabilities Catalog, provide real-time insights into emerging attack techniques, helping security teams prioritize defenses accordingly [9, 20].

- Virtualization and Isolation: Sandboxing and virtualized environments, such as Virtual Desktop Infrastructure (VDI) and Remote Browser Isolation, help mitigate zero-click exploits by executing potentially malicious code in controlled environments. Organizations can use disposable virtual machines to test untrusted files or messages before they reach critical systems. This strategy limits malware persistence and prevents lateral movement in case of infection. Zero-Trust Architecture (ZTA): Implementing Zero-Trust principles ensures that all network activities are continuously verified, and access is granted on a need-to-know basis. By enforcing multi-factor authentication (MFA), least privilege access, and micro segmentation, organizations can limit the potential damage caused by zero-click exploits [2, 20].

### 3.2 Reactive and Detective Security Measures

Since zero-click attacks often bypass traditional security measures, it is essential to have robust detection and response mechanisms to identify and contain threats at an early stage. Key reactive and detective strategies include:

- Advanced Endpoint Security: Deploying next-generation antivirus (NGAV), Endpoint Detection and Response (EDR), and behavior-based anomaly detection is crucial. Traditional signature-based security tools are ineffective against zero-day exploits, whereas AI-driven behavioral analytics can detect abnormal system activities that may indicate an attack [2, 20].
- Content Filtering and Email Security: Zero-click exploits often leverage messaging apps, emails, and multimedia files as initial attack vectors. Organizations should implement email filtering solutions, file format validation, and malicious link detection to block phishing attempts and suspicious attachments. Additionally, strict email policies (e.g., disabling automatic link previews or restricting the execution of embedded scripts) can mitigate risks [20].
- Intrusion Detection and Network Security: Using Intrusion Detection/Prevention Systems (IDS/IPS), Next-Generation Firewalls (NGFW), and Secure Web Gateways (SWG) helps identify and block suspicious network traffic associated with zero-click exploits. Network segmentation further restricts an attacker's ability to move laterally across systems, minimizing the blast radius of an attack [20].
- Incident Response and Recovery Planning: Despite preventive measures, some attacks may succeed. Organizations must establish a well-defined incident response framework, ensuring rapid detection, containment, eradication, and recovery. This includes forensic analysis, threat hunting, and system restoration protocols to mitigate potential damage and prevent future incidents [9, 20].

### 3.3 Why Are Zero-Click Attacks Particularly Difficult to Defend Against?

Zero-click attacks pose significant challenges to individuals and organizations due to several unique characteristics that complicate their detection [2], prevention, and mitigation. The primary factors contributing to the difficulty in defending against zero-click attacks include:

- Absence of User Interaction: Unlike traditional cyberattacks that often rely on user manipulation, such as phishing emails or malicious downloads, zero-click attacks require no user action [18]. Because these attacks do not depend on user mistakes or interactions, detecting and tracing their origin becomes considerably more challenging. Additionally, zero-click attacks typically provide no visible signs of compromise, making timely identification and remediation difficult [2].

- Capability for Automated Execution: Zero-click attacks often utilize automation to execute rapidly and propagate across multiple systems simultaneously. The automated nature of these attacks enables attackers to scale their operations significantly, complicating defensive strategies [22]. Defenders face the dual challenge of responding rapidly and the need for scalable solutions to counter the speed and reach of these automated attacks.
- Utilization of Zero-Day Vulnerabilities: A critical aspect of zero-click attacks is their frequent reliance on zero-day vulnerabilities—previously undisclosed software or hardware flaws that are unknown to developers and vendors, for which patches do not yet exist. As these vulnerabilities remain unknown to vendors, defenders lack immediate solutions to prevent exploitation [23]. Consequently, systems are vulnerable to compromise until a security update is developed and deployed, limiting the effectiveness of proactive defense measures.

## 4 Developing a Conceptual Framework for Enhanced Cybersecurity Defense

Given the increasing prevalence and complexity of zero-click exploits, there is a critical need for a novel conceptual framework that integrates advanced cybersecurity practices to detect, prevent, and respond to these threats. Unlike traditional attacks, zero-click exploits operate silently, often leveraging unknown vulnerabilities without requiring user interaction, which makes their detection and mitigation particularly difficult [2, 6].

The proposed framework addresses these challenges by combining several core components: advanced threat detection and analytics, threat intelligence integration, proactive vulnerability management, dynamic incident response, and secure communication. It relies on emerging technologies, such as artificial intelligence (AI), machine learning (ML), blockchain, and quantum cryptography, to form a scalable, adaptive, and proactive cybersecurity defense mechanism [5, 24], as illustrated in Fig. 1.

Threat Detection and Analytics form the foundation of the framework. AI and ML are utilized to monitor behavioral patterns, detect anomalies in network traffic, and provide real-time identification of zero-click attack vectors [32, 39]. These systems are supported by continuous monitoring and logging mechanisms, enabling the rapid detection of suspicious activity without relying on signature-based detection methods.

Threat Intelligence and Identification involve collecting and analyzing structured and unstructured data from multiple sources, including global threat feeds and previous attack histories. This intelligence enables predictive modelling of threat behavior and improves situational awareness for more targeted defense strategies [24].

Vulnerability assessment and management practices are conducted through routine vulnerability scanning, automated penetration testing, and comprehensive risk assessments. These measures collectively facilitate the identification, evaluation, and prioritization of system vulnerabilities. The prompt deployment of patches and regular software

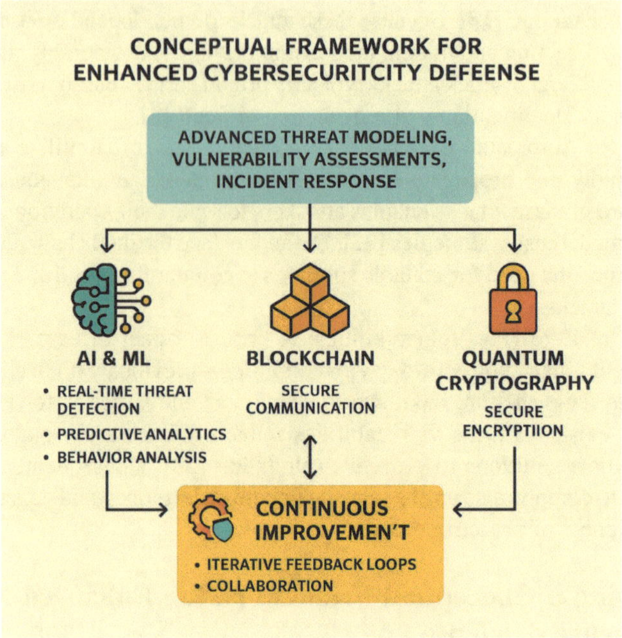


**Fig. 1:** Conceptual Framework for Enhanced Cybersecurity

updates further reduces exposure to known vulnerabilities, effectively minimizing the potential attack surface leveraged by zero-click exploits [31].

Incident Response and Mitigation mechanisms are embedded in the framework to ensure rapid containment and recovery. A tailored incident response plan for zero-click scenarios outlines specific procedures, including system isolation, root-cause analysis, remediation steps, and post-incident reporting. Collaboration with internal and external stakeholders facilitates coordinated responses and resilience [2].

Secure Communication underpins the entire framework. Blockchain is utilized for immutable logging and secure communication channels, while quantum cryptography ensures the confidentiality of sensitive transmissions against both classical and future quantum computing threats [28, 39].

A distinguishing feature of the proposed framework is its emphasis on continuous improvement. Feedback loops from each component feed into a central knowledge base, refining detection algorithms, updating intelligence, and optimizing response protocols. This iterative process ensures the framework remains responsive to evolving threat landscapes and technological shifts [30].

By holistically integrating these components, the proposed conceptual framework provides a resilient and future-proof approach to defending against zero-click and other advanced cyber threats.

### 4.1 Threat Detection & Analytics

Threat detection and analytics are indispensable for identifying cybersecurity challenges and formulating effective countermeasures. In this component, artificial intelligence (AI) and machine learning (ML) algorithms help recognize patterns in user behavior, device activity, and network traffic [5, 26]. When suspicious activity is detected, threats can be flagged in real-time. Behavioral analysis is also employed to continuously monitor the normal functioning of systems and internal processes, enabling the detection of potential anomalies and insider threats [27].

Anomaly detection techniques, powered by both statistical models and machine learning (ML)-based algorithms, are used to identify novel or deviant behavior patterns that may indicate an ongoing or imminent attack [31]. These approaches are beneficial in identifying sophisticated or zero-day attacks that do not follow known signatures. Furthermore, semantic techniques for analyzing system call patterns can enhance host-based intrusion detection, offering high precision in threat detection through both contiguous and discontinuous pattern analysis [32].

### 4.2 Intelligence & Threat Identification

The Intelligence and Threat Identification section is dedicated to recognizing specific threats and profiling them. Sophisticated AI and ML systems are deployed to identify patterns in both known and previously unseen threats, thereby providing a proactive security posture [5, 26]. Predictive algorithms are essential for detecting patterns that may indicate malicious intent [32]. Historical data analysis further contributes by analyzing previously collected threat data to anticipate future attack trends [23]. Additionally, global threat intelligence sources are integrated to provide contextual awareness and comprehensive visibility into evolving threat landscapes [33].

### 4.3 Vulnerability Assessment & Management

Vulnerability Assessment and Management focuses on identifying and mitigating weaknesses in systems before they are exploited. Automated scanning tools are frequently employed to probe systems for vulnerabilities, ensuring ongoing monitoring [31]. Techniques such as red teaming and penetration testing help simulate attacks and highlight weaknesses [25]. Risk assessments evaluate the potential impact of those vulnerabilities on operations. Patch management ensures timely remediation of identified flaws, minimizing the exposure window [34].

### 4.4 Incident Response & Mitigation

This component addresses activities involved in managing security breaches detected. Organizations implement structured incident response plans that define roles, escalation procedures, and communication protocols [35]. Isolation techniques are deployed to contain attacks and minimize propagation during active incidents [36]. Post-incident forensics help in identifying the source and nature of the attack, while recovery mechanisms focus on restoring normal operations with minimal disruption [37].

### 4.5 Continuous Improvement

The cybersecurity framework must evolve through continuous improvement to remain resilient. Feedback loops from incidents, detection systems, and post-mortem reviews are essential for iterative enhancement [30]. Regular system updates, patch cycles, and fine-tuning of detection algorithms are critical to adapting to emerging threats [38]. Moreover, information sharing across organizations enhances threat awareness and enriches collective defense [39].

### 4.6 Secure Communication

Secure communication forms the bedrock of the entire cybersecurity infrastructure. Blockchain technologies ensure immutability and authenticity in communication through private key encryption and distributed consensus [39]. Meanwhile, quantum cryptography introduces theoretically unbreakable encryption, ensuring confidentiality even in a post-quantum era [28]. Together, these technologies safeguard communication against interception and tampering, maintaining the integrity of sensitive data exchanges.

## 5 Discussion

Despite the claims by the NSO Group regarding the undetectable nature of its Pegasus spyware, recent research has identified viable methodologies to detect compromised devices. For instance, analyzing network communication patterns linked to known NSO-related domains, such as free247 downloads, or tracking device interactions with suspicious domains like nomodes.com can effectively reveal spyware activity indicative of Pegasus intrusion [18]. Additionally, specific forensic artifacts, such as processes labelled "bh" (bridgehead) within the SQLite databases of infected iOS devices and the disabling of crash log reporting via modifications to the com. apple.CrashReporter.plist file, represents notable indicators of potential malware compromise [19]. Acknowledging the inherent difficulty in consistently identifying subtle indications of spyware infection, Amnesty International introduced the Mobile Verification Toolkit (MVT), a specialized Python-based tool explicitly designed to detect known indicators associated with Pegasus spyware [19]. Nevertheless, the adaptive and rapidly evolving characteristics of Pegasus, particularly its frequent changes to domains, processes, and naming conventions, pose significant challenges to detection methodologies, highlighting the critical need for continuously evolving cybersecurity tools and defensive strategies [17].

Addressing these challenges, the proposed framework integrates advanced analytical approaches, including anomaly detection utilizing k-means clustering, behavioral analytics employing moving averages, and comprehensive integration with updated threat intelligence databases. Collectively, these techniques considerably enhance the capability to detect anomalous behaviors typical of zero-click spyware intrusions. Such an integrative approach markedly surpasses conventional methods reliant on historical data analysis, which may overlook emerging or nuanced threats [2]. Moreover, the inclusion of blockchain technology for secure and immutable logging strengthens the framework's cybersecurity posture. This approach effectively prevents unauthorized alterations and potential leaks of sensitive forensic data, thereby reinforcing the integrity and reliability of incident investigations and legal responses [20]. Blockchain-based architectures have proven effective in mitigating advanced cyber threats in IoT sensor networks, supporting their broader applicability for enhancing system resilience and ensuring data integrity in diverse cybersecurity environments [40]. However, the effectiveness of such advanced analytical methods is contingent on the availability, consistency, and completeness of network data. In practice, datasets often suffer from incompleteness, inconsistencies, or inaccuracies, which can significantly impair the precision and reliability of anomaly detection models. Given the continuous and dynamic evolution of spyware capabilities, it remains imperative to regularly update global threat intelligence repositories and consistently refine detection algorithms. Such ongoing efforts are essential for sustaining robust cybersecurity defenses against sophisticated and evolving threats like zero-click exploits [13].

## 6 Conclusion

The increasing sophistication and prevalence of zero-click exploits pose a critical challenge in modern cybersecurity, primarily due to their covert nature, lack of user interaction, and exploitation of zero-day vulnerabilities. To address these complex threats, this study introduced a novel, integrated conceptual framework designed to effectively detect, mitigate, and respond to zero-click cyber intrusions. Our proposed framework leverages advanced methodologies such as anomaly detection through machine learning algorithms, behavioral analytics, historical traffic analysis, and secure blockchain-based logging for forensic integrity. The incorporation of blockchain technology within the framework notably enhances the reliability and immutability of event logs, ensuring credible forensic analyses and significantly augmenting defensive capabilities against advanced persistent threats, such as Pegasus spyware. Furthermore, by employing unsupervised and interpretable artificial intelligence models, our approach offers robust, real-time threat detection capabilities that are suitable for dynamic and complex environments, including IoT and cloud infrastructures.

Despite the promising potential demonstrated, several inherent limitations remain pertinent. The effectiveness of the developed framework significantly depends upon the availability and quality of complete, accurate datasets and timely threat intelligence. Challenges such as noisy, incomplete, and manipulated data pose significant hurdles, potentially compromising detection accuracy and efficiency. Therefore, continuous refinement and adaptation of detection algorithms, coupled with regular updating of threat intelligence databases, are essential components to sustain and enhance the effectiveness of the proposed framework. Looking forward, it is imperative that future research endeavors prioritize the enhancement of real-time adaptive detection mechanisms capable of responding swiftly to evolving attack vectors. Equally critical is the promotion of extensive global intelligence-sharing platforms and comprehensive zero-trust strategies to enforce rigorous access controls within hybrid technological ecosystems. Ultimately, an adaptive, collaborative, and proactive cybersecurity posture grounded in automation, behavioral analytics, and strategic cross-sector cooperation remains the most effective strategy to counteract the continuously evolving and stealthy nature of zero-click exploits and other sophisticated cyber threats.

## References


1. Nisha, T.N., Shailendra Kulkarni, M.: Zero click attacks – a new cyber threat for the e-banking sector. J. Finan. Crime. **30**(5), 1150–1161 (2023). https://doi.org/10.1108/JFC-06-2022-0140
2. Younis, A.A., Daher, Z., Martin, B., Morgan, C.: Mapping zero-click attack behavior into MITRE ATT&CK Mobile: a systematic process. In: Proceedings - 2022 International Conference on Computational Science and Computational Intelligence, CSCI 2022, January, pp. 890–896 (2022). https://doi.org/10.1109/CSCI58124.2022.00160
3. Di Salvo, P.: We have to act like our devices are already infected. Invest. Journal. Inter. Surveil. Journal. Pract. **16**(9), 1849–1866 (2021). https://doi.org/10.1080/17512786.2021.2014346
4. Singh, A., Tanha, M., Girdhar, Y., Hunter, A.: Interpretable android malware detection based on dynamic analysis. In: Proceedings of the 10th International Conference on Information Systems Security and Privacy - Volume 1: ICISSP.; ISBN 978-989-758-683-5, pp. 195–202. SciTePress (2024). https://doi.org/10.5220/0012415800003648
5. Jain, D., Choudhary, D., Anand, A., Trivedi, N.K., Gautam, V., Mohapatra, S.K.: Cybersecurity solutions using AI techniques. In: 2022 10th International Conference on Reliability, Infocom Technologies and Optimization (Trends and Future Directions) (ICRITO), pp. 1–8 (2022). https://doi.org/10.1109/ICRITO56286.2022.9965045
6. Prabith, G.S., Abhishek, S., Anjali, T., Ravindran, R.: Zero-click exploits and malware: an in-depth analysis and case studies. In: 2023 16th International Conference on Security of Information and Networks (SIN), pp. 1–9 (2023). https://doi.org/10.1109/SIN60469.2023.10474959
7. Mustafa Kareem, K.: A comprehensive analysis of Pegasus spyware and its implications for digital privacy and security. Int. J. Intell. Syst. Appl. Eng. **12**(3), 1360–1373 (2024) https://ijisae.org/index.php/IJISAE/article/view/5527
8. Rudie, J., Katz, Z., Kuhbander, S., Bhunia, S.: Technical analysis of the NSO Group's Pegasus Spyware. In: 2021 International Conference on Computational Science and Computational Intelligence (CSCI), Las Vegas, NY, USA, pp. 747–752 (2021). https://doi.org/10.1109/CSCI54926.2021.00188
9. Yasmeen, K., Adnan, M.: Zero-day and zero-click attacks on digital banking: a comprehensive review of double trouble. Risk Manage. **25**(4), 1–24 (2023). https://doi.org/10.1057/s41283-023-00130-4
10. Karimipour, H., Dehghantanha, A., Parizi, R.M., Choo, K.-K.R., Leung, H.: A deep and scalable unsupervised machine learning system for cyber-attack detection in large-scale smart grids. IEEE Access. **7**, 80778–80788 (2019). https://doi.org/10.1109/ACCESS.2019.2920326
11. Kim, P.: The Hacker Playbook 3: Practical Guide to Penetration Testing, pp. 328–362. Secure Planet LLC, South Carolina (2014)
12. Pashentsev, E., Bazarkina, D.: Malicious Use of Artificial Intelligence and International Psychological Security in Latin America, vol. 18, pp. 154–177. ICSPSC, Moscow (2020)
13. Ahmed, U., Nazir, M., Sarwar, A., et al.: Signature-based intrusion detection using machine learning and deep learning approaches empowered with fuzzy clustering. Sci. Rep. **15**, 1726 (2025). https://doi.org/10.1038/s41598-025-85866-7
14. Kovács, A.: Ransomware: a comprehensive study of the exponentially increasing cybersecurity threat. Insights Region. Dev. **4**(2), 96–104 (2022)
15. Yazdinejad, A., Parizi, R.M., Dehghantanha, A., Karimipour, H.: Cryptojacking detection in IoT using learning techniques. Appl. Soft Comput. **96**, 106630 (2020). https://doi.org/10.1016/j.asoc.2020.106630
16. Conti, M., Mancini, L.V., Spolaor, R., Verde, N.V.: iOS Mobile malware analysis: a state-of-the-art. J. Comput. Virol. Hack. Tech. **19**, 123–139 (2023). https://doi.org/10.1007/s11416-023-00477-y

17. Kareem, K.: A comprehensive analysis of pegasus spyware and its implications for digital privacy and security. arXiv preprint arXiv:2404.19677 (2024)
18. Zúquete, A., Gomes, R., Ferreira, P.: The current state and future of mobile security in the light of the Pegasus case. Multimed. Tools Appl. **82**, 12345–12367 (2023). https://doi.org/10.1007/s11042-023-14400-6
19. Cinar, A.C., Kara, T.B.: The current state and future of mobile security in the light of the recent mobile security threat reports. Multimed. Tools Appl. **82**, 20269–20281 (2023). https://doi.org/10.1007/s11042-023-14400-6
20. Stafford, V.: Zero Trust Architecture, NIST Special Publication 2020, pp. 1–59. https://doi.org/10.6028/NIST.SP.800-207. (Accessed: Jan. 2025)
21. Durr-E-Shahwar, M., Imran, A.B., Altamimi, W., Khan, S.H., Alsaffar, M.: Quantum cryptography for future networks security: a systematic review. IEEE Access. **12**, 180048–180078 (2024). https://doi.org/10.1109/ACCESS.2024.3504815
22. Enoch, S.Y., Huang, Z., Moon, C.Y., Lee, D., Ahn, M.K., Kim, D.S.: HARMer: cyber-attacks automation and evaluation. ArXiv. **8**, 129397–129414 (2020). https://doi.org/10.1109/ACCESS.2020.3009748
23. Bilge, D., Dumitras, T.: Before we knew it: an empirical study of zero-day attacks in the real world. In: Proceedings of 2012 ACM Conf. Computer and Communications Security (CCS), pp. 833–844. https://doi.org/10.1145/2382196.2382284
24. Schlette, D.: Cyber threat intelligence sharing. In: Encyclopedia of Cryptography, Security and Privacy, pp. 522–524 (2025). https://doi.org/10.1007/978-3-030-71522-9_1717
25. Kotwani, B., Sawant, M., Chopra, D.: Red teaming vs. blue teaming: a comparative analysis of CyberSecurity strategies in the digital battlefield. Int. J. Sci. Res. Eng. Manag. **07**, 1–11 (2023). https://doi.org/10.55041/IJSREM27675
26. Rigaki, M., Garcia, S.: Bringing a GAN to a knife-fight: Adapting malware communication to avoid detection. In: Proceedings of IEEE European Symposium on Security and Privacy Workshops (EuroS&PW), pp. 70–75 (2018). https://doi.org/10.1109/SPW.2018.00019
27. Guin, U., DiMase, D., Turner, J.A., Tehranipoor, M., Ginwala, A.: Counterfeit integrated circuits: detection, avoidance, and the challenges ahead. J. Electron. Test. **30**(1), 9–23 (2014). https://doi.org/10.1007/s10836-013-5430-8
28. Gisin, N., Thew, R.: Quantum communication. Nat. Photonics. **1**(3), 165–171 (2007). https://doi.org/10.1038/nphoton.2007.22
29. Acarturk, C., Ulubay, M., Erdur, E.: Continuous improvement on maturity and capability of Security Operation Centres. IET Inf. Secur. **15** (2020). https://doi.org/10.1049/ise2.12005
30. Holm, H.: Signature based intrusion detection for zero-day attacks: (not) a closed chapter? In: Proceedings of 47th Hawaii International Conference on System Sciences (HICSS), pp. 4895–4904 (2014). https://doi.org/10.1109/HICSS.2014.600
31. Creech, G., Hu, J.: A semantic approach to host-based intrusion detection systems using contiguous and Discontiguous system call patterns. IEEE Trans. Comput. **63**(4), 807–819 (2014). https://doi.org/10.1109/TC.2013.13
32. Muthusubramanian, M., Mohamed, I.A., Pakalapati, N.: Machine learning for cybersecurity threat detection and prevention. Int. J. Innov. Sci. Res. Technol. **9** (2024). https://doi.org/10.5281/zenodo.10776751
33. Al-Ayed, A., Furnell, S., Zhao, D., Haskell-Dowland, P.: An automated framework for managing security vulnerabilities. Inf. Manag. Comput. Secur. **13**, 156–166 (2005). https://doi.org/10.1108/09685220510589334
34. Dorofee, A.J., Killcrece, G., Ruefle, R.M., Zajicek, M.T.: Incident Management Capability Metrics Version 0.1. Defense Technical Information Center (2007) https://resources.sei.cmu.edu/asset_files/TechnicalReport/2007_005_001_14873.pdf

35. Alejandro, M.C., Andrés, G.H., Ricardo, V.F.: Constructing an architecture-based cybersecurity solution for a system. MethodsX. **9**(10), 102010 (2023). https://doi.org/10.1016/j.mex.2023.102010. PMID: 37424761; PMCID: PMC10326440
36. Alhidaifi, S.M., Asghar, M.R., Ansari, I.S.: A survey on cyber resilience: key strategies, research challenges, and future directions. ACM Comput. Surv. **56**(8), Article 196 (2024). https://doi.org/10.1145/3649218
37. Jazairy, A., Brho, M., Manuj, I., Goldsby, T.: Cyber risk management strategies and integration: toward supply chain cyber resilience and robustness. Int. J. Phys. Distrib. Logist. Manag. **54**, 1–29 (2024). https://doi.org/10.1108/IJPDLM-12-2023-0445
38. Buczak, A., Guven, E.: A survey of data mining and machine learning methods for cyber security intrusion detection. IEEE Commun Surv Tutor. **18**(2), 1153–1176 (2016). https://doi.org/10.1109/COMST.2015.2494502
39. Zheng, Z., Xie, S., Dai, H., Chen, X., Wang, H.: An overview of blockchain technology: architecture, consensus, and future trends. In: 2017 IEEE International Congress on Big Data (BigData Congress), Honolulu, HI, USA, pp. 557–564 (2017). https://doi.org/10.1109/BigDataCongress.2017.85
40. Arachchige, K.G., Murtaza, M., Cheng, C.T., Albahlal, B.M., Lee, C.C.: Blockchain-enabled mitigation strategies for distributed denial of service attacks in IoT sensor networks: an experimental approach. Comput. Mater. Cont. **81**(3), 3679–3705 (2024)

# A Scalable Cybersecurity Model for Shared SOCs in SMEs

Eleftherios Zacharioudakis[1(✉)] and Elena Kakoulli[2,3]

[1] Igor Sikorsky Kyiv Polytechnic Institute, National Technical University of Ukraine, Kyiv, Ukraine
5b4agl@gmail.com

[2] Intelligent Systems Laboratory, Department of Computer Science, Neapolis University Pafos, Pafos, Cyprus
e.kakoulli@nup.ac.cy

[3] Electrical Engineering and Computer Engineering and Informatics, Cyprus University of Technology, Limassol, Cyprus

**Abstract.** As cyber threats rise against Small and Medium Enterprises (SMEs) they find themselves unable to afford specialized Security Operations Centers (SOCs). The study introduces a conceptual framework for a collaborative SOC model which empowers SMEs to fulfill regulatory requirements such as the NIS2 Directive and simultaneously reduce cyber risks and optimize security expenditures. The proposed framework consists of a multi-tenant architecture centralized for continuous threat detection and incident response which supports regulatory requirements and addresses data privacy and scalability issues. The model enables enterprises to access advanced cybersecurity functionalities through shared resources and collaborative efforts. While this work remains conceptual, it lays the theoretical groundwork for future empirical validation through real-world pilot testing. The research examines the theoretical framework of shared SOC models and highlights their benefits while preparing for upcoming implementation and evaluation processes.

**Keywords:** Conceptual Framework for SOCs · Shared Security Operations Center (SOC) · SME Cybersecurity Model · NIS2 Directive Compliance · Collaborative Cybersecurity Infrastructure · Multi-Tenant Architecture · AI-Driven Threat Detection · Cost-Effective Cybersecurity · Cyber Risk Mitigation · Centralized Cybersecurity Solutions

## 1 Introduction

Small and medium enterprises (SMEs) form a vital part of the global economy while facing constant threats from advanced cyberattacks. SMEs do not have enough financial and technical capabilities to establish strong cybersecurity defenses compared to large enterprises which makes them susceptible to security breaches and noncompliance with regulations [1].


K. Daimi and A. Alsadoon (Eds.): ICR 2025, LNNS 1487, pp. 257–269, 2025.
https://doi.org/10.1007/978-3-031-95652-2_22

The NIS2 Directive requires more stringent cybersecurity protections for sensitive information which becomes enforceable in 2027. SMEs face serious compliance obstacles because they typically work with limited budgets and scarce expertise which puts them at risk for legal and financial problems.

This study introduces a conceptual framework which enables a shared Security Operations Center (SOC) to serve SMEs. The collaborative model facilitates resource sharing and access to expert security teams while providing continuous threat monitoring to make sophisticated cybersecurity accessible and cost-effective for all organizations while maintaining regulatory compliance.

Key contributions of this work include:

1. **Cost Efficiency**: A shared SOC model helps SMEs overcome financial obstacles.
2. **Regulatory Compliance**: Integrated support for NIS2 Directive adherence.
3. **Collaborative Resilience**: Strengthening cybersecurity through collective defense.

## 2 Background

Businesses today experience unprecedented opportunities for innovation and growth through digital transformation which especially benefits SMEs. The digital transformation journey for SMEs has led to a rising number of cybersecurity threats. The financial constraints and limited technical expertise of SMEs prevent them from establishing strong cybersecurity defenses compared to larger enterprises that possess dedicated teams and resources.

### 2.1 Evolution of Cybersecurity Threats

The last ten years have seen cyberattacks become more sophisticated and extensive as they attack businesses regardless of their size. Due to their basic cybersecurity infrastructure small businesses which used to be seen as less attractive targets now face frequent cyber exploitation. Research shows that every year a large percentage of SMEs suffer cyberattacks while many cannot recover from significant breaches [2]. These attacks take advantage of weak security detection systems which emphasize the critical requirement for scalable cybersecurity solutions that work effectively.

### 2.2 Regulatory Landscape

Governmental and regulatory bodies have established strict compliance rules to tackle these vulnerabilities and strengthen cybersecurity resilience. The European Union's NIS2 Directive which will become effective by 2027 marks a significant step towards boosting cybersecurity capabilities of organizations including SMEs [3]. The directive requires organizations to implement strong risk management procedures along with secure supply chain practices and incident reporting mechanisms [4]. The new security measures establish a safer digital ecosystem but impose considerable difficulties for SMEs with limited resources which could result in their non-compliance. SMEs require a clear cybersecurity governance framework which enables them to meet regulatory demands through structured risk mitigation and compliance processes.

### 2.3 The Case for Shared SOCs

The development of shared SOCs represents a viable approach to resolve these existing challenges. Shared SOCs allow SMEs to access advanced cybersecurity capabilities through joint resource and expertise sharing. Dimitrov et al. [5] present a shared SOCs conceptual framework centered around centralized monitoring and proactive threat detection with incident response capabilities that allows SMEs to access advanced security solutions while maintaining manageable expenses.

The adoption of Cyber Threat Intelligence (CTI) platforms like Malware Information Sharing Platform (MISP) allows shared SOCs to improve situational awareness while enabling coordinated responses among multiple SMEs [6]. SMEs encounter difficulties with CTI platform adoption because of data privacy worries along with expertise deficits and interoperability problems [7]. The fundamental principles of collaborative network theories such as trust and shared responsibility guide these platforms' alignment with data privacy standards to create strong cybersecurity frameworks [8].

The paper advances these security developments by introducing a conceptual framework for shared SOCs specifically designed for SME requirements. This framework combines theoretical knowledge about multi-tenant structures with cooperative cybersecurity models and regulatory requirements to establish a foundation for upcoming research initiatives and practical applications.

## 3 Related Work

Current research demonstrates multiple approaches to strengthen SME cybersecurity with shared models and advanced frameworks which establish a solid basis for the new framework.

1. **Collaborative Cybersecurity Frameworks**: Shared SOCs among SMEs boost security maturity through combined resources and expert knowledge. Armenia et al. [9] introduced dynamic simulation approaches in their study. They demonstrate through dynamic simulation the cost-benefit analysis of collaborative cybersecurity partnerships which positions them as attractive options for SMEs.
2. **Cyber Threat Intelligence (CTI)**: The work by Van Haastrecht et al. [6] demonstrates how shared CTI solutions such as MISP can boost the cybersecurity capabilities of SMEs. Specifically, it highlights how shared CTI solutions such as MISP strengthen cybersecurity measures for SMEs. The proposed shared SOC depends on these tools to establish its data-sharing capabilities.

3. **Security Maturity Models**: The situational awareness model from Renaud and Ophoff [10] delivers valuable understanding about SME cybersecurity control adoption and prediction which is vital for the proposed framework.
4. **Cost-Effective Cybersecurity Solutions**: Dimitrov et al. [5] demonstrate shared SOCs as an economical cybersecurity strategy for SMEs which helps in lowering both financial and operational burdens.
5. **Comparative Frameworks**: Simola's study [8] examines information sharing models in cybersecurity which reveals the strengths and weaknesses of collaborative networks while offering essential guidance for shared SOC development.

These works demonstrate how shared SOCs can effectively solve cybersecurity problems faced by SMEs. The conceptual framework uses previous research findings as its base to demonstrate theoretical benefits while setting up future empirical tests.

# 4 Methodology

The following section presents the conceptual framework and theoretical method for creating a shared SOC designed to meet SME-specific requirements. The methodology developed three main components that include framework design followed by theoretical evaluation and planning for future validation.

## 4.1 Framework Architecture and Core Components

The proposed shared SOC framework adopts a multi-tenant, cloud-native architecture tailored for SMEs to balance security needs with affordability. The layered architecture is logically divided into five integrated components that collectively deliver enterprise-grade cybersecurity functionalities.

At the foundation lies the *Data Collection Layer*, where distributed agents, sensors, and log forwarders are deployed across SME environments to collect raw security events. These events are then forwarded securely to the central SOC.

Above this is the *Data Processing and Analytics Layer*, which employs real-time preprocessing pipelines powered by a Kafka-like stream ingestion mechanism. This layer cleans and normalizes incoming data while simultaneously enabling high-throughput processing. Machine learning models—such as supervised classifiers (e.g., Random Forest) and unsupervised algorithms for anomaly detection—evaluate the events, assign threat scores, and generate contextualized alerts. This core analytical functionality is further illustrated in Algorithm 1.

The *Security Operations Layer* manages real-time monitoring and incident handling. Here, both human analysts and automated playbooks triage alerts, investigate threats, and orchestrate coordinated responses. The 24/7 nature of this layer ensures persistent threat vigilance and quick containment.

Compliance obligations are addressed through the *Compliance and Reporting Layer*, which automates policy enforcement, audit readiness, and log retention.

Compliance outputs are mapped to industry standards, such as NIS2, providing SMEs with evidence for regulators and internal audits.

To protect tenant data integrity, the *Access and Segmentation Layer* enforces strict logical separation among participating SMEs using RBAC (role-based access control), encryption-at-rest and in-transit, and container-level isolation techniques.

Collectively, these components enable each SME to benefit from: centralized AI-powered detection, incident response coordination, elastic resource scaling, and continuous compliance monitoring—all within a secure, segmented multi-tenant SOC environment.

Figure 1 provides an overview of the architectural components, their data flows, and operational interactions.

**Algorithm 1.** Live Event Stream Processing

```
INPUT: Live event stream from sensors/agents
PROCESS:
for each incoming event do
    features = EXTRACT_FEATURES(event)
    score = DETECTION_MODEL.predict(features)
    if score indicates malicious then
        ALERT = createAlert(event, score)
        INCIDENT_RESPONSE.handle(ALERT)
    end if
end for
CONTINUOUS LEARNING:
- Incorporate feedback (true positives, false positives)
- Periodically retrain DETECTION_MODEL
```

### 4.2 Theoretical Evaluation

Existing literature and frameworks serve as the basis for a theoretical evaluation of the proposed framework's benefits.

- **Cost-Effectiveness**: The study compares shared SOCs with traditional in-house SOCs through financial modeling [5].
- **Compliance Readiness**: The framework maintains alignment with NIS2 compliance milestones to minimize the risk of non-compliance [4].
- **Collaborative Benefits**: This research investigates how shared threat intelligence platforms such as MISP influence situational awareness capabilities [6].

### 4.3 Future Validation Planning

This paper does not include a working framework but it provides guidance on future validation steps. Framework validation refers to assessing performance through real-world pilot deployments that will measure scalability, incident response improvements, cost savings, and compliance effectiveness.

- **Pilot Testing**: The shared SOC will be tested with select SMEs to determine its performance and improve the model.
- **Metrics for Success**: Key performance indicators to focus on include cost savings measures, reductions in incident response times, and improvements in compliance readiness evaluations.

**Scalability Objectives:** To ensure the shared SOC framework can adapt to diverse operational needs, scalability will be evaluated across several technical dimensions during pilot deployments:

- **Concurrent SME Support**: The number of SMEs that can be simultaneously supported without performance degradation.
- **Log Ingestion Rate**: The volume of event logs that can be processed per second from distributed endpoints.
- **Detection Latency**: Time delay between event ingestion and classification by the AI model.
- **Incident Response Throughput**: Number of security alerts triaged and handled in real time.

The deployment will leverage cloud-native technologies such as **Docker** and **Kubernetes** to enable elastic resource scaling based on workload demands. These tools will support dynamic container orchestration and resource isolation across SME tenants. Monitoring these parameters will provide insights into the framework's operational efficiency, growth potential, and infrastructure needs.

- **Scalability Testing**: The next step involves gradually onboarding more SMEs to evaluate the architecture's ability to maintain stability and performance under increased load.

### 4.4 Tools and Technologies

The proposed framework leverages state-of-the-art technologies:

- **Artificial Intelligence (AI)**: Automated threat detection and risk prediction [2].
- **Cyber Threat Intelligence (CTI) Platforms**: Real-time data sharing and collaboration.
- **Cloud Computing**: Ensuring accessibility and scalability for participating SMEs.

### 4.5 Comparative Analysis

The comparative cost analysis presented in Table 1 reflects expected operational and strategic benefits derived from findings in existing literature on shared SOC models [11–16]. These theoretical estimates provide a foundational comparison in terms of cost, expertise, compliance support, and scalability. Real-world cost effectiveness and return on investment (ROI) will be further quantified during future pilot deployments using empirical deployment data.

The comparative analysis in Table 1 draws from relevant studies on SOC design and SME implementations. Key features were categorized thematically under four domains: Cost, Expertise, Compliance Support, and Scalability. This thematic classification enables a more structured comparison of shared versus in-house SOC models, emphasizing operational and regulatory trade-offs SMEs must consider.

The analysis in Table 1 contrasts shared and in-house SOCs by identifying their principal characteristics.

**Table 1.** Comparative Analysis of Shared SOCs vs. In-House SOCs.

| Feature | Shared SOC Model | In-House SOC |
|---|---|---|
| Cost | Shared among SMEs [11,12] | Entirely borne by individual SME [11] |
| Expertise | Centralized, high-level expertise [13,14] | Limited by SME resources [13,14] |
| Compliance Support | Integrated tools for NIS2 adherence [12,15] | SME-specific efforts required [11,15] |
| Scalability | Flexible and adaptable to new SMEs [11,16] | Fixed infrastructure limits [11,16] |

The shared SOC model achieves cost reduction by combining resources from multiple organizations but in-house SOCs require each SME to bear the complete financial burden alone. The shared model grants organizations access to centralized top-tier expertise and advanced threat intelligence resources that they could not afford separately but in-house solutions rely only on what internal resources they already have. Shared SOCs offer integrated compliance tools and procedures which simplify regulatory adherence including the NIS2 Directive and remove repetitive tasks SMEs encounter when handling compliance alone. Shared SOCs benefit from multi-tenant architecture flexibility to grow by incorporating new members whereas in-house SOCs experience significant expenditures and technical obstacles when trying to scale their established infrastructures.

## 5 Conceptual Framework

The conceptual framework presented provides an adaptable and cooperative SOC solution specifically designed to meet the challenges SMEs encounter. The framework utilizes a centralized system design along with multi-tenancy and collective intelligence strategies to deliver strong cybersecurity protection while optimizing costs and meeting regulatory requirements.

Figure 1 illustrates the conceptual model which includes the multi-tenant architecture and essential cybersecurity components. The diagram exhibits how SMEs connect with the shared SOC and its operational elements. The diagram maps out information flow beginning with data collection and analysis and progresses through to response coordination and compliance support.

For a detailed explanation of the underlying AI-driven threat detection processes and streaming data architecture, refer to Sect. 4.1.

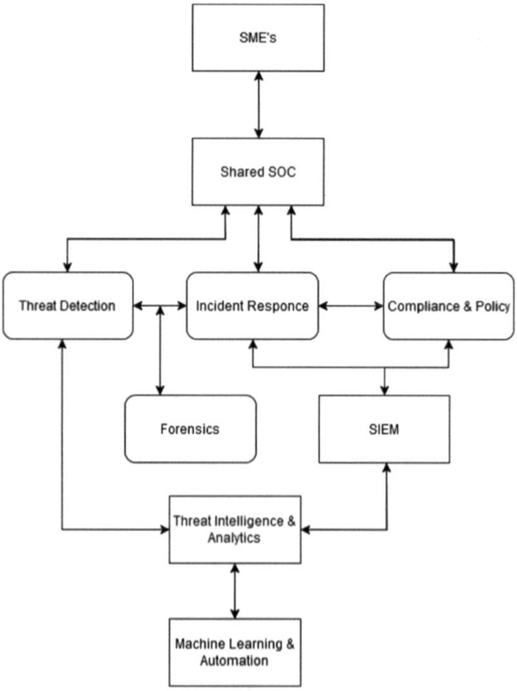


**Fig. 1.** Conceptual Model of the Shared SOC.

### 5.1 Implementation Roadmap

To operationalize the proposed framework, this paper outlines a staged roadmap beginning with targeted pilot deployments. Selected SMEs from various sectors will participate in early trials to assess architectural performance, validate threat detection accuracy, and test compliance automation features.

During these pilots, key performance indicators (KPIs) will include metrics such as incident response time—from detection to containment—compliance readiness scores based on benchmark frameworks like CIS, and projected cost savings versus conventional in-house SOC setups.

Following validation, iterative refinements will be applied based on feedback loops. These may include tuning machine learning thresholds, improving user interfaces for SOC analysts, or enhancing interoperability with existing SME IT systems.

Finally, the framework will undergo full-scale rollout across a broader SME ecosystem. Dynamic resource scaling using Docker/Kubernetes-based cloud orchestration will support operational elasticity as tenant numbers grow. The overall goal is to move from conceptual prototype to a scalable, production-grade shared SOC for real-world SMEs.

## 6 Anticipated Benefits and Challenges

The shared SOC model delivers a revolutionary solution for SME cybersecurity through efficient cost management and scalable operations that adhere to regulatory standards. This section explains how SMEs benefit from shared SOC participation and outlines the associated challenges along with possible mitigation approaches.

### 6.1 Anticipated Benefits

The shared SOC framework offers several key advantages that make it particularly suitable for SMEs. First, it delivers cost efficiency by allowing multiple organizations to pool financial and technical resources. Instead of each SME investing in separate hardware, security analysts, and compliance tools, the shared model spreads those costs across participants—improving affordability and return on investment.

Second, compliance with cybersecurity regulations such as the NIS2 Directive becomes more accessible. The SOC provides integrated reporting dashboards, automated audit mechanisms, and pre-configured compliance templates aligned with established standards like the CIS Benchmarks. This streamlines governance and reduces the internal burden on SMEs.

Another benefit is improved cyber resilience. The centralized threat monitoring infrastructure enables faster incident detection and response across tenants. Shared intelligence feeds and collective situational awareness further strengthen defense postures.

Finally, the scalable design allows SMEs to grow into the framework without architectural bottlenecks. Elastic cloud infrastructure ensures that adding new tenants, increasing log volumes, or adjusting policies does not compromise performance or security guarantees.

Together, these benefits demonstrate how the shared SOC approach democratizes cybersecurity capabilities that were once reserved for large enterprises.

### 6.2 Challenges and Mitigation Strategies

While a shared SOC model offers numerous benefits organizations can leverage, its implementation encounters multiple obstacles which need resolution before full adoption becomes feasible.

1. **Data Privacy and Trust Concerns**: SMEs often show reluctance to participate in shared cybersecurity models because they worry about maintaining data confidentiality and protecting sensitive information. *Mitigation:* The deployment of strict data segmentation rules together with end-to-end encryption and role-based access controls allows each SME to protect its data fully while gaining access to shared resources.
2. **Scalability and Performance**: The system performance and resource allocation must be managed effectively as additional SMEs join the shared SOC. *Mitigation:* The implementation of dynamic resource allocation through scalable cloud-based infrastructure allows the SOC to support more participants without experiencing performance issues.
3. **Compliance Complexity**: The diverse regulatory frameworks across SMEs prevent the development of a universal compliance solution. *Mitigation:* The shared SOC features customizable compliance modules which enable SMEs to adjust their security monitoring and reporting to match specific industry regulations.
4. **Resistance to Adoption**: There exists hesitation among SMEs when asked to move away from their conventional solitary cybersecurity approaches to adopt a shared model. *Mitigation:* Implementing awareness programs alongside training sessions and case studies showing shared SOCs' effectiveness can reduce resistance while promoting adoption.

The shared SOC framework provides SMEs with a sustainable and scalable cybersecurity solution that maintains cost efficiency while meeting current and future regulatory standards.

## 7 Future Work

The shared SOC framework's theoretical basis requires further research and practical implementation to determine its functional validity and effectiveness. Key directions include:

- **Pilot Deployment**: A small-scale pilot program incorporating various SMEs from different industries will test the framework's validity. Performance metrics including cost reduction achievements and incident response efficiency alongside compliance preparedness will serve as measures of success.
- **Integration of Advanced Technologies**: The incorporation of advanced technologies serves as a critical development for improving the shared SOC framework's capabilities. Advanced automation through AI integration in future framework iterations will enhance predictive threat analysis and speed

**Table 2.** Future Research Directions for Shared SOC Framework

| **Focus Area** | **Objective** |
|---|---|
| Pilot Deployment | Validate the framework with real-world data and assess its effectiveness. |
| Advanced Technologies | Integrate AI, blockchain, and CTI platforms to enhance automation and security. |
| Scalability Testing | Ensure the framework can accommodate varying SME sizes and geographies. |
| Socio-Technical Analysis | Address cultural and organizational barriers to adoption. |
| Regulatory Evolution | Adapt the framework to comply with changing cybersecurity regulations. |

up response times to new threats. Blockchain technology enables secure data sharing that remains unchanged and transparent between SMEs involved in the partnership fostering trust and collaboration. CTI platforms need integration to link SMEs with worldwide intelligence networks which helps develop proactive security measures and a unified strategy for tackling advanced cyber threats. The integration of advanced technologies will significantly boost the framework's operational efficiency and expand its capacity to scale and withstand disruptions.

- **Scalability Testing**: Testing the framework's ability to scale in various SME ecosystems and geographic regions will demonstrate its capability to adapt to distinct business conditions.
- **Socio-Technical Analysis**: Research going forward needs to explore the organizational and social elements involved in establishing a shared SOC by focusing on cultural resistance to team-oriented models and on fostering trust and transparency among SME partners.
- **Regulatory Evolution**: The framework requires updates to integrate new compliance requirements with the evolution of cybersecurity regulations. Investigating modular and adaptive compliance systems will help maintain the framework's relevance.

Table 2 details the primary research objectives for each identified future research focus area.

## 8 Conclusion

The paper introduces a shared SOC framework that serves to tackle cybersecurity challenges which SMEs frequently encounter. The model utilizes centralized resources and advanced analytics together with shared threat intelligence to deliver scalable and cost-effective cybersecurity solutions that maintain regulatory compliance.

The shared SOC framework provides all businesses with enterprise-level security capabilities and promotes teamwork in identifying threats and managing incidents. The combination of AI-driven threat intelligence with the platform enables SMEs to improve their cyber defense mechanisms while simultaneously cutting expenses and simplifying compliance tasks.

This paper establishes a theoretical basis that will guide subsequent validation efforts and practical implementation through real-world testing and iterative refinement to prove practical feasibility.

## References

1. Ntingi, N., du Toit, J., von Solms, S.: A community security operations centre (ComSOC) model for SMMEs in developing countries. In: Arai, K. (ed.) Intelligent Computing, pp. 443–456. Springer, Cham (2024)
2. de Arroyabe, J.F., Arroyabe, M., Fernandez, I., Arranz, C.: Cybersecurity resilience in SMEs. A machine learning approach. J. Comput. Inf. Syst., 1–17 (2023)
3. Wang, W., Sadjadi, S.M., Rishe, N.: A survey of major cybersecurity compliance frameworks. In: 2024 IEEE 10th Conference on Big Data Security on Cloud (BigDataSecurity), pp. 23–34 (2024). https://doi.org/10.1109/BigDataSecurity62737.2024.00013
4. Azinheira, B., Antunes, M., Maximiano, M., Gomes, R.P.: Information security and cybersecurity assessment in SME-an implementation methodology. J. Glob. Bus. Technol. **19**(1) (2023)
5. Dimitrov, W., Dimitrov, G., Spasov, K., Syarova, S.: Conceptual model for a shared cybersecurity operations center for ICS. In: Proceedings of the Computational Methods in Systems and Software, pp. 493–503. Springer (2021)
6. Van Haastrecht, M., et al.: A shared cyber threat intelligence solution for SMEs. Electronics **10**(23), 2913 (2021)
7. Rifa, M.: Challenges to small and medium businesses for cyber threat intelligence sharing (2024)
8. Simola, J.: Comparative research of cybersecurity information sharing models (2019)
9. Armenia, S., Angelini, M., Nonino, F., Palombi, G., Schlitzer, M.F.: A dynamic simulation approach to support the evaluation of cyber risks and security investments in SMEs. Decis. Support Syst.**147**, 113,580 (2021)
10. Renaud, K., Ophoff, J.: A cyber situational awareness model to predict the implementation of cyber security controls and precautions by SMEs. Organ. Cybersecur. J. Pract. Process People **1**(1), 24–46 (2021)
11. Bhavsar, R., Thakar, V.: Design and implementation of an open-source security operations center for effective cyber threat detection and response (2025)
12. Bassey, C., Chinda, E.T., Idowu, S.: Building a scalable security operations center: a focus on open-source tools. J. Eng. Res. Rep. **26**(7), 196–209 (2024)
13. Wang, J., et al.: A distributed framework for security operation center in the application of institute of high energy physics. In: International Symposium on Grids and Clouds (ISGC), vol. 19 (2023)
14. Mocanu, F., Scripcariu, L.: Implementation of a security operation center-an essential cybersecurity solution for organizations. In: 2023 27th International Conference on System Theory, Control and Computing (ICSTCC), pp. 539–544. IEEE (2023)

15. Brett, M.: An approach to establishing a multi-organisational public sector security operations centre. Cyber Secur. Peer-Rev. J. **6**(4), 373–383 (2023)
16. Fysarakis, K., Mavroeidis, V., Athanatos, M., Spanoudakis, G., Ioannidis, S.: A blueprint for collaborative cybersecurity operations centres with capacity for shared situational awareness, coordinated response, and joint preparedness. In: 2022 IEEE International Conference on Big Data (Big Data), pp. 2601–2609. IEEE (2022)

# Computer Science and Computer Engineering Education

# Enhancing SQL Learning with Large Language Models: Generating Translations and Explanations for Educational Use

Samira Moser and Ela Pustulka(✉)

The University of Applied Sciences and Arts Northwestern Switzerland FHNW, School of Business, Olten, Switzerland
samira.moser@gmx.ch, elzbieta.pustulka@fhnw.ch

**Abstract.** We explore the potential of large language models (LLMs) to help business users to understand SQL, with a view to include such techniques in teaching and programming support tools. We propose a new method which uses LLMs in two stages: content creation and content evaluation. Our method was tested with 32 SQL queries from Spider and five LLMs. We discovered that using RAG is not beneficial. Human evaluation showed that our method successfully generates quality outputs which can be used in teaching or business. Our students showed a preference for short structured explanations and found both the explanations and translations to be useful.

**Keywords:** SQL translation generation · SQL explanation generation · database education · Retrieval Augmented Generation (RAG) · SQL2Text · Large Language Model (LLM)

## 1 Introduction

Large Language Models (LLMs) [1,2] are increasingly being used by our students and by business but they currently lack quality controls and may lead to erroneous solutions. We want to use LLMs to provide extra learning support. In particular, we would like to use LLMs reliably to enhance our SQL learning game [3] and to support students and business users in the use of database development tools by providing high quality SQL translations and explanations.

LLM business scenarios include data warehousing, online data processing, data science and data analysis [4]. Current research on the boundary of SQL and AI focuses on text to SQL translation (Text2SQL) [5]. Translation accuracy depends on the method used and the test dataset (query specifications, sample schema and SQL), with the highest accuracy just over 70% on SPIDER [6]. There is little research devoted to SQL2Text as highlighted by [7–9]. Particularly, translation and explanation quality has not been investigated, and correctness and usefulness to learners or business people with limited database knowledge is unclear. As providing quality assurance (QA) in LLM use could lead to reliable


K. Daimi and A. Alsadoon (Eds.): ICR 2025, LNNS 1487, pp. 273–282, 2025.
https://doi.org/10.1007/978-3-031-95652-2_23

business and educational solutions, we aim to create a reliable LLM use scenario including both generation and QA.

We investigated the following questions. First, what is the quality of SQL to NL translation and of SQL explanation. Second, what is the best prompting strategy (pure SQL, or retrieval augmented generation RAG [10]). Third, how do LLMs compare in terms of quality. Fourth, do our students find the solution acceptable and, fifth, what are the cost implications.

Our new method includes automated quality control. Our experiment used 32 SPIDER queries and several LLMs to translate SQL to text, explain SQL, and assess the quality. Our prompts were: a simple one using only the SQL and an instruction, and two prompts with RAG. In the quality evaluation, LLMs graded outputs on a scale 1 to 4 (low to high) and scores below 3 were examined by eye. The method was verified by our students who rated the outputs and filled in a survey.

We present the following contributions. First, we present a method which uses LLMs in two steps to produce good quality SQL to natural language (NL) translations and explanations. Second, we verify our method using human verification. Our experiment makes a strong business case for using LLMs in both educational and business SQL solutions.

This paper continues as follows. Section 2 presents related work. Section 3 details our experiment and Sect. 4 presents the results. We discuss and conclude in Sect. 5.

## 2 Related Work

Large Language Models (LLMs) [11] are complex software systems based on very large matrices of token probabilities which can be used to generate text and other media. Their purpose is to produce the most probable outcome of tokens, given a prompt. Recent surveys include work by Yang et al. [12] which looks at the LLMs from the perspectives of models, data, and downstream tasks such as natural language understanding, generation, knowledge-intensive tasks, reasoning, and supporting humans in situations where actionable plans need to be developed to cope with poorly specified real-world scenarios. As most LLMs are generic, one of the approaches is to engineer the prompt given to the LLM. For instance, retrieval augmented generation (RAG) [10] can provide an LLM with additional information.

Katsogiannis and Koutrika [4] said that SQL to text translation is under researched, which directly inspired our work. Mitsopolu and Kutrika [5] analysed almost 30 Text-to-SQL benchmarks and proposed a new evaluation methodology with an error analysis method for SQL query categorisation. The analysis included: structural and operator variety, operator, schema usage and content usage, schema complexity and quality, database size. In the NL specifications they analysed schema linkage, lexical and syntactic complexity, and readability. Spider [6] and KaggleDBQA [13] have the highest structural variety. Spider has a low operator use and most queries cover less than 10 columns while Atis [14] uses the most conditions on data values. Spider has medium structural variety, lexical complexity and schema quality, high schema linkage, syntactic complexity and readability and is low in all other measures.

Al-Lawati et al. [9] developed a complex NL utterance generation strategy which creates NL variants for the same SQL. They used a Graph Neural Network (GNN) and the SQL syntax tree. The evaluation used three smaller LLMs and GPT-4 [15] and discovered that the method improves performance for smaller language models but does not help with GPT-4. Sandkuhl [16] investigated whether LLMs can be used for QC of LLM output and concluded that LLMs can support quality control, but cannot fully substitute human experts. Hamzic et al. [17] performed QC on text generation from 20 LLMs and created guidelines for selecting the most suitable LLMs for complex RAG applications. There are no other relevant publications for SQL and no further reports directly in this area.

Zhang [18] reports using AI in a database technology course for case study generation, entity relationship (ER) modelling, test data design, generating SQL, and business performance analysis. Students feel that AI tools help them understand tables/attributes, support critical thinking, and help with creativity and learning, i.e. with higher-level cognitive skills. Students also said that AI tools help when they apply concepts to business problems like problem solving, business case generation and generating SQL code.

Wanjiru et al. [19] investigated automated SQL grading. They proposed a model for defining correctness levels used by a grading system. By increasing the number of properties and the number of outcomes in the model, they achieved a better differentiation of incorrect answers, which might lead to more objective grading. Jury et al. [20] investigated using LLMs to get programming help for students. They reported that prompt chaining and one-shot learning are useful strategies for optimising the output of an LLM. The students found LLMs to be a useful source of learning guidance.

## 3 Methods

Figure 1 shows the experiment consisting of generation and evaluation. The left hand side shows content generation (three LLMs generating translations and explanations) and the right hand side shows the evaluation: cosine similarity, prompts asking LLMs for accuracy, understandability and alignment with the query, students ranking the outputs and taking a survey, and ourselves scoring outputs below 3.

The query set consisted of 32 Spider queries with SQL, NL specification, and schema. Table 1 shows two queries and makes it clear that even the shortest query we selected would not be easy for our students. For each query, the NL specification is also shown. Two specifications are given for the second query, of which we used the first one. Figure 2 shows query length distribution in words. All queries are included in at least one of the categories shown in Table 2 which shows the percentage of queries in each category; on average, the queries use operations from three categories.

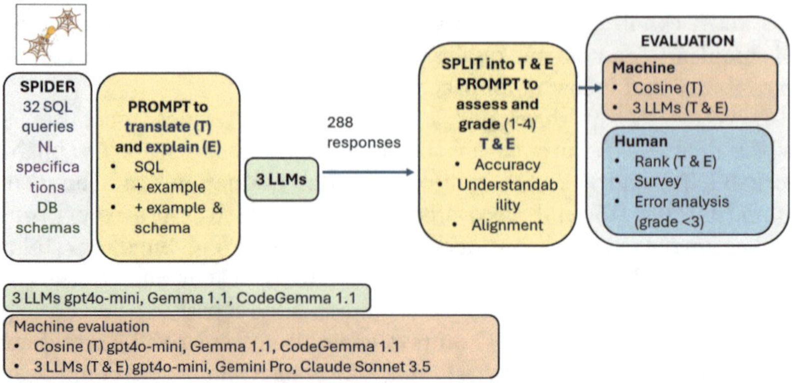


**Fig. 1.** Experiment overview: translation and explanation generation and evaluation.

**Table 1.** The shortest and longest query and NL questions.

| SQL Query | NL Question(s) |
|---|---|
| SELECT document_name, template_id FROM Documents WHERE Document_Description LIKE "%w%" | What is the document name and template id for document with description with the letter 'w' in it? |
| SELECT T1.fname, T1.age FROM student AS T1 JOIN has_pet AS T2 ON T1.stuid=T2.stuid JOIN pets AS T3 ON T3.petid=T2.petid WHERE T3.pettype='dog' AND T1.stuid NOT IN (SELECT T1.stuid FROM student AS T1 JOIN has_pet AS T2 ON T1.stuid=T2.stuid JOIN pets AS T3 ON T3.petid= T2.petid WHERE T3.pettype='cat') | 1. Find the first name and age of students who have a dog but do not have a cat as a pet.<br>2. What is the first name of every student who has a dog but does not have a cat? |

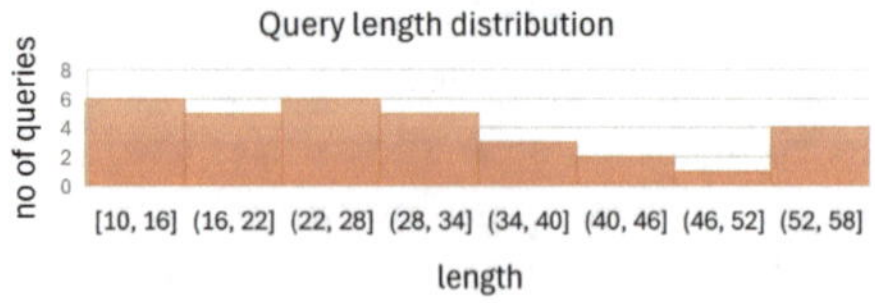


**Fig. 2.** Query length distribution, lengths ranging from 10 to 58 query terms.

We tested five Large Language Models (LLMs) [21] which became available in 2024. In content creation we used: OpenAI's GPT-4o-mini [22], Google's Gemma 1.1 [23] and CodeGemma 1.1 [24] with seven billion parameters each and in the assessment OpenAI's GPT-4o-mini, Google's Gemini Pro 1.5 [25] and Anthropic's Claude Sonnet 3.5 [26].

**Table 2.** Percentage of queries in each category.

| Category | % of Queries |
|---|---|
| Calculation (i.e. sum, avg., count) | 78 |
| Group By | 47 |
| Natural Join | 44 |
| Greater/Smaller/AND/OR/Equal | 41 |
| Other Join | 34 |
| Subquery | 34 |
| Order By | 22 |
| Not in | 16 |
| Intersect | 16 |
| Like | 9 |

**Table 3.** Prompt template for gpt4o-mini.

| |
|---|
| Provide first a natural language translation followed by an explanation of the SQL query. Go through it step by step and output the result in simple and concise language. Use the information of the context as examples for the translation and the schema to get the names of tables and columns. Keep the output in line with the length number. |
| **Context:** `// SQL example queries`<br>**Schema:** `// DB schema information`<br>**Query:** `// SQL query`<br>**output_length:** `// query_length *3` |

We used GTE-large [27] to vectorise Spider inputs used in RAG and to calculate cosine similarity of translations. Prompt design was inspired by [28,29], with three variants: (1) SQL with an instruction to translate and explain, (2) SQL, the instruction and the example query and translation pairs, and (3) SQL, the example query and translation pairs and the DB schema. Table 3 shows the prompt template.

Table 4 shows example translation prompt and the output for a query giving low scores. The LLM gives a low score and justifies its decision by pointing out the translation problems. The automated part of the evaluation included, first, splitting the output into translation and explanation and then, for the translation, cosine similarity with GTE-large [27]. Then, for both translation and explanation, we carried out LLM evaluation with three LLMs, to be graded on a scale 1 to 4. All outputs scoring below 3 were examined by eye. Selected outputs were given to our students for rating. Students worked in small teams (2 to 3 people) and in each case rated three translations and then three explanations, for a number of queries.

**Table 4.** Example translation examined by hand.

| |
|---|
| *Spider SQL*: SELECT T2.name , T2.capacity from concert AS T1 JOIN stadium AS T2 ON T1.stadium_id = T2.stadium_id WHERE T1.year ≥ 2014 GROUP BY T2.stadium_id ORDER BY count(*) DESC LIMIT 1 |
| *Spider NL*: Show the stadium name and capacity with most number of concerts in year 2014 or after. |
| *LLM Translation*: The query wants to find the name of the stadium that hosted the most events in a particular year. |
| *Accuracy*: - The translation correctly identifies that the query is about finding a stadium. However, it incorrectly states "in a particular year" when the query is actually looking at all years from 2014 onwards. It misses mentioning that the query is also retrieving the capacity of the stadium. It uses the term "events" instead of "concerts," which is less precise. It doesn't mention that the query is selecting only one stadium (the one with the most concerts). *Understandability*: - The translation is simple and easy to understand. However, it lacks important details that are present in the SQL query. *Comparison* with the given question: - The question "Show the stadium name and capacity with most number of concerts in year 2014 or after" is actually a more accurate representation of the SQL query than the given translation. *Assessment scores*: **Accuracy: 2 (Major errors)** *Understandability*: 3 (Minor errors) *Overall score*: **2 (Major errors)** The translation has significant omissions and one incorrect statement. While it captures the general idea of finding a stadium based on event frequency, it misses crucial details about the time frame, the specific type of events (concerts), and the additional information being retrieved (capacity). The translation is easy to understand, but its lack of precision and completeness makes it potentially misleading. |

## 4 Results

The cosine similarity, between the NL query and LLM translations ranged from 0.49 to 0.95. Average scores per prompt type/LLM combination are shown in Fig. 3. The highest avg. score, 0.85, was for gpt4o-mini with the RAG prompt including example query. When we group the averages by prompt type, we see the average cos similarity of 0.78 for both RAG prompts and 0.82 for pure SQL (SD<1), which shows that using RAG leads to more variety in translations.

Figure 4 shows translation and explanation scores averaged per prompt type. Overall, we see a higher score for the prompt-only type. The translation and explanation evaluation scores are similar, but explanation scores were usually higher.

Nine students, ages 22–27 (seven male, two female), were present in class (class size 19, attendance not mandatory) and took part in an experiment which involved ranking and survey. They ranked the translations and explanations for understandability, accuracy and general preference. For each assessment, we showed the SQL, NL and the LLM outputs. The students ranked the answers from best to worst. There were no significant differences. The survey asked the

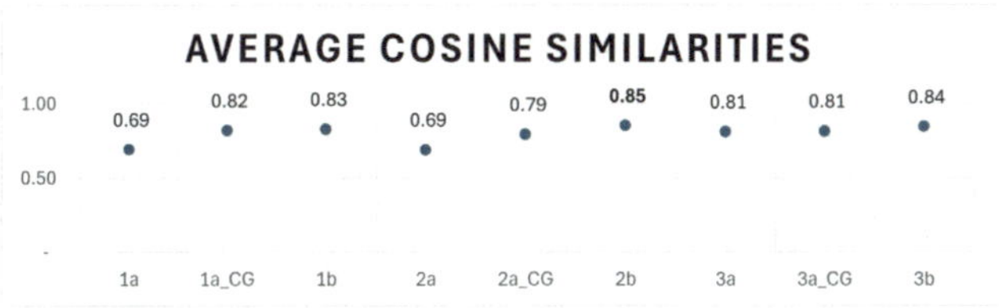


**Fig. 3.** Cosine similarity scores for three LLMs and three prompt types.

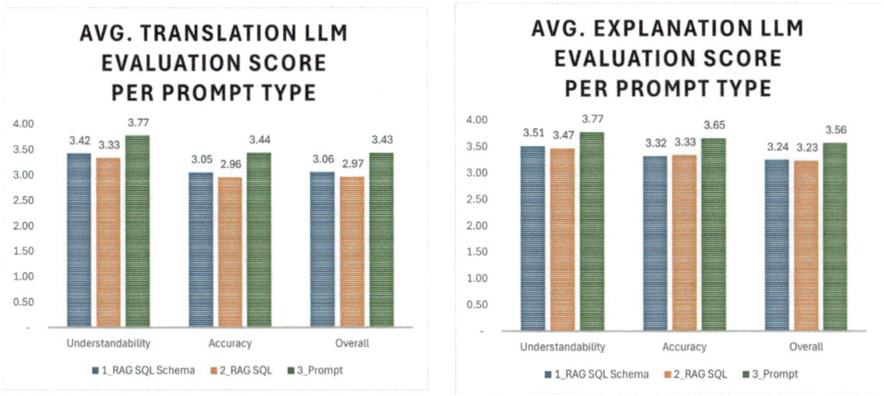


**Fig. 4.** Average translation and evaluation scores per prompt type.

students seven questions to cover correctness, clarity, understandability, and usefulness, based on [20]. The students liked the application and appreciated its use in supporting learning. Figure 5 shows the survey results grouped by assessment area. It turned out the students prefer shorter outputs, like to see the explanations numbered, and prefer explanations with no code.

We analysed the LLM outputs scoring below 3 by hand: 94 translations and 71 explanations (29% of all outputs). Figure 6 shows errors for all variants. We observe RAG confusion for Gemma (1a, 2a), less for Code Gemma (2a, 2a_CG) and the least for gpt (1b, 2b, 3b). The best outcomes are for 3a (Gemma), 3a_CG (Code Gemma) and 3b (gpt) with a pure SQL prompt which is the most robust. Of the three LLMs, gpt (3b) has the best performance with 4 errors which we classified as misunderstanding. Some SQL queries turned out to be a challenge for all LLMs both in translation and explanation. Misunderstandings are more prevalent in translations than explanations. The number of hallucinations, where information was fabricated, was low (1 % of translation errors and 1.4 % for explanations).

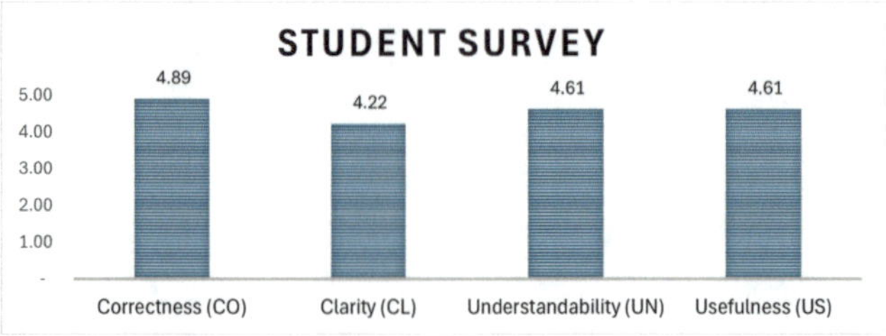


**Fig. 5.** Survey Outcomes.

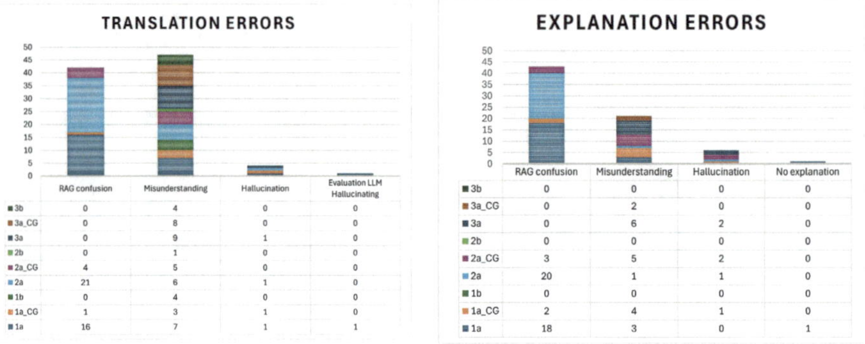


**Fig. 6.** Manual error analysis shows RAG confusion.

We used two types of LLMs: one hosted by the owner, OpenAI, and the other as a local LLM model on Google Colab, for the two Gemma versions. Table 5 shows the costs we incurred.

**Table 5.** Experiment costing.

| Cost Type | OpenAI GPT-4o-mini | Google (Code)Gemma |
|---|---|---|
| API Calls | USD 2.16 | n/a |
| Online Processing (Google Colab) | n/a | 40 € |
| Total | USD 2.16 | 40 € |

## 5 Discussion and Conclusion

We have designed a robust solution allowing us to generate supporting materials for teaching, including our SQL game [3]. Our solution is reusable [30]. The most important observations are as follows. Prompt-only applications perform best for SQL2Text and GPT-4o-mini was the best overall. There were very few hallucinations (1%). We used LLMs successfully to provide quality control. Our students confirmed the usefulness of this solution. Other business contexts would require rerunning our experiment with a different benchmark.

Future work will include application to real business problems in collaboration with our business partners, for instance in data integration. We will directly generate SQL translations and explanations in our teaching game and the class examples. We will investigate other QC control frameworks and model fine tuning.

In summary, we have produced a method which can weed out poor LLM output automatically and is applicable in teaching and business. The solution can now be automated and will include voting on outputs, either based purely on the rating provided by the LLMs or some other measures of goodness which could supplement LLM judgments.

## References


1. Vaswani, A., et al.: Attention is all you need. In: NeurIPS '17, pp. 5998–6008 (2017)
2. Devlin, J., Chang, M., Lee, K., Toutanova, K.: BERT: pre-training of deep bidirectional transformers for language understanding. In: Proceedings of the NAACL-HLT 2019, vol. 1, pp. 4171–4186. ACL (2019)
3. Pustulka, E., Krause, K., de Espona, L., Kennel, A.: SQL scrolls - a reusable and extensible DGBL experiment. In: CSERC '21, pp. 39–48. ACM (2022)
4. Katsogiannis-Meimarakis, G., Koutrika, G.: A survey on deep learning approaches for text-to-SQL. VLDB J. **32**(4), 905–936 (2023)
5. Mitsopoulou, A., Koutrika, G.: Analysis of text-to-SQL benchmarks: limitations, challenges and opportunities. In: Proceedings of the EDBT 2025, pp. 199–212. OpenProceedings.org (2025)
6. Yu, T., et al.: Spider: a large-scale human-labeled dataset for complex and cross-domain semantic parsing and text-to-SQL task. In: EMNLP '18, pp. 3911–3921. ACL (2018)
7. Kokkalis, A., Vagenas, P., Zervakis, A., Simitsis, A., Koutrika, G., Ioannidis, Y.: Logos: a system for translating queries into narratives. In: Proceedings of the 2012 ACM SIGMOD, pp. 673–676. ACM (2012)
8. Eleftherakis, S., Gkini, O., Koutrika, G.: Let the database talk back: natural language explanations for SQL. In: SEA-Data '21, vol. 2929, pp. 14–19. CEUR-WS.org (2021). https://ceur-ws.org/Vol-2929/paper3.pdf
9. Al Lawati, A., Lucas, J., Mitra, P.: Semantic captioning: benchmark dataset and graph-aware few-shot in-context learning for SQL2Text. In: COLING '25, pp. 8026–8042. ACL (2025)
10. Salemi, A., Zamani, H.: Evaluating retrieval quality in retrieval-augmented generation. In: SIGIR '24, pp. 2395–2400. ACM (2024)
11. McDonough, M.: Large Language Model. Encyclopædia Britannica, Inc. (2025). https://www.britannica.com/topic/large-language-model
12. Yang, J., et al.: Harnessing the power of LLMs in practice: a survey on ChatGPT and beyond. ACM Trans. Knowl. Discov. Data **18**(6) (2024)
13. Lee, C., Polozov, O., Richardson, M.: KaggleDBQA: realistic evaluation of text-to-SQL parsers. In: ACL/IJCNLP 2021, vol. 1, pp. 2261–2273. ACL (2021)
14. Hemphill, C.T., Godfrey, J.J., Doddington, G.R.: The ATIS spoken language systems pilot corpus. In: Speech and Natural Language: Proceedings of a Workshop Held at Hidden Valley, Pennsylvania, June 24–27, 1990 (1990)

15. Achiam, J., et al.: GPT-4 technical report. arXiv preprint arXiv:2303.08774 (2023)
16. Sandkuhl, K.: LLM-assistance for quality control of LLM output. In: Perspectives in Business Informatics Research, pp. 36–50. Springer, Cham (2024)
17. Hamzic, D., Wurzenberger, M., Skopik, F., Landauer, M., Rauber, A.: Evaluation and comparison of open-source LLMs using natural language generation quality metrics. In: BigData '24, pp. 5342–5351. IEEE (2024)
18. Zhang, X.: Teaching tip: incorporating AI tools into database classes. J. Inf. Syst. Educ. **36**(1), 37–52 (2025)
19. Wanjiru, B., van Bommel, P., Hiemstra, D.: Sensitivity of automated SQL grading in computer science courses. In: ICR'24, pp. 283–299. Springer Nature (2024)
20. Jury, B., Lorusso, A., Leinonen, J., Denny, P., Luxton-Reilly, A.: Evaluating LLM-generated worked examples in an introductory programming course. In: ACE '24, pp. 77–86. ACM (2024)
21. Auffarth, B.: Generative AI with LangChain: Build Large Language Model (LLM) Apps with Python, ChatGPT and Other LLMs. Packt Ltd, 1st edn. (2023)
22. OpenAI: GPT-4o mini 10.2024 [large lanaguage model]. https://openai.com/index/gpt-4o-mini-advancing-cost-efficient-intelligence/
23. Gemma Team: Mesnard, T., et al.: Gemma 1.1 [large language model] (2024). https://www.kaggle.com/m/3301
24. CodeGemma Team, Hartman, A.J., et al.: Codegemma: open code models based on gemma - codegemma 1.1 [large language model] (2024). https://goo.gle/codegemma
25. Google: Gemini 1.5 pro-001 [large language model]. https://gemini.google.com/u/2/app/74678e68630afef0
26. Anthropic: Claude 3.5 sonnet. https://docs.anthropic.com/en/docs/about-claude/models, large language model]. Anthropic
27. Li, Z., Zhang, X., Zhang, Y., Long, D., Xie, P., Zhang, M.: Towards general text embeddings with multi-stage contrastive learning. arXiv:2308.03281v1
28. Wei, J., et al.: Chain-of-thought prompting elicits reasoning in large language models. In: NeurIPS '22, vol. 35, pp. 24824–24837 (2022)
29. Zhang, D., et al.: SpeechGPT: empowering large language models with intrinsic cross-modal conversational abilities. In: EMNLP '23 (2023)
30. Moser, S.: Repository (2024). https://github.com/Sammynmo/MT_RAG_LLM

# Teaching Abstraction in Computer Science Courses

Neelam Soundarajan(✉)

Computer Science and Engineering Department, The Ohio State University, Columbus, USA
neelam@cse.ohio-state.edu

**Abstract.** A number of authors have stressed the importance of *abstraction* in Computer Science. Over the last thirty years or so, colleges and universities and even high schools have developed CS courses, using *object-oriented* languages such as *Java*, *Python*, etc., that attempt to teach abstraction from the start. In spite of this, many students do not develop adequate abstraction skills. They are able to write code in their particular language but because it is not well-designed from the point of view of abstraction, it tends to be brittle and difficult for others to build on or modify, etc. In this paper, we develop a way based on the idea of *reflective abstraction* to effectively address the problem so that a greater number of students will be able to develop good quality code that is extendible and can be used by other software engineers in their own systems.

**Keywords:** STEM Education · OO Programming · Learning Paradox · Reflective Abstraction · Constructivism

## 1 Introduction

A number of authors have stressed the importance of *abstract thinking* in computer science (CS); see, e.g., [1–5]. Kramer [6] argues that abstraction is the *key* to computing. He states that better students are able to deal with complexity, are able to come up with clean designs, and are able to deal with involved distributed algorithms, systems, etc.; on the other hand, other students find distributed algorithms incomprehensible and often cannot identify what is important in a problem and what is not; their solutions tend to be relatively complex. The reason for this difference between the two groups, according to Kramer, is the difference in their abilities to engage in abstract thinking.

Kramer further claims that the difference between these two groups of students is *innate* and that there is no effective way to teach students in the less capable group in such a way that they are able to engage in abstract thinking. The author further suggests that the appropriate course of action is to ensure that students who are not able to engage in abstract thinking be identified using a suitable test, such as the one described by Annas *et al.* [7], and ensure that


K. Daimi and A. Alsadoon (Eds.): ICR 2025, LNNS 1487, pp. 283–293, 2025.
https://doi.org/10.1007/978-3-031-95652-2_24

students who are not able to engage in abstract thinking are not admitted to computing programs even if their grades in prerequisite courses are very good. If we accept the claim that there is no effective way to teach students abstract thinking, this seems to be an appropriate course of action.

Our goal in this paper is to *solve* the problem of enabling students to engage in abstract thinking. We describe a method that will help students develop abstraction skills rather than simply giving up on those whose abstraction abilities are deemed insufficient. However, it is too late to try to do this in CS courses, especially, at the college-level. The problem develops earlier in the curriculum in math courses and, specifically, in Algebra courses, at the middle and high school levels. It is in the algebra course that students first encounter abstraction. It is where, for example, they first come across the novel idea that a *variable* such ss $X$ may be used to denote *any* integer. We also show how our approach will help students later when they take CS courses.

To see how novel the idea of variables may seem upon first encounter, see the paper by Sfard [8] which provides a fascinating account of how many *centuries* it took mathematicians to develop idea of variable *after* the essential ideas of algebra had been well understood. Many students in the algebra course do not understand abstract notions such as variables and get into the habit of simply *memorizing* and mechanically applying rules such as *cross-multiplication* according to which an equation such as $(A/B = X/Y)$ may be rewritten as $(A * Y = X * B)$ with no understanding of *why*, in terms of the underlying properties of numbers, such an equation makes sense.

There are, of course, a large number of middle and high schools in most countries around the world. These schools, typically, employ a number of teachers to teach their algebra courses. The teachers go through a number of years of education and training. Thus, in the US, algebra teachers typically complete a four-year degree program in *Math Education* followed by a year or more of *in-the-field* training where the teacher is considered an apprentice teacher and is supervised by an experienced teacher while teaching their classes. This means that any changes we propose should *not* require retraining the teachers. Hence our solution is an online system that is designed to be used by individual students or small groups of students *outside* regular school hours in order to help them improve their understanding of the topics discussed by their school teachers in the classroom as well as to prepare for topics yet to be discussed during regular class meetings.

## 2 Literature Review

In this section, we review three different approaches, Explicit Instruction, Constructivism, and Guided Discovery, that have been used in schools and colleges to teach various STEM topics. Next, we discuss the notion of *learning paradox* which is concerned with the difficulty of learning new *concepts* such as *variables* or *abstract data types*.

### 2.1 Explicit Instruction

Explicit Instruction is the standard approach used in schools. The teacher lectures to a class full of students on the topic(s) of the day and students are expected to take notes and study them, along with their textbook(s). The teacher demonstrates how specific problems related to the topic may be solved. Students may be asked, during the class period, to work individually or in small groups to solve similar problems. Students are also expected to work on their own to solve problems that, typically, appear in each chapter of the book.

Students are, typically, assigned a number of homework problems, similar to the ones seen in the class, that they have and submit their solutions for evaluation and feedback. Questions and problems that are posed in the midterm and final examinations for the course tend to be similar to the ones demonstrated by the teacher and to the homework problems. The same students who paid careful attention during the lectures and worked diligently generally do well on these exams and their course grades will, correspondingly, be good. These students are assumed to have a good grasp of the techniques *and concepts* that are considered most important in the topic(s) of the course. However, Gray and Tall [9] argue that while a student who is able to solve standard textbook problems effectively may have developed *procedural fluency*, there is no guarantee that the student has also developed deep *conceptual* understanding of the topic.

A number of educational video games have been developed over the years that are intended to help students with their school work. One of the popular games in the case of algebra is *DragonBox Algebra* [10, 11]. These games present a number of problems, similar to the homework and textbook problems set in a playful or otherwise engaging environment. As a result, students playing these games enjoy working on the problems presented by the game and improve their skills in solving such problems. Many of these same students hate working on standard homework problems. Thus, these games enable even such students to develop the ability to solve homework and exam problems resulting in improved grades in their courses. But they do not contribute to developing students' conceptual understanding.

### 2.2 Constructivism

Proponents of *constructivism* [12, 13] argue that in order to *truly* understand an idea, the learners must *construct* it for themselves. Although constructivism is typically discussed in the context of topics such as physics, it applies to mathematics as well. Thus, in the case of algebra, the learners must, for example, construct the idea of *variable* for themselves.

While there is no question that students who are able to construct, by themselves, the idea of variable will have a superb understanding of the idea, hardly *any* student will succeed in doing so. The approach of guided discovery is a compromise, and we turn to it next.

### 2.3 Guided Discovery

An example from the physics education literature will help clarify what is meant by "*conceptual understanding*". An important topic in high school and first year college physics courses is Newton's Laws of Motion. It is also one for which students have difficulty internalizing the underlying concepts and applying them correctly to situations that may arise in practice but are not typical textbook-type problems. "Concept inventories" [14,15] have been created in order to pin down such misconceptions. These are multiple-choice tests administered after students have successfully completing the relevant courses. Nieminen *et al.* [16], in their test, posed a scenario in which an 18-wheeler truck and a subcompact car collide head-on at high speed and the question concerned the force exerted by each on the other. Newton's Third Law of Motion which states that the force exerted by an object $A$ on a second object $B$ is equal and opposite to the force exerted by $B$ on $A$. In the test, the student had to choose from among a number of alternatives ranging from the correct one, that they are equal and opposite; to one that sounds more intuitive, that the truck exerts much greater force on the car than does the car on the truck; to a ridiculous one, "neither exerts a force on the other, the car gets smashed simply because it gets in the way of the truck". While a number of students did pick the correct answer, a surprising number chose one of the wrong answers, including the ridiculous one. What this demonstrates is that while their course grades may indicate that these students may have learned the mechanics of applying Newton's Laws to compute, say, the acceleration given the mass of an object and the force acting on it, they had not really internalized its *conceptual* underpinnings. Gray and Tall [9] and Sfard [17,18] discuss the importance of conceptual understanding but they do not offer any guidance on how we may help students achieve conceptual understanding.

The essence of the *guided discovery* approach is to help students develop conceptual understanding without expecting them to *discover* the concepts by themselves as is the case with constructivism. The teacher *guides* the student in the quest to arrive at the concept in question. Guided discovery may be difficult to implement in a classroom since different students may require different levels of guidance. Hence, there are video games. e.g., those developed by the *Virtual Reality* company, *Prisms of Reality, Inc.*, [19], for such topics as linear functions, exponential growth, etc. The idea is that, as students play these games on their VR headsets, the game will guide them to "discover" the underlying concepts.

While that is reasonable in principle, in practice there is a potential problem. The student may get so engaged in the story and the visuals that he or she does not really comprehend the underlying concept. Precisely this happened at Metro Middle School, an urban school in Columbus, Ohio, where eighth grade students were working on understanding slope, linear functions and exponential functions. After playing the VR games from *Prisms* on these topics, discussions among the students as well as between the students and their teacher suggested that they had picked up some wrong ideas. Thus, many students seemed to think that exponential functions are similar to quadratic or cubic functions in their rate of growth. This is not entirely surprising since the game, of necessity, can only have the student go through a small number of instances. Thus in the case of exponential growth, the Prisms game uses the example of infection spreading among a population due to a virus with each person infecting, say, three others. When the student player sees what happens to the number of people infected over, say, five cycles, they see that the corresponding graph rises in a non-linear manner, similar to a quadratic or cubic function. They cannot imagine that after, say, one hundred cycles, the exponential growth would have grown far, far beyond cubic functions, etc.

### 2.4 Learning Paradox

The fundamental problem in learning any new concept is explained by the *learning paradox* [20–22]. Cognitive theories assert that learners actively construct knowledge and mental structures based on knowledge and mental structures they *already* possess. The paradox is, in that case, how can anyone acquire a *new* concept which is not anything like what they already possess? How can a middle school student understand *variables* or *derivatives* of functions when they don't already possess knowledge or mental structures that are similar? This is why the eighth graders playing the *Prisms* VR game did not acquire the idea of *exponential growth* since they didn't already possess this concept.

## 3 Our Approach

The solution to the paradox lies in the concept of *reflective abstraction.* We start by considering two examples.

### 3.1 Two Examples

Consider a simple expression such as $3 + 4$. For many Algebra students, this expression is an *instruction* to add 3 and 4. But when they come across an expression such as $3 + X$ in their algebra course, what do they do? How can you add 3 to $X$ when you do not know what $X$ is? Or when asked to simplify the expression $3 + 4X - 2Y + X$, how can they proceed? Or when asked to solve the equation $5X - 3 = X + 5$? For these students, algebra becames a symbol manipulation game and to play the game, they must memorize rules such as "change sides, change signs" and apply them.

Or-Bach and Lavy [23] report on third-year CS students who had taken two courses on object-oriented programming and design; a year-long course on OOP with implementation in Java; and a one semester course on Software Engineering with emphasis on Object Oriented Analysis and Design (OOAD). They were given a relatively standard OO design task related to a company with monthly employees and hourly employees with monthly employees being rewarded for extra hours worked and everyone who has worked at the company for three more years receiving a present during the holidays. Total costs of salaries and presents is managed and processed by the HR department. The students were asked to schematically describe the relevant classes and connections between them including design details of the components of the classes such as class names, attributes, methods and their purposes, using OOP principles. They were also asked to list the OO concepts and principles they used. A correct answer should include the class `Employee` as a base class with two derived-classes for the two types of employees. The base class should include an abstract method for calculating salary, and concrete methods for calculating length of employment and for deciding eligibility for the holiday present. A separate class for HR should be included.

Several of the thirty three students in the Or-Bach and Lavy study included irrelevant classes such as one representing the entire company as well as classes that should have been integrated as methods or attributes of the other classes. Other students included classes for special procedures such as calculating eligibility for a present. Some students even included a class corresponding to holiday present. Clearly, these students, despite several years of study of OO programming and OOAD, still had difficulty with abstraction.

The primary question being addressed in our work is, "how do we help students develop abstraction skills in the Algebra course in middle and high schools as well as in Computer Science courses in college?

### 3.2 Reflective Abstraction

Our approach, based on the concept of *reflective abstraction* [24,25], helps address the learning paradox. Explicit instruction, constructivism and guided discovery, are often ineffective in helping students develop an understanding of *abstract* ideas. Instead, students should *arrive* at the idea via *reflection*, i.e., carefully thinking about the presented examples, constructing their *own* examples *and* counterexamples, analyse others' work to identify flaws or especially interesting twists, etc., [26].

One important consideration is that, from the point of view of high school teachers, it is critical that students develop good procedural abilities, even more than conceptual understanding. The reason is that, in much of the US, during their junior or senior year in high school, all students are required to go through state-mandated *proficiency exams* on these topics. These exams are designed to assess the students' *procedural* skills based on courses such as Algebra 1 and the performance of the student in these exams determine whether or not the student successfully graduates from high school and receives a diploma so that they can go on to STEM careers and/or enter STEM college programs; or, if the student's performance is inadequate, they are forced to drop out of high school.

Hence our approach *cannot replace* standard classroom instruction. At the same time, it cannot be an additional set of activities in the classroom since there will not be enough time during the school day for that purpose. Therefore, we plan to build an online system that may be used over the web by students during after-school hours.

# 4 Results and Discussion

## 4.1 Middle/High School Algebra

The author is working with algebra teachers at the Metro Middle and High School in Columbus, Ohio, to develop a set of activities and exercises involving linear algebraic expressions such as $3 + 4X - 2Y + X$ and linear equations such as $5X - 3 = X + 5$. Once these have been developed and tested with volunteer students, they will be fine-tuned and made available to the entire class. These will then be extended to deal with quadratic, cubic and exponential expressions and to solving more complex equations.

These activities will share some key features. Each will present a set of examples and a set of counterexamples *without* any indication of which ones fall into each category. The students will be challenged to classify them appropriately and provide an intuitive explanation –not a formal proof– in each case of their choice. For instance, students may be asked to consider each of the following rules: $X * A = Y * B$ may be rewritten as $X + B = Y + A$; or as $X - B = Y - A$; or as $B - X = A - Y$; and classify each as an example of a *valid* or *invalid* rule, along with an intuitive justification. In addition, as part of the same activity, students may be asked to construct their own rules and have *other* students in the class classify them appropriately and provide intuitive explanations.

This is the essence of reflective abstraction. When students engage in such constructive activities, they develop deep conceptual understanding. This is *not* the same as *constructivism.* Constructivism does not, for instance, require students to come up with *counterexamples.* It simply asserts that students should, on their own, construct knowledge without offering guidance on *how.*

## 4.2 Abstraction in CS Courses

The author regularly teaches an undergraduate course on programming languages with a focus on OO principles. The course is taken by third and fourth year CS students. These are students who have gone through a rigorous one-year long sequence focusing on developing OO software following the principles of encapsulation, abstraction, precise specification of the interface provided by a class, separation of concerns, etc. The students have also completed a one-semester long course on software engineering where they design and develop an application software according to given (informal) specifications.

The main programming project in the author's course requires students to design and implement an *interpreter* for a simple imperative language named *Core.* During the lectures, the author presents details of how the parsing, printing and execution of various parts of Core may be implemented using pseudo-code. Crucially, this discussion completely ignores the OO principles and practices that students have studied in great detail in their earlier courses. But semester after semester, almost no student in the course notices this. Even when the author explicitly poses the question, "What is wrong with what we have been doing thus far?", many students will claim that there was nothing wrong or point to minor issues such as the fact that size of the representation we were using for the abstract parse tree of the program being interpreted might be insufficient. No student ever raises the issue that our parse and execute procedures are tightly interwoven with the details of our particular representation of the abstract parse tree rather than having a separate class that encapsulates those details and provides a suitable interface that the parse and execute procedures can make use of.

Why is this? The answer is that those courses use the *Explicit Instruction* approach to teach these new ideas and Explicit Instruction does not work when trying to learn new ideas. This is also students in Or-Bach and Lavy's study [23] failed to apply the OO principles that they had learned in earlier courses.

The answer is an approach based on *reflective abstraction.* However, given the length of a semester, we cannot expect students to analyze a number of software projects and classify them as examples or counterexamples of abiding by good OO principles. Instead, the author has developed a set of multiplechoice questions similar to questions in concept inventories that probe the student's grasp of these principles. During the presentation at the conference, the author will'discuss some of these questions and seek feedback from the audience.

### 4.3 Contributions

To summarize, we have considered four approaches, these being Explicit Instruction, Constructivism, Guided Discovery and Reflective Abstraction. We now discuss their relative strengths, weaknesses and relevance for learning abstraction. The primary strength of *Explicit instruction* is that is helps students to develop procedural knowledge. By the same token, it is generally ineffective in developing conceptual understanding. The main strength of *Constructivism* is that, when it works, it is very effective in developing conceptual understanding. Unfortunately, it often does not work. *Guided discovery* tries to help students arrive at conceptual understanding but sometimes students end up developing incorrect ideas. *Reflective abstraction* pushes the students toward arriving at conceptual understanding by considering a number of examples and classifying each as valid or invalid along with intuitive explanations; and constructing their own examples and counterexamples and providing intuitive explanations in each case. This approach can be extremely effectiveand is far more likely to work than either Constructivism or Guided discovery in helping students develop conceptual understanding. Its primary weakness is that it is extremely difficult to implement in the classroom.

Table 1 provides a tabular comparison of the strengths, weaknesses and relevance for abstraction learning of each approach. It also includes a brief description of each approach.

**Table 1.** Comparison of Approaches

| Approach | Description | Strengths | Weaknesses | Relevance for Abstraction Learning |
|---|---|---|---|---|
| Explicit Instruction | Teacher-led lectures and problem solving exercises | High usability in classroom, develops procedural knowledge | Limited in developing deep conceptual understanding | Limited |
| Constructivism | Students, with no assistance, construct knowledge and concepts | Very effective when it works | Often does not work | Very High |
| Guided Discovery | Teacher guides the student to help them arrive at concepts | Can be effective | Difficult to implement in classrooms | High |
| Reflective Abstraction | Students arrive at concepts via examples, counterexamples, etc. | Very effective | Difficult to implement in classrooms | Very High |

Next, we turn, in Table 2, to a comparison of traditional classrooms and the proposed *online system* based on reflective abstraction along a number of other dimensions. Accessibility for the classroom is limited to school hours whereas the online system will be accessible 24/7. Scalability for the classroom is very low since the only way to cater to a very large number of students is to build new schools, train new teachers, hire them, etc. By contrast, scalability for the online system is achieved at almost zero cast.

**Table 2.** Comparison of Classroom vs. Online System

| Feature | Traditional Classroom | Online System based on Reflective Abstraction |
|---|---|---|
| Accessibility | Limited to scheduled hours | Available anytime anywhere |
| Scalability | Very Low | Very High |
| Interactivity | Varies from limited to high | Varies from limited to high |
| Feedback | High | Varies from limited to high |
| Empirical Support | Limited | Very Limited |

Interactivity in the classroom depends on the individual teacher. For the online system, interactivity will depend on the details of the implementation. Empirical support for effectiveness of classrooms for developing procedural knowledge is high and for conceptual knowledge is very low as shown by work on concept inventories. Empirical support for effectiveness of the online system based on reflective abstraction does not yet exist since our system seems to be the first of its kind; but Piaget's work shows that it should be very effective for developing conceptual knowledge. Table 2 provides a summary of these aspects.

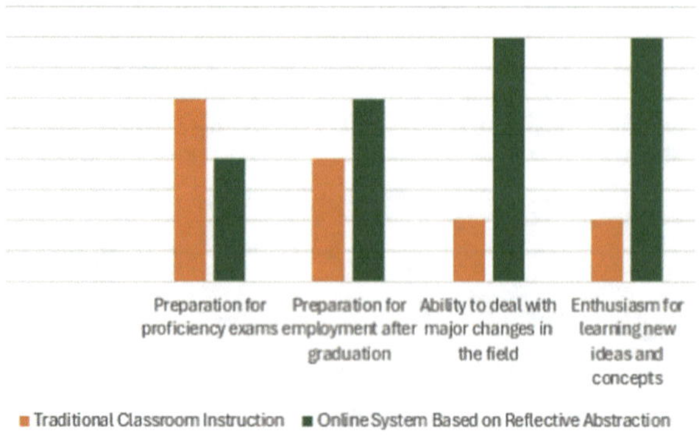


**Fig. 1.** Reflective Abstraction-Based Online System vs. Traditional Classroom

Figure 1 shows the strengths and weaknesses of our approach and the traditional classroom in the form of a chart.

## 5 Conclusions

Although the weakness of traditional classroom instruction in helping students develop conceptual understanding has been known for decades, the approach continues to persist. The main reason for this is the difficulty of changing such a well-established system. Further, traditional classrooms do help students develop procedural knowledge which is the starting point for conceptual understanding. Finally, classroom instruction prepare students for proficiency exams they must successfully complete in order to graduate from high school whereas developing reflective abstraction abilities do not, usually, contribute to this preparation. But when it comes to preparing students for employment after graduation, ability to deal with major changes in a given field or to enter new technical fields and enthusiasm for learning new ideas and concepts, students who develop good reflective abstraction abilities will excel.

The unique strength of reflective abstraction is its focus on conceptual understanding. And, indeed, that is what most STEM teachers would *want* their students to develop. Surprisingly, though, although much research in such fields as psychology has explored the ramifications of reflective abstraction, STEM educators seem to have ignored it. Our work is an attempt to fill this gap in this important domain.

## References

1. Kramer, J.: Abstraction in computer science & software engineering: a pedagogical perspective. Syst. Des. Front. J. **3**(12), 1–9 (2006)
2. Liskov, B., Snyder, A., Atkinson, R., Schaffert, C.: Abstraction mechanisms in CLU. Commun. ACM **20**(8), 564–576 (1977)

3. Statter, D., Armoni, M.: Teaching abstraction in computer science to 7th grade students. ACM Trans. Comput. Educ. (TOCE) **20**(1), 1–37 (2020)
4. Wing, J.: Computational thinking. Commun. ACM **49**(3), 33–35 (2006)
5. Koppelman, H., Van Dijk, B.: Teaching abstraction in introductory courses. In: Proceedings of the Fifteenth Annual Conference on Innovation and Technology in Computer Science Education, pp. 174–178 (2010)
6. Kramer, J.: Is abstraction the key to computing? Commun. ACM **50**(4), 36–42 (2007)
7. Annas, S., Hasma, S., et al.: The abstraction ability in constructing relation within triangles by the seventh grade students of junior high school. J. Phys. Conf. Ser. **954**, 012029 (2018)
8. Sfard, A.: The development of algebra: confronting historical and psychological perspectives. J. Math. Behav. **14**(1), 15–39 (1995)
9. Gray, E.M., Tall, D.O.: Duality, ambiguity, and flexibility: a "proceptual" view of simple arithmetic. J. Res. Math. Educ. **25**(2), 116–140 (1994)
10. Gibbs, P.: Game based learning: the effects of "DragonBox" 12+ on algebraic performance of middle school students. University of Baltimore (2020)
11. Chan, J.Y.C., Closser, A.H., Ngo, V., Smith, H., Liu, A.S., Ottmar, E.: Examining shifts in conceptual knowledge, procedural knowledge and procedural flexibility in the context of two game-based technologies. J. Comput. Assist. Learn. **39**, 1274–1289 (2023)
12. Cobern, W.: Constructivism. J. Educ. Psychol. Consult. **4**(1), 105–112 (1993)
13. Onuf N.: Constructivism. In: World of Our Making, pp. 35–65. Routledge (2012)
14. Ibrahim Abou Halloun and David Hestenes: The initial knowledge state of college physics students. Am. J. Phys. **53**(11), 1043–1055 (1985)
15. Hestenes, D., Wells, M., Swackhamer, G.: Force concept inventory. Phys. Teach. **30**(11), 141–158 (1992)
16. Nieminen, P., Savinaninen, A., Viiri, J.: Force concept inventory=based multiple-choice test. Phys. Rev. Sp Tpcs-Phys Educ. Res. **6**(2), 020109 (2010)
17. Sfard, A.: On the dual nature of mathematical conceptions: Reflections on processes and objects as different sides of the same coin. Educ. Stud. Math. **22**(1), 1–36 (1991)
18. Sfard, A., Linchevski, L.: The gains and the pitfalls of reification-the case of algebra. Educ. Stud. Math. **26**, 191–228 (1994)
19. Prisms of Reality Inc.: Virtual reality games for math (2024)
20. Fodor, J.: Fixation of belief and concept acquisition. In: Language and Learning: The Debate Between Jean Piaget and Noam Chomsky, pp. 142–149, Harvard University Press (1980)
21. Bereiter, C.: Toward a solution of the learning paradox. Rev. Educ. Res. **55**(2), 201–226 (1985)
22. Bratianu, C.: The learning paradox and the university. J. Appl. Quant. Methods **2**(4), 375–386 (2007)
23. Or-Bach, R., Lavy, I.: Cognitive activities of abstraction in object orientation: an empirical study. ACM SIGCSE Bull. **36**(2), 82–86 (2004)
24. Piaget, J., Campell, R.: Studies in Reflecting Abstraction. Psychology Press (2014)
25. Beth, E.W., Piaget, J.: Strict demonstration and heuristic procedures. In: Mathematical Epistemology and Psychology, pp. 86–100. Springer (1966). https://doi.org/10.1007/978-94-017-2193-6_4
26. Mason, J., Watson, A.: Mathematics as a constructive activity: exploiting dimensions of possible variation. Making Connection Res. Teach. Undergraduate Math. Educ. **73**, 191–204 (2008)

# Enhancing VR Education through AI-Driven Emotional Adaptation: A Survey on Emotion-Centric VFX and Adaptive Learning Environments

Sobia Kousar[1(✉)], Farnaz Farid[2], Mukta D. O. Dinesh Kumar[1], Somesh S. O. Guljari Lal[1], and Mahmoud Bekhit[3,4]

[1] Asia Pacific International College, Sydney, Australia
[2] School of Social Sciences, Western Sydney University, Sydney, Australia
farnaz.farid@westernsydney.edu.au
[3] Peter Faber Business School, Australian Catholic University (ACU), North Sydney, NSW, Australia
mahmoud.bekhit@acu.edu.au
[4] Faculty of Engineering and Information Technology, University of Technology Sydney (UTS), Sydney, Australia

**Abstract.** Virtual reality (VR) is transforming education through completely immersive environments in which students can interact with content in dynamic and meaningful ways. The future of education lies in leveraging immersive technologies to build highly engaging and interactive learning environments. Integrating visual effects (VFX), such as lighting, colors, and animations, is essential in building emotional engagement and fostering impactful learning experiences. Despite these advancements, integrating artificial intelligence (AI) to adapt VFX in response to the user's emotions has not been widely explored. This survey investigates the potential of AI-driven emotion recognition and adaptive VFX to enhance engagement, motivation, and learning retention in VR education. This survey reviews the latest developments in AI, VFX, and VR technologies, highlighting the significant gaps, such as a lack of frameworks that combine these elements for emotionally responsive educational tools. While this study does not involve direct experimentation or implementation, it aims to offer valuable recommendations and insights for researchers, educators, and developers. The goal is to guide the development of inclusive VR learning environments that serve the diverse emotional and educational needs of the learners.

**Keywords:** Virtual Reality (VR) · Artificial Intelligence (AI) · Adaptive Visual Effects (VFX) · Emotion Recognition · Immersive Learning · Personalized Education · Engagement and Motivation · Multisensory Experiences


K. Daimi and A. Alsadoon (Eds.): ICR 2025, LNNS 1487, pp. 294–308, 2025.
https://doi.org/10.1007/978-3-031-95652-2_25

## 1 Introduction

Technological innovations have continuously shaped the evolution of education, but few will have the potential to be as transformational as VR. This breakthrough medium is changing everything from how learners approach content to utterly immersive environments unhindered by the constraints of legacy approaches to education. By replicating real-world scenarios and abstract concepts, VR can achieve unprecedented interaction and understanding [8]. However, VR's true potential lies in its ability to respond dynamically to the emotional and cognitive needs of learners, a true strength of VR that has not yet been utilized within today's educational frameworks [35].

Within such environments, VFX becomes an essential influence on emotional appeal and learning outcomes. Lights, color schemes, animations, and soundscapes are just some elements that would provoke emotional responses and enforce learning objectives. Despite their potential, most VR and VFX applications for education are static and fail to adapt to the fluctuating emotional states of students. This creates a disconnect between the learner and the immersive environment. The integration of AI addresses this gap: it can detect variations in the emotional state in real-time and further triggers the adaptation of VFXs into environments that would be both immersive and emotionally responsive [24]. These are theoretical possibilities rather than assertions of experimentation or real-world use in this survey. For example, an AI system integrated with emotion recognition could analyze a learner's facial expressions and physiological cues to detect disengagement or dissatisfaction. Based on this data, the system may provide a more personalized and encouraging learning experience by changing the VR environment's lighting to a soothing blue tone or adding inspirational noises to re-engage the student.

Recent research has extensively examined the significance of adaptive and personalized learning systems. The optimization of virtual learning environments (VLE) has been emphasized using multimodal emotion classification [16]. It has also been highlighted how wearable technology can record emotional states in real-time for VR-based instruction [26]. Nevertheless, there is still a significant gap in how these technologies might be integrated with coherent frameworks to produce instructional resources that are emotionally adaptive. Figure 1 illustrates a conceptual framework with VR as a core element incorporating AI, emotion recognition, adaptive VFX and adaptive personalization. It shows how feedback mechanisms such as eye tracking, facial expressions and physiological responses, all based on emotions, enable AI to adapt learning content in real-time with VFX for emotionally engaging and personalized learning environments in VR.

The main objective of this survey is to establish comprehensive knowledge of how AI-driven emotion recognition and adaptive VFX can transform VR education. The study reviews recent technological developments while pointing out critical gaps in research and practice. The absence of cohesive frameworks that integrate AI, VFX, and VR into emotionally adaptive learning systems presents a serious barrier to genuinely personalized education. The findings of this paper provide actionable insights for the people who work in the field of education, research and development to design inclusive and engaging learning experiences that meet the diverse needs of learners. To guide this investigation, this survey addresses the following research question: "How can AI-driven

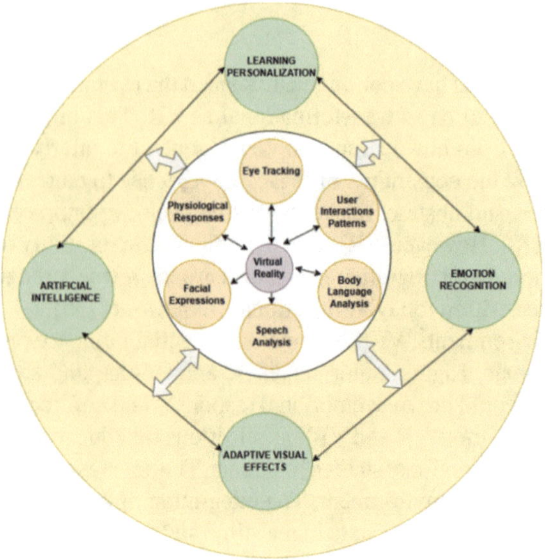


**Fig. 1.** The interconnected focus areas of this survey: Emphasizing the alignment of VR, AI, and VFX to create emotionally responsive learning environments

emotion recognition and adaptive VFX enhance engagement and learning outcomes in virtual reality (VR) education?"

This survey is organized into sections that outline the integration of VR, AI, and VFX for emotionally adaptive learning systems. Section 1 introduces the transformative role of VR in education and highlights the importance of emotionally responsive environments. Section 2 details VR's current applications, benefits, and educational challenges. Section 3 explores how VFX facilitates emotional involvement and how it aligns with learning objectives. Section 4 focuses on AI-powered emotion recognition algorithms and their implementation in VR learning settings. Section 5 covers adaptive visual effects technologies and their effect on learner experience optimization. Section 6 offers suggestions and future possibilities for developing emotionally adaptive VR systems. Finally, Section 7 concludes the survey and outlines future research directions.

## 2 Transformative Potential and Challenges of VR in Education

This section lays the foundation for how VR and related immersive technologies can transform educational settings. VR has grown so fast that it has become metamorphous in education, bringing immersion into the learning curve of subjects worldwide. Its applications range from traditional classroom settings to specialized domains like engineering and medical education, providing students with exceptional experiential learning opportunities in virtual settings. There have been instances where virtual laboratories successfully replaced mechanical laboratories, enabling the trainees to perform experiments conveniently in a well-controlled interactivity environment [1]. Similarly, in medical education, VR headsets introduce complex surgical procedures, showing safe and engaging use: the practice students should perform joyfully while developing their skills [21]. Furthermore, VR has been demonstrated to enhance group learning across multi-person competitive environments, a concept presently used in anatomy education, leveraging the problem-solving contributions of several students as they work in a group [10]. The collaborative potential of VR is further increased by cloud-based platforms such as V-Social, which give students with special needs greater access to tailored learning experiences [20]. The increased integration of VR for immersive learning into higher education institutions, with the emergence of other technologies like the Metaverse, will increase its potential to bring a revolution in the field of education [14].

The main advantage of VR is the possibility to create immersive learning activities that improve students' engagement, motivation, and retention. Immersive VR settings allow students to actively interact with complicated subjects, resulting in more significant learning and knowledge retention. From this, it was learned that situated activities in VR greatly enhance learning outcomes, at least in STEM education [6]. Moreover, features like the personalization of VR scenarios, adapted to the preferences of individuals, have been proven to enhance both learner satisfaction and effectiveness [30]. Personalization provides individualized learning pathways, making educational information more accessible and inclusive. Another critical component of VR's success is interactivity. This embodied learning, in which the user interacts physically within the virtual space, strengthens cognitive and emotional connections to the object [13]. Additionally, it opens broader perspectives on collaborative learning opportunities because, in VR, students work in a team and socially interact with their peers, which is especially highly valued in areas such as music education, where collaboration is very essential [11]. These cooperative and immersive experiences demonstrate VR's ability to produce emotionally compelling and productive learning settings.

The main advantage of VR is the possibility to create immersive learning activities that improve students' engagement, motivation, and retention. Immersive VR settings allow students to actively interact with complicated subjects, resulting in greater learning and retention of knowledge. From this, it was learned that situated activities in VR greatly enhance learning outcomes, at least in STEM education [6]. Moreover, features like the personalization of VR scenarios, adapted to the preferences of individuals, have been proven to enhance both learner satisfaction and effectiveness [30]. Personalization provides individualized learning pathways, making educational information more accessible and inclusive. Another critical component of VR's success is interactivity. This embodied learning, in which the user interacts physically within the virtual space, strengthens cognitive and emotional connections to the object [13]. Additionally, it opens broader perspectives on collaborative learning opportunities because, in VR, students work in a team and socially interact with their peers, which is especially highly valued in areas such as music education, where collaboration is essential [11]. These cooperative and immersive experiences demonstrate VR's ability to produce emotionally compelling and productive learning settings.

Despite VR's revolutionary potential, several obstacles prevent its broad use in educational contexts. For instance, the high cost of VR equipment and software remains very high, especially for underfunded institutions [2]. These limitations prevent the general adoption of VR, particularly in areas with limited resources and technological assistance. The effectiveness of organizing VR content for pedagogical means or noting the importance of teacher presence within virtual rooms is not yet recognized [1],[21]. These challenges signify the importance of incorporating emotionally engaging elements, discussed in-depth in Sect. 3, to overcome barriers to the adoption of VR.

Table 1 highlights the transformative potential of VR in education, such as enhancing engagement, collaboration and personalization, along with key challenges, such as high costs and limited pedagogical integration. It shows the main areas where VR technologies can be revolutionary in education, the main challenges for adoption and solutions to overcome these obstacles. The classification highlights specific areas such as application, engagement, personalization, pedagogical integration, and technological innovation, and it shows the potential of VR for improving immersive learning, collaboration, and adaptation. However, the barriers highlighted, from prohibitively high costs to scalability issues and lack of integration framework, strengthen the case for comprehensive, adaptive frameworks that utilize AI-infused solutions and adaptive VFX.

The suggestions, from leveraging low-cost VR tools to integrating AI for real-time personalization to designing modular architectures, offer real-world guidance for overcoming such barriers. These findings are in line with the overarching theme of this section, which emphasizes VR's revolutionary potential in education and the need for innovative approaches to ensure seamless adoption.

## 3 Harnessing VFX for Emotional Engagement in VR Education

In VR education, lighting, color, movements, and music are essential factors that affect both emotional and cognitive reactions. These components influence students' perspectives and encourage more in-depth participation. Color-filtered lighting has proved to be very influential in research on visual and emotional experiences in learning systems [25], hence making it possible to create specific atmospheres that enhance focus and engagement. The interrelation between light and color affects both emotion and performance and physiological well-being and supports a holistic design approach in educational fields [4]. Apart from the significant influence of visual components, audio factors are essential for developing learning experiences that are emotionally and entirely immersive. To provide multimodal experiences that increase immersion and connection with learning materials, sound and audio effects are essential for improving emotional involvement in virtual reality and substantially contributing to emotional engagement. Well-designed audio in VR has the potential to enhance it even more by coupling it with visual effects, creating multisensory experiences that would further solidify emotional connections to the learning material.

Animations are an essential part of VR that enhances sound and visual effects, which can improve focus and reduce cognitive overload. They provide dynamic storytelling and successfully communicate complex concepts to keep users' attention and emotional engagement and act as the bedrock of visual storytelling in VR. Dynamic animations maintain user interest and convey abstract ideas effectively [33]. Motion and visual dynamics can play a significant role in the affective impression of users,

**Table 1.** Key Transformations and Barriers in VR Education

| Classification | Ref. | Potential for Transformation | Challenges | Strategies for Overcoming Challenges |
|---|---|---|---|---|
| Application Areas | [1, 3] | Enables practical learning in technical and medical training through virtual laboratories and simulations. | The high cost of VR equipment and software makes it inaccessible to underfunded institutions. | Develop cost-effective VR hardware and software solutions and utilize open-source VR tools. |
| Engagement and Collaboration | [20, 13] | It improves student engagement through immersive experiences and promotes collaborative learning in virtual spaces. | Requires extensive technical infrastructure and user training, which limits scalability. | Invest in cloud-based VR platforms such as V-Social to support collaborative and scalable VR systems. |
| Personalization | [30, 26] | Customizable VR experiences, improve satisfaction and success by tailoring content to individual needs. | There is a lack of adaptive real-time frameworks and integration with recognized learning theories | Integrate AI and adaptive VFX to enable real-time personalization based on learners' emotional state. |
| Pedagogical Integration | [8, 10] | Supports immersive learning with STEM and interdisciplinary areas such as music and anatomy lessons. | Limited framework for effectively integrating VR into traditional pedagogy or ensuring teacher presence. | Develop structured frameworks for integrating VR into the curriculum and train teachers for hybrid virtual-physical instruction. |
| Technological Advancements | [16, 24] | Advances such as haptic feedback and dynamic VFX enrich multi-sensory experiences for deeper emotional engagement. | High demands for computing power and power consumption for real-time dynamic rendering. | Optimize VR systems with scalable architectures and low-latency rendering techniques to reduce resource requirements. |

and it is said that changes in illuminance and color temperature can provoke specific reactions; thus, the role of personalized lighting design in VR space is manifested [19].

Expanding on the fundamental function of animations and customized visual effects in promoting emotional involvement, a case study offers a more in-depth understanding of how these components might be strategically employed to affect perception and judgment in immersive settings. By dynamically manipulating lighting and animations, it was possible to simulate realistic environments that were emotionally engaging yet educationally effective. Integrating dynamic lighting and animations enables learners to engage with virtual scenarios, emulating real-life challenges and enhancing their decision-making skills [12]. These VFX features collaboratively facilitate the establishment of compelling learning environments that motivate instructors and engage learners [30]. Despite the advancements in VFX, a critical gap remains in achieving real-time emotional adaptability.

Table 2 illustrates some key VFX elements in VR education: their emotional impact, applications, challenges, and prospects. It provides an overview of the key VFX elements that define emotional immersion in VR learning, their emotional impact, learning applications and potential challenges. Each aspect, lighting, sound, animation, and dynamic rendering, is critical to creating immersive environments that increase focus, elicit emotional responses and simplify complex ideas through dynamic storytelling. The table lists the practical challenges of these elements, such as the computational cost of real-time dynamic rendering, the complexity of coordinating multisensory inputs, and the need for adaptive systems that respond to learners' emotional states. These challenges align with the broader theme of Sect. 3, namely the challenge of developing scalable and adaptable VFX solutions for VR education. The observations in Table 2 highlight the need to overcome these obstacles to realize VFX's emotional and cognitive benefits in educational environments.

## 4 AI-Driven Adaptive VFX in VR Education

The discussion of emotion recognition and adaptive VFX investigates their possible collaboration for individualized, emotionally responsive VR learning environments. These technologies increase student engagement and improve learning results by rapidly responding to their emotional states. Adaptive VFX allows VR systems to dynamically modify visual and auditory elements such as lighting, soundscapes, and animations to foster a personalized, immersive experience.

Incorporating adaptive VFX is a logical step in building on the developments in emotion recognition technologies, allowing VR environments to react dynamically to learners' emotional states. Studies have demonstrated how AI-driven systems can modify lighting, soundscapes, and animations to support emotional engagement [7]. For example, adjusting the brightness and color tones of the lighting can have a calming or stimulating effect, depending on whether the learner is under stress or not. Similarly, auditory elements such as soundscapes and background music play a crucial role in enhancing immersion by adjusting the pace and volume to the learner's emotional feedback [29]. Animations, including transitions and visual feedback, sustain engagement by creating dynamic and responsive interactions. AI-powered adaptive VFX holds promise for improving learning outcomes in VR education. By creating emotionally immersive environments tailored to individual learners, these systems promote more

**Table 2.** Summary of VFX Elements and their Impact on VR Education

| VFX Element | Reference | Emotional Impact | Applications for VR Education | Challenges | Future Potential |
|---|---|---|---|---|---|
| Lighting and Colors | [25] | Enhances focus, sets mood, and evokes emotional responses | Used in virtual labs to simulate real-life environments for STEM education. | High computational resources for real-time changes. | AI-driven lighting for real-time emotion adaptation |
| Sound and Audio | [29] | Create immersive multisensory learning experiences. | Enhance engagement in VR music and language education. | It isn't easy to synchronize with emotional states. | Real-time sound modulation based on emotional feedback |
| Animations | [33] | Simplifies complex concepts through dynamic storytelling. | Visualizing abstract scientific concepts like molecular structures. | Significant design expertise required | Personalized AI-driven animations for adaptive learning, |
| Dynamic VFX Rendering | [19] | Provides immersive experiences through real-time visual updates. | Gamified learning to maintain motivation. | High processing and power consumption | Scalable systems for seamless dynamic rendering |
| Multisensory Integration | [18] | Combines visual, auditory, and tactile stimuli for holistic engagement | Applied in medical simulations for surgery and diagnosis. | Complex synchronization of multiple sensory inputs. | Enhanced multisensory synchronization for deeper immersion. |

profound engagement, improve motivation and enhance long-term retention by reinforcing emotional connections with the material. As shown in Fig. 2, the continuous feedback loop remains directions.

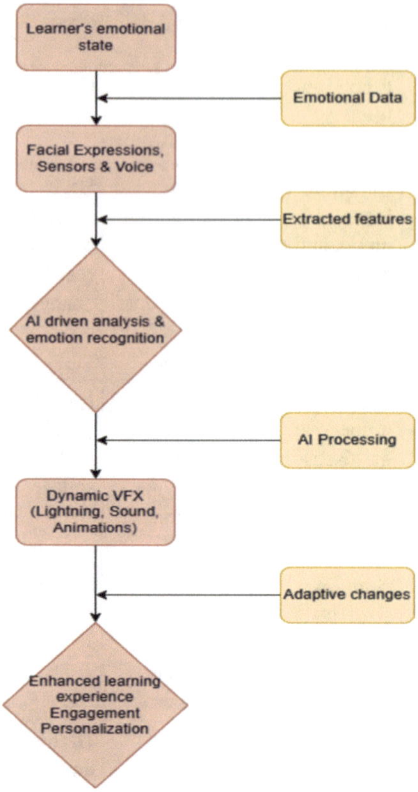


**Fig. 2.** AI-powered adaptive workflow that demonstrates how to assess students' emotional states and modify visual effects in real-time to improve personalization and engagement.

## 5 Technological Frontiers and Challenges in Emotionally Adaptive VR Learning

Recent developments in VR, AI, and VFX technology have greatly aided the establishment of immersive learning environments. The development of sophisticated hardware, such as haptic feedback systems and sophisticated headgear, has made more realistic and captivating educational experiences possible in virtual reality (VR) [28]. AI has made significant strides in emotion identification, with real-time monitoring of physiological data, voice modulation, and facial expressions becoming more accurate [27].

At the same time, VFX technologies, including real-time rendering and dynamic lighting modifications, have enriched the immersive quality of VR environments by providing multimodal learning experiences [5]. Despite these developments, various technological issues exist in integrating AI, VFX, and VR into a combined adaptive learning system. One key research gap is the lack of a framework incorporating these technologies into an emotionally adaptive learning system. Although AI and VR are individually leveraged to improve learning, they are not often combined with adaptive

VFX, frequently leading to fragmented and subpar experiences [30]. Furthermore, existing solutions lack real-time adaptive frameworks capable of dynamically responding to learners' emotional and cognitive states [23]. Current emotion recognition systems, while improving, still struggle with real-time accuracy, synchrony of multimodal data, and computational efficiency.

The survey aims to emphasize the importance of bridging these gaps to provide inclusive and fully customized learning environments. However, a significant obstacle to creating learning environments that are individualized and adaptive is the lack of unified frameworks integrating various technologies. Interdisciplinary cooperation is required to bridge these gaps by creating AI-driven adaptive visual effects frameworks. In addition, scalability and accessibility remain significant challenges. Most current VR learning platforms are not designed for emotionally adaptive learning because real-time adaptation requires computationally demanding AI model innovations such as reinforcement learning-based adaptation [9], and compact AI models can facilitate real-time emotional adaptation without requiring upper-level computing capabilities. Furthermore, brain-computer interfaces (BCIs) introduce a novel gateway for promoting adaptive learning environments [3].

Table 3 summarizes the technological framework for education in virtual reality, including haptic feedback systems, AI-driven emotion recognition, dynamic lighting, multimodal emotion recognition and scalable VR solutions. It provides an overview of the technological frameworks driving emotionally adaptive VR systems, including their applications, benefits, and challenges, and highlights their contribution to immersive learning. While the section addresses broader challenges, the table outlines practical observations, including the promise of multimodal emotion recognition for personalized learning and the need for scalable VR solutions to improve accessibility. These observations underpin the survey's call for innovative, inclusive and adaptable solutions to overcome technological limitations and optimize VR learning environments.

# 6 Findings and Future Directions in Adaptive VR Learning Systems

This study emphasizes the transforming possibilities of integrating VR, VFX, and artificial intelligence technology to provide emotionally flexible learning surroundings. Significant analysis shows that real-time emotional responsiveness improves learner engagement, retention, and accessibility, which AI-driven frameworks enable. But present systems have notable flaws: Rule-based adaptation mechanisms lack the dynamic flexibility required for complex learning scenarios; existing emotion recognition models often rely on unimodal data (e.g., facial expressions or physiological signals), leading to misclassification errors and reduced personalizing; and disjointed workflows between AI, VR, and VFX pipelines introduce latency, undermining real-time adaptability [9, 23]. These constraints draw attention to how urgently coherent, multimodal systems that give technical accuracy priority, as well as instructional effectiveness, are needed.

To realize the full potential of emotionally intelligent VR learning systems, the following interdisciplinary challenges must be addressed.

**Table 3.** Summary of Technological Frontiers and Challenges in VR Education

| Technological/ Framework | Ref. | Learning Type | Used for | Commonly Used Method | Positives | Negatives |
|---|---|---|---|---|---|---|
| Haptic Feedback Systems | [28] | Simulation Training | Advanced hardware that allows for haptic feedback. | Practical simulations for hands-on learning. | Provides realistic, immersive training that improves engagement and retention. | Implementation is costly; complex hardware is required, along with continuous maintenance. |
| AI-Driven Emotion Recognition | [27] | Adaptive Learning | Real-time analysis of physiological data. | Physiological and Facial Data Input. | It allows personalized learning, which increases emotional and cognitive engagement. | Inaccuracies are common among varied populations; high-quality sensor data is essential. |
| Dynamic Lighting and Rendering | [5] | Visual Enhancement | Real-time changes in lighting and texture adjustment. | Designing immersive, mood-enhancing VR settings | Multisensory stimulation improves attention and emotional involvement. | High computational resource demands may lead to system lags in low-budget setups |
| Multimodal Emotion Recognition | [9] | Emotion Analysis | Extensive evaluation of emotional states. | Combining Physiological, verbal, and facial information. | Offers comprehensive emotional feedback and facilitates immediate environmental adaptation. | Implementation is complex because of data synchronization issues. |
| Scalable VR Solutions | [17] | Inclusive Education | Making VR accessible in underdeveloped areas. | Cloud-based virtual reality platforms. | Reduces cost hurdles and boosts VR use in varied educational states. | Limited effectiveness in areas with inadequate internet and infrastructure. |

One of the most significant obstacles to deploying these systems is the demand for accurate multimodal fusion concurrently processing emotional data from multiple sources (e.g., EEG, heart rate, facial expressions) with low latency. Future research must prioritize improving the synchronization of multimodal data and fine-grained tuning of AI models to minimize misclassification errors in emotion classification. Reinforcement learning (RL) presents a promising approach to enhance real-time adaptability in complex learning scenarios. Reinforcement learning can allow AI to refine adaptation mechanisms iteratively by learning from user interactions, making VFX adaptations more context-aware and improving long-term user engagement. Unlike traditional rule-based models, RL enables AI to refine adaptation mechanisms based on dynamic user interactions. This can significantly reduce the need for manual adjustments in VR learning environments while improving the accuracy of VFX-driven emotional adaptations [9]. However, for RL to be effective in VR learning, it must be trained on diverse user interactions to ensure adaptability across different learning contexts.

Developing coherent frameworks that seamlessly combine AI, VR, and VFX technologies for emotionally responsive learning environments should remain a top priority for future research. These frameworks must guarantee smooth real-time adaptation, where emotional states are continuously tracked and utilized to modify the learning environment [34] dynamically. For instance, AI-driven emotion recognition that uses physiological signals and facial and speech patterns could create highly personalized user experiences [9, 23]. Real-time VFX changes in response to AI-processed emotional states depend on the interaction of more exact subsystems. AI-driven emotion detection, for example, must interact dynamically with VR rendering engines to change surrounding stimuli (e.g., lighting and avatar interactions) without compromising immersion. Although industry-wide cooperation is required to build universal protocols, standardized APIs and middleware solutions might help to close these gaps.

Beyond technological challenges, emotional computing in education raises ethical questions that deserve examination. While biased artificial intelligence models might support inequality, over-reliance on emotion-aware systems risks lowering learner autonomy. To ensure these technologies complement rather than replace human teachers, multidisciplinary research must set standards for open emotion labelling, user permission, and algorithmic responsibility.

Offering direct neural input to AI-driven adaptive systems [3], integrating brain-computer interfaces (BCIs) marks a revolutionary horizon for personalized learning. BCIs might capture delicate cognitive and emotional states that conventional sensors would overlook, enabling hitherto unheard-of degrees of personalization. Developers must prioritize user-friendly and scalable technology to democratize access to emotionally sensitive VR settings. By streamlining the integration of VFX and artificial intelligence technologies, modular frameworks—such as those using Raspy Control [32], laying the groundwork for affordable and flexible systems—can help to reduce costs.

To provide inclusion for students with different cognitive and emotional demands, efforts should be made to design VR systems that meet diverse learning needs. VR settings can be customized to offer individualized learning experiences by including multimodal data, such as physiological signs and speech patterns [17]. This integrated data enables the creation of collaborative virtual environments where students can interact socially, communicate and solve problems together. This is a key feature of modern educational paradigms that emphasize teamwork and social learning [28]. These improvements will be essential to developing inclusive and emotionally compelling learning environments. In addition, the combination of environmental information and sensor data with advanced AI-driven algorithms can enhance real-time adaptations to provide unprecedented educational solutions. These improvements will enable the development of versatile and truly immersive learning experiences [27].

Dealing with these issues calls for coordinated efforts across groups in VR, artificial intelligence, and educational research. Priority one consists of three phases: deploying hybrid artificial intelligence models for interpretable adaptations combining data-driven RL with explainable rule-based reasoning; validating systems utilizing longitudinal research assessing emotional well-being and learning results; and establishing open-source criteria for VR multimodal emotion identification to hasten repeatability.

By integrating these cutting-edge approaches, next-generation research can fill existing gaps in adaptive learning technology and provide a strong foundation for the future of VR education systems. These advancements will require a multidisciplinary effort from researchers, educators, policymakers, and technology experts. Collaboration is essential for securing funding, establishing ethical AI-driven education standards, and ensuring that emotionally adaptive VR learning systems remain innovative and inclusive.

## 7 Conclusion

This survey covers the revolutionary role of VR in education, leading to emotionally adaptive learning experiences through the integration of AI-driven emotion recognition and adaptive VFX. By dynamically responding to learners' emotional and cognitive states, these technologies promote engagement, motivation and content retention, offering a new paradigm for immersive learning. Although VR-based education has immense potential, challenges such as the lack of standard frameworks, exorbitant computational costs and the complexity of real-time customization continue to prevent widespread adoption. This study highlights the importance of VFX in driving emotional responses and the need for AI-driven emotion recognition as a key enabler for real-time adaptive learning systems. Despite these innovations, the lack of multimodal integration frameworks and the technological limitations of real-time AI adaptation remain significant challenges. Future research needs to focus on scalable AI architectures, virtual collaborative learning spaces and emotionally adaptive VR systems that personalize learning experiences in real-time. Through the development of brain-computer interfaces, reinforcement learning and multimodal AI models, researchers can develop emotionally intelligent, inclusive and adaptive educational systems that intelligently adapt learning environments to cognitive and affective feedback. The future of AI-driven VR learning lies in developing intelligent, data-driven and emotionally engaging systems that improve personalization, engagement and accessibility, paving the way for the next generation of immersive education.

## References


1. Abbas Shah, S.F., Ahmad, I., Raza, M., Khalid, A., Hussain, T.: Integrating educational theories with virtual reality: enhancing engineering education and VR laboratories. Soc. Sci. Human. Open. **10**, 101207 (2024). https://doi.org/10.1016/j.ssaho.2024.101207
2. Al-Ansi, A.M., Al-Kinani, M.A., Al-Mashhadani, H.S., Rahman, A.A.: Analyzing augmented reality (AR) and virtual reality (VR) recent developments in education. Soc. Sci. Human. Open. **8**(1), 100532 (2023). https://doi.org/10.1016/j.ssaho.2023.100532

3. Álvarez Ariza, J., Nomesqui Galvis, C.: RaspyControl Lab: a fully open-source and real-time remote laboratory for education in automatic control systems using Raspberry Pi and Python. HardwareX. **13**, e00396 (2023). https://doi.org/10.1016/j.ohx.2023.e00396
4. Barbato, G., Bellia, L., Morone, A.: How the colours of objects and light affect human emotions, performance and health. The need for a holistic approach to designing indoor environments. Color Cult. Sci. **11**(01), 67–73 (2019)
5. Burton, S.L.: Advancements in AI-driven education: transforming learning and training with intelligent technologies. World J. Busi. Res. **4**(1), 9 (2024)
6. Chiou, H.-H.: The impact of situated learning activities on technology university students' learning outcome. Educ. Train. **63**(3), 440–452 (2020). https://doi.org/10.1108/ET-04-2018-0092
7. Dalvi, C., Churi, P., Desai, K., Patil, P.: A survey of AI-based facial emotion recognition: features, ML & DL techniques, age-wise datasets and future directions. IEEE Access. **9**, 165806–165840 (2021). https://doi.org/10.1109/ACCESS.2021.3131733
8. Devassy, S.M., Thomas, J., Nair, R., Menon, S.: Development of immersive learning framework (ILF) in achieving the goals of higher education: measuring the impact using a pre–post design. Sci. Rep. **13**(1), 17692 (2023)
9. Dumitru, C.: Future of learning: adaptive learning systems based on language generative models in higher education. In: Impact of Artificial Intelligence on Society, pp. 31–42. Chapman and Hall/CRC (2025)
10. Du, Y.-C., Fan, S.-C., Yang, L.-C.: The impact of multi-person virtual reality competitive learning on anatomy education: a randomized controlled study. BMC Med. Educ. **20**(1), 343 (2020). https://doi.org/10.1186/s12909-020-02155-9
11. Sánchez-Jara, J.F.M., et al.: Artificial intelligence-assisted music education: a critical synthesis of challenges and opportunities. Educ. Sci. **14**(11), 1171 (2024). https://doi.org/10.3390/educsci14111171
12. Kim, H., Lee, J., Park, S., Choi, Y.: The impacts of visual effects on user perception with a virtual human in augmented reality conflict situations. IEEE Access. **9**, 35300–35312 (2021). https://doi.org/10.1109/ACCESS.2021.3062037
13. Khorasani, S., et al.: Hands-on or hands-off: deciphering the impact of interactivity on embodied learning in VR. Comput. Educ. X Real. **3** (2023). https://doi.org/10.1016/j.cexr.2023.100037
14. Kshetri, N., Rojas-Torres, D., Grambo, M.: The Metaverse and higher education institutions. IT Professional. **24**(6), 69–73 (2022). https://doi.org/10.1109/MITP.2022.3222711
15. Lai, J.W., Cheong, K.H.: Educational opportunities and challenges in augmented reality: featuring implementations in physics education. IEEE Access. **10**, 43143–43158 (2022). https://doi.org/10.1109/ACCESS.2022.3166478
16. Lima, R., Costa, P., Almeida, J., Ferreira, M.: Multimodal emotion classification using machine learning in immersive and non-immersive virtual reality. Virtual Reality. **28**(2) (2024). https://doi.org/10.1007/s10055-024-00989-y
17. Liu, P.Z.Y., Chen, X., Wang, J., Zhang, H.: Rapid distortion correction enables accurate magnetic resonance imaging-guided real-time adaptive radiotherapy. Phys. Imag. Radiat. Oncol. **25**, 100414 (2023). https://doi.org/10.1016/j.phro.2023.100414
18. Lopes, C.R., Silva, F.A., Pereira, J.L., Costa, M.F.: PerceptSent: exploring subjectivity in a novel dataset for visual sentiment analysis. IEEE Trans. Affect. Comput. **14**(3), 1817–1831 (2023). https://doi.org/10.1109/TAFFC.2022.3225238
19. Mostafavi, A., Xu, T.B., Kalantari, S.: Effects of illuminance and correlated color temperature on emotional responses and lighting adjustment behaviors. J. Build. Eng. **86**, 108833 (2024)
20. Nuguri, S.S., Kumar, A., Patel, H., Reddy, V.: vSocial: a cloud-based system for social virtual reality learning environment applications in special education. Multimed. Tools Appl. **80**(11), 16827–16856 (no date). https://doi.org/10.1007/s11042-020-09051-w

21. Ojala, S., Rantala, A., Virtanen, T., Karjalainen, T.: The impact of teacher's presence on learning basic surgical tasks with virtual reality headset among medical students. Med. Educ. **27**(1) (2022). https://doi.org/10.1080/10872981.2022.2050345
22. Shomoye, M., Zhao, R.: Automated emotion recognition of students in virtual reality classrooms. Comput. Educ. X Real. **5**, 100082 (2024). https://doi.org/10.1016/j.cexr.2024.100082
23. Solanki, A.: Advancements in artificial intelligence: a comprehensive review and future prospects. Int. J. Artif. Intell. Res. Dev. (IJAIRD). **2**(1), 53–64 (2024)
24. Somarathna, R., Bednarz, T., Mohammadi, G.: Virtual reality for emotion elicitation—a review. IEEE Trans. Affect. Comput. **14**(4), 2626–2645 (2023). https://doi.org/10.1109/TAFFC.2022.3181053
25. Suh, J.K., Park, E.K., Iwamoto, D.: Color-filtered lighting: visual and emotional impact in learning environments. Int. J. Architect. Spat. Environ. Design. **14**(1), 41–55 (2020)
26. Suhaimi, N.S.S., Mountstephens, J., Teo, J.: A dataset for emotion recognition using virtual reality and EEG (DER-VREEG): emotional state classification using low-cost wearable VR-EEG headsets. Big Data Cogn. Comput. **6**(1), 16 (2022). https://doi.org/10.3390/bdcc6010016
27. Subramanian, B., Kim, J., Maray, M., Paul, A.: Digital twin model: a real-time emotion recognition system for personalized healthcare. IEEE Access. **10**, 81155–81165 (2022)
28. Theebanraj, U., Kanishkar, R., Gunathilake, C.D., Hennayake, H.M.G.J., Karunathilaka, S.: Empowering virtual education and lecturing through AI and ML advancements. Int. Res. J. Innov. Eng. Technol. **7**(10), 57 (2023)
29. Turchet, L., Hamilton, R., Camci, A.: Music in extended realities. IEEE Access. **9**, 15810–15832 (2021). https://doi.org/10.1109/ACCESS.2021.3052931
30. Valmorisco, S., Raya, L., Sanchez, A.: Enabling personalized VR experiences: a framework for real-time adaptation and recommendations in VR environments. Virtual Reality. **28**(3) (2024). https://doi.org/10.1007/s10055-024-01020-0
31. Vistorte, A.O.R., Silva, M.R., Andrade, T.P., Costa, L.D.: Integrating artificial intelligence to assess emotions in learning environments: a systematic literature review. Front. Psychol. **15** (2024). https://doi.org/10.3389/fpsyg.2024.1387089
32. Vladimirovich Kotov, E., Mallikarjuna Raju, K.: Real-time adaptive control of electric vehicle drives using artificial neural networks. MATEC Web Conf. **392** (2024). https://doi.org/10.1051/matecconf/202439201178
33. Xie, X., Cai, J., Fang, H., Tang, X., Yamanaka, T.: Effects of colored lights on an individual's affective impressions in the observation process. Front. Psychol. **13**, 938636 (2022)
34. Yang, H., Han, X.: Face recognition attendance system based on real-time video processing. IEEE Access. **4**, 159143–159150 (2020). https://doi.org/10.1109/ACCESS.2020.3007205
35. Maghool, S.A.H., Moeini, S.H.I., Arefazar, Y.: An educational application based on virtual reality technology for learning architectural details: challenges and benefits. Archnet-IJAR Int. J. Arch. Res. **12**(3), 246 (2018)
36. Zhang, Z., Fort, J.M., Giménez Mateu, L.: Facial expression recognition in virtual reality environments: challenges and opportunities. Front. Psychol. **14**, 1280136 (2023). https://doi.org/10.3389/fpsyg.2023.1280136

# Enhancing Technical Education for Students and People with Disabilities Through Virtual Reality: A Case Study Using a CNC Device

Mario Covarrubias[1(✉)], Makam Ramachandra Gupta Shashank[1], Nicolás Norambuena[2], Felipe Muñoz[2], Cristobal Galleguillos[2], and Jose Valin[2]

[1] Department of Mechanical Engineering, Politecnico di Milano, Milan, Italy
mario.covarrubias@polimi.it, shashank.makam@mail.polimi.it
[2] Pontificia Universidad Católica de Valparaíso, Valparaíso, Chile
nicolas.norambuena.o@mail.pucv.cl,
{felipe.munoz,cristobal.galleguillos,jose.valin}@pucv.cl

**Abstract.** Virtual Reality (VR) is currently one of the most influential technological trends and is projected to grow significantly in the coming years. A defining feature of VR is its ability to fully immerse users in a digital environment, eliminating real-world distractions and enabling focused engagement with virtual processes. This study presents the design and implementation of a VR-based training application for the Charly4U CNC milling machine. Developed using the Unity3D engine, the tool offers an interactive, step-by-step simulation aimed at enhancing technical education and improving accessibility for users with limited machining experience. The application was tested with two user groups: engineering students and adolescents with cognitive disabilities from the ASPOC Onlus Lab. Usability was evaluated through the System Usability Scale (SUS), with results showing high user satisfaction and strong usability scores across both groups (SUS scores of 81 and 87, respectively). The findings support the effectiveness of immersive VR environments for skill development and inclusive education, demonstrating the potential of this approach to complement traditional CNC training methods in a safe and engaging way.

**Keywords:** Virtual Reality · Education · Special Education · People with disabilities · Social equity

## 1 Introduction

Over the last ten years, Virtual Reality (VR) has emerged as a powerful tool across a wide range of sectors, with education standing out as one of the most promising areas of application [5,8]. VR involves the use of computer-generated simulations that users can interact with in real time through specialized hardware, such as head-mounted displays (HMDs), motion-sensitive controllers, and


K. Daimi and A. Alsadoon (Eds.): ICR 2025, LNNS 1487, pp. 309–318, 2025.
https://doi.org/10.1007/978-3-031-95652-2_26

spatial tracking systems. These immersive technologies substitute the physical world with a fully synthetic environment, fostering deep engagement by removing external distractions.

In educational settings, VR is increasingly recognized for its potential to revolutionize how students learn, [10,11] offering experiential and interactive opportunities that traditional classroom methods cannot easily replicate. For instance, students can perform virtual experiments, navigate simulated environments, or explore mechanical systems from a first-person perspective, all within a controlled and safe space [6,7].

Institutions like the Politecnico di Milano have incorporated VR into their academic programs, enabling learners to participate in activities such as digital prototyping, process visualization, and system interaction. These VR-based experiences help students build a deeper understanding of technical subjects by allowing them to directly manipulate virtual representations of real-world tools and procedures.

The project presented in this study centers on the design and implementation of a VR application for training in CNC milling operations. The aim is to provide a realistic, yet completely safe environment where users—particularly those without prior hands-on experience—can familiarize themselves with the processes involved in operating a CNC machine. This approach mitigates safety risks and helps build user confidence before interacting with the actual equipment.

Unlike AR and MR, which maintain some connection with the real world, VR excels in creating entirely self-contained experiences. This makes it especially well-suited for training scenarios that demand full attention and immersion, such as those involving complex machinery, hazardous procedures, or remote or costly equipment. VR's ability to simulate these environments enables safe exploration, repeated practice, and a learner-centered approach to skill development.

The structure of this paper is as follows. Section 2 outlines the educational rationale for using VR in technical training. Section 3 describes the application's technical specifications, while Sect. 4 details the user interface and interaction design. Section 5 explains the usability evaluation method, followed by Sect. 6, which defines the target users. Section 7 presents the test results, and Sect. 8 concludes the study with final remarks and future directions.

## 2 Virtual Reality in Education

The main goal of this project is to utilize VR technology to enhance learning experiences, particularly for engineering students. Gaining hands-on experience is crucial for comprehending intricate processes and tasks. CNC milling machines, while essential in the field of manufacturing, can often seem intimidating to students due to their complexity and the potential hazards associated with improper handling. Traditional educational approaches require an experienced instructor to guide students through the operation process, which can sometimes pose limitations in terms of accessibility and learning pace. VR effectively addresses these challenges by allowing students to engage in realistic simulations of CNC machining operations in a safe and controlled environment. By interacting with a virtual replica of the machine, learners can practice various procedures, from setup to execution, without the risk of damaging physical equipment or causing injury.

Virtual Reality (VR) allows undergraduate students to independently explore and interact with all necessary instructional content through an intuitive interface. The application provides access to detailed 3D models and step-by-step procedures within a secure, immersive environment—eliminating the immediate need for direct supervision from instructors [3,12]. All required resources are embedded within the application, enabling learners to complete tasks autonomously and effectively. To contextualize this approach, it is useful to examine previous research efforts in the field of Augmented Reality (AR) in education and understand the contributions made thus far by the academic community [13].

Additionally, previous studies have highlighted the effectiveness of such technologies in helping learners visualize abstract concepts and phenomena that would otherwise be difficult to perceive—such as those that are extremely small, large, rapid, or slow for the human eye to detect [9].

## 3 Technical Specifications of the Application

Upon launching the application, users are introduced to the system through a preliminary scene that shows the project's name and its collaborating partners. The next phase provides a detailed overview of the Charly4U CNC milling machine, including its technical specifications, operational characteristics, and manufacturer information. Users can then navigate through various interactive menus that allow them to access different training modules.

Each module presents a structured, step-by-step training sequence using VR-based interactions, ensuring users gain a thorough understanding of the CNC machining process before transitioning to real-world applications.

FROM THIS LINK [2], REVIEWERS CAN DOWNLOAD a VIDEO OF THE VR APPLICATION.

## 4 Menu and Scenes

The VR application was developed using the Unity3D game engine, chosen for its cross-platform capabilities, integrated physics engine, and strong support for VR development through packages such as XR Interaction Toolkit. Following the initial scene—where the project's title and partner institutions are introduced—the application transitions to a second environment that presents key technical information about the Charly4U CNC milling machine. This includes specifications such as machine dimensions, axis travel ranges, and operational capabilities. On the opposite side of the interface, additional details about the manufacturer are provided, along with a clickable link beneath the company's logo that directs users to the official website. This section serves as an introductory overview of the CNC machine's features, construction, and performance characteristics. Figure 1 illustrates the physical Charly4U milling device.

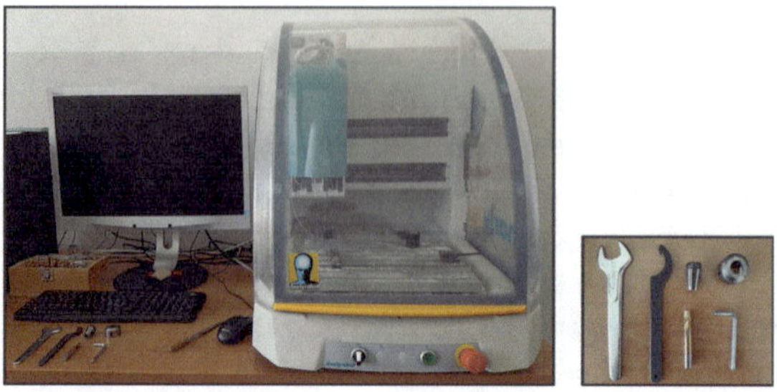

**Fig. 1.** The CNC Milling Device (Charly4U from Mecanumeric) [4]

Figure 2 illustrates the virtual environment designed for the training application. The scene replicates a simplified factory setting, where the 3D model of the Charly4U CNC milling machine is accurately positioned. This virtual space serves as the main interactive area in which users can navigate around the machine, view it from different angles, and engage with its components. By simulating a realistic workshop layout, the environment enables full virtual immersion, helping users build spatial awareness and familiarity with the machine's structure before operating real equipment. This design enhances both the learning experience and user engagement.).

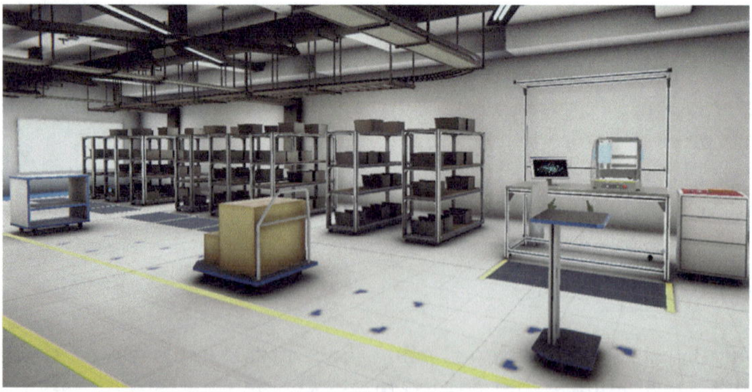

**Fig. 2.** Virtual Environment for the Charly4U training application

Figure 3 illustrates the virtual environment specifically designed to deliver an immersive static experience. This setup allows users to engage with the simulated CNC milling machine environment without the need for physical movement, making it ideal for seated interactions or limited mobility scenarios

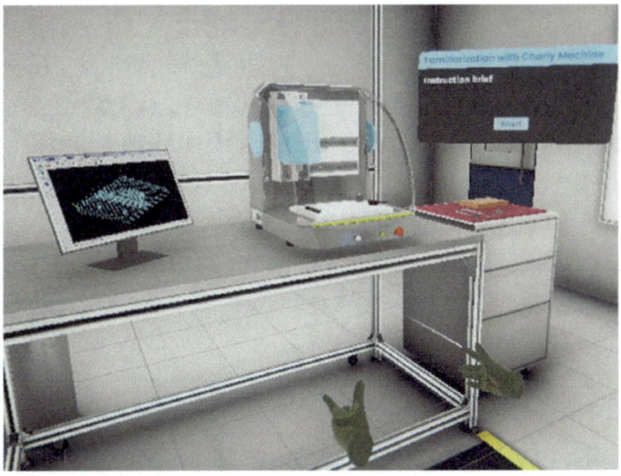

**Fig. 3.** Application designed for static experience.

### 4.1 Hand Interactions

Hand representation within virtual reality environments is a key component in shaping the quality and intuitiveness of user interaction, as can be seen from Fig. 4. A well-designed hand model should be anatomically accurate, with smooth and natural animations that mimic real-life movement. Finger gestures and physics-based interactions should be seamless to enhance realism and usability. Additionally, providing clear and responsive feedback during actions such as grabbing, releasing, and triggering objects is essential for an intuitive and immersive experience. Well-implemented hand interactions can significantly improve user engagement, making virtual environments feel more natural and interactive.

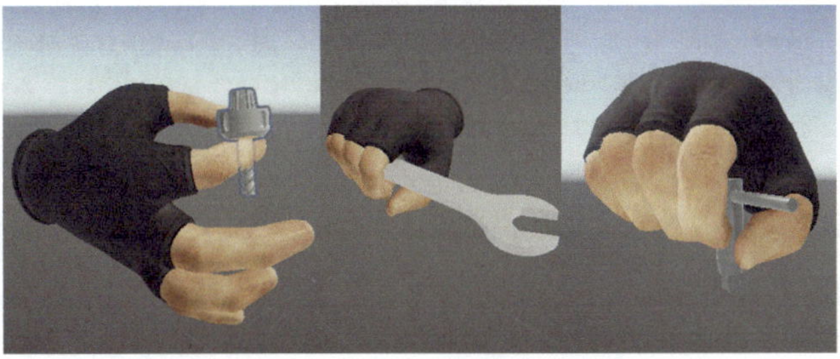

**Fig. 4.** Virtual hands interactions.

### 4.2 Haptic Feedback in Virtual Reality

Haptic feedback serves as a critical bridge between human sensory perception and digital interactions, making it an essential component of VR experiences. By simulating tactile sensations, haptic feedback contributes to a deeper sense of immersion by simulating tactile sensations, enabling users to perceive physical contact during actions like grasping or interacting with virtual elements. This is typically achieved through vibrations or force feedback in handheld controllers, providing a more realistic and engaging experience. A common example of haptic feedback in everyday technology is the slight vibration a smartphone emits when a user long-presses the touchscreen to activate a feature.

In the developed application, handheld controllers deliver haptic feedback when an object is grabbed, released, or triggered, enhancing user interaction and engagement within the virtual space.

### 4.3 Instruction Panel in Virtual Reality

Reading long passages of text in Virtual Reality is not ideal, which is why typography does not play a dominant role in VR design. However, since VR relies on a visual user interface, text remains an essential component of the experience. The way text is integrated into a virtual environment significantly impacts readability and user interaction.

One key consideration is when and how text should be displayed. Should it always remain visible, appear only when needed, or be used specifically for critical notifications or warnings? Understanding these requirements helps in selecting the appropriate display method and typography for a VR interface.

**Anchored to Head Display.** In this approach, text moves along with the user's head movements, ensuring that it remains within their field of view at all times. While this method keeps important information readily accessible, it can be intrusive and, in Augmented Reality (AR), may obstruct visibility of the real world. Therefore, it is best suited for displaying crucial notifications or short messages rather than extended content.

However, since our heads naturally move by a few degrees even when focusing, reading head-anchored text can result in slight jitter, causing discomfort and making it harder to read. Due to this, head-anchored text is not recommended for long-form content or detailed instructions.

### 4.4 Visual Highlighters/Markers

In Virtual Reality (VR) environments, visual aids and highlights play a crucial role in providing guidance and enhancing user interaction. In the application, an outline shader is implemented to help users identify objects they need to pick up or interact with at each step. Additionally, a Fresnel shader has been developed to assist users in correctly positioning and aligning objects, ensuring a more intuitive and seamless experience.

## 5 Usability Test

To evaluate the application's usability, the System Usability Scale (SUS), developed by John Brooke in 1986, was adopted. Before delving into the specifics of

SUS, it is essential to consider the broader concept of usability. Usability cannot be meaningfully assessed without taking into account the context in which a system is employed and the characteristics of its intended users.

Collecting both qualitative and quantitative feedback from users is essential for refining the application's design and functionality. Participants provide valuable insights into their preferences, challenges, and suggestions for improvement, helping to enhance usability and overall user experience.

A key aspect of usability testing is assessing the learnability factor—determining how easily participants can understand and follow the processes involved in operating the Charly4U CNC machine.

The primary objectives of usability testing were to improve user experience, identify and resolve usability issues, gather user feedback, iteratively refine the design, make informed design decisions, and evaluate performance metrics and learnability factors in a VR environment.

At the time of this report, the application was tested with five individuals from both design and engineering backgrounds. Among them, three had prior experience with VR, while the remaining two were first-time users. To familiarize them with the VR environment, those new to VR first interacted with the Oculus First Hands app before using this application.

## 6 Target Population

Once the System Usability Scale (SUS) test was established, the next step was to define the target population. As previously mentioned, this Virtual Reality (VR) application for the Charly4U CNC milling machine was developed to assist students in learning how to operate the machine. Given this objective, the primary target audience for the usability test consisted of undergraduate engineering students, particularly those enrolled in mechanical and industrial production courses. Bachelor's degree students were chosen over master's students since, at the undergraduate level, there is often limited access to hands-on CNC machine training, with most learning being theoretical. These courses provide foundational knowledge of machining processes, making them ideal for evaluating the effectiveness of the VR application.

Over a period of several days, 22 individuals with diverse backgrounds participated in the testing. Some had prior experience working with the CNC machine and were already familiar with its operation. Others had only received theoretical instruction, making it particularly interesting to observe their interaction with the application. Finally, a subset of students and technical staff had never operated a CNC machine before, making their feedback especially valuable in assessing the accessibility and effectiveness of the VR training tool.

Furthermore, the application was tested with students from the ASPOC Onlus Lab, an organization dedicated to supporting teenagers with cognitive disabilities such as Down Syndrome, Autism, and intellectual disabilities. ASPOC (Associazione per lo Sviluppo del Potenziale Cognitivo) [1] was founded by parents of these teenagers and focuses on developing meaningful learning environments that enhance their cognitive and motor skills. The goal was to evaluate whether the VR-based training could provide an engaging and accessible learning experience for students with disabilities, offering them an opportunity to interact with complex machinery in a safe and controlled virtual environment.

## 7 Test Results

The VR application, optimized for use with the Quest 3 headset, was tested with students enrolled in two academic courses at the School of Design at Politecnico di Milano: CAD Models and Design for Interaction. These courses, as their titles suggest, are closely aligned with themes related to CAD-CAM technologies. Given this alignment, the decision to involve these students in the testing phase was particularly relevant. The evaluation was conducted remotely, without the presence of the physical CNC machine, allowing students to gain preliminary exposure to the Charly4U CNC milling device in a virtual environment. A total of 61 students participated in this phase, providing a robust data set for assessing the usability of the desktop version of the application (Table 1).

**Table 1.** System Usability Scale (SUS) results for the VR-based version of the application. Polimi Students.

| # | **Statement** | Likert Scale (1–5) | Normal Mean (0–4) | **Std. Dev.** |
|---|---|---|---|---|
| 1 | I would like to use this application frequently. | 4.51 | 3.52 | 0.92 |
| 2 | I found the application unnecessarily complex. | 2.10 | 3.12 | 1.75 |
| 3 | I thought the application was easy to use. | 4.65 | 3.76 | 0.68 |
| 4 | I would need assistance from a technical person to use this application. | 2.10 | 3.12 | 1.37 |
| 5 | The various functions in this application were well integrated. | 4.5 | 3.68 | 0.52 |
| 6 | I noticed significant inconsistencies within the application. | 1.47 | 3.55 | 0.71 |
| 7 | Most users would learn to use this application quickly. | 4.72 | 3.68 | 0.53 |
| 8 | I found the application cumbersome to use. | 1.97 | 3.20 | 1.49 |
| 9 | I felt confident using the application. | 4.36 | 3.76 | 0.49 |
| 10 | I needed to learn many things before I could use this application. | 1.78 | 3.36 | 1.19 |
| **Overall SUS Score (0–100)** | | | **87** | **19.8** |

Thirteen ASPOC students participated in the evaluation (Table 2). To ensure effective comprehension, the testing began with a collective instructional session using a projector to explain the application's purpose and features. Subsequently, each student had the opportunity to interact individually with both the tablet and desktop versions of the application. From a subjective standpoint, the experience was met with high enthusiasm. The opportunity to interact with a dynamic virtual environment was both novel and stimulating for the participants. Notably, some students—despite challenges with motor skills—interacted with the application more fluidly and effectively than some engineering students or staff, particularly in gesture-based input tasks.

Following these hands-on sessions, all students completed a ten-question usability questionnaire. Using a five-emoticon Likert scale converted into numerical values, the results indicated an average score above 4, reflecting very positive user feedback regarding the VR application's performance and accessibility.

**Table 2.** System Usability Scale (SUS) results for the VR-based version of the application. Aspoc Students.

| # | **Statement** | Likert Scale (1–5) | Normal Mean (0–4) | **Std. Dev.** |
|---|---|---|---|---|
| 1 | I would like to use this application frequently. | 4.10 | 3.28 | 1.57 |
| 2 | I found the application unnecessarily complex. | 2.19 | 2.91 | 2.99 |
| 3 | I thought the application was easy to use. | 4.51 | 3.51 | 1.16 |
| 4 | I would need assistance from a technical person to use this application. | 2.19 | 2.91 | 2.34 |
| 5 | The various functions in this application were well integrated. | 4.22 | 3.43 | 0.89 |
| 6 | I noticed significant inconsistencies within the application. | 1.52 | 3.31 | 1.21 |
| 7 | Most users would learn to use this application quickly. | 4.19 | 3.43 | 0.91 |
| 8 | I found the application cumbersome to use. | 2.00 | 2.98 | 2.55 |
| 9 | I felt confident using the application. | 4.00 | 3.51 | 0.84 |
| 10 | I needed to learn many things before I could use this application. | 1.75 | 3.13 | 2.03 |
| **Overall SUS Score (0–100)** | | | **81** | **16.5** |

## 8 Conclusions

This work can be summarized in three main parts: the first is related with Inventor and 3ds MAX. In this context all the 3D models and the animations were created and then converted in a file format that can be used in Unity3D. The second is related to the application development with Unity3D game engine in two different configurations. The third and last part concerns the analysis of the tests results both on university students as well as on the ASPOC team. It has been proved that augmented reality can be used in different sectors, from educational to industrial one, allowing the user to interact with the environment in a completely new way. The proposed work is mainly focused on educational field, proposing a VR application that helps non skilled people on working with a

CNC milling machine. This was mainly done for students of Politecnico di Milano – Lecco campus where the Charly4U CNC machine is present. Many students, especially those without prior experience, reported feeling more confident in their ability to operate the real Charly4U CNC machine after using the VR application. Furthermore, instructors noted a reduction in hesitation and error rates during subsequent in-person lab sessions following the VR experience In this context this application was developed, to help students on working on the machine in safety.

## References


1. ASPOC association (2021). http://www.aspoc.it/index.aspx
2. For reviewers (2021). https://www.youtube.com/watch?v=HZsLeJfOH84, month=mar,lastaccessed=
3. Antonietti, A., Imperio, E., Rasi, C., Sacco, M.: Virtual reality and hypermedia in learning to use a turning lathe. J. Comput. Assist. Learn. **17**(2), 142–155 (2001)
4. Aruanno, B., et al.: Enhancing inclusive education for young students with special needs through mixed reality: exploring the potential of CNC milling machine application **21**(3), 522–535 (2024). all Open Access, Gold Open Access
5. Rajan, M.H., Herbert, C., Polly, P.: A synthetic review of learning theories, elements and virtual environment simulation types to improve learning within higher education. Thinking Skills Creativity **56**, 101732 (2025)
6. Jiang, X., Zhou, W., Sun, J., Chen, S., Fung, A.: Empathy enhancement through VR: a practice-led design study. Int. J. Hum. Comput. Stud. **194**, 103397 (2025)
7. Ka, J., Kim, H., Kim, J., Kim, W.: Analysis of virtual reality teaching methods in engineering education: assessing educational effectiveness and understanding of 3D structures. Virtual Real. **29**(1) (2025). https://doi.org/10.1007/s10055-024-01081-1. all Open Access, Gold Open Access
8. Magaña, E.C., Ariza, A.C., Ruiz-Palmero, J., Guillén-Gámez, F.D.: Virtual, augmented, and mixed reality in the university environment: an analysis of scientific production. J. New Approaches Educ. Res. **14**(1), 8 (2025)
9. Nor Farhah Saidin, N.D.A.H., Yahaya., N.: A review of research on augmented reality in education: advantages and applications. Int. Educ. Stud. **8**(13), 1–8 (2015)
10. Oje, A.V., Hunsu, N.J., Fiorella, L.: A systematic review of evidence-based design and pedagogical principles in educational virtual reality environments. Educ. Res. Rev. **47**, 100676 (2025)
11. Santilli, T., Ceccacci, S., Mengoni, M., Giaconi, C.: Virtual vs. traditional learning in higher education: a systematic review of comparative studies. Comput. Educ. **227**, 105214 (2025). all Open Access, Hybrid Gold Open Access
12. Vieira, C.B., Seshadri, V., Oliveira, R., Reinhardt, P., Calazans, P., Filho, J.: Applying virtual reality model to green ironmaking industry and education: 'a case study of charcoal mini-blast furnace plant'. Mineral Process. Extract. Metall. **126**(1–2), 116–123 (2017)
13. Wu, H.K., Lee, S., Chang, H.Y., Liang, J.C.: Current status, opportunities and challenges of augmented reality in education. Comput. Educ. **62**, 41–49 (2013)

# Enhancing Academic Advising Through AI Chatbots: A Smart Support System for Students

Wasin Alkishri[1](✉), Mahmood Al-Bahri[2], and Yousuf Al Husaini[1]

[1] Arab Open University, Seeb, Oman
{Wasan.k,yousufnaser}@aou.edu.om
[2] Sohar University, Sohar, Oman
Mbahri@su.edu.om

**Abstract.** The Arab Open University, Oman is one of the premier institutions in the rapidly evolving educational landscape that embraces technology to assist students with support services. Artificial intelligence-driven chatbots are game changers as they can be used for customized guidance and support to change learning processes. However, recently, some studies have also focused on their ability to promote student engagement and self-directed learning and enhance academic performance. Approaching the problem traditionally sometimes leads to issues such as a lack of available advisors, inconsistency with information dissemination, and managing many students. These drawbacks complicate decision-making, course selection and academic performance. To meet this challenge, AOU started developing an AI chatbot-based student support academic advising system as the need for efficiency, responsiveness, and personalization of student support is growing. This project focuses on building an AI chatbot for an academic advisor. With state-of-the-art natural language processing (NLP), the bot will improve the advising experience for students and staff. For context-aware conversational interactions, we used the GPT API in the project and a simple Python script to make the local web interface for integrating the API. Because it is open-source, customizable, and scalable while also supporting individual user login, the customizability of OpenWebUI was highly attractive. We employed the AYA model from Cohere, which achieved 94% outstanding performance in serving queries on advising topics with the lowest resource utilization in Arabic and English.

**Keywords:** AI chatbot · academic advising · natural language processing · student engagement · self-directed learning · GPT API · OpenWebUI · AYA model · educational technology

## 1 Introduction

Generally Artificial Intelligence (AI) transforms how students interact with digital learning environments, from human-led assistance to AI-powered solutions. In addition, real-time support in educational contexts could be made through AI-powered virtual assistants, also known as intelligent conversational agents, designed to process and simulate human-like interactions [1]. They are thus becoming increasingly popular among several


K. Daimi and A. Alsadoon (Eds.): ICR 2025, LNNS 1487, pp. 319–329, 2025.
https://doi.org/10.1007/978-3-031-95652-2_27

mega domains such as customer service, healthcare, and e-learning due to their ability to provide instant feedback, work in a 24/7 manner, and speak naturally [2, 3]. With the help of these AI-driven systems, students are getting help for their academic-related queries, assignments, and course recommendations, which is reducing the burden on human instructors and the administrative staff. Educational institutions are leveraging virtual assistants to increase learning accessibility, improve student engagement, and take academic processes out of human hands. Student learning support is an essential part of the Higher Education Institutions (HEIs) that has been acknowledged as a critical element in enhancing academic performance, retention, and satisfaction [4–6]. One of the most prominent difficulties and challenges faced by most students is accessing relevant academic information at the right time, which is essential for continuing their education. However, the demand for personalized guidance exceeds what traditional academic support systems can provide due to the limited availability of faculty members compared to the huge student body and limited resources [7]. Students' expectations of immediate and interactive assistance have been growing in line with reliance on digital technologies. Concerning this, AI-powered virtual assistants have sound potential. Such intelligent systems help students and institutions bridge communication gaps with student support that can be delivered at an individual student level, addressing frequently asked questions and bringing greater depth to the learning process anytime and from anywhere. The global chatbot market was valued at $15.57 billion in 2024 and will grow by $46.64 billion by [8]. The chatbots are widely used with more than 987 million users across the globe and are used for answering student questions and academic support. The development costs range from $5,000 to $500,000 which allows institutions to develop solutions that are tailored to the needs and budgets. See Fig. 1.

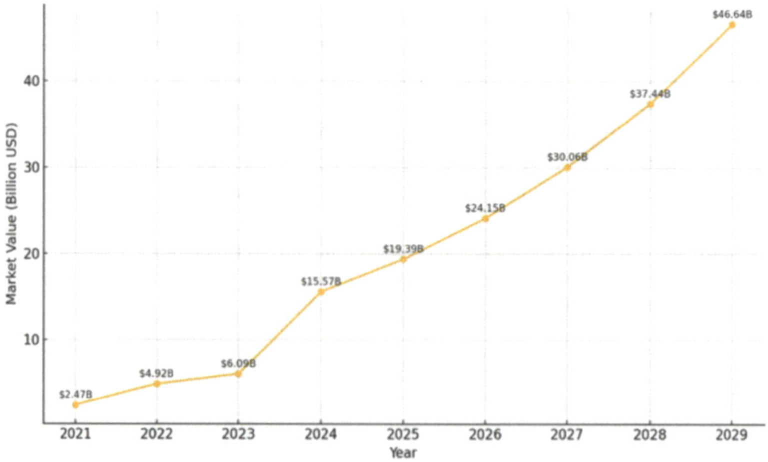


**Fig. 1.** Global chatbot market value (2021–2029)

Integrating AI-powered virtual assistants into the academic learning environment of universities can produce a responsive and supportive learning environment, which can lead to student success. This research aims to develop a chatbot to aid students within the Arab Open University, Oman, especially in the Faculty of Computer Studies. Its programmes include three undergraduate programmes, three diploma programmes and one master's programme. The IT faculty has an approximate population of 950 students, and there are nine faculty members whose classes consist of around 100 students each semester. With this high student-to-advisor ratio, having enough time for advisors to address the student quizzes and provide personalized academic guidance is challenging. Thus, students face difficulties getting timely information regarding the institutes' registration procedures, prerequisites, course requirements.

In particular, this study intends to design and implement a chatbot to help students examine their academic and administrative issues by alleviating the stress on faculty advisors. The chatbot will be an interactive support system that enhances access to critical information while enabling advisors to work on more strategic responsibilities, such as targeted academic planning. This paper contributes the novel integration of the GPT-based Aya model with OpenWebUI for providing bilingual (Arabic and English) academic support for students of the Arab Open University. It will be developed using neural networks and NLP technologies to improve its conversational capabilities and accuracy of sounding responses. By bringing at least two sides of stakeholders together – students and faculty – this innovative bilingual chatbot is a game changer that bridged the gap between them and help them advise each other any time within an instant AI-driven response. The rest of this paper will be structured as follows: Section 2 provides a literature review on chatbot applications in education and how related research progresses towards AI-driven academic support. The research methodology for Sect. 3 is the development process and the implementation framework of the chatbot. The efficacy of the chatbot is evaluated in Sect. 4, and the study results are presented. The paper concludes in Sect. 5 with key findings, conclusions, and study significance.

## 2 Literature Review

One of the newest trends in educational practice is artificial intelligence, which offers many innovative solutions for academic support services. Recently, chatbots have been of interest because they can facilitate academic advising processes. Firstly, this paper reviews the theoretical background, technological aspects, and gaps of previous works in the area of chatbots for academic advising, and it serves as a basis for the present study.

### 2.1 Overview of Chatbots

Natural language processing is applied to machines learning to have conversations similar to those of humans. They are suitable for the advisory role as they can process, understand, respond to, and answer real-time queries [9]. Chatbots are developed into three main types: task-oriented, data-driven, predictive, and generative AI. Each type has its own usage and uses different technological frameworks with varying levels of complexity and functionality. One of the defining characteristics of task-oriented chatbots is that they are rule-based systems meant to do predefined tasks. Natural Language

Processing (NLP) systems translate the user input and generate responses through structured rules or scripts [10]. Most of their enquiries or judgements, for instance, supplying business hours, making trades or satisfying regularly requested questions. Despite being simple, these chatbots are extremely effective in demand in the chatbot in customer service and support settings where interactions are predictable and have limited scope. Unlike personalization, deeper contextual understanding, or understanding of complex queries, task-oriented chatbots cannot understand novel user requests or adapt to changing user needs [11]. Virtual or digital assistants do better than task-oriented chatbots, also called data-driven chatbots. To understand context and predict user needs, we used sophisticated NLP, Natural language understanding (NLU) and machine learning (ML) [12]. They can offer personalized recommendations (and even strike up conversations reactively) based on historical data and user behaviour. Examples are Siri of Apple and Alexa of Amazon, and predictive analytics are used to provide assistance tailored to the person's desire. Unlike task-oriented, data-driven chatbots improve their accuracy and relevance with time. Nevertheless, they suffer from the scalability constraints faced by organizations with limited infrastructure due to their dependence on large datasets and computational resources. The most advanced technology of conversational AI is the Generative AI chatbots, which are based on deep learning models like GPT (Generative Pretrained Transformer) to develop dynamic contextual responses [13]. Generative AI chatbots are unlike task-oriented or data-driven systems wherein the responses or workflows are already defined. Instead, they learn to generate text in response to the conversational context and can handle open-ended queries, engage in deep conversational passages, and mimic human-like conversational patterns. One of the best qualities these chatbots possess is their ability to be creative and adaptive, thus being perfect for use in education, content creation, and customer conversation. However, their reliance on such advanced AI models results in significant computational overhead, leading to serious ethical issues, biases and misinformation.

## 2.2 Chatbots in Academic Settings

AI chatbots have been widely used to help students and educators in educational environments in multiple ways. [14] mention usage in tutoring, answering frequently asked questions (FAQs), and giving feedback on the assignments. Chatbots also help language learning by allowing interactive conversations. They also manage administrative tasks such as class scheduling and tracking student progress.

In a potential study, researchers created an informed chatbot for university resources called BARKPLUG V.2. A retrieval augmented generation pipeline along with large language models (LLMs) was used to create the proposed chatbot. Requiring retrieval for the large model to work also allows it to be augmented with domain-specific data that is contextually accurate and appropriate in real-time. According to an average RAGAS score of 0.96, BARKPLUG V.2 generated relevant and accurate responses very well. The applications include both student support and administrative assistance and faculty resource management, which is why its applications to boosting information access and operational efficiency in academic institutions are both broad and promising. This study [15] develops an application to enhance higher education learning through the generation capability of ChatGPT by embedding it into an information retrieval-based framework.

This hybrid architecture brings novelty in that ChatEd manages to capture ChatGPT's flexibility and conversational depth while keeping the precision and domain specificity of information retrieval systems. The systematic view of AI chatbots in education was conducted by [13], specifically to see the relationship of these AI chatbots with student engagement and personalized learning. Many studies have chosen to analyze how chatbots can help improve learning efficiency through real-time feedback, reduce student anxiety, and increase motivation in such online learning environments. In a study on chatbots in language learning, [16] looked more specifically at using chatbots in interactive conversations. Therefore, the study reported that chatbots significantly increase students' speaking and understanding skills due to their providing instant feedback, easing pronunciation, and adjusting for students' progress [17]. Examined AI chatbots as multi-functional teaching assistants in computer science education. Chatbots can be used as virtual tutors and problem-solving guides, thereby assisting students in grasping complex topics through interactive engagement and supporting collaborative learning. In their work, [18] focused on ChatGPT introduced to higher education through a student survey. Some students liked its ability to clarify concepts and receive quick answers, while others disliked its generic responses. They called for making upgrades in order to make chatbots more reliable. [19] explored the impact of chatbot design on student engagement. This study found that features of chatting that are more human, such as personalized greetings and natural conversation styles, improved satisfaction of the student and also increased interaction time, meaning that chatbots should be more relatable to improve learning outcomes. [20] analyzed the efficiency benefits of AI chatbots in higher education. The idea behind the study was to use chatbots to do automatic repetition tasks like grading, attendance tracking, and addressing FAQs, enabling educators to pay more attention to interactive teaching. The study of how chatbots aid students with disabilities was investigated by [21]. It indicated how such speech-to-text and text-to-speech features helped make educational content more accessible and inclusive, increasing engagement and inclusivity for visually and hearing-impaired students. [22] addressed the ethical challenges of AI chatbots in education. The paper stressed the need for algorithmic fairness, reduced bias, and the risk of poorly trained chatbots perpetuating discrimination. It said that ethical AI ought to be practised, and there should be greater transparency and regular audits. In the course of doing a comprehensive evaluation of artificial intelligence in the field of education, [23] pay much attention to learning analytics. The students were informed that by analyzing the patterns of data and how they relate with student performance, and how specific students could be managed, it was easy for the teachers to make judgment. In order to conduct meta-analysis, [24] gathered statistical data about the effectiveness of chatbots from a number of studies. The findings, on the other hand, proved that AI chatbots significantly improve student engagement and motivation as they provide timely support and an interactive learning experience.

Although many AI-based chatbots are available that can assist students in academic fields, they are not intended for academic tutoring and are not linked to the Arab Open University's information. Furthermore, most chatbots do not understand Arabic or the Gulf linguistic dialect and culture.

## 3 Proposed System

This research follows a structured methodology of collecting, preprocessing, integrating the model, its deployment to develop an AI powered assistant for academic purposes.

### 3.1 Data Collection

The first phase was data collection where various academic resources were collected including student plans, university registration details and institutional policies. These data sources were important to structure a base of knowledge about universities that allows the AI assistant to generate accurate answers regarding university or university related queries. Finally, the stored information was fed into a relational database (SQLite), allowing for structured retrieval and efficient processing. These categories are Academic and Behavioral questions, General questions, Student performance questions, Admission requirements questions, Subject registration questions, Facility and service questions, Academic advisors and teachers' questions, General questions, General questions, and Follow-up and Evaluation questions.

### 3.2 Preprocessing

The next phase involved applying preprocessing techniques to clean and organize the data. This included text extraction (PDFs), language filtering, tokenization and structuring user records. Python scripts like PDFAR2EN.py helped preprocess Arabic text, transforming students' information into structured datasets, and PushData2DB.py to integrate the data into the database. It also used natural language understanding (NLU) techniques in order to recognize features for key entities and intent from student queries in order to help the system deal with a wide variety of academic queries.

### 3.3 Implementation

In the implementation stage, Fig. 2, we integrated both part API based services and part AI-based processing. For communication with the backend, the system used Flask APIs, and the model is a hybrid one that also included integration with external API-based AI services. The Google Search API was used to safeguard external academic references, and advanced text summarization and intent classification were performed through Cohere AI models. In the meantime, the AYA AI model served as the centerpiece in making sense of and producing human-like responses in Arabic and English, hence giving a smooth and native fluent user experience between the lines of languages. With real-time translation between Arabic and English, the FilterAREN.py script facilitated the creator's accessibility for users. Inside the AI assistant, the decision module handled queries entering the system, classifying intent, retrieving information relevant to the request from the database and generating an appropriate reply. To allow those session-based interactions (conversation continuity), the AI memory module (EnableMemoryUSERS.py) was incorporated. Text-to-image generation and AI-assisted PDF processing using FilterMakePicture.py and PDF2AI.py – the users could visualize data or find insights in uploaded documents.

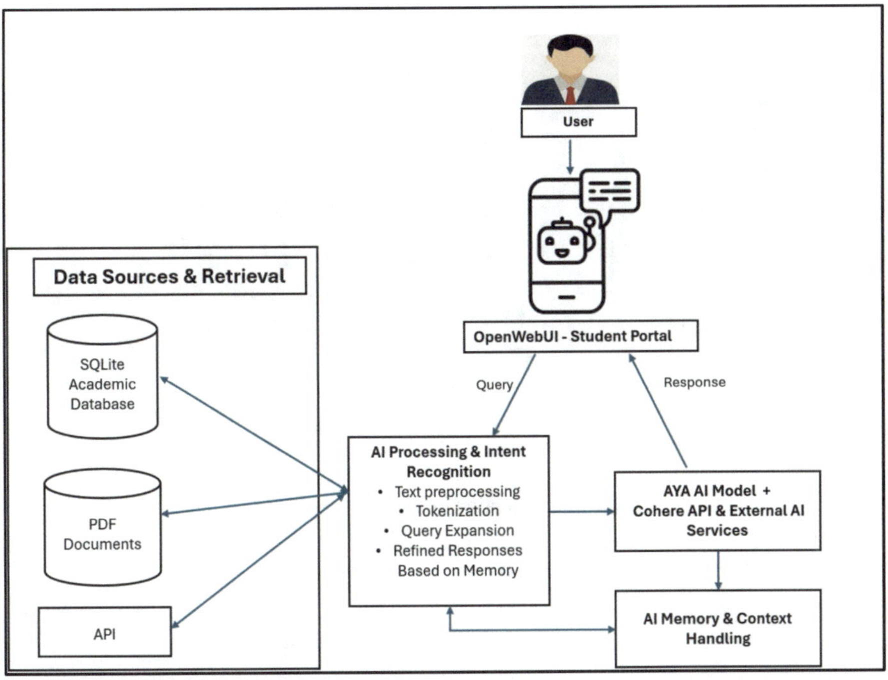


**Fig. 2.** Chatbot Model Development Process

# 4 Results and Discussion

We conducted a validation and testing phase to validate the developed chatbot and test its efficacy and accuracy. It was tested on 11 categories ranging from different aspects of university-related queries. See Fig. 3, The chatbot asked 10 questions for each category, and the following criteria rated their answers:

- Fully Correct and Complete Answer: 100%
- Answer Contains Details but Not Complete: 75%
- Answer Contains Part of the Required Information Only: 50%
- Answer Very Incomplete or Incorrect: 25%
- No Answer or Completely Incorrect Answer: 0%.

After the chatbot generated answers, they were manually evaluated according to the criteria listed above. See Table 1.

Across all categories, the average accuracy and reliability of the chatbot were at 94%. The test was made in Arabic and English, as represented in Figs. 4 and 5. It could answer an input in the correct language, meaning it responded to bilingual interaction correctly. For instance, if a user were to ask about what to do after they received a low GPA, the chatbot answered in Arabic with a detailed and clear structure on what to do. The chatbot also answered the same question in English and offered accurate and context-relevant guidance. Results confirm the reliability of the chatbot's support to students and

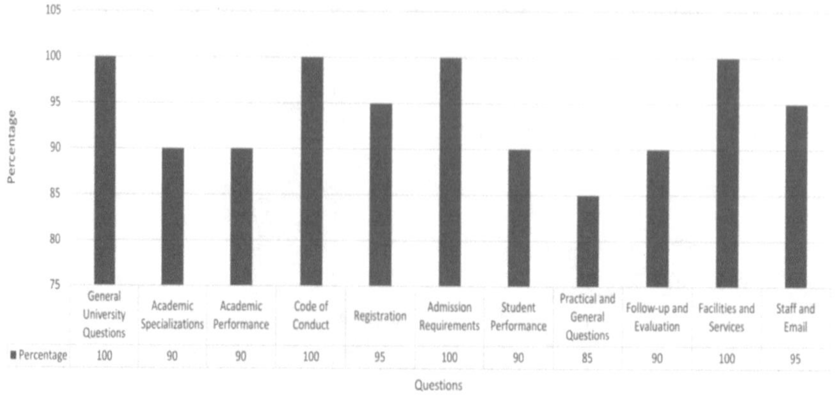


**Fig. 3.** Result of benchmark questions

**Table 1.** Evaluation criteria of the chatbot

| Question Group | Accuracy | Remarks |
|---|---|---|
| General University Questions | 100% | Answers are accurate and comprehensive for all questions. |
| Academic Specializations | 90% | Answers are clear, with minor missing details in some subpoints. |
| Academic Performance | 90% | Accurate responses, but some points need more clarification. |
| Code of Conduct | 100% | All answers are complete and correct. |
| Registration | 95% | Generally accurate, with minor exceptions in some details. |
| Admission Requirements | 100% | Answers are comprehensive and meet all required criteria. |
| Student Performance | 90% | Accurate, but some answers need additional details. |
| Practical and General Questions | 85% | Most answers are correct, but some lack context or detail. |
| Follow-up and Evaluation | 90% | Accurate, but some need clarification on specific conditions. |
| Facilities and Services | 100% | Responses are accurate and fully cover the topic. |
| Staff and Email | 95% | High accuracy, covering all listed employees effectively. |

its adaptation to any language. However, there is still room for improvement in response speed and/or deeper contextual understanding.

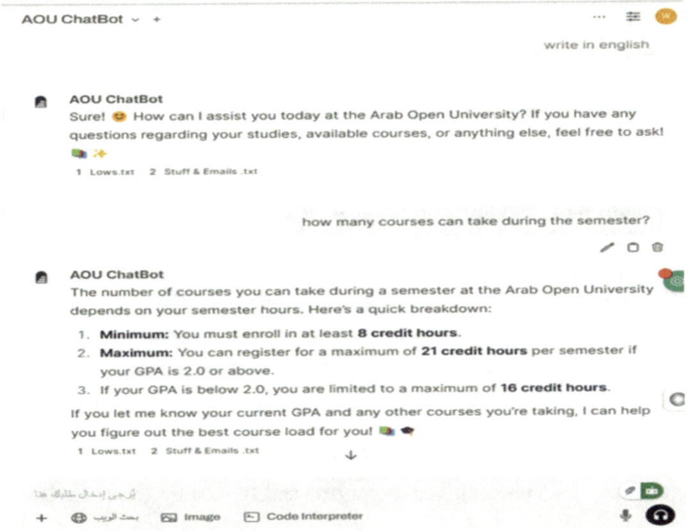


**Fig. 4.** Sample chatbot conversation in English

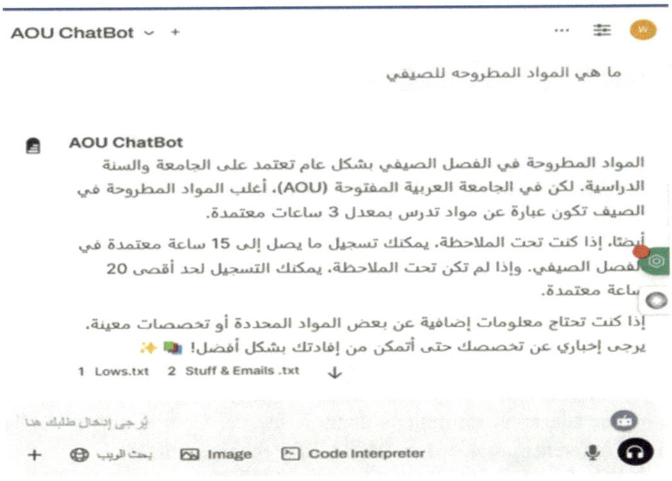


**Fig. 5.** Sample chatbot conversation in Arabic

## 4.1 Limitations and Future Work

A limitation observed in testing is that the chatbot responds slightly slowly, which may impact the user experience. Although it gives the correct answers, it has issues regarding response speed and how to handle the questions better. In the future, reducing latency, context understanding, and supporting multiple languages, mainly Arabic, would improve the system's usability and accessibility for a broader set of students.

## 5 Conclusion

The world has recently witnessed tremendous developments in artificial intelligence technologies. One of the most notable developments is the emergence of generative AI, which has transformed the way humans interact with intelligent systems. One of its most prominent applications is conversational generative AI, where machines are now able to understand and respond to natural language in a way that mimics real human interaction. In this project, it was demonstrated that the chatbot could answer diverse university-related questions with high accuracy and effectiveness. It proved a reliable tool for supporting students in various educational categories with an overall accuracy of 94%. Conversely, there are still some inadequacies on response time and understanding of context. To address these limitations, as well as further increasing language support, its functionality would be further enhanced, and it would help even more effectively with first-year students in the future.

**Acknowledgements.** This research was supported and funded by the Arab Open University, Oman.

**Declaration.** The authors declare that the research was conducted in the absence of any commercial or financial relationships that could be construed as a potential conflict of interest.

## References

1. Gubareva, R., Lopes, R.P.: Virtual assistants for learning: a systematic literature review. Proc. CSEDU. **1**, 97–103 (2020)
2. Yusuf, H., Money, A., Daylamani-Zad, D.: Pedagogical AI conversational agents in higher education: a conceptual framework and survey of the state of the art. Educ. Technol. Res. Dev. **73**, 1–60 (2025)
3. Wu, R., Yu, Z.: Do AI chatbots improve students' learning outcomes? Evidence from a meta-analysis. Br. J. Educ. Technol. **55**(1), 10–33 (2024)
4. Winkler, R., Söllner, M.: Unleashing the potential of chatbots in education: A state-of-the-art analysis. Acad. Manag. Proc. **2018**(1), 15903 (2018)
5. Niyozov, N., Saburov, S., Ganiyev, S., Olimov, S.: AI-powered learning: revolutionizing technical higher education institutions through advanced power supply fundamentals. In: E3S Web of Conferences, vol. 461, p. 01092. EDP Sciences (2023)
6. Yu, C., Yao, G.: Enhancing student engagement with AI-driven personalized learning systems. Int. Trans. Educ. Technol. (ITEE). **3**(1), 1–8 (2024)
7. F. Pedro, M. Subosa, A. Rivas, and P. Valverde, Artificial Intelligence in Education: Challenges and Opportunities for Sustainable Development, 2019
8. Exploding Topics, "Chatbot statistics," 2024. [Online]. Available: https://explodingtopics.com/blog/chatbot-statistics [Accessed: Mar. 25, 2025]
9. Gangal, A., et al.: Natural language processing: A review. AIP Conf. Proc. **2771**(1) (2023)
10. Hussain, S., Ameri Sianaki, O., Ababneh, N.: A survey on conversational agents/chatbots classification and design techniques. In: Web, Artificial Intelligence and Network Applications: Proc. Workshops of the 33rd Int. Conf. on Advanced Information Networking and Applications (WAINA-2019), vol. 33, pp. 946–956 (2019)
11. Gunnam, G. R.: The Performance and AI Optimization Issues for Task-Oriented Chatbots. Ph.D. dissertation, The University of Texas at San Antonio (2024)

12. Neupane, S., et al.: From questions to insightful answers: Building an informed chatbot for university resources. arXiv preprint arXiv:2405.08120. (2024)
13. Hwang, G.J., Chang, C.Y.: A review of opportunities and challenges of chatbots in education. Interact. Learn. Environ. **31**(7), 4099–4112 (2023)
14. Wijayanti, L.I., Sanyata, S.: Challenges and opportunities for adult education in the digital era: the role of guidance and counseling. Jurnal Bimbingan dan Konseling Terapan. **8**(2), 304–313 (2024)
15. Wang, K., Ramos, J., Lawrence, R.: ChatEd: A chatbot leveraging ChatGPT for an enhanced learning experience in higher education. arXiv preprint arXiv:2401.00052. (2023)
16. Pérez, J.Q., Daradoumis, T., Puig, J.M.M.: Rediscovering the use of chatbots in education: a systematic literature review. Comput. Appl. Eng. Educ. **28**(6), 1549–1565 (2020)
17. Cao, C.C., Ding, Z., Lin, J., Hopfgartner, F.: AI chatbots as multi-role pedagogical agents: Transforming engagement in CS education. arXiv preprint arXiv:2308.03992. (2023)
18. Song, X., et al.: Integrating AI in college education: positive yet mixed experiences with ChatGPT. Meta-Radiol. **2**(4), 100113 (2024)
19. Araujo, T.: Living up to the chatbot hype: the influence of anthropomorphic design cues and communicative agency framing on conversational agent and company perceptions. Comput. Hum. Behav. **85**, 183–189 (2018)
20. Khanna, P., Jha, S.: AI-based digital product 'robo-advisory' for financial investors. Vision. **09722629241298399** (2024)
21. Shelton, A., Gezer, T.: Investigating the educational experiences of students with disabilities during the COVID-19 school disruption: an international perspective. Large Scale Assess. Educ. **11**(1), 34 (2023)
22. V. Dignum, Responsible Artificial Intelligence: Designing AI for Human Values. 2017
23. Zawacki-Richter, O., Marín, V.I., Bond, M., Gouverneur, F.: Systematic review of research on artificial intelligence applications in higher education—where are the educators? Int. J. Educ. Technol. High. Educ. **16**(1), 1–27 (2019)
24. Huang, G., Wang, S.: Is artificial intelligence more persuasive than humans? A meta-analysis. J. Commun. **73**(6), 552–562 (2023)

# Optimizing Learning Experiences: MVC BLAZOR Components and Emerging Educational Technologies in LMS Development

Krenar Huseini, Agon Memeti(✉), Florinda Imeri, and Shkurte Luma-Osmani

Department of Computer Sciences, Faculty of Natural Sciences and Mathematics, University of Tetova, Tetovo, North Macedonia
{k.huseini3615111010,agon.memeti,florinda.imeri, shkurte.luma}@unite.edu.mk

**Abstract.** Rapid developments in the educational landscape make the use of Learning Management Systems (LMS) ideal for organising and conducting the learning process. This paper focuses on describing a strategic framework by which the performance of the University Learning Management System can be improved using MVC architecture with Blazor. These strategies are organized into four subsections, each addressing an important part of the system. The initial focus is on gaining performance insights which are gained through thorough responsiveness and load time monitoring and analysis. Then the Resource Loading Performance Analysis section will cover how to efficiently load assets to decrease page load times and reduce the load on the server. Next, optimization of data transfer between the server and Blazor components, emphasizing techniques like data compression and smart batching are shown. Lastly, the study of caching strategies is revealed, explaining how frequently accessed data is cached strategically and the setting up of expiration policies. This systematic approach to optimization aims to elevate the LMS of the University of Tetova, promising a more responsive, efficient, and enriched learning experience for both educators and students.

**Keywords:** LMS · MVC Blazor · Optimization · Educational technologies · Web Application Performance · Higher Education Systems

## 1 Introduction

Learning Management Systems are digital platforms designed to facilitate the administration, documentation, tracking, and delivery of educational courses or training programs. They provide teachers and students with an online classroom that reinforces learning processes [1, 2]. As in [4] most learning management systems contain a standard set of tools that are used to facilitate learning and discussion in an online environment. In the field of web development, developers have a multitude of frameworks and technologies at their disposal to create powerful and engaging applications. Also the .NET ecosystem includes specific implementations of the MVC pattern, such as ASP.NET MVC, which is a framework that uses this pattern for building web applications. Therefore, while MVC


K. Daimi and A. Alsadoon (Eds.): ICR 2025, LNNS 1487, pp. 330–338, 2025.
https://doi.org/10.1007/978-3-031-95652-2_28

(Model-View-Controller) as a notion is broadly applicable, ASP.NET MVC is a specific implementation within the .NET framework. Anyway, both of them have garnered substantial popularity in recent times. A well-optimized LMS can pointedly improve the educational process, while poor system performance can have disadvantageous effects on educational results.

The research aims to this paper aims to improve the performance of a university LMS through specific optimization strategies using MVC Blazor, moreover the idea of this paper delineates a strategic framework for optimizing the performance of University of Tetova - Learning Management System (LMS) developed under the MVC (Model-View-Controller) architecture with Blazor; optimizing learning experiences by holding paramount significance in fostering effective and efficient educational outcomes. By tailoring learning experiences to individual needs, preferences, and learning styles, optimization ensures that students or learners engage more deeply with the content, next the paper measures performance metrics, optimizing data transfer between the server and Blazor components and caching strategies. This personalized approach enhances understanding, retention, and application of knowledge.

The paper is organized as follows: The first section deals with introductory concepts of the topic, followed by the literature review as the second chapter. The third chapter deals with emerging educational technologies, as well as optimization strategies, concluding with a summary.

## 2 Literature Review

A literature review will be used to study various emerging technologies, LMS developments, existing optimization approaches, MVC architecture, and the integration of Blazor components with potential challenges. Also, the example of the implemented system at the University of Tetova will be shown and evaluated.

The demands of the global world urge the world of education and academics to constantly adapt to technological developments, especially adaptation to the use of ICTs in the learning process [5]. As in [7] a learning management system (LMS) is a software application or Web-based technology used to plan, implement, and assess a specific learning process. Typically, an LMS provides an instructor with a way of creating and delivering content, monitoring student participation, and assessing student performance. The same author] noted that the LMS supports teachers in their work by providing access to teaching material and assignments. It is common to use an LMS for purely online study (distance courses/e-learning) or as a supplement to classroom teaching.

Before delving into the actual coding of application logic and the design of its interface, an examination of the system's architecture is required. Equally important is ensuring that the system is not only capable of adeptly executing all its necessary functions but also possesses inherent flexibility for potential expansions and modifications to its functionality. Similar research [8] proposes embedding smart technology to boost the learning involvement and organizational efficacy through data-driven decision-making, automation, and tailored learning. It offers two models: the SmartQuiz integration module, which personalizes assessments, built on learner performance, and a dynamic dashboard for real-time progress tracking.

If the initial assumption is that the project will have extensive functionality, it is worth considering using patterns and frameworks. Application of design patterns and frameworks will keep flexibility and structure in the application, accelerating the development process [3]. The use of patterns and frameworks will make the application flexible and well-structured, as well as accelerate its development [3].

The Model-View-Controller (MVC) is a foundational programming pattern that segregates an application's business logic from its graphical interface. This separation facilitates a clear and organized structure, through which efficient management of both the underlying functionality and the user interface components can be performed.

Sandnes and Eika [9] introduce a streamlined Model-View-Controller (MVC) framework realized in Excel that permits educators to accomplish day-to-day tasks more proficiently. This system accomplishes the easy generation of lecture plans, student presentation agendas, and peer-review plans. Correspondingly, the MVC framework, serves as the industry standard for online application development by clearly defining the roles of the Model, View, as well as Controller to shorten testing and preservation, while also addressing critical gaps in online learning and educational technology over advanced solutions provided by the ASP.NET MVC framework [10].

The impact of technology on learning and teaching is often at the forefront of demands, particularly from those who dictate the funding available to pay for technology within education systems. However, this is not an unreasonable request as there is merit in impact evaluations of educational technologies, including of emerging technologies [6]. The concept of effectiveness and the need for some form of tangible proof that something 'works' means that some form of influence or impact of educational technology on its users needs to be demonstrated. As in [6], evaluating the impact of emerging technologies is even more challenging. Educational Technologies (ETs) have drawn the interest of researchers and educators in formal education because of the persistent and future challenges anticipated within the educational sphere in society.

According to the Online Learning Consortium, high-quality digital learning experiences are founded based on principles of equitable, inclusive, and accessible learning environments for every student. One key strategy involves using technology to create interactive and personalized learning environments. Incorporating educational software, virtual simulations, and online resources allows learners to engage with the content at their own pace and tailored to their individual needs. Adaptive learning platforms, for example, dynamically adjust the difficulty level of content based on a student's performance, ensuring a customized learning path that maximizes comprehension and retention.

Further, real-life examples and practical applications deepen students' understanding of the subject while making it more relevant and engaging. The development of an LMS using MVC architecture with Blazor holds significant potential for positively impacting learning experiences. By adopting the MVC pattern, the separation of concerns between the application's components allows for a clear organization of the system's architecture.

This structural clarity not only facilitates development, but also easier maintenance and scaling of the LMS. The use of Blazor enables the development of interactive and dynamic web applications using C# and .NET which can enhance the user interface and user experience within the LMS.

# 3 Optimization Strategies

For ensuring the seamless function of the University LMS it is essential to require extended performance insights, which means close monitoring and analysis of responsiveness, load times, and other efficiency aspects of the LMS.

The process of optimizing a higher education LMS will involve a comprehensive analysis of resource loading performance. Efficient transfer of data is highly important for the smooth operation of a Blazor-based University LMS. Interactions between the server and Blazor components involve data exchange. Optimizing this data exchange is important in order to reduce latency and enrich responsiveness for the user. Techniques which can be employed to streamline communication include data compression, smart batching, i.e. sending multiple operations or requests as a single one to minimize as much as possible the number of network calls, and the minimization of unnecessary data transfers.

Through the caching of frequently accessed data, such as user profiles, commonly used resources, and other course materials, administrators will be able to reduce the load on the server and enhance response times. Client-side caching of static assets and server-side caching of dynamic data can create a more efficient and responsive learning environment.

## 3.1 Performance Insights of the University LMS

The efficiency and user experience of an online platform, especially one as crucial as a Learning Management System (LMS), rely significantly on its loading speed and visual stability. By employing performance metrics gathered from Chrome DevTools, a comprehensive understanding of the LMS's performance can be obtained.

**Data Collection Methodology**

- **Tools Used:** Performance metrics were collected using Chrome DevTools, which allows for comprehensive analysis of web performance, including detailed insights into rendering times and layout shifts as shown in Fig. 1.
- **Frequency of Collection:** Metrics were gathered during multiple testing sessions to ensure consistency and reliability. Each session included both initial load tests and repeated load tests under various conditions, such as different device types to capture a more broad view of performance.
- **Comparison Approach:** Data from each session was compiled and analyzed over time. This comparison allowed us to assess the effectiveness of optimizations made to the LMS, ensuring that enhancements led to measurable improvements in loading speeds and visual stability.

**Performance Metrics Overview**

- First Contentful Paint (FCP): The LMS does very impressively with an FCP of 0.64 seconds reflecting significant optimization efforts that have reduced loading times by 20% compared to the previous measurement of 0.8 seconds, giving users an accelerated loading of content when opening the platform. This fast display of the first content elements contributes greatly to the positive user experience through reduced perceived loading times.

- DOMContentLoaded (DCL): The reported DCL of 0.68 seconds means that the core structure of the LMS, which includes the basic HTML document, becomes available for user interaction in a very short period of time. This faster readiness improves the user's ability to interact with it immediately upon their arrival which represents an improvement from 0.9 seconds in earlier testing.
- Largest Contentful Paint (LCP): The reported LCP of 0.96 seconds describes how long it takes to have the most significant content element on the page rendered fully. This metric has improved from 1.3 seconds and is important because it shows the speed at which users are able to view the primary content of the platform, determining how quickly the user can access resources or other important information.
- Cumulative Layout Shift (CLS): The measured CLS value of 0.0144 represents a high visual stability within the LMS.This improvement is critical, as earlier measurements showed a CLS of 0.04, highlighting the effective mitigation of unexpected shifts during loading. A minimal number of unexpected shifts or movements of page elements during loading contribute to a smooth and uninterrupted user experience, improving ease of navigation and comprehension.

Collectively, these performance metrics not only underpin the user-centric design and efficiency of the University's LMS but also demonstrate tangible improvements resulting from our optimization efforts. The quick loading times (denoted by FCP, LCP, and DCL), along with minimal layout shifts (CLS), demonstrate a commitment to providing an optimal learning environment. The platform's capability to swiftly deliver content while maintaining visual stability enhances accessibility and usability, positively impacting the overall user experience for students, educators, and administrators.

```
public async void UploadProfilePicture()
{
    try
    {
        await fileUploader.Upload(RPATH_PROFILEPICTURE);
        var filepath = fileUploader.FilePaths;
        profdata.image = filepath[0].RelativePath;
        await _profprofiledata.UploadProfilePicture(profdata);
        this.ImageModalVisibility = false;
        this.StateHasChanged();
        await ShowNotification("Success", "Profile picture successfuly updated!", "e-toast-success");
    }
    catch (Exception ex)
    {
        await ShowNotification("Warning", "Upload failed, please check the document you attached!", "e-toast-danger");
        Console.WriteLine(ex.Message);
    }
}
```

**Fig. 1.** Code Extract of the Main Functions

## 3.2 Resource Loading Performance Analysis of the University LMS

For educational platforms like an LMS, fast loading times are extremely important. Quicker loading times improve user engagement and accessibility, creating a positive learning experience for students. This analysis is conducted on the resource loading optimizations identified within our LMS, analysing how they contribute to an efficient learning environment.

Promising Performance: Our analysis reveals several positive insights that pave the way for a smooth user experience:

- **Lightning-Fast Essentials**: Critical CSS files like free.min.css and free v4 shims.min.css load within milliseconds, ensuring users see the core page layout instantly. Similarly, JavaScript libraries like popper.min.js and bootstrap.min.js follow suit, enabling rapid interaction with UI elements. This swift rendering sets the stage for a positive first impression.
- **Minimizing Bottlenecks:** We identified resources like jquery-3.6.1 almumin.js and lottle-player.js as potential bottlenecks due to their size. However, by using minification, compression, and asynchronous loading we significantly reduced their load times without compromising functionality. This proactive approach ensured smooth sailing for even the most resource-intensive elements.
- **Continuous Improvement:** Analysing resources like Inte-players and PCard.pg allowed us to proactively address any minor performance hiccups. By investigating their usage patterns and exploring optimization strategies, we refined the LMS's efficiency, ensuring a consistently smooth experience for all users.

Impacting the Learning Journey: These optimizations translate into real-world benefits for our students:

- **Reduced Frustration:** Fast loading times minimize waiting periods and frustration, allowing students to focus on learning, not technology. This fosters a more engaging and productive learning environment.
- **Increased Accessibility:** Improved performance ensures the LMS remains accessible to students with diverse needs and varying internet connection speeds. This promotes inclusivity and ensures everyone has equal access to educational resources.
- **Enhanced Engagement:** A seamless user experience keeps students on track and immersed in their learning journey. This translates to higher engagement levels and improved learning outcomes.

### 3.3 Optimizing Data Transfer Between the Server and Blazor Components

We have used multiple strategies and methods to enhance the efficiency of our system for example: minimizing initial loads, SignalR communication, component-level state management, caching strategies, data binding optimization which includes techniques used to increase the effectiveness of data synchronization amid a user interface (UI) and the underlying data model in applications so it suits more approachable and performs better, also lazy loading, image and asset optimization and many more, as explained briefly below.

In the example above in Fig. 1 we have provided a code snippet from our LMS for a method named 'UploadProfilePicture' that contains 'StateHasChanged' which is called after certain changes have been made to the component's state.

Blazor components often work with asynchronous operations, such as file uploads, API calls, or other data retrieval processes. After the asynchronous operations complete and data changes occur (like updating the profdata.image path), Blazor might not automatically detect these changes because they occur asynchronously.

When we call the UploadProfilePicture method from the profprofiledata service, the parent component re-renders but not the child, who is not aware that his state has changed. In order to make the child aware that his state has changed and that it should re-render, we call the StateHasChanged() method.

After updating the profdata.image and hiding the image modal, calling StateHasChanged() ensures that any changes to the component's state are immediately reflected in the UI. This guarantees that users see the updated profile picture or any UI changes associated with the upload process promptly after they occur.

### 3.4 Caching Strategies

Storing certain information locally in the browser alleviates the need for repeated server requests to fetch the same data. By utilizing client-side storage and accessing stored data via BrowserStorage .GetAsync<int>("lendaID"), our system reduces server load and enhances the overall system efficiency, especially in scenarios like this where frequent data retrieval is required.

Client-side caching benefits include:

1. **Reduced Server Load:** By retrieving data from the client's browser storage, we reduced the number of requests sent to the server, leading to faster load times for users.
2. **Improved User Experience:** Data can be accessed instantly, enabling quick re-rendering and personalized adjustments, like scrolling straight to the user's last viewed course.
3. **Offline Access:** Some client-side caches persist across sessions, allowing users to continue where they last left off even if they lose connection temporarily.

In contrast, *server-side caching* stores frequently accessed data on the server itself, although it minimizes repetitive computations and speeds up data retrieval, server-side caching always requires network requests, which can bring latency compared to instant local access on the client. Additionally, server-side caching is less effective for scenarios where a user's preferences or data (such as in our case the last viewed course) are individualized and need to be updated frequently.

Therefore, in our system, we decided to go for a client-side caching strategy to handle the specific needs of fast re-rendering, user personalization, and efficiency which improved the cache hit rate from 75% to 90% indicating that the majority of data retrieval requests are successfully served from local storage.

What this block of code in Fig. 2 does is check if the app is used from mobile: The first line public bool EnableMobileUI; defines a boolean variable called EnableMobileUI. The following line, // Check if the app is used from mobile, suggests there's code somewhere that sets the value of this variable based on whether the app is running on a mobile device. This information might be used later to adjust the UI or behavior for mobile users.

```
public bool EnableMobileUI;
// Check if the app is used from mobile
protected override async Task OnAfterRenderAsync(bool firstRender)
{
    if (firstRender)
    {
        //stored lenda id
        var resultofstoredlendaid = await BrowserStorage.GetAsync<int>("lendaID");
        storedlendaid = resultofstoredlendaid.Success ? resultofstoredlendaid.Value : 0;
        await IJS.InvokeVoidAsync("ScrollToElement", "#course-" + storedlendaid.Value);
        EnableMobileUI = await IJS.InvokeAsync<bool>("isMobile");
        this.StateHasChanged();
    }
}
```

**Fig. 2.** Code Extract of the Mobile Usage Check

The next section checks if it's the first time the app is rendering (if (firstRender)) and then tries to retrieve a value called "lendaID" from the browser storage using the BrowserStorage.GetAsync<int>("lendaID") call. This function attempts to get an integer value associated with the key "lendaID" from the browser's storage.

If the "lendaID" value is not found in the storage (resultofstoredlendaid.Success ? resultofstoredlendaid.Value: 0), the code sets the storedlendaid variable to 0. This suggests that "lendaID" might be an identifier for something important in the app, and if it's not stored yet, the app uses a default value of 0.

Overall, this code snippet demonstrates how the app uses browser storage to cache the user's progress and preferences. It remembers which course the user was viewing and adjusts the UI based on whether they're using a mobile device. This caching can help improve the user experience by making the app feel faster and more personalized.

## 4 Conclusion

These optimization strategies for the University LMS are a testament to a framework focused on performance improvement in the use of the platform for the enhancement of the learning process for its users. This study on optimisation of performance insights, caching strategies, and data transfer optimisation has shown a clear process through which the University LMS can be transformed into a more responsive and efficient platform.

The results obtained from performance analysis give the grounding for effective improvements, ensuring that everything in the LMS will run smoothly. Resource loading performance analysis outlines the need for optimization in asset loading, which will improve page load times and prevent overloaded conditions of server resources. Optimization of data transfer between the server and Blazor components allows for fast and consistent interactions, creating a more seamless user experience. Finally, the strategic implementation of caching strategies is guaranteed to reduce server load and enhance response times. User feedback collected through surveys post-optimization indicated a 30% increase in user satisfaction ratings, reflecting the tangible benefits of these enhancements on the learning experience. Additionally, empirical data revealed a 10% improvement in course grading rates among students, suggesting that quicker access to resources facilitates better user experience.

The use of Blazor in our LMS is not merely a technical choice, it represents a shift toward more interactive and dynamic learning experiences. By leveraging Blazor's capabilities, we can provide features such as component-based architecture and seamless client-server interactions, which are not typically available in conventional LMS platforms. This innovative approach positions our LMS as a forward-thinking solution in the field of educational technology.

## References

1. Association of Public Land-Grant Universities. Optimizing High-Quality Digital Learning Experiences - A Playbook for Faculty
2. Bradley, V.M.: Learning management system (LMS) use with online instruction. Int. J. Technol. Educ. (IJTE). **4**(1), 68–92 (2021). https://doi.org/10.46328/ijte.36
3. Erich, G., et al.: Design Patterns - Elements of Reusable Object-Oriented Software. Addison Wesley (1977)
4. K-12 Blueprint: Learning Management System (LMS) Guide. Clarity Innovations (2014)
5. Munir, T., Suyitno, M.: Development of learning management system-based blended learning model using Claroline in higher education. Int. J. Interact. Mob. Technol. (2020)
6. Mutlu, C., et al.: Measuring the impact of emerging technologies in education: a pragmatic approach. In: Second Handbook of Information Technology in Primary and Secondary Education (2018)
7. Torsten, A.: Learning Management Systems. Master Thesis (2019)
8. Memeti, A., Nuhi, A.: Embedding Smart Tech: MVC Blazor Learning Management System with Embedded Computing. In: 2024 13th Mediterranean Conference on Embedded Computing (MECO), Budva, Montenegro, vol. 2024, pp. 1–4. https://doi.org/10.1109/MECO62516.2024.10577895
9. Sandnes, F.E., Eika, E.: A simple MVC-framework for local management of online course material. In: Uskov, V., Howlett, R., Jain, L. (eds.) Smart Education and e-Learning 2017. SEEL 2017. Smart Innovation, Systems and Technologies, vol. 75. Springer, Cham (2018). https://doi.org/10.1007/978-3-319-59451-4_15
10. Priyanka, D.: Educational technology and libraries supporting online/digital learning with the ASP. NET MVC framework. In: AI-Assisted Library Reconstruction, pp. 191–208. IGI Global (2024)

# Feasibility Study on Leveraging Proof Assistants for Educational Purposes

Fernand Dubler(✉), Ulrich Ultes-Nitsche, and Dorian Guyot

University of Fribourg, Fribourg, Switzerland
{fernand.dubler,ulrich.ultes-nitsche,dorian.guyot}@unifr.ch

**Abstract.** This paper evaluates the educational impact of proof assistants in computer science education through a feasibility study. We developed a methodology using interactive theorem proving to measure students' understanding of computer science concepts, focusing on instruction set architectures within the Coq proof assistant. Through pre/post assessments and structured learning tasks, we evaluated both our testing framework and students' learning outcomes, providing insights for classroom integration of proof assistants.

**Keywords:** proof assistant · education · instruction set architecture · assembly · Coq

## 1 Introduction

Formal methods, while fundamental to computer science curricula, have seen limited industry adoption outside safety-critical systems and high-stakes applications. Our research explores new applications of formal methods, specifically investigating proof assistants as teaching tools in computer science education. Our hypothesis is that student learning improves when they both implement and prove properties about new concepts, encouraging deeper engagement and independent discovery of edge cases. While unit tests can verify implementation correctness, proving theorems provides a richer learning experience through self-directed exploration. Therefore, our research question can be formulated as follows: *Can proof assistants be leveraged as an educational tool for teaching the practical applications of computer science and does their use have an observable effect on students' learning?* The use of proof assistants in a teaching context is promoted in various publications. Some prominent examples are the books by Pierce et al. [1,2] that cover the proof assistant Coq [3] and the functional programming language Gallina. To this end, other closely related topics from the domains of logic, theoretical computer science, and mathematics are covered. Many similar projects with educational goals exist, of which some are mentioned in the bibliography [4–6]. Our study differs from these works in that its goal is not only to explore the usage of interactive theorem proving in teaching, but to test whether this practice has a positive impact on the students' progress. Our


K. Daimi and A. Alsadoon (Eds.): ICR 2025, LNNS 1487, pp. 339–349, 2025.
https://doi.org/10.1007/978-3-031-95652-2_29

aim is also to investigate the applicability of proof assistants as a tool for the teaching of practical computer science concepts that do not classically involve the formulation and proving of mathematical theorems. In order to leverage proof assistants as a learning tool, students must have the necessary skills to use them. For this reason, we decided to conduct the study within a graduate course in which students' prior knowledge about functional programming is refreshed and the necessary skills in interactive theorem proving are acquired during the first half of the semester. The study is then conducted in the second half of the semester whose curriculum does not traditionally involve the use of proof assistants. Students will be working through an interactive set of tutorials which also includes small implementation tasks in self-study sessions. The gained knowledge is then consolidated and tested during classroom sessions where students have to prove their implementations correct. In order to detect whether the act of developing interactive proofs has a beneficial effect on students' understanding, we test the mental model of the concepts that they acquired during the self-study sessions (before proving) and after the classroom sessions (after proving). As a testing method, we decided to include test questions into the "self-study" as well as the "in-classroom" tutorials. To ensure the rigor of our key contribution, namely the developed data collection and testing method, we undertook a feasibility study, which is the subject of this paper.

## 2 Feasibility Study: Design and Implementation

As outlined in the previous section, we developed a novel data collection and testing method, whose intended use is to make the impact of proof assistants on students' learning observable. To ensure the rigor of this method, we undertook a feasibility study aimed at assessing it on a small scale. The results may not only help us refine the methodology for the larger-scale study but also provide valuable insights on how to design the learning materials and the overarching course in which it will be embedded.

*Participant Recruitment.* A significant initial challenge was recruiting participants for this preliminary study. The main constraint was the requirement for participants to understand and implement basic definitions and proofs in the Coq proof assistant. The prerequisite of having attended the previous semester's systems verification course limited the pool of potential participants considerably. Furthermore, many course participants had completed their studies at the end of the past semester, making them less accessible. However, given the exploratory nature of this feasibility study, and the fact that it will be followed by a larger scale study, we did not require a large number of participants. We thus considered the three students who volunteered sufficient to test our approach in this feasibility study.

*Study Methodology.* The experiment designed for the feasibility study closely mirrored the one planned for the larger-scale study. The writing of tutorials, code examples, implementation and proving tasks, as well as test questions all followed the same style. However, there are a few aspects specific to the feasibility study. In the main study, the experiments will be conducted immediately following a half-semester introduction to the Coq proof assistant, and participants will possess the necessary skills. Additionally, the main study may be conducted over multiple course executions and may involve a comparison between two groups of students: one that learns through a combination of implementation and proof-based tasks, and another that focuses solely on implementation. In contrast, the feasibility study focused on refining the data collection process and therefore concentrated on the former approach. Also, the three participants had not used Coq in five to six months, which we had to account for when designing the tutorial. We aimed to maintain simplicity in the implementation tasks and proof complexity, while introducing unfamiliar concepts to reliably measure a learning effect. Having worked with the students, we knew of their limited exposure to instruction set architectures, which is why we designed the tutorial as an introduction to this subject.

*Assessor Role.* In addition to these measures, we observed the students during the experiment and guided them through the proving challenges regarding syntax, the use of proving tactics, and pointing out existing lemmas that could be used to complete a proof. This approach not only allowed us to execute the experiment in an acceptable amount of time but also to collect information that would otherwise be lost. These observations are reflected in the experiment protocols as "Assessor Comment" (see Table 2) and helped shape the interpretation of the collected "hard data". We understand that in the main study, it will not be possible to observe students this closely during the experiments. Therefore, we aimed to learn enough from this preliminary study to design a rigorous testing framework that does not require additional manual observation to be viable.

*Tutorial Structure.* The tutorial serves as an introduction to instruction set architectures (ISA). It begins with a concise definition of the term, followed by guidelines on how to navigate and engage with the material. Subsequently, it introduces fundamental vocabulary and concepts, interspersed with code segments demonstrating their implementation in Coq. The tutorial also presents essential helper functions and proofs. This initial section aims to equip students with the understanding to comprehend the instruction descriptions that follow. The instruction descriptions are adapted from the AVR® Instruction Set Manual [7] and are included in the tutorial as shown in Listing 1. The students are introduced to three basic instructions from the aforementioned ISA. Each section contains code samples and proofs that showcase the instructions' behavior, following a consistent structure (outlined in Table 1). Having worked with the material ourselves, we were aware of potential misunderstandings in the instructions behavior. We designed the implementation and proof challenges to guide students through these pitfalls subtly, without explicit highlighting. This approach aims to facilitate a learning effect that we hope to measure in this study.

We anticipate that additional such pitfalls may be uncovered in the larger scale main study.

**Table 1.** Structure of Tutorial Sections

| | |
|---|---|
| Description | A modified excerpt from the actual instruction set manual describing an instruction |
| Implementation | The instruction is implemented in code |
| Questions | One or more questions test student understanding. Each question presents an initial state, and students provide the resulting state after executing one or two instructions. Solutions depend on instruction behavior. Students indicate their confidence and may leave comments |
| Example execution | An example execution of the instruction showcases how it operates |
| Proof | One or more theorems are proven about the instruction |
| Questions | Additional questions assess changes in student understanding between coding and theorem proving |

*NOP Tutorial Section.* We chose to start with the `nop` instruction as its behavior is very simple and thus serves as a good introductory example. The instruction literally does nothing; its only effect on the state is that the program counter is incremented by one. The implementation is provided by the tutorial and serves as an example that students can use as a template for subsequent instructions, which they are going to implement themselves. One simple question asks about the state before and after executing a `nop` instruction. We test whether students understand that the only observable state change is the program counter being incremented by one. The first example execution gives students instant feedback on their answer. In this case, the state change is correctly reflected by the example, which is why we expect students to either become more confident about their answer or change their mind if their answer is incorrect. Students must then fill in a simple proof that shows that the given implementation of `nop` is consistent with the description. This exercise primarily serves as a warm-up for students who haven't been in contact with a theorem prover for a while. We do not expect a significant difference in the answers to the following test questions compared to before. The behavior of the nop instruction is clear from the description and the given implementation. The only expected difference is an increase in reported confidence. We are well aware that this increase in confidence might be due to both the sample instruction and the proven lemma.

*LDI Tutorial Section.* We felt, that `ldi` is a good choice for a follow-up. The instructions' behavior is easy to grasp while containing a few caveats that might challenge students inexperienced with instruction sets. The instruction `ldi` loads a value into a register. Note the caveat that the value must be between 0 and 255. Another caveat would be that the instruction does not operate on all registers. The latter has however been purposefully overlooked in the tutorial for the sake of simplicity. As with most instructions, the program counter is incremented by one. For this instruction, students are tasked with its implementation (ldi_impl). Note that (ldi_impl) and similar notations refer to the corresponding entries in the 'Assignment' column of Table 2. In designing this task, we were particularly interested in observing how students would handle the aforementioned caveat. Since they had access to the relevant information in the instruction description, they might implement it correctly. However, it's also possible they might overlook this detail, as they weren't given explicit instructions regarding this aspect. After the implementation students answer two questions. The first question (ldi_q1_bp) asks students to correctly predict the state change with a legally formed `ldi` instruction. In the second question (ldi_q2_bp), students encounter an `ldi` instruction with a value exceeding 255, rendering it malformed. This tests whether students are aware of this caveat. We were concerned that if both questions were nearly identical, differing only in the input value, students might become aware of the caveat. To avoid this, as the question's purpose is to assess current knowledge rather than extend it, we added a `nop` instruction to the initial state. Students aware of the caveat should answer correctly, while others might be distracted by this small addition and fail to question the large input value. In this instance, the example executions might provide students with a false sense of security, as the success of the execution depends on their implementation of the instruction. Students then do two proofs. First they prove that their implementation works in the happy path. *If on any given state, `ldi r i` is executed, where `r` is a register and `i` a value between 0 and 255 then, in the resulting state, the register `r` contains the value `i`.* With the second lemma students prove that their implementation correctly handles the case where the input value is out of bounds. *If on any given state, `ldi r i` is executed, where `r` is a register and `i` a value greater than 255 then, the resulting state is considered erroneous.* We then ask the same questions (ldi_q1_ap and ldi_q2_ap) as before and expect students that implement `ldi` correctly, to keep their previous answer and have a raise in confidence. Students that did not consider the bounds are expected to change their answers accordingly.

*ADD Tutorial Section* Finally, students are introduced to the `add` instruction. On a superficial level it's behavior is easy to understand, however it is conceptually more complex than the `ldi` instruction. This is why the tutorial provides more explicit guidance, allowing students to complete the experiment within the allotted time frame with greater ease. The instruction adds the values contained in two registers `Rd` and `Rr` and stores the result in `Rd`. Other than the previously discussed instructions, `add` also has an effect on the status register (SREG). To keep things simple, we decided to only cover the zero (`Z`) and (`C`) flag in this tutorial and omit the others. This is also reflected in the excerpt of the instruction set manual shown in Listing 1. The `Z` flag is set to `1` when the result of the operation equals the value `0`, otherwise it is set to `0`. The `C` flag is set to `1` if the

```
(*
  ADD - Add without Carry
  ------------------
  Description: Adds two registers Rd and Rr and places the result
  in the destination register Rd.
  Operation: Rd ← Rd + Rr
  Syntax: ADD Rd,Rr
  Operands: -
  Program Counter: PC ← PC + 1

  Status Register (SREG) and Boolean Formula:
  Z: ¬R7 ∧ ¬R6 ∧ ¬R5 ∧ ¬R4 ∧ ¬R3 ∧ ¬R2 ∧ ¬R1 ∧ ¬R0
  C: Rd7 ∧ Rr7 ∨ Rr7 ∧ ¬R7 ∨ ¬R7 ∧ Rd7
*)
```

Listing 1: ISA excerpt of the ADD instruction

addition yields a result greater than 255 otherwise it is set to `0`. Naturally, the program counter is incremented by one. The code which implements the behavior of the instruction according to the description is provided by the tutorial. This, to allow the experiment to proceed faster. In the larger scale study we will expect students to implement such instructions on their own. The instruction set manual does not describe certain subtleties about the behavior of the instruction. This allowed us to include a naive implementation of the instruction, that follows the description of the instruction set manual but does not always behave as expected. The result being computed by the assignment `r := (m + n)` is not correct in all cases. The instruction set manual does not specify what happens when the result of the addition is greater than 255. Experienced programmers might expect the result to be truncated to 8 bits, but this is not specified at this position in the manual. The following test question (add_q1_bp) addresses a peculiar situation where the registers `Rd` and `Rr` contain out-of-bound values. Note that in a correct implementation of the ISA, this scenario should not occur, as a register's size is one byte and thus cannot contain values greater than 255. However, in this tutorial, we are implementing a mathematical model where abstracting such constraints may be beneficial, allowing registers to contain natural numbers. When considering the instruction set manual, a correct answer would be, that there is no way to predict the outcome of the operation. The example execution then shows however, that given the current implementation, the correct answer would be, that register `16` contains the value `2048`. The zero flag therefore is set because the eight first bits of its binary representation (`1000 00000000`), considered by the boolean formula for `Z` (see Listing 1) are zero. The carry flag is not set for the same reason. All three lemmas cover the happy path of the `add` instruction. The first two are provable with the current implementation and we expect students to be able to do so. The third and last lemma however, states that *if on any given state,* `add` *r1 r2 is executed, where r1 and r2 are registers containing the values* `m` *and* `n` *respectively, then in the resulting state, the carry flag is set if the sum of* `m` *and* `n` *is greater than 255.* This is not provable with the current implementation. Consider the case where the numbers 200 (`11001000` in binary) and 100 (`01100100`) are added. The resulting value 300 (`1 00101100`) is out of bound. According to the boolean formula of the instruction set manual $Rd7 \wedge Rr7 \vee Rr7 \wedge \neg R7 \vee \neg R7 \wedge Rd7$. The carry flag should be set, but it is not in this implementation which blindly follows the description of the instruction set manual. Students are therefore expected to recognize the issue and state so. The question that follows (add_q2_ap) tests whether students understood this fact. It is about the (realistic) case where the result of the addition is greater than 255. In this case, the boolean formulas from the instruction set manual for the flags work as intended. The zero flag is unset, and the carry flag is set. The same applies to our implementation as it correctly implements the ISA. However, when considering the result stored in `r16`, the implementation stores the value `300`. What should happen, is that the result should be truncated to fit the 8-bit size of the register. Together with the additional carry flag, this would yield the correct value of the computation `300 (1 00101100)`, but the register itself should contain the value `44 (101100)`. Unlike before, the questions posed before (add_q1_bp) and after (add_q2_ap) the proving tasks are now different. This deliberate change is part of an experiment to determine the most reliable method. Our concern was that using the same question could influence students' responses, a phenomenon known as priming. On the other hand, using different questions might make it more challenging to accurately measure any learning effects that occur.

## 3 Results

Table 2 summarizes the results for the LDI and ADD instructions. The NOP instruction, which served as a warm-up exercise, is not included. Proofs are also omitted, as the outcomes were as expected. The table includes the following columns: "Student" lists the non-identifying student names; "Assignment" refers to the implementation task or question they were required to solve; the therein appended strings "bp" and "ap" indicate whether a question was asked before or after the proof; "Response", categorizes the students' answers as "Naive", "Informed", or "Partial"; and "Assessor Comment" provides additional context for the results. The presence of a learning effect is assessed through the observation of students' responses to the questions before proof (bp) to after proof (ap).

*General Effectiveness of Approach.* Our testing approach, generally proved effective. In multiple instances, we were able to observe a learning effect, as evidenced by changes in students' responses. For example, Student Blues' response changed from "Naive" in ldi_q2_bp to "Informed" in ldi_q2_ap. However, we discovered that its reliability depends on the careful design of the test questions as well as the implementation and proving challenges. The following considerations should therefore be taken into account for the design of the main study.

**Table 2.** Results Overview

| Student | Assignment | Response | Confidence | Assessor Comment |
|---|---|---|---|---|
| Red | ldi_impl | Naive | | No input checking |
| Red | ldi_q1_bp | Informed | 4 | |
| Red | ldi_q2_bp | Naive | 5 | High confidence probably due to previous example execution |
| Red | ldi_q1_ap | Informed | 5 | |
| Red | ldi_q2_ap | Informed | 4 | Student recognized that instruction is malformed and assumed it to not execute |
| Red | add_q1_bp | Naive | n/a | |
| Red | add_q2_ap | Informed | 3 | Student recognized that there must be an overflow and assumed it to have the highest possible value (255) |
| Blue | ldi_impl | Naive | | No input checking |
| Blue | ldi_q1_bp | Informed | 4 | |
| Blue | ldi_q2_bp | Naive | 5 | Students confidence in their incorrect answer was emboldened by the compute statement of the previous question |
| Blue | ldi_q1_ap | Informed | 5 | |
| Blue | ldi_q2_ap | Informed | 1 | Student recognized that the execution would fail and behavior is unknown or undefined |
| Blue | add_q1_bp | Partial | 2 | Naive with respect to register value. Informed with respect to status register |
| Blue | add_q2_ap | Naive | 3 | Student shows that they understood the problematic in the comment |
| Green | ldi_impl | Naive | | No input checking |
| Green | ldi_q1_bp | Informed | 4 | |
| Green | ldi_q2_bp | Naive | 5 | The question was answered just after executing the example code for the previous question |
| Green | ldi_q1_ap | Informed | 5 | |
| Green | ldi_q2_ap | Naive | 5 | Student answered in reference to their own implementation and not the ISA definition. They would have changed their answer otherwise. This can be confirmed by assessor observation and the student comment on the previous proof that failed |
| Green | add_q1_bp | Partial | 3 | Naive with respect to register value. Informed with respect to status register |
| Green | add_q2_ap | Naive | 4 | The proof that the student did covered the case of too large numbers as input parameters. It also did not make any statement about the size of the result but on the carry flag. It also did not cover overflows occurring when adding two numbers within bounds |

*Ambiguity of Test Questions.* Firstly, it is essential to ensure that test questions are answered by students with respect to the specification rather than their own implementation. The purpose of the questions is after all to test the students mental model of the subject matter not their own (potentially faulty) implementation. This is especially relevant after the solving of the proving challenge. The test questions should therefore be designed in such a way that there is no ambiguity in this regard.

*Priming Effect of Questions.* Contrary to our initial concerns, using the same question before and after the proving challenge did not seem to have a negative impact on the tests validity. In fact, measuring the change in students' opinions and confidence was easier when the questions were identical. Our fear that the question might influence students' responses before attempting the proof proved unfounded. Concretely, we are more satisfied with the design of the LDI challenge than the ADD challenge, despite the latter being a more interesting problem with greater learning opportunities. Additionally, we observed that the ADD instruction covered too many learning units. This made it challenging to determine what students had learned and what they had not through the test questions. There should be at least one question per learning unit, each testing a specific aspect of the implementation.

*Effect of Sample Executions.* Finally, we found that executing instructions after answering the questions could have an effect on students mental model. It illustrates misconceptions in case their answer does not align with the execution result. On the other hand, it reinforces a students mental model if they align. In both cases the effect depends however on the students implementation of the specification. Therefore a sample execution may only challenge a student with respect to their implementation and uncover an discrepancy between their mental model and their own implementation.

## 4 Conclusion and Outlook

While our small sample size of three participants prevents conclusions about proof assistants' effectiveness for learning, the study demonstrates the viability of our measurement approach. This validation provides a solid foundation for our upcoming large-scale study. It will therefore involve a series of exercises where students implement functions in a tutorial-style exercise, followed by test questions to gauge their initial understanding. They will then prove properties related to their implementation during class, and answer the same test questions again to assess their learning progress. Naturally we also plan to address the key issues of our approach that we discovered in the feasibility study. We will use identical questions before and after the proving challenge to measure changes in students' opinions and confidence, as this approach proved effective in our initial study. Additionally, we will ensure that each learning unit is covered by at least one specific question, and consider breaking down complex challenges into multiple parts to facilitate more accurate assessment of student learning. In the larger study, assessors won't be able to observe students directly due to simultaneous task completion in class and partially outside of class. To maintain reliable results, assessor intervention will be minimized. However, students will be better prepared with an introduction to Coq at the start of the semester, reducing the need for guidance. With more relaxed time constraints, students will be required to provide explanations and comments for their answers, which will help compensate for the lack of live observation and provide insight into their motivation and knowledge state.

## Notes on the use of tools and generative AI

This paper was written with the assistance of multiple large language models. Specifically, we utilized Anthropic's Claude 3.5 [8] as well as the Llama 3.1 70B [9] model. These models were employed as writing aids to refine grammar, syntax, and text optimization, but did not contribute to the content or substance of the paper. All scientific content, methodology, and conclusions were developed independently by the authors.

## References

1. Pierce, B.C., et al.: Logical Foundations, vol. 1. Software Foundations. Version 6.7. Electronic textbook (2025). http://softwarefoundations.cis.upenn.edu
2. Pierce, B.C., et al. Programming Language Foundations, Vol. 2. Software Foundations. Version 6.7. Electronic textbook (2024). http://softwarefoundations.cis.upenn.edu
3. The Coq Development Team. The Coq Reference Manual. Version Release 8.20.1 (2025). https://github.com/coq/coq/releases/download/V8.20.1/coq-8.20.1-reference-manual.pdf. Accessed Jan 2025
4. Steen, A., Wisniewski, M., Benzmüller, C.: Einsatz von Theorembeweisern in der Lehre. In: Schwill, A., Lucke, U. (eds.) Hochschuldidaktik der Informatik: HDI2016 - 7. Fachtagung des GI-Fachbereichs Informatik und Ausbildung/- Didaktik der Informatik, vol. 10, pp. 81–92. Commentarii informaticae didacticae (CID). Am Neuen Palais 10, 14469 Potsdam: Universitätsverlag Potsdam (2016). isbn: 978-3-86956- 376-3
5. Karsten, N., et al.: ProofBuddy: a proof assistant for learning and monitoring. In: Machkasova, E. (ed.) Proceedings of the Twelfth International Workshop on Trends in Functional Programming in Education, vol. 382, pp. 1–21. Electronic Proceedings in Theoretical Computer Science. Open Publishing Association (2023). https://doi.org/10.4204/EPTCS.382.1
6. Keenan, M., Omar, C.: Learner-centered design criteria for classroom proof assistants. https://hazel.org/papers/learnercenteredproofshatra2024.pdf

7. Microchip Technology Incorporated. AVR® Instruction Set Manual. Version Rev. DS40002198A - 05/2020. U.S.A. (2020). https://ww1.microchip.com/downloads/en/DeviceDoc/AVR-Instruction-Set-Manual-DS40002198A.pdf
8. Anthropic. The Claude 3 Model Family: Opus, Sonnet, Haiku (2024). https://assets.anthropic.com/m/61e7d27f8c8f5919/original/Claude-3-Model-Card.pdf. Accessed Jan 2025
9. Meta. Model Information (2024). https://github.com/meta-llama/llama-models/blob/main/models/llama3_1/MODELCARD.md. Accessed Jan 2025

# Key Determinants for Successful Digital Transformation: Insights from Content Analysis and Educational Implications

Ana Kutnjak(✉) and Igor Pihir

University of Zagreb Faculty of Organization and Informatics, Varaždin, Croatia
{akutnjak,ipihir}@foi.unizg.hr

**Abstract.** An era of unpredictable market conditions demands digital transformation (DT) for modern organization success. DT is not merely a technological shift but a comprehensive redefinition of business strategies, processes, and models. To navigate this complex transformation, organizations must focus on key DT determinants, including Strategy orientation; Customer centricity; ICT and process infrastructure; Talent, capability and capacity strengthening; and Innovation culture and organizational commitment. As DT requires adaptability, innovation, and cross-disciplinary expertise, strengthening talent and fostering a culture of knowledge sharing is essential. DT professionals must acquire different skills in the fields of computer science, strategic management, information systems, emerging technologies, and agile methodologies to enable sustainable transformation. Research fosters literature review, content analysis, and validation of existing determinants by linking them to education in information systems, computer science, and engineering. The findings highlight the need for a minor adaptation of the determinants and need for ongoing education and training to ensure DT experts are equipped to drive and sustain DT initiatives.

**Keywords:** Successful Digital Future · Determinants · Digital Transformation · Content Analysis · Preliminary Investigation

## 1 Introduction

We are in an era of rapid technological advancement and organizations must embrace digital transformation to stay competitive amid growing market pressures. Digital transformation, as a shift in mindset, goes beyond merely adopting new technologies. It requires a fundamental rethinking of organizational strategies, processes, and business models [1–3]. While contemporary technologies and innovation are essential for digital transformation, the change is not only technological but also organizational, ultimately leading to business transformation [4]. By leveraging digital technologies, organizations can enhance operational efficiency, foster innovation, and create new revenue streams [5]. Digital transformation is a challenging and rigorous process that requires the engagement of all enterprise resources - human, technological, physical, organizational and financial [6].


K. Daimi and A. Alsadoon (Eds.): ICR 2025, LNNS 1487, pp. 350–361, 2025.
https://doi.org/10.1007/978-3-031-95652-2_30

Although it offers numerous benefits, digital transformation comes with substantial challenges. Organizations struggle with insufficient digital skills, cultural resistance, legal constraints, inadequate funding, and infrastructure limitations [7]. Furthermore, balancing technological advancements with organizational readiness and market demands remains a complex task. A successful transformation requires mastering multi-channel interactions, fostering organizational agility, and aligning with customer expectations [8]. Additionally, changes in organizational culture, resource allocation, and leadership approaches are essential for long-term digital success [9, 10]. While many organizations recognize the importance of transformation, only a fraction effectively integrate digital strategies into their operations [11, 12].

To navigate challenges, organizations must identify key determinants that facilitate digital transformation. This study builds on the research of Pihir et al. [5, 13], who identified five essential determinants of DT: (i) *Strategy orientation (SO)*; (ii) *Customer centricity (CC)*; (iii) *ICT and process infrastructure (ICTP)*; (iv) *Talent, capability and capacity strengthening (TCCS)*; and (v) *Innovation culture and organizational commitment (ICOC)*. Applied cohesively, these determinants influence the success of an organization's digital transformation. To analyze them, this study employs qualitative content analysis, a method that provides systematic, reliable, and reproducible insights from textual data [14, 15]. Content analysis is particularly suitable for assessing key themes within a specific research context, making it an appropriate method for this study [16–18]. It is a research technique that follows a set of well-defined procedures to derive valid, systematic, credible, and replicable conclusions from textual data [16]. Additionally, it is used to uncover latent content within textual sources, allowing for a deeper understanding of underlying themes and structures [19]. A deductive coding approach is applied, using themes derived from existing empirical research, particularly from Pihir et al. [5, 13] and Roche [20]. By analyzing determinants in the collected data, this research aims to validate their relevance and assess the potential need for modification, providing a structured approach to enhancing digital transformation strategies. Additionally, this study seeks to conduct a systematic, structured, and comprehensive review of determinants, which has not been previously undertaken in existing research. Furthermore, it aims to bridge the gap in the insufficient focus of published studies on educating young professionals in digital transformation, identifying the knowledge, skills, and experience crucial for digital transformation education in informatics, computer science, and engineering, extending the findings of [21, 22].

This study represents an initial exploration and forms part of a larger doctoral dissertation research. It is driven by two research questions: *Which (additional) determinants do scholars consider essential for the effective implementation of digital transformation? Which knowledge, skills, and experience are crucial in the education of future experts needed for DT*? The primary study objective is to examine existing determinants and assess whether modifications or refinements are necessary. This paper begins with an introductory chapter, followed by a methodology section. The results section presents findings, while discussion and conclusion provide an in-depth interpretation of results.

## 2 Methodology

Previous research showed that scholars define determinants of digital transformation differently, using terms like drivers, enablers, factors, pillars, and others. To capture this diversity, the methodology follows three steps: (1) literature review, (2) content analysis, and (3) validation of existing determinants by linking them to education in information systems, computer science, and engineering.

To ensure that this study resulted in the analysis of relevant papers, first step was conducted using the scientific databases Scopus (S) and Web of Science (WoS; W). The authors of this paper searched the scientific databases using a query that included the term digital transformation and the terms *determinant* or driver* or enabler* or factor* or pillar* or catalyst* or element* or component* or lever* or condition* or requirement* or antecedent* or essential* or prerequisites* or foundation* or influencer* or facilitator* or criteria*, focusing on article title or abstract or keywords. This yielded 14,697 papers from Scopus and 8,196 from WoS, but the query was found to be too broad. Refining the search to titles only reduced results to 717 (S) and 400 (W) papers. Further narrowing based on title and keywords resulted in 242 (S) and 102 (W) papers. To ensure relevance, the query was adjusted to include key terminology in the title, keywords, and abstract, yielding 213 (S) and 97 (W) papers. For the final selection, only papers with 5 or more citations in both databases were considered. This threshold ensured the selection of impactful papers, filtering out less influential studies and enhancing analysis reliability. Applying this criterion reduced the pool to 77 (S) and 40 (W) papers, with 39 WoS papers overlapping, leaving 78 papers for analysis. A final relevance check based on titles, keywords, and abstracts led to the exclusion of 40 misaligned papers, resulting in a final selection of 38 papers for content analysis. Figure 1 illustrates the research procedure used to narrow results and focus on key studies in the field.

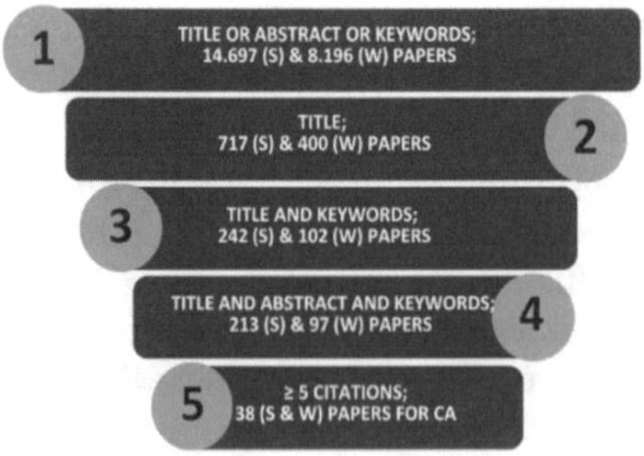


**Fig. 1.** Steps of bibliographical research conducted in this study.

## 3 Research Findings

In line with the research question and objective, the following section presents the research findings. As mentioned earlier, the central method of this study is content analysis, with key elements including: (i) the unit of analysis, referring to the content of

38 selected papers, (ii) the meaning unit, which can be a word, sentence, paragraph, or other analytical unit that helps uncover answers to the research question, (iii) condensed meaning unit, which simplifies and captures the essential meaning of the meaning unit, (iv) codes, representing keywords that encapsulate the content of the condensed meaning unit, and (v) themes, which operate at an abstract level, capturing the latent content of the unit of analysis [15, 17].

Figure 2 illustrates the content analysis approach and the application of method to 38 papers narrowed down in the previous step. These papers are analyzed to identify key meanings, codes, and themes extracted by the authors from existing knowledge.

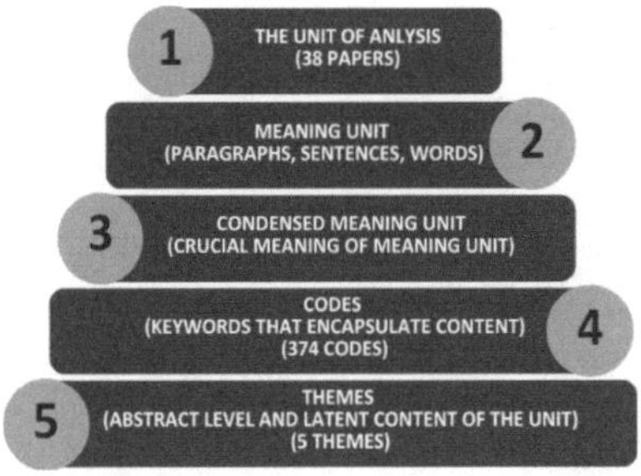


**Fig. 2.** Steps conducted in this study in content analysis.

Content analysis was conducted in several steps. In the first step, sections of the papers describing the determinants (in any terminological variant, such as drivers, enablers, factors, etc.) of digital transformation were selected, and their content was transformed into condensed meaning units, which were subsequently converted into codes. The structured extraction of sentences demonstrates how key meaning units were condensed into codes, ensuring that only the most relevant content was retained, most often in the form of a few key words, as shown in Table 1.

**Table 1.** Findings from the first step of content analysis.

| **Meaning unit** [23] |
|---|
| There are seven key resources for digital transformation across three categories: technology (IT infrastructure; IT management capacity), organization (digital strategy; top management; employee skills), environment (government support; partnerships). |
| **Condensed meaning unit** |
| Seven key resources: IT infrastructure, IT management capacity, digital strategy, top management, employee skills, government support and partnerships. |
| **Codes** |
| IT infrastructure; IT management capacity; digital strategy; top management; employee skills; government support; partnerships. |

After the initial analysis, the research process required additional steps relevant to content analysis, as presented in Tables 2 and 3.

**Table 2.** Findings from the second step of content analysis.

| Code no. | Codes | Themes [5, 13] | | | | |
|---|---|---|---|---|---|---|
| | | SO | CC | ICTP | TCCS | ICOC |
| 1. | data | | | x | | |
| 2. | process automation | | | x | | |
| 3. | customer-oriented approach | | x | | | |
| ... | ... | | | | | |
| 372. | enhancement of employee skills | | | | x | |
| 373. | leader's adaptability in management | x | | | | |
| 374. | flexibility enabled by technology | | | x | | |

The content analysis led to the detection of 374 codes, which, in the next step, had to be analyzed and assigned to corresponding themes/determinants of digital transformation (see Table 2), using a deductive coding approach. This classification was conducted in alignment with previous research [5, 13], to confirm the validity of existing determinants or identify the need for their modification. Consequently, this step is crucial for refining theoretical models used in this research and ensuring their applicability across different domains. To ensure coding reliability, the authors independently coded the data and assigned codes to themes, resolving discrepancies through discussion and consensus, while a predefined classification framework maintained transparency and reproducibility of the results.

After identifying and defining all codes in the analyzed papers, the third step of the analysis required grouping the codes into themes (Table 3). Since some codes were not adequately represented in the existing themes' titles and structures, three themes had to be modified, while the remaining two remained unchanged. Compared to existing models of digital transformation determinants [5, 13], which relied on a smaller number of scientific papers to identify determinants, this study utilizes a larger set of carefully selected papers and confirms the relevance of core themes while identifying the need for modification in three areas - *Strategy orientation, ICT and process infrastructure* as well as *Innovation culture and organizational commitment*. These findings enable the authors to address the research questions. On one hand, the results highlight the need to modify existing determinants, while on the other, the analysis of keywords and themes in the reviewed papers reveals the necessity to align competencies in information systems, computer science, and engineering with the evolving demands of digital transformation.

**Table 3.** Findings from the third step of content analysis.

| Themes/most common codes | No of codes per theme |
|---|---|
| ***Strategic orientation and leadership*** | 93 |
| strategic leadership and managerial support in digital transformation; strategic planning and digital strategy; strategic partnership and ecosystems [3, 8, 12, 23–52] | |
| ***Customer centricity*** | 28 |
| customer orientation; focus on customers; customer satisfaction; user experience [8, 24, 25, 27–32, 39–41, 43, 45, 53–56] | |
| ***Technical, technological, data, and process infrastructure*** | 90 |
| compatibility of integrated technologies and implementation of new ones; data management, analytics, and security; integration of technologies with business processes [8, 23–26, 29–34, 36–57] | |
| ***Talent, capability and capacity strengthening*** | 76 |
| strengthening and adapting employees' knowledge and skills; collaborative work environment and knowledge sharing; promotion of interdisciplinary teams; empowerment and autonomy of employees [8, 12, 23, 24, 26, 28–47, 49–52, 55] | |
| ***Organizational commitment and innovation development culture*** | 58 |
| appropriate organizational structure; organizational agility, flexibility, and dynamism; innovation management and an innovative organizational culture; strengthening a culture of commitment to change [8, 12, 24, 26, 28, 29, 31–33, 35–38, 40, 42, 43, 45–51, 53, 56] | |
| ***External factors (not relevant for the research)*** | 29 |
| financing digital initiatives through funds and government subsidies; regulatory frameworks for digital transformation; appropriate legislative frameworks [23, 27, 29, 30, 32, 34, 35, 37, 39, 42–47, 49, 51, 54, 55] | |
| ***SUM*** | **374** |

## 4 Discussion

The unchanged themes, or determinants of digital transformation, are *Customer centricity* (CC) and *Talent, capability and capacity strengthening* (TCCS) indicating that their content and titles fully covered the identified codes in this research. On the other hand, the themes *Strategy orientation, ICT and process infrastructure* as well as *Innovation culture and organizational commitment* have been modified based on the identified codes within each theme.

In *Strategy orientation*, besides digital strategy, it is important to highlight the significance of leadership and managerial support for digital transformation. Furthermore, strategic partnerships and resource sharing within the ecosystem are inevitable activities in digital transformation initiatives, which is why this theme has been renamed *Strategic orientation and leadership*. Earlier studies [5, 13] fail to adequately highlight the crucial role of strategic collaborations and resource sharing within the ecosystem as one of the fundamental parts of digital transformation. This research bridges that gap, offering a deeper understanding of their significance, emphasizing the role of management in these activities. Similarly, *ICT and process infrastructure* has been deconstructed into key thematic units, explicitly addressing the technical, technological, data, and process aspects that earlier research often treated as a single construct [5, 13]. By introducing *Technical, technological, data, and process infrastructure* as a revised theme, this study provides a more granular perspective, ensuring a clearer understanding of the interaction and alignment of these components in digital transformation. In this way, this study not only emphasizes the importance of selecting compatible technologies for business processes but also contributes to recognizing the significance of data and data analytics for business improvement and strengthening digital transformation initiatives. Finally, the modification of *Innovation culture and organizational commitment*, underscores the importance of an appropriate organizational structure, as well as the need for agility and flexibility, which serve as the foundation for fostering innovation and advocating a culture of change. Prior research overlooked the importance of organizational structure and agility in fostering innovation [5, 13], focusing mainly on innovation as a goal rather than as a process facilitated by flexibility and adaptability. Consequently, the theme, or determinant of digital transformation, has been slightly modified to *Organizational commitment and innovation development culture,* emphasizing the structural and cultural enablers of innovation in digital transformation. These findings contribute to a more nuanced and applicable theoretical framework, directly answering the first research question. This research confirms the significance of key digital transformation determinants, aligning with prior studies [5, 13], yet also reveals gaps and necessary modifications. Unlike previous research, which primarily concentrated on individual factors, this study integrates them into a more interconnected framework, reinforcing the multifaceted nature of digital transformation.

In reference to the second research question, it is essential to accentuate that digital transformation experts must possess a broad spectrum of knowledge, skills, and experience [21]. However, prior models lack a structured breakdown of competencies needed for effective digital transformation implementation. This study addresses this gap by systematically categorizing the essential capabilities in several key areas. First, establishing the conditions for strategic orientation, implementing an effective digital strategy, and advocating for resource sharing within the ecosystem are crucial skills for leaders who recognize digital transformation as an opportunity. Additionally, identifying internal infrastructure capacities and enhancing them with new technologies, data policies, expertise development, and a culture of knowledge sharing among employees are indispensable elements of transformation. Flexibility and agility, along with an innovation driven culture, are key enablers of successful digital transformation, making it essential for experts to establish the necessary development conditions within their organizations. As customers are central to an organization's business model, experts must understand customer needs, assess satisfaction in a timely manner, and identify potential opportunities arising from unmet demands.

## 5 Conclusion

This study contributes to a deeper understanding of digital transformation requirements while also providing a foundation for future research and educational improvements in informatics, computer science, and engineering. The findings demonstrate that while some existing determinants remain relevant, others require modification to better align with evolving digital transformation demands. This study's key contribution lies in its refinement of existing classification models and its broader, more comprehensive analysis of digital transformation determinants. Unlike previous studies, which relied on narrower sets of analyzed papers and often treated determinants in isolation, this research systematically integrates them into an interconnected framework, improving their applicability across various domains. By providing a more structured classification, it enhances the theoretical foundations of digital transformation and offers a clearer roadmap for its successful implementation. By systematically analyzing a larger and more carefully selected dataset, this research overcomes the limitations of previous studies, which resulted in less refined classifications of determinants. Furthermore, the study highlights the crucial skills, knowledge, and experience necessary for digital transformation experts, particularly in areas such as strategic orientation, leadership, infrastructure management, and innovation driven adaptability. These insights help bridge the gap between academic research and practical application, ensuring that future professionals are better equipped to navigate digital transformation challenges.

## References


1. Albukhitan, S.: Developing digital transformation strategy for manufacturing. Proc. Comp. Sci. **170**, 664–671 (2020). https://doi.org/10.1016/j.procs.2020.03.173
2. Kutnjak, A.: Covid-19 accelerates digital transformation in industries: challenges, issues, barriers and problems in transformation. IEEE Access. **9**, 79373–79388 (2021). https://doi.org/10.1109/ACCESS.2021.3084801
3. Petrova, L.A., Niyazbekova, S.U., Kuznetsova, T.E., Sarbassova, S.B., Baymukhametova, K.I.: Digital Transformation as a Strategic Direction Business Development in Modern Conditions Lecture Notes in Networks and Systems, vol. 245, pp. 183–192. Springer International Publishing (2022). https://doi.org/10.1007/978-3-030-77000-6_22
4. Westerman, G., Bonnet, D., McAfee, A.: Leading Digital: Turning Technology into Business Transformation. Harvard Business Review (2014)
5. Pihir, I., Tomičić-Pupek, K., Tomičić Furjan, M.: Digital transformation playground: literature review and framework of concepts. J. Inform. Organ. Sci. **43**, 33–48 (2019). https://doi.org/10.31341/jios.43.1.3
6. Kutnjak, A., Pihir, I., Furjan, M.T.: Digital transformation case studies across industries—literature review. In: 2019 42nd International Convention on Information and Communication Technology, Electronics and Microelectronics (MIPRO), pp. 1293–1298 (2019). https://doi.org/10.23919/MIPRO.2019.8756911
7. Kutnjak, A., Pihir, I.: Challenges, issues, barriers and problems in digital transformation—systematic literature review. In: Proceedings of the 30th International Scientific Central European Conference on Information and Intelligent Systems, pp. 133–140. University of Zagreb, Faculty of Organization and Informatics, Varaždin (2019)

8. Brkić, L., Tomičić Pupek, K., Bosilj Vukšić, V.: A framework for bpm software selection in relation to digital transformation drivers. Tehnicki Vjesnik. **27**, 1108–1114 (2020). https://doi.org/10.17559/TV-20190315193304
9. Bennett, E.E., McWhorter, R.R.: Virtual HRD's role in crisis and the post Covid-19 professional lifeworld: accelerating skills for digital transformation. Adv. Dev. Hum. Resour. **23**, 5–25 (2021). https://doi.org/10.1177/1523422320973288
10. Sá, M.J., Serpa, S.: The covid-19 pandemic as an opportunity to foster the sustainable development of teaching in higher education. Sustainability. **12**, 1–16 (2020). https://doi.org/10.3390/su12208525
11. Calabrese, M., La Sala, A., Fuller, R., Laudando, A.: Digital platform ecosystems for sustainable innovation: toward a new meta-organizational model? Admin. Sci. **11**, 119 (2021). https://doi.org/10.3390/admsci11040119
12. Wolf, M., Semm, A., Erfurth, C.: Digital transformation in companies – challenges and success factors. Commun. Comput. Inform. Sci. **863**, 178–193 (2018). https://doi.org/10.1007/978-3-319-93408-2_13
13. Pihir, I., Tomičić-Pupek, K., Tomičić Furjan, M.: Digital transformation insights and trends. In: Proceedings of the 29th Central European Conference on Information and Intelligent Systems, p. 9. Faculty of Organization and Informatics, University of Zagreb, Varaždin (2018)
14. Drisko, J.W., Maschi, T.: Content Analysis. Oxford University Press (2016)
15. Elo, S., Kyngäs, H.: The qualitative content analysis process. J. Adv. Nurs. **62**, 107–115 (2008). https://doi.org/10.1111/j.1365-2648.2007.04569.x
16. Bengtsson, M.: How to plan and perform a qualitative study using content analysis. NursingPlus Open. **2**, 8–14 (2016). https://doi.org/10.1016/j.npls.2016.01.001
17. Graneheim, U.H., Lindgren, B.-M., Lundman, B.: Methodological challenges in qualitative content analysis: a discussion paper. Nurse Educ. Today. **56**, 29–34 (2017). https://doi.org/10.1016/j.nedt.2017.06.002
18. Vaismoradi, M., Turunen, H., Bondas, T.: Content analysis and thematic analysis: implications for conducting a qualitative descriptive study. Nurs. Health Sci. **15**, 398–405 (2013). https://doi.org/10.1111/nhs.12048
19. Cho, J.Y., Lee, E.-H.: Reducing confusion about grounded theory and qualitative content analysis: similarities and differences. Qualit. Rep. (2014)
20. Roche, B.: The 4 Key Drivers for Digital Transformation in the Enterprise (an excerpt of a chapter from my forthcoming ebook on Digital Transformation) | LinkedIn, https://www.linkedin.com/pulse/4-key-drivers-digital-transformation-enterprise-excerpt-brian-roche/, last accessed 3 Mar 2025
21. Kutnjak, A., Križanić, S., Pihir, I.: Educational and practical view of knowledge, skills and experience needed by a chief digital officer. In: Presented at the 11th Annual International Conference of Education and New Learning Technologies (EDULEARN19) (2019). https://doi.org/10.21125/edulearn.2019.1389
22. Pejić Bach, M., Šebalj, D., Garbin Praničević, D., Pihir, I.: Employment of business informatics graduates: preliminary results. In: Presented at the Central European Conference on Information and Intelligent Systems (2018)
23. Zhang, X., Xu, Y., Ma, L.: Research on successful factors and influencing mechanism of the digital transformation in SMEs. Sustainability (Switzerland). **14** (2022). https://doi.org/10.3390/su14052549
24. Muehlburger, M., Rueckel, D., Koch, S.: A framework of factors enabling digital transformation. In: Presented at the 25th Americas Conference on Information Systems, AMCIS 2019 (2019)
25. Schallmo, D., Williams, C.A., Boardman, L.: Digital transformation of business models-best practice, enablers, and roadmap. Int. J. Innov. Manag. **21**, 1740014 (2017). https://doi.org/10.1142/S136391961740014X

26. Jafari-Sadeghi, V., Amoozad Mahdiraji, H., Alam, G.M., Mazzoleni, A.: Entrepreneurs as strategic transformation managers: exploring micro-foundations of digital transformation in small and medium internationalisers. J. Bus. Res. **154**, 113287 (2023). https://doi.org/10.1016/j.jbusres.2022.08.051
27. Tangi, L., Janssen, M., Benedetti, M., Noci, G.: Barriers and Drivers of Digital Transformation in Public Organizations: Results from a Survey in the Netherlands. Lecture Notes in Computer Science (including subseries Lecture Notes in Artificial Intelligence and Lecture Notes in Bioinformatics). 12219 LNCS, 42–56 (2020). https://doi.org/10.1007/978-3-030-57599-1_4
28. Koseoglu, O., Keskin, B., Ozorhon, B.: Challenges and enablers in BIM-enabled digital transformation in mega projects: the Istanbul new airport project case study. Buildings. **9**, 1–24 (2019). https://doi.org/10.3390/buildings9050115
29. Jonathan, G.M.: Digital transformation in the public sector: identifying critical success factors. In: Information Systems. EMCIS 2019 Lecture Notes in Business Information Processing. 381 LNBIP, pp. 223–235. Springer, Cham (2020). https://doi.org/10.1007/978-3-030-44322-1_17
30. Tarute, A., Duobiene, J., Kloviene, L., Vitkauskaite, E., Varaniute, V.: Identifying factors affecting digital transformation of SMEs. In: Presented at the Proceedings of the International Conference on Electronic Business (ICEB) (2018)
31. Morakanyane, R., O'Reilly, P., McAvoy, J.: Determining digital transformation success factors. In: Presented at the Proceedings of the Annual Hawaii International Conference on System Sciences (2020)
32. Van Dyk, R., Van Belle, J.-P.: Factors influencing the intended adoption of digital transformation: A South African case study. In: Presented at the Proceedings of the 2019 Federated Conference on Computer Science and Information Systems, FedCSIS 2019 (2019). https://doi.org/10.15439/2019F166
33. Rueckel, D., Muehlburger, M., Koch, S.: An updated framework of factors enabling digital transformation. Pacific Asia J. Assoc. Inf. Syst. **12**(1–26) (2020). https://doi.org/10.17705/1pais.12401
34. Wang, Y., Su, X.: Driving factors of digital transformation for manufacturing enterprises: a multi-case study from China. Int. J. Technol. Manag. **87**, 229–253 (2021). https://doi.org/10.1504/ijtm.2021.10045161
35. Li, H., Han, Z., Zhang, J., Philbin, S.P., Liu, D., Ke, Y.: Systematic identification of the influencing factors for the digital transformation of the construction industry based on LDA-DEMATEL-ANP. Buildings. **12** (2022). https://doi.org/10.3390/buildings12091409
36. Lammers, T., Tomidei, L., Trianni, A.: Towards a novel framework of barriers and drivers for digital transformation in industrial supply chains. In: Presented at the PICMET 2019 - Portland International Conference on Management of Engineering and Technology: Technology Management in the World of Intelligent Systems, Proceedings, Portland, United States (2019). https://doi.org/10.23919/PICMET.2019.8893875
37. Jović, M., Tijan, E., Vidmar, D., Pucihar, A.: Factors of digital transformation in the maritime transport sector. Sustainability (Switzerland). **14** (2022). https://doi.org/10.3390/su14159776
38. Kostakis, P., Kargas, A.: Big-data management: A driver for digital transformation? Information (Switzerland). **12** (2021). https://doi.org/10.3390/info12100411
39. Xiao, J., Han, L., Zhang, H.: Exploring driving factors of digital transformation among local governments: foundations for smart city construction in China. Sustainability (Switzerland). **14** (2022). https://doi.org/10.3390/su142214980
40. Escobar, F., Almeida, W.H.C., Varajão, J.: Digital transformation success in the public sector: a systematic literature review of cases, processes, and success factors. Information Polity. **28**, 61–81 (2023). https://doi.org/10.3233/IP-211518

41. Hrustek, L., Tomicic Furjan, M., Pihir, I.: Influence of digital transformation drivers on business model creation. In: Presented at the 2019 42nd International Convention on Information and Communication Technology, Electronics and Microelectronics, MIPRO 2019 - Proceedings (2019). https://doi.org/10.23919/MIPRO.2019.8756666
42. Zhang, G., Wang, T., Wang, Y., Zhang, S., Lin, W., Dou, Z., Du, H.: Study on the influencing factors of digital transformation of construction enterprises from the perspective of dual effects—a hybrid approach based on PLS-SEM and fsQCA. Sustainability (Switzerland). **15** (2023). https://doi.org/10.3390/su15076317
43. Ta, V.A., Lin, C.-Y.: Exploring the determinants of digital transformation adoption for SMEs in an emerging economy. Sustainability (Switzerland). **15** (2023). https://doi.org/10.3390/su15097093
44. Chandrayan, B., Gupta, S., Kumar, R., Dangayach, G.S., Jagtap, S.: Modelling and analysis of key enablers of digital transformation in food SMEs using ISM and MICMAC approach. Int. J. Intell. Enterp. **10**, 419–444 (2023). https://doi.org/10.1504/IJIE.2023.133826
45. Sergei, T., Arkady, T., Natalya, L., Pathak, R.D., Samson, D., Husain, Z., Sushil, S.: Digital transformation enablers in high-tech and low-tech companies: a comparative analysis. Aust. J. Manag. **48**, 801–843 (2023). https://doi.org/10.1177/03128962231157102
46. Alshehab, A., Alfozan, T., Gaderrab, H.F., Alahmad, M.A., Alkandari, A.: Identifying significant elements of the digital transformation of organizatios in Kuwait. Indo. J. Electr. Eng. Comput. Sci. **26**, 318–325 (2022). https://doi.org/10.11591/ijeecs.v26.i1.pp318-325
47. Saihi, A., Ben-Daya, M., As'ad, R.: A survey of the underlying success factors of maintenance digital transformation. Presented at the IFAC-PapersOnLine. **55**, 2944–2949 (2022). https://doi.org/10.1016/j.ifacol.2022.10.179
48. Kryvovyazyuk, I., Britchenko, I., Smerichevskyi, S., Kovalska, L., Dorosh, V., Kravchuk, P.: Digital transformation and innovation in business: the impact of strategic alliances and their success factors. Ikonomicheski Izsledvania. **32**, 3–17 (2023)
49. Liu, H., Yu, H., Zhou, H., Zhang, X.: Research on the influencing factors of construction enterprises' digital transformation based on DEMATEL-TAISM. Sustainability (Switzerland). **15** (2023). https://doi.org/10.3390/su15129251
50. Laorach, C., Tuamsuk, K.: Factors influencing the digital transformation of universities in Thailand. Int. J. Innov. Res. Sci. Stud. **5**, 211–219 (2022). https://doi.org/10.53894/ijirss.v5i3.646
51. Mihu, C., Pitic, A.G., Bayraktar, D.: Drivers of digital transformation and their impact on organizational management. Stud. Busi. Econ. **18**, 149–170 (2023). https://doi.org/10.2478/sbe-2023-0009
52. Zakharov, V., Ludushkina, E., Kislinskaya, M., Kornilova, E., Novikov, A.: Digital transformation of enterprise trends, factors, results. Nexo Rev. Cient. **35**, 133–145 (2022)
53. Ebert, C., Duarte, C.H.C.: Requirements engineering for the digital transformation: industry panel. Presented at the Proceedings - 2016 IEEE 24th International Requirements Engineering Conference, RE 2016 (2016). https://doi.org/10.1109/RE.2016.21
54. Werth, O., Schwarzbach, C., Rodríguez Cardona, D., Breitner, M.H., von der Schulenburg, J.-M.G.: Influencing factors for the digital transformation in the financial services sector. Zeitschrift fur die gesamte Versicherungswissenschaft. **109**, 155–179 (2020). https://doi.org/10.1007/s12297-020-00486-6
55. António Porfírio, J., Augusto Felício, J., Carrilho, T.: Factors affecting digital transformation in banking. J. Bus. Res. **171**, 114393 (2024). https://doi.org/10.1016/j.jbusres.2023.114393

56. Levkovskyi, B., Betzwieser, B., Löffler, A., Wittges, H.: Why do organizations change? a literature review on drivers and measures of success for digital transformation. In: Presented at the 26th Americas Conference on Information Systems, AMCIS 2020 (2020)
57. Dokuchaev, V.A.: Digital transformation: New drivers and new risks. In: Presented at the 2020 International Conference on Engineering Management of Communication and Technology, EMCTECH 2020 - Proceedings (2020). https://doi.org/10.1109/EMCTECH49634.2020.9261544

# Education vs. Earnings: An Analytical Perspective on Fields of Study and Salaries Using Python

Kirtankumar Patel, Leela Avula, and Samah Senbel(✉)

Sacred Heart University, Fairfield, CT, USA
{patelk31,avula1}@mail.sacredheart.edu, senbels@sacredheart.edu

**Abstract.** This research paper presents a comprehensive data analysis of study fields, employment, and salaries, containing information on academic majors, employment rates, gender distributions, and salary metrics. The study explores the relationship between academic disciplines and employment outcomes using techniques such as data cleaning, preprocessing, exploratory data analysis (EDA), and visualization. Key metrics, including employment rates, full-time employment rates, unemployment rates, and median salaries, were computed and compared across major categories. For instance, the analysis revealed that engineering majors exhibit an 83% full-time employment rate and command the highest median salaries, while arts majors show a full-time employment rate of just 63% with significantly lower earnings. By employing visualizations like heatmaps, scatter plots, and bar plots, the study provides a detailed understanding of employment trends. These findings highlight substantial variations in employment outcomes by field of study. This analysis offers valuable insights to students, educators, and policymakers, enabling them to align educational pathways with labor market needs. The results emphasize the importance of STEM and technical fields, which offer stronger job prospects and financial rewards, compared to fields such as arts and humanities. Challenges such as missing data and multicollinearity were also addressed, ensuring the robustness of the findings.

**Keywords:** Employment outcomes · academic majors · STEM majors · Python analysis · salary trends

## 1 Introduction

In today's increasingly complex and competitive job market, the relationship between an individual's field of study and their employment outcomes has become crucial for students, educators, and policymakers alike. Choosing an academic major is a pivotal decision that has far-reaching implications on career stability, job satisfaction, and lifetime earnings. As industries evolve, shaped by rapid technological advancements and shifting economic demands, aligning educational choices with market needs is essential for maximizing employability and financial success. Students, in particular, benefit from a nuanced understanding of how specific academic disciplines correlate with employment prospects and salary potential, enabling them to make data-informed decisions that align with their career aspirations and financial goals.


K. Daimi and A. Alsadoon (Eds.): ICR 2025, LNNS 1487, pp. 362–372, 2025.
https://doi.org/10.1007/978-3-031-95652-2_31

This study presents a comprehensive data analysis exploring the relationship between academic fields, employment outcomes, and salary metrics. The dataset used in this research includes diverse fields of study, with detailed data on employment rates, gender distribution, and salary metrics across multiple academic disciplines. By leveraging data cleaning, preprocessing, exploratory data analysis (EDA), and visualization techniques, this research delves into key indicators such as full-time employment rates, unemployment rates, and median salaries. Through bar plots, scatter plots, and heatmaps, the study seeks to provide a visual and statistical examination of how specific academic fields impact employment outcomes.

The objectives of this research are two-fold: to evaluate the economic value of different academic disciplines and to highlight trends in employment outcomes across fields of study. This paper seeks to assist students and advisors by identifying academic areas with high employment stability and competitive salary potential, thus aiding in effective educational planning and workforce readiness. Additionally, the study provides valuable insights for policymakers to guide future educational reforms that align with labor market dynamics and address gaps in high-demand sectors.

While this research provides a significant perspective on the connection between academic choices and career outcomes, it also addresses certain challenges encountered during the analysis. These include handling missing data, managing multicollinearity issues, and interpreting the impact of demographic factors such as gender. By addressing these challenges, the study presents a balanced view of the complexities involved in analyzing the interplay between education and employment.

Ultimately, this research contributes to a deeper understanding of how academic fields shape employment opportunities and economic outcomes, underscoring the need for data-driven decision-making in education and career planning. The results are anticipated to empower students, educators, and policymakers with actionable insights to align educational pathways with emerging workforce needs, fostering a generation better prepared for long-term career success.

The findings from this analysis reveal notable disparities in employment success based on the academic major chosen. For example, majors within the arts and humanities tend to yield lower employment rates and salaries, highlighting a mismatch between these fields and current labor market demands. Conversely, disciplines such as engineering, healthcare, and business exhibit high employment rates and robust salary prospects, suggesting that technical and industry-aligned majors offer more stable career paths and financial advantages. These insights underscore the importance of aligning educational programs with job market needs, particularly in fields where technological and industry trends drive high demand for specialized skills.

## 2 Background

Several researchers studied the effect of the job market and the different fields of study for undergraduates in the USA. In our study we concentrate on measuring the effect of the breadth of a field of study (number of different majors within the field) and the resulting employment rate and median salary. For example the major category "Engineering" has majors such as Architecture, Aeronautical engineering, etc.

Emanuel Melichar's studies for the American Economic Association [1] on economists' salaries in the 1960s identify experience, employer type, and educational attainment as significant salary determinants, with industry roles offering the highest salary progression [2]. He finds that while advanced degrees, especially Ph.D.'s, increasingly impact earnings, the influence of experience has slightly declined, as education gains prominence in differentiating salaries among economists.

Sullivan et al. [4] and Maisel & Gaddy [8] examine how education affects career outcomes, noting that graduates from elite institutions, particularly in fields like computer science, tend to achieve higher earnings. Sullivan et al. highlight the enhanced salary potential for graduates of prestigious programs, while Maisel & Gaddy find that recent computer science doctorates enjoy high employment rates, especially in competitive industry roles. Both studies emphasize strategic educational choices as crucial for long-term career success.

In "Male-Female Pay Differentials in Professional Employment," Burton G. Malkiel and Judith A. Malkiel [5] address gender-based salary disparities within corporations, showing that factors like education, experience, and job assignments influence pay outcomes. Similarly, Dorceta Taylor [3] explores how race, gender, and field shape job and salary expectations among U.S. science and engineering students. Both studies underscore how demographic and structural influences on employment perpetuate salary disparities.

Eleanor L. Babco's [7] "Salaries of Scientists, Engineers, and Technicians: A Summary of Salary Surveys" (1987) compiles data from 1986–1987, revealing rising starting salaries in technical fields despite reduced job offers. Trends by field, gender, and employment type highlight broader economic shifts affecting demand for specific professions. Zhang and Cheng's [6] "Study of Employment Salary Forecast using KNN Algorithm" (2019) uses 2018 data to predict Java back-end salaries, achieving 88.1% accuracy. Their findings suggest a misalignment between graduates' expectations and market salaries, advocating for better alignment to improve employment outcomes.

Lastly, Gishkayeva, Aziyeva, and Abubakarov's [9] "Employment and Salary as Indicators of Social Quality of Life" (2019) examine labor relations in Russia, tracing shifts from state-controlled to market-driven systems post-1990s. They find persistent wage disparities and low labor productivity affecting quality of life and argue that wage levels play a critical role in access to essential services and public trust.

## 3 Methodology

This study's methodology encompasses a structured approach to examining employment outcomes across academic majors, organized into several core stages:

**Data Collection:** The dataset contains comprehensive information on academic majors, employment status (full-time, part-time, seasonal), unemployment rates, and median salaries. Each major is categorized under broader academic fields to facilitate aggregate comparisons. The dataset is from the USA Census bureau [10] and is published as part of the USA census public datasets.

**Data Preprocessing:** Basic data cleaning and standardization were conducted to ensure data integrity: several duplicate data columns were removed, and new metrics were created, including employment rates, full-time employment ratios, and unemployment rates. These were calculated mathematically from the employment raw numbers. There was no missing or incorrect data in our dataset. The dataset was also transformed and grouped by major categories to enable cross-disciplinary comparisons.
**Exploratory Data Analysis (EDA):** EDA was employed to identify significant trends and variations across fields of study. Descriptive statistics provided a summary of central tendencies and variability, while data visualizations like bar plots, scatter plots, and heatmaps highlighted relationships between variables and identified majors with higher or lower employment stability.
**Key Metric Calculations:** Key indicators, such as overall employment rate, full-time employment rate, and unemployment rate, were calculated to assess the impact of academic majors on job market outcomes. Salary percentiles were also computed to capture income potential within each field.
**Visualization and Interpretation:** Various visualizations, including heatmaps and bar plots, illustrated employment and salary patterns by academic major, supporting interpretation of complex data. Each visualization provided insights into how different majors correlate with employment success and earnings potential.
**Conclusion and Recommendations:** Based on analysis and visualization findings, recommendations were developed for students and educators. Insights into fields with higher job security and salary prospects were highlighted to assist in data-driven educational planning.

# 4 Results

## 4.1 Statistical Analysis

Figure 1 shows the total number of individuals employed across different major categories. Business leads with the highest number of employed individuals, followed by Education, Engineering, and Humanities & Liberal Arts. Computers & Mathematics ranks ninth, while fields such as Arts, Biology & Life Sciences, and Agriculture & Natural Resources appear lower on the employment scale.

This distribution underscores the influence of academic choices on employment outcomes, with Business and Engineering graduates enjoying strong demand due to their broad applicability and technical expertise. Lower-ranked majors often align with more specialized industries, where graduates may pursue non-traditional career paths, resulting in fewer full-time employment opportunities.

Figure 2 shows unemployment rates across various academic majors, with Business majors experiencing the highest unemployment, likely due to field saturation. Humanities & Liberal Arts and Engineering also have high unemployment, despite their skill advantages. Computers & Mathematics fare better, indicating higher demand for tech skills, unlike the arts, social sciences, and education, which see greater unemployment. Fields like Agriculture and Interdisciplinary Studies show the lowest unemployment, suggesting niche markets with fewer graduates. This trend implies that broader fields face more competition, while specialized majors offer stronger employment prospects.

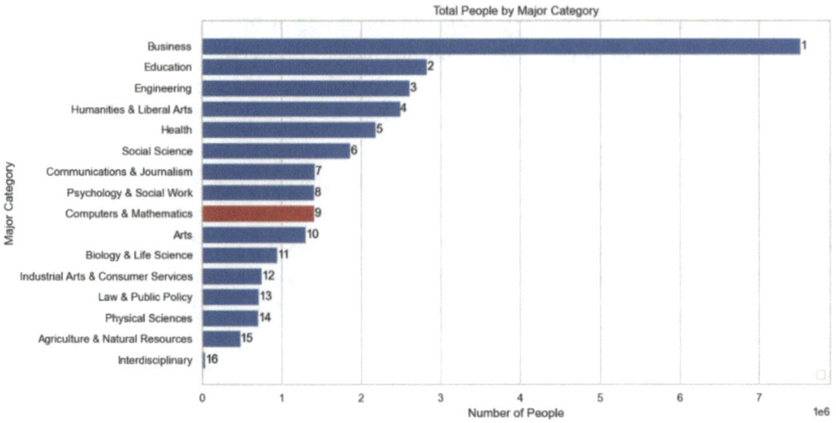


**Fig. 1:** Total Employed by Major

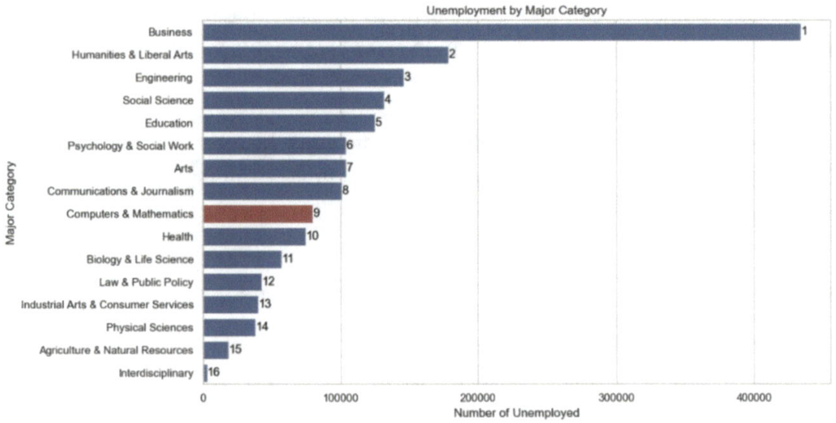


**Fig. 2:** Unemployment by Major Category

Figure 3 shows that Engineering, Computers & Mathematics, and Business majors earn the highest median salaries, reflecting the strong market demand for technical and managerial skills. Physical Sciences and Agriculture & Natural Resources also offer competitive wages, though not as high as these top fields. In contrast, Humanities & Liberal Arts, Arts, Psychology & Social Work, and Education rank lower, with Education earning the lowest median salary. The salary gap highlights the financial advantage of technical fields, where specialized skills align with industry demand. This data suggests that while lower-salary majors may offer fulfilling careers, they often come with non-financial rewards.

To summarize, we observe that the Computer Science and mathematics major is relatively low in numbers compared to the other majors (ranked 9th), and that its unemployment rate matches the employment rate in rank. However, the median salary for

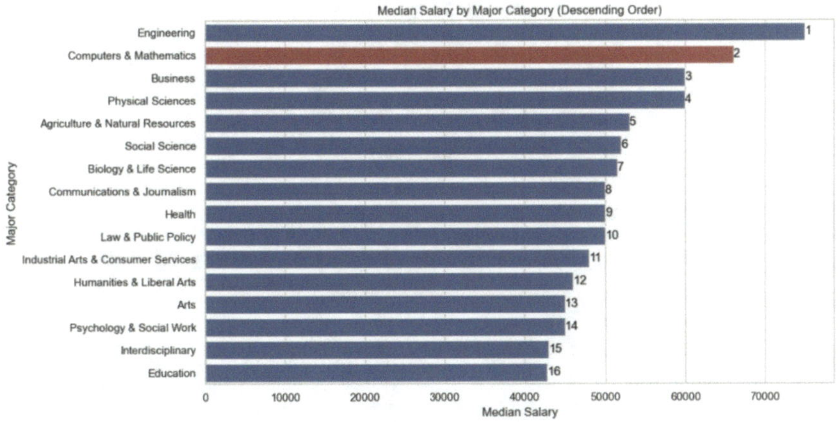


**Fig. 3:** Median Salary by Major Category

this major ranks 2nd, making it a worthwhile major to pursuit. The reason for the higher salary is both demand by industry and the relatively low number of graduates in the field.

## A. **Employment Rate Analysis**

Figure 4 highlights employment rates by academic major, with Computers & Mathematics leading at 80%, followed by Communications & Journalism and Business at 79%, reflecting strong demand in technology, media, and business sectors. Education ranks lowest at 63%, suggesting job market challenges, possibly due to regional teacher shortages or demand fluctuations. Social Science, Psychology & Social Work, and Humanities & Liberal Arts also show lower employment rates (around 68%–69%), likely reflecting fewer positions in these specialized fields. Majors like Engineering, Health, and Agriculture & Natural Resources have moderate employment rates (72%–76%), indicating steady demand. Overall, technical fields tend to offer higher employment rates, while niche or public sector majors may face more variability.

Figure 5 compares full-time employment rates across academic fields, showing significant variations based on majors. Engineering leads with an 83% full-time employment rate, followed by Business, Computers & Mathematics, and Agriculture & Natural Resources, each exceeding 81%, indicating strong job stability in technical and vocational fields. Arts has the lowest full-time employment rate at 63%, underscoring challenges in creative fields, while Education, Health, and Humanities & Liberal Arts hover around 67–68%, reflecting moderate job stability. Fields like Communications & Journalism (75%) and Social Sciences (76%) offer balanced opportunities but often require specialization. Overall, STEM-B fields tend to secure higher full-time employment, contrasting with more niche fields like Arts and Humanities, which face competitive job markets and lower full-time employment prospects.

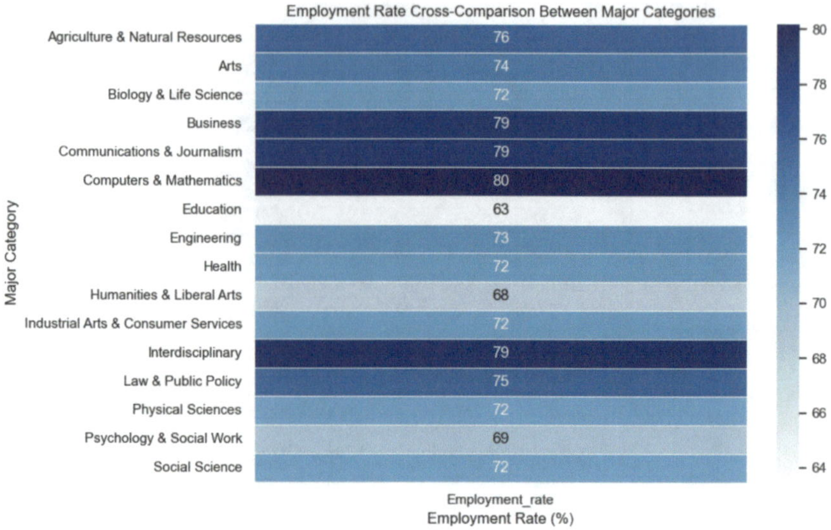


**Fig. 4:** Employment Rate Cross-Comparison Between Major Categories

## B. **Analysis of Specializations within Majors**

Table 1 shows the number of major specializations in each major. We note the large number of specializations in the engineering field in particular, due to its specialized nature. Computer science and mathematics is in the mid-range with 11 sub-categories.

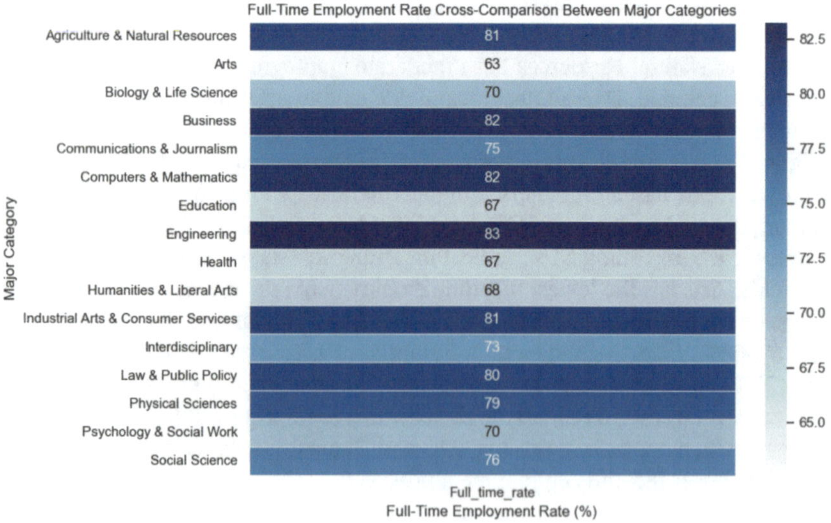


**Fig. 5:** Full-Time Employment Rate by Major Categories

**Table 1:** Major Category and Major Counts

| Category | Major Counts |
|---|---|
| Engineering | 29 |
| Education | 16 |
| Humanities & Liberal Arts | 15 |
| Biology & Life Science | 14 |
| Business | 13 |
| Health | 12 |
| Computers & Mathematics | 11 |
| Agriculture & Natural Resources | 10 |
| Physical Sciences | 10 |
| Psychology & Social Work | 9 |
| Social Science | 9 |
| Arts | 8 |
| Industrial Arts & Consumer Services | 7 |
| Law & Public Policy | 5 |
| Communications & Journalism | 4 |
| Interdisciplinary | 1 |

Figure 6 illustrates the relationship between the number of academic majors and their average unemployment rates across various categories. Engineering, with nearly 30 majors, boasts the lowest unemployment rate below 3%, highlighting strong demand for technical graduates. Business, with around 13 majors, follows closely at approximately 4%, reflecting its competitive nature and broad applicability.

In contrast, the Arts category, despite fewer majors, experiences high unemployment rates exceeding 7%, indicating significant challenges for creative graduates, while Interdisciplinary studies also struggle with over 6% unemployment. Fields like Health, Education, and Agriculture & Natural Resources, which offer moderate major numbers, maintain lower unemployment rates around 3–4%, suggesting stable demand. Overall, this analysis emphasizes that selecting a major with a technical or vocational focus, such as Engineering or Business, is likely to lead to better employment outcomes compared to creative or interdisciplinary fields.

The pie chart in Fig. 7 depicts the distribution of individuals across various academic disciplines, highlighting significant disparities in educational focus. Business is the largest field, accounting for 24.7% of the total population, followed by Psychology & Social Work (11.8%) and Social Science (9.0%), indicating a strong preference for business education likely driven by market demand. STEM fields collectively represent a smaller portion, with Engineering at 6.7%, Computers & Mathematics at 4.5%, and Biology & Life Science at 2.6%, raising concerns about workforce development in these high-employability areas. Humanities-related disciplines, such as Arts

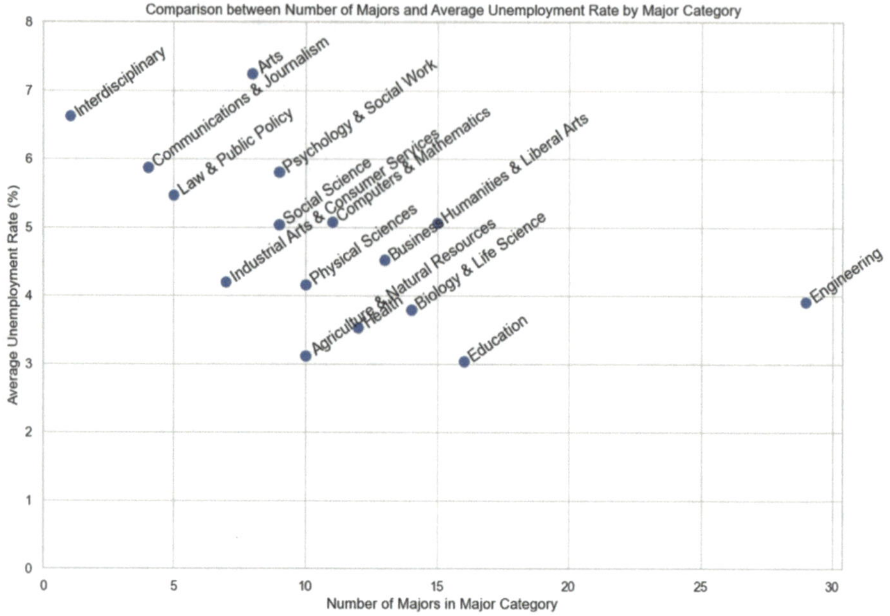


**Fig. 6:** Number of Majors and Unemployment Rate

(9.4%) and Humanities & Liberal Arts (4.5%), remain popular, while Agriculture & Natural Resources (7.4%) and Health (1.6%) have modest representation despite their societal importance. This distribution suggests a potential misalignment between educational choices and market needs, highlighting the importance of workforce planning and educational policy to address skills gaps in critical sectors.

We observe an interesting almost linear relationship between the number of majors and the unemployment rate. We conclude that the more a field had specific subfields, the more there is demand for it from the market, and this could be due to the large breadth and depth of the field.

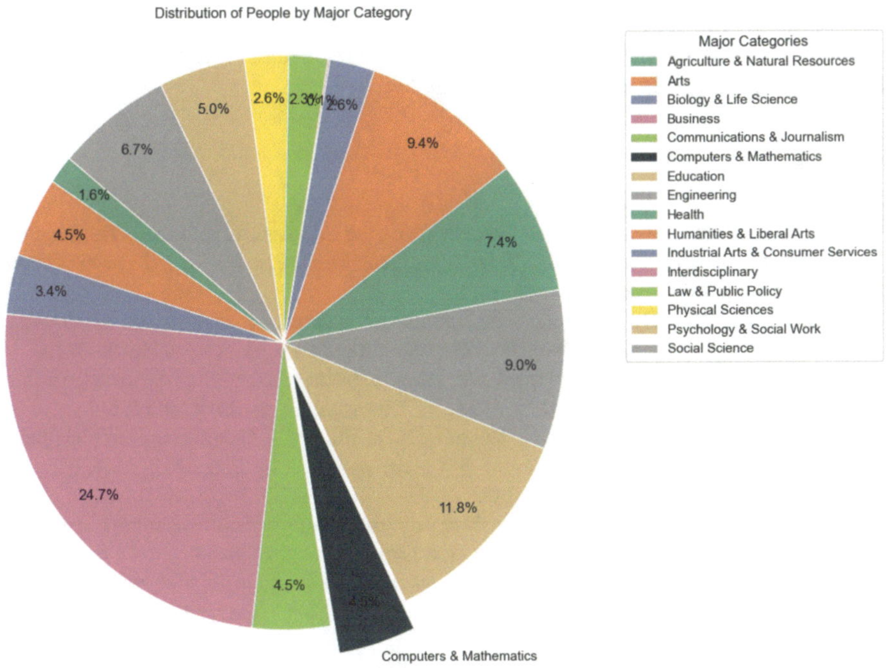


**Fig. 7:** Distribution Analysis by Major Categories

## 5 Conclusion

In conclusion, the findings of this study provide a comprehensive view of the relationship between academic disciplines, employment outcomes, and salaries. STEM and business majors emerge as clear leaders in employment stability and financial returns, reflecting the high market demand for specialized technical and managerial skills. Fields like engineering, computers, and mathematics command the highest median salaries and exhibit robust employment rates, positioning them as attractive choices for students prioritizing career stability and growth. Conversely, the arts, humanities, and interdisciplinary studies face more significant challenges, with lower employment rates and median earnings highlighting the competitive nature of these fields.

This analysis underscores the importance of aligning academic programs with labor market demands. For students, it emphasizes making informed decisions based on their career aspirations and the economic viability of their chosen field. For educators and policymakers, the insights offer guidance for tailoring curricula and resource allocation to meet industry needs and close skill gaps in critical sectors like technology and healthcare. Addressing challenges like missing data and demographic disparities remains essential for refining future analyses and ensuring a fair representation of all fields. Future work in this area would be to study the trends in growth of the different fields to be able to predict where the employement market will be in the future, thus helping students better choose a major.

Ultimately, the study advocates for a data-driven approach to educational planning, enabling students to achieve meaningful careers and policymakers to foster a workforce that aligns with evolving economic priorities.

## References


1. Committee on the National Science Foundation on the Economics Profession: The structure of economists' employment and salaries, 1964. Am. Econ. Rev. **55**(5), 1–98 (1965) http://www.jstor.org/stable/1802489
2. Melichar, E.: Study III: changes in the structure of economists' salaries and employment 1964–1966. Am. Econ. Rev. **58**(5), 70–122 (1968) http://www.jstor.org/stable/1808918
3. Taylor, D.: Employment preferences and salary expectations of students in science and engineering. BioScience. **57**(2), 175–185 (2007). https://doi.org/10.1641/B570212
4. Sullivan, A., Parsons, S., Green, F., Wiggins, R.D., Ploubidis, G.: Elite universities, fields of study and top salaries: which degree will make you rich? Br. Educ. Res. J. **44**, 663–680 (2018). https://doi.org/10.1002/berj.3453
5. Malkiel, B.G., Malkiel, J.A.: Male-female pay differentials in professional employment. Am. Econ. Rev. **63**(4), 693–705 (1973) http://www.jstor.org/stable/1808858
6. Zhang, J., Cheng, J.: Study of employment salary forecast using KNN algorithm. In: Proceedings of the International Conference on Modeling, Simulation, and Big Data Analysis. Atlantis Press (2019)
7. Babco, E.L.: Salaries of Scientists, Engineers and Technicians. A Summary of Salary Surveys, 13th edn, https://eric.ed.gov/?id=ED292625
8. Maisel, H., Gaddy, C.: Employment and salaries of recent doctorates in computer science. Commun. ACM 40, 9. **1997**, 90–93 (1997). https://doi.org/10.1145/260750.260778
9. Gishkayeva, L., Aziyeva, R., Abubakarov, M.: Employment and salary as indicators of social quality of life. In: Bataev, D.K. (ed.) Social and Cultural Transformations in the Context of Modern Globalism European Proceedings of Social and Behavioural Sciences, vol. 58, pp. 2048–2057. Future Academy (2019). https://doi.org/10.15405/epsbs.2019.03.02.238
10. US census website, https://www.census.gov/data.html, last accessed on 3 Feb 2025

# Exploring Embedded Computing Integration in MVC Blazor-Based Learning Management Systems

Agon Memeti[1](✉), Neshat Ajruli[1], Ibrahim Neziri[2], and Shkurte Luma-Osmani[1]

[1] Department of Computer Sciences, Faculty of Natural Sciences and Mathematics, University of Tetova, Tetovo, North Macedonia
{agon.memeti,n.ajruli3192026,shkurte.luma}@unite.edu.mk
[2] Department of Psychology, Faculty of Philosophy, University of Tetova, Tetovo, North Macedonia
ibrahim.neziri@unite.edu.mk

**Abstract.** Learning Management System developed with embedded computing involves considering the communication between the web-based application and the embedded systems. The aim of this paper is integrating embedded computing in MVC Blazor - based LMS of University of Tetova using GraphQL to create Smart Learning Ecosystems. The objective is to enhance the educational experience by leveraging advanced technologies, fostering seamless interaction, and optimizing learning processes through the integration of embedded computing and GraphQL in the Blazor framework. The approach embraces GraphQL as optimal solutions for constructing interfaces that facilitate seamless data interchange. This technology forms a robust foundation for creating modern and agile systems that prioritize communication and interoperability in the ever-evolving landscape of web development.

**Keywords:** LMS · MVC Blazor · Embedded computing · GraphQL · Smart Learning Ecosystems · Agile systems

## 1 Introduction

Emerging new pedagogies with technologies, such as design-based learning, have the ability and potential to revolutionize formal teaching processes [1]. The notion of Smart Education is grounded on smart learning through, but not constrained, IoT devices and additional Information and Communication Technologies (ICT), and it is thoroughly associated with the literature on Smart Cities [2]. Based on [3] Smart Learning as a new educational paradigm is centered around smart devices and technologies, enabling personalized learning experiences for students. This approach is referred to in the literature as Technology-Enhanced Learning (TEL).

This integration enhances the educational experience by enabling seamless interaction between the LMS and embedded systems, optimizing learning processes through real-time data exchange. Unlike existing solutions, this approach leverages GraphQL's


K. Daimi and A. Alsadoon (Eds.): ICR 2025, LNNS 1487, pp. 373–382, 2025.
https://doi.org/10.1007/978-3-031-95652-2_32

flexibility to construct agile interfaces that facilitate efficient communication and interoperability. By combining embedded computing and GraphQL in the Blazor framework, the paper presents a novel solution for creating modern, dynamic, and responsive learning environments that address the evolving needs of web-based education systems.

This paper introduces a design-based case study implemented at the University of Tetova, utilizing Blazor components in conjunction with GraphQL for embedded computing. We propose a flexible and responsive web application capable of seamlessly interacting with embedded devices, such as QR codes, to display real-time attendance data for all university staff. The approach involves combining Blazor, a web framework, with GraphQL, a query language for APIs, so this integration enhances real-time communication and data exchange between the Blazor components and embedded computing devices.

Current LMS solutions often rely on traditional RESTful APIs and lack integration with embedded systems, which can lead to several limitations: Performance and Scalability Issues, Limited Real-Time Capabilities, ack of Seamless Integration with Embedded Devices, inflexibility in Data Handling. By highlighting these shortcomings and demonstrating how our approach effectively addresses them, we provide a clearer understanding of the research gap and the specific advantages of our solution.

GraphQL is well known for the Efficiency and Flexibility, Real-Time Data Handling and Schema Definition and on the other side Blazor has strong points the Integration with. NET Ecosystem, it's Component-Based Architecture as well as C# and. NET Usage. While RESTful APIs are a common choice for data communication, they were not selected due to their limitations in efficiency and the complexity of managing multiple endpoints.

The paper is organized as mentioned: the next section is literature review and recent related works, the third section deals with embedded computing integration, while the last one deals with the platform design and development.

## 2 Literature Review

As in [4], a Learning Management Systems (LMS) presents a joint station of communication to all the partakers of the course; this is a main motive to use them as the channel to demonstrate various visualizations.

Learning Management Systems (LMS) offer both sides, including teachers and students with an online virtual classroom that reinforces the processes of learning. In such online classroom surroundings, Learning Management Systems (LMS) reinforce all the participants in the learning process [5].

As technology continues to advance and educational paradigms shift towards greater student-centered approaches, the Learning Management System (LMS) of the future is poised to transcend its role as a mere administrative tool. The evolving landscape of education demands a dynamic LMS that not only streamlines administrative tasks but also seamlessly integrates cutting-edge pedagogical tools and adaptive learning technologies [6].

The future LMS must be a hub of innovation, fostering collaborative and interactive learning experiences tailored to individual student needs. It will serve as a catalyst for personalized education, leveraging artificial intelligence and data analytics to provide insightful feedback, track progress, and offer customized learning pathways. In essence, the LMS of tomorrow will be a transformative force, redefining the way education is delivered and experienced in the digital age. Also there has been a great effort in predicting student performance by analyzing their academic scores, demographics, as well as extracurricular activities [11].

## 2.1 Embedded Computing in Education

The embedded system is a mixture of computer software and hardware, and possibly supplementary mechanical or electronic elements, that are built to perform one or more dedicated roles, either individualistically or as fragments of a greater system [6]. Among the first studies on embedded systems topic was published in 2000 [7] and emphasized that it is essential for future embedded systems designers to be trained accordingly and to have knowledge about the whole design process in order to make global instead of local decisions. The researchers claim that they believe that next - generation courses in embedded computing ought to move away from the conversation of components and toward the discussion of design and analysis of the systems".

Embedded computing plays a pivotal role in modern education by seamlessly integrating technology into the learning environment. The use of embedded systems in interactive whiteboards and smart classrooms is more than mandatory. These systems enable teachers to create dynamic and engaging lessons, incorporating multimedia elements, interactive activities, and real-time collaboration. Students benefit from a more immersive and interactive learning experience, as these embedded technologies cater to diverse learning styles and foster student engagement [6].

Additionally, embedded computing facilitates the integration of educational software, enabling personalized learning paths that cater to individual student needs, thereby enhancing the overall effectiveness of instruction. Furthermore, the adoption of embedded computing in education extends beyond the classroom. Online learning platforms and educational apps leverage embedded systems to provide students with accessible and interactive content, fostering self-directed learning. Embedded systems also contribute to the development of educational robotics, enhancing hands-on learning experiences in science, technology, engineering, and mathematics (STEM) subjects [7]. By incorporating embedded computing into educational tools and resources, institutions can equip students with the digital literacy skills necessary for the twenty-first century, preparing them for a technology-driven future.

### 2.2 MVC Blazor Framework

Blazor is a web framework developed by Microsoft that allows developers to build interactive web applications using C# and. NET instead of relying solely on JavaScript.

The Model-View-Controller (MVC) pattern is a key architectural concept in software development, and Blazor, particularly in its server-side variant, aligns with this pattern [12].

Below are some features of MVC in the context of the Blazor framework: Model-View-Controller Architecture; Component-Based Architecture; Razor Syntax; Data Binding; Dependency Injection; Routing; Event Handling; Code Separation and Server-Side and WebAssembly Hosting Models [12].

## 3 Proposed Methodology

### 3.1 Embedded Computing Integration in MVC Blazor - Based LMS

The main University e-Services that are used by our university are Learning Management Systems, e-Library and e-Administrative solutions. These services include all forms of electronically supported learning and teaching.

The information and communication systems, whether network learning or not, serve as specific media to implement the learning process. There are different functional requirements that e-services are supporting, starting from the basic ones which are; course registration, supplying computer accessories and communication technologies; range of communications options; and also different other solutions but with isolated support [8].

The existing LMS implemented at University of Tetova is using MVC Blazor framework (DFD model below).

The embedded model that we are proposing and implementing is for flexible REST Services, using GraphQL - a dynamic and responsive web application that can seamlessly interact with and display real-time data from embedded devices (QR Code) for all the University staff attendance.

We have successfully implemented the entire Learning Management System (LMS) using Blazor MVC applications. This technology stack has provided a robust and interactive user interface, enhancing the overall user experience. To further augment the capabilities of the LMS, my next step involves integrating embedded computing.

This integration will enable the LMS to leverage the power of embedded systems, offering enhanced performance and functionality. The use of embedded computing within the LMS will open up new possibilities for real-time data processing, enabling quicker and more efficient responses to user interactions.

In addition to incorporating embedded computing, we optimize data exchange within the LMS by implementing GraphQL. By adopting this modern and versatile technology, we establish seamless communication channels between different components of the system. The use of GraphQL empowers the LMS with a flexible and efficient query language, enabling clients to request precisely the data they need. This strategic combination of embedded computing and GraphQL is poised to elevate the functionality and connectivity of the LMS, ultimately delivering a more dynamic and responsive learning platform.

Through GraphQL, the smart learning ecosystem becomes a hub of efficient data exchange, ensuring that learners and educators can access and share information effortlessly. This strategic integration aligns with the vision of a smart learning ecosystem, where technological innovation converges with educational excellence, fostering a holistic and personalized learning experience for users.

### 3.2 Technical Implementation

The integration is done through: GraphQL Approach; Develop Blazor Components; Implemented GraphQL Server for Embedded Computing; Use GraphQL Queries from Blazor; Integrate GraphQL Client in Blazor and Have Real-time Updates.

## 4 Results and Discussion: Platform Design and Implementation

The proposed platform offers significant potential for improving staff attendance management across specific courses at the university, streamlining the process and saving considerable time (see Fig. 1). By utilizing advanced technologies and automation, the system ensures more efficient and accurate tracking of student attendance, reducing the administrative workload for institutions and providing valuable insights into attendance patterns and trends (Fig. 2).

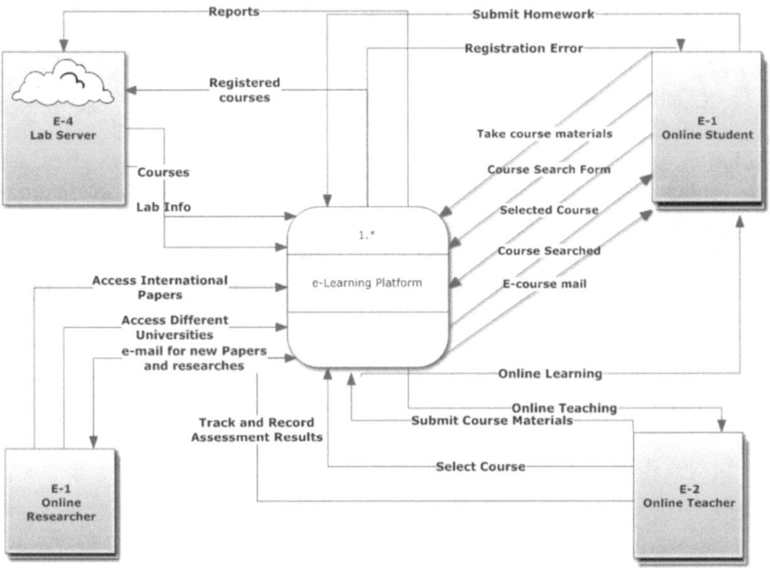


**Fig. 1.** University of Tetova LMS - DFD Diagram [9]

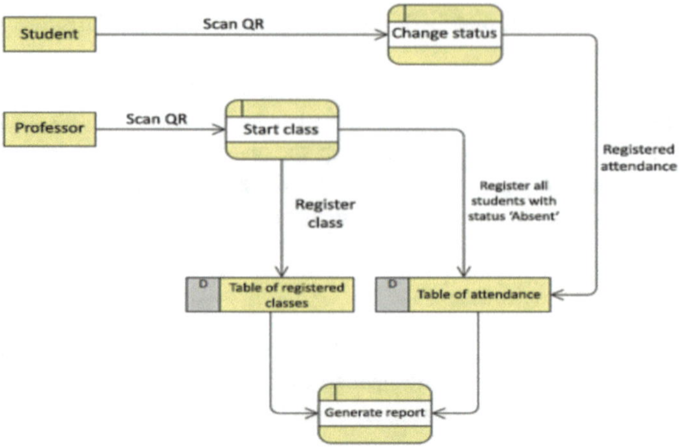


**Fig. 2.** Proposed Platform Design [10]

In the pursuit of seamlessly integrating Blazor components with embedded computing systems, we will leverage GraphQL as the communication bridge between the device and the Blazor component. The decision to employ GraphQL is grounded in its superior efficiency compared to RESTful APIs, particularly in the context of embedded devices grappling with resource limitations.

Our choice for implementing a GraphQL server in this paper centers on Hot Chocolate, a powerful and feature-rich GraphQL library for. NET. Hot Chocolate stands out for its comprehensive support for the GraphQL specification, enabling seamless integration and efficient data querying. Its extensibility, performance optimizations, and intuitive syntax make it an ideal choice for building robust and scalable GraphQL APIs.

Hot Chocolate's ability to seamlessly integrate with existing. NET applications and its strong community support further solidify its position as our preferred GraphQL server solution. Its developer-friendly features and continuous updates align perfectly with our project requirements, ensuring a smooth and effective implementation of GraphQL capabilities.

After adding Hot Chocolate we need to define the types our GraphQL schema should contain. These types and their fields define what consumers can query from our GraphQL API.

```
public class Employee
{
public int employee_id { get; set; }
public string personal_number { get; set; }
public DateOnly birthdate { get; set; }
public string sex { get; set; }
public string phone { get; set; }
public string status { get; set; }
public string country_code { get; set; }
public string nationality_code { get; set; }
public string image { get; set; }
public string employee_type { get; set; }
public int bank_id { get; set; }
public double account_number { get; set; }
public int personal_digits { get; set; }
public EmployeeTranslations employee_translation { get; set; }
}
public class EmployeeTranslations
{
public int employee_translation_id { get; set; }
public int employee_id { get; set; }
public string first_name { get; set; }
public string last_name { get; set; }
public string address { get; set; }
public string city { get; set; }
public string language { get; set; }
}
public class EmployeeAttendance
{
public int attendance_id { get; set; }
public int employee_id { get; set; }
public Employee employee { get; set; }
```

```
public DateOnly attendance_date { get; set; }
public TimeOnly entry_time { get; set; }
public TimeOnly exit_time { get; set; }
}
```

We define the GraphQL query we want to perform, for example fetching a list of all employee's attendance, but only the information we need, not all the properties we have declared above.

```
query {
allEmployeeAttendance {
attendance_date
entry_time
exit_time
employee {
email
employee_translation
{
first_name
last_name
}}}}
```

After that we define the necessary services that will fetch the data we need using Dapper, also the query resolvers which are important because it determines how the GraphQL server interacts with and invokes resolver functions during the execution of a GraphQL query.

```
var translations =
result.Read<EmployeeTranslations>().ToList();
var attendances = result.Read<EmployeeAttendance>().ToList();
// Link EmployeeTranslations to Employees
foreach (var employeeTranslation in translations)
{
var employee = employees.FirstOrDefault(e => e.employee_id ==
employeeTranslation.employee_id);
if (employee is not null)
{
employee.employee_translation = employeeTranslation;
}}
// Link EmployeeAttendance to Employees
foreach (var attendance in attendances)
{
var employee = employees.FirstOrDefault(e =>e.employee_id ==
attendance.employee_id);
if (employee is not null)
{
attendance.employee = employee;
}}
return attendances;
}}}
```

```
public class EmployeeService : IEmployeeService
{
private readonly IConfiguration _configuration;
private IDbConnection Connection
{
get
{
return new
SqlConnection(_configuration.GetConnectionString("LmsDbConnecti
on"));
}}
public EmployeeService(IConfiguration configuration)
{
_configuration = configuration;
}
public List<EmployeeAttendance>
GetAllEmployeeAttendance()
{
using (var conn = Connection)
{
var query = @"SELECT * FROM employee
SELECT * FROM employee_translations WHERE language = 'shq';
SELECT * FROM employee_attendance";
var result = conn.QueryMultiple(query);
var employees = result.Read<Employee>().ToList();
```

And those below are the query resolvers that we mentioned above.

When all this is ready now we can use these services to show the data in a Blazor component like below:

```
<h1>Employee attendance</h1>
<UseGetEmployeeAttendance Context="result">
<ChildContent>
@foreach (var item in result.AllEmployeeAttendance!)
{
var translation = item?.Employee?.Employee_translation;
<li>@translation?.First_name @translation?.Last_name
(@item?.Employee?.Email) [@item?.Attendance_date:
@item?.Entry_time - @item?.Exit_time]</li>
}
</ChildContent>
<ErrorContent>
Something went wrong …<br />
@result.First().Message

</ErrorContent>
<LoadingContent>
Loading ...
</LoadingContent>
</UseGetEmployeeAttendance>
```

The paper contributions include specific improvements that our method brings to the LMS performance include the following:

- **Reduced Latency**: By integrating GraphQL with the embedded systems, the method optimizes real-time data querying and minimizes redundant data retrieval, resulting in faster response times and reduced latency during interactions with the LMS.
- **Improved Data Accuracy**: The use of GraphQL allows for precise data queries, ensuring that only the required data is retrieved, reducing the likelihood of errors and improving overall data accuracy within the system.
- **Seamless Real-Time Data Exchange**: The integration of embedded computing with the LMS enables real-time communication between the LMS and embedded devices (e.g., QR codes), allowing for immediate updates on attendance and other data-driven tasks.
- **Enhanced System Responsiveness**: The combination of embedded computing and GraphQL in the Blazor framework creates a more dynamic and responsive user interface, which improves overall system performance and user experience.

The results highlight how GraphQL, particularly through the use of Hot Chocolate, provides superior efficiency in data querying compared to RESTful APIs. This directly ties to the research question concerning the effectiveness of GraphQL in resource-constrained environments. The choice of Hot Chocolate and its seamless integration with .NET applications addresses the objective of ensuring compatibility and performance within the existing technology stack. The process of defining GraphQL types and queries, as well as the implementation of Dapper for data fetching, directly responds to the research question about optimizing data retrieval and interaction between the GraphQL server and the Blazor components.

## 5 Conclusions

This paper presented the incorporation of a Learning Management System (LMS) with embedded computing, focusing on effective communication between the web-based application and embedded systems. The primary goal was to integrate embedded computing into the MVC Blazor-based LMS of the University of Tetova by utilizing GraphQL, for staff attendance. The overarching objective was to establish Smart Learning Ecosystems that enhance the educational experience by incorporating advanced technologies. Through the integration of embedded computing and RESTful APIs in the Blazor framework, the paper aims to foster seamless interaction and optimize learning processes.

The chosen approach emphasizes the use of GraphQL as optimal solutions for constructing interfaces that facilitate smooth data interchange. The integration of embedded computing and GraphQL in the Blazor framework showcases a forward-thinking approach to building Smart Learning Ecosystems that align with the demands of the ever-evolving field of education and technology.

## References

1. Erkki, R., et al.: Creating smart connected learning ecosystems: a hybrid model for design-based learning. Interact. Design Archit. J. **52** (2022)
2. Lee, J., Zo, H., Lee, H.: Smart learning adoption in employees and HRD managers. Br. J. Educ. Technol. **45**(6), 1082–1096. https://doi.org/10.1111/bjet.12210
3. Stavropoulos, P., et al.: A Smart Learning Model targeting regional SME ecosystems: a conceptual framework. In: 11th Conference on Learning Factories (2021)
4. Leony, D., et al.: Learning analytics in the LMS: Using browser extensions to embed visualizations into a Learning Management System. In: 7th European Conference on Technology Enhanced Learning (EC-TEL 2012) (2012)
5. Bradley, V.M.: Learning management system (LMS) use with online instruction. Int. J. Technol. Educ. (IJTE). **4**(1), 68–92 (2021). https://doi.org/10.46328/ijte.36
6. Pasricha, S.: Embedded systems education in the 2020s: challenges, reflections, and future directions. In: Proceedings of the Great Lakes Symposium on VLSI 2022, p. 2022
7. Wolf, W., Madsen, J.: Embedded systems education for the future. In: Proceedings of the IEEE, pp. 23–30 (2000)
8. Memeti, A., et al.: Coordinating service resources: an architecture for REST service collaboration. In: International Scientific Conference Computer Science (2015)
9. Memeti, A., Cico, B.: Supporting content and learner collaboration and interaction through cloud computing models. In: Sixth International Conference on Computational Intelligence, Communication Systems and Networks. IEEE (2014)
10. Nuhi, A., et al.: Smart attendance system using QR code. In: Proceedings of 9th Mediterranean Conference on Embedded Computing (2020)
11. Nadar, N.: Enhancing student performance prediction through stream-based analysis dataset using modified XGBoost algorithm. Int. J. Inform. Technol. Sec. **15**(2), 75–86 (2023). https://doi.org/10.59035/KNUG1085
12. Microsoft: .Net. https://dotnet.microsoft.com/en-us/apps/aspnet/web-apps/blazor. Accessed 26 August 2024

# Health Informatics and Biomedical Imaging

# Urban Technologies for Sustainable Aging: Addressing Vision Impairments in Older Populations

Gema Martinez-Navarrete[1], Vanessa Zorrilla-Muñoz[2,3](✉), Eduardo Sáenz-de-Cabezón[4], Nicanor Morales-Delgado[1], Ramon Peral-Orts[5], María Silveria Agulló-Tomás[2,6], Nicolas Garcia Aracil[1], Jose Maria Sabater-Navarro[1], and Eduardo Fernandez[1,7]

[1] Department of Anatomy and Human Embriology, Miguel Hernandez University, San Joan, Spain
{gema.martinen,nmorales,nicolas.garcia,j.sabater, e.fernandez}@umh.es
[2] Bioengineering Institute, Miguel Hernandez University, Elche, Spain
vzorrilla@umh.es, msat.polsoc@uc3m.es
[3] University Institute on Gender Studies, University Carlos III of Madrid, Madrid, Spain
[4] Department of Mathematics and Computation Department, University of La Rioja, Logroño, Spain
eduardo.saenz-de-cabezon@unirioja.es
[5] Department of Applied Mechanical Engineering, Miguel Hernandez University, Elche, Spain
ramon.peral@umh.es
[6] Social Sciences Department, University Carlos III of Madrid, Madrid, Spain
[7] Networking Research Centre of Bioengineering, Biomaterials and Nanomedicine (CIBER-BBN), Madrid, Spain

**Abstract.** According to the WHO, over 1 billion people worldwide experience moderate to severe visual impairment. A significant majority of these people are aged 50 or older. Urban areas often concentrate environmental factors such as pollution, toxic gases and chemicals, which contribute to the development of visual impairments and exacerbate eye health issues. Unfortunately, these conditions are frequently irreversible, subjecting affected individuals to these challenges as they age. In addition, there is a digital divide among people in terms of using mobile Apps and wearables which becomes more evident the older they get. This article analyses the digital divide experienced by individuals aged over 50 with visual impairments, investigating this disparity through the perspective of technology user perception. This chapter specifically aimed to explore individuals' perceptions on how technology has contributed to enhancing various aspects of their daily lives; alongside evaluating the effectiveness of solutions they have adopted to overcome challenges through technology use. The data was sourced from the questionnaire 'Encuesta de Discapacidad, Autonomía personal y Situaciones de Dependencia, EDAD (2020)' carried out in Spain among people with disabilities. Among the 2,405 participants who addressed the question related to visual impairments, 74 individuals reported retinitis pigmentosa, 257 magna myopia, 367 age-related macular degeneration, 150 diabetic retinopathy, 345 glaucoma


K. Daimi and A. Alsadoon (Eds.): ICR 2025, LNNS 1487, pp. 385–396, 2025.
https://doi.org/10.1007/978-3-031-95652-2_33

and 1,207 were affected by cataracts. The results indicate a prevailing negative perception among individuals concerning the use of technology, particularly in relation to aspects of vision, self-care and domestic life. However, a positive trend was evident among people with visual impairments, as they recognize the potential of technology to provide valuable assistance. Consequently, there is a growing emphasis on supportive technologies designed to prevent dangerous situations and enhance safety during urban public transport use. Further improvements in these technologies hold the potential to create safer and more sustainable urban environments. Additionally, exploring quantum computing optimization could enhance the design of these technologies by efficiently correlating user perception data with functional variables.

**Keywords:** Sustainable ageing · older people · visual impairments · mobility · technology · intersectional · gender · quantum computing

# 1 Introduction

More than 1 billion people worldwide suffer from moderate to severe visual impairment, according to data from the World Health Organization (WHO) [1]. This significant demographic primarily consists of individuals aged 50 and older [*íbid*]. Vision-related challenges are particularly prevalent among adults and older individuals, often stemming from conditions such as cataracts, diabetic retinopathy, glaucoma, and age-related macular degeneration [2]. In many cases, environmental factors contribute to the development of these diseases and exacerbate eye health issues, particularly in urban areas where exposure to and concentration of air pollution, toxic gases, and chemicals are more pronounced [3, 4]. The progression of these vision problems is typically irreversible, forcing affected individuals to cope with these challenges throughout their adult and later years. Emerging technologies, such as microarrays [5], visual prosthesis [6] and navigation systems (i.e. EGARA) [7], offer promising tools for restoring vision or assisting adults and older persons dealing with visual impairments or blindness. While prior research has advanced assistive technologies for visual impairments (such as visual prosthesis, microarrays), it often overlooks how older adults perceive usability and adoption, leaving a gap in understanding the digital divide's human factors. For example, the significant digital divide persists in the use of mobile apps and wearables, a gap that becomes more evident as individuals age get [7], more for older women [8]. This disparity is compounded by factors such as limited accessibility, lack of digital literacy, and socioeconomic barriers, which further hinder the adoption of these technologies among vulnerable populations. Moreover, emerging computational approaches may offer future solutions to scale technology design, addressing these adoption gaps.

This article analyses the digital divide experienced by people with visual impairments aged over 50, focusing on their perceptions as technology users. We specifically investigated how individuals perceive the impact of technologies on various aspects of their daily lives, including mobility, communication, and self-care, as well as the effectiveness of the strategies they have employed to overcome challenges through the use of these technologies. Through this analysis, we aim to assess how assistive technologies can address the digital divide—specifically in terms of access, usability, and acceptance—among adults over 50 with visual impairments, while pinpointing gaps in current solutions and proposing innovative approaches to enhance their quality of life. Moreover, past research has rarely examined how visually impaired adults over 50 perceive technology usability, often prioritizing clinical outcomes over lived experiences, thus limiting insights into adoption barrier.

## 2 Method

The study employed the secondary database "Encuesta de Discapacidad, Autonomía personal y Situaciones de Dependencia, EDAD (2020)" [9] which covers all Spanish provinces. Several items were selected of the database: The 6 vision-related items were chosen to reflect common functional challenges reported by participants, such as reading fine print and recognizing faces across a distance, which are essential for maintaining social engagement and independence among visually impaired adults over 50. Similarly, the 14 self-care items were selected to encompass a broad yet practical range of autonomy tasks—such as washing, dressing, and eating—representing critical aspects of personal care and well-being captured within the dataset's scope. This approach ensured that the analysis focused on difficulties most pertinent to the target population's lived experiences while aligning with the database's comprehensive coverage of disability-related domains.

The sample comprised 9,658 individuals aged 50 or older, including 3,732 men and 5,926 women. The mean age of the participants was 73.71 years, with a standard error of $\pm 0.128$ ($71.62 \pm 0.201$ for men and $75.03 \pm 0.163$ for women). Table 1 presents the diagnoses for men and women, highlighting the most prevalent disabilities. These included osteoarthritis (14.33% of men, 37.53% of women) and arthritis (7.24% of men, 20.66% of women), followed by diabetes (9.63% of men, 13.88% of women). Among the total sample, 2,405 individuals (24.91% of the 9,658 participants) aged 50 and above reported visual impairments. Specifically, 74 individuals were diagnosed with retinitis pigmentosa, 257 with high myopia (magna myopia), 367 with age-related macular degeneration, 150 with diabetic retinopathy, 345 with glaucoma, and 1,207 with cataracts. These findings underscore the significant burden of visual and musculoskeletal conditions within this demographic, with notable gender differences in prevalence.

To assess the internal consistency of the scales used in this study, Cronbach's alpha was calculated for each set of items. This statistical measure evaluates the reliability of the scales by determining how well the items within each domain correlate with one another, with values of 0.7 or higher indicating acceptable reliability. The analysis itself was performed using Pearson correlation tests, with significance thresholds set at $p < 0.01$ and $p < 0.05$. All variables were measured on a Likert Scale. The independent variables were collected from individuals aged 50 and older with disabilities and included 6 items related to vision challenges, 14 items concerning self-care, and 6 items about domestic life, each rated on a 4-point scale (1 = minimal difficulty, 4 = maximum difficulty). The dependent variable, 'How would you describe your overall health?', was scored on a 5-point scale, where 1 represented very good health and 5 denoted very poor health. Additionally, the question 'Do you feel that new technologies have improved aspects of your daily life?' was rated on a 4-point scale, with 1 indicating significant improvement and 4 suggesting a negative impact.

**Table 1.** Diseases diagnosed by sex and persons with 50 and more years based on the database of EDAD (2020) [9].

| Diagnosed disease | Total N=(9658) | Freq. | Men (n=3732) | Freq. Men | Women (n=5926) | Freq. Women |
|---|---|---|---|---|---|---|
| Down Syndrome | 22 | 0.23% | 10 | 0.10% | 12 | 0.12% |
| Autism Spectrum Disorders | 37 | 0.38% | 24 | 0.25% | 13 | 0.13% |
| Amyotrophic Lateral Sclerosis | 63 | 0.65% | 22 | 0.23% | 41 | 0.42% |
| Hydrocephalus/Spina Bifida | 65 | 0.67% | 14 | 0.14% | 51 | 0.53% |
| Retinitis pigmentosa | 74 | 0.77% | 33 | 0.34% | 41 | 0.42% |
| Cerebral Palsy | 88 | 0.91% | 52 | 0.54% | 36 | 0.37% |
| Laryngectomy | 118 | 1.22% | 53 | 0.55% | 65 | 0.67% |
| Schizophrenia | 138 | 1.43% | 66 | 0.68% | 72 | 0.75% |
| Brain Damage from Head Trauma | 139 | 1.44% | 79 | 0.82% | 60 | 0.62% |
| Diabetic retinopathy | 150 | 1.55% | 69 | 0.71% | 81 | 0.84% |
| Bipolar Disorder | 184 | 1.91% | 73 | 0.76% | 111 | 1.15% |
| Epilepsy | 198 | 2.05% | 92 | 0.95% | 106 | 1.10% |
| Multiple Scleroris | 211 | 2.18% | 50 | 0.52% | 161 | 1.67% |
| Agenesis/Amputations | 221 | 2.29% | 116 | 1.20% | 105 | 1.09% |
| *Magna myopia | 257 | 2.66% | 73 | 0.76% | 84 | 0.87% |
| Rare Disease | 262 | 2.71% | 106 | 1.10% | 156 | 1.62% |
| Spinal Cord Injury | 344 | 3.56% | 179 | 1.85% | 165 | 1.71% |
| Glaucoma | 345 | 3.57% | 143 | 1.48% | 202 | 2.09% |
| Parkinson | 360 | 3.73% | 167 | 1.73% | 193 | 2.00% |
| Age-related macular degeneration | 367 | 3.80% | 110 | 1.14% | 257 | 2.66% |
| Fibromyalgia | 593 | 6.14% | 68 | 0.70% | 525 | 5.44% |
| Alzheimer | 630 | 6.52% | 190 | 1.97% | 440 | 4.56% |
| Muscular Dystrophy | 672 | 6.96% | 259 | 2.68% | 413 | 4.28% |
| Chronic Kidney Disease | 699 | 7.24% | 311 | 3.22% | 388 | 4.02% |
| Heart Attack | 754 | 7.81% | 424 | 4.39% | 330 | 3.42% |
| Brain Damage from Stroke | 902 | 9.34% | 422 | 4.37% | 480 | 4.97% |

*(continued)*

**Table 1.** (*continued*)

| Diagnosed disease | Total N=(9658) | Freq. | Men (n=3732) | Freq. Men | Women (n=5926) | Freq. Women |
|---|---|---|---|---|---|---|
| Cancer/Malignancy | 1085 | 11.23% | 454 | 4.70% | 631 | 6.53% |
| Cataracts | 1207 | 12.50% | 398 | 4.12% | 809 | 8.38% |
| Other disease associated with the disability | 1459 | 15.11% | 594 | 6.15% | 865 | 8.96% |
| Chronic Anxiety | 1644 | 17.02% | 452 | 4.68% | 1192 | 12.34% |
| Chronic Depression | 1836 | 19.01% | 499 | 5.17% | 1337 | 13.84% |
| Diabetes | 2271 | 23.51% | 930 | 9.63% | 1341 | 13.88% |
| Arthritis | 2694 | 27.89% | 699 | 7.24% | 1995 | 20.66% |
| Osteoarthritis | 5009 | 51.86% | 1384 | 14.33% | 3625 | 37.53% |
| Total diseases/diagnostic | 9658 | 100% | 3732 | 38.64% | 5926 | 61.36% |

*Magna myopia refers to severe nearsightedness.

## 3 Results

The results are presented in Table 2, encompassing all diagnosed conditions (N = 9,658), including visual impairments such as retinitis pigmentosa, high myopia (magna myopia), age-related macular degeneration, diabetic retinopathy, glaucoma, and cataracts. The table shows the correlations between the main variables and the two key questions: 'How would you rate your overall health?' and 'Do you believe that the use of new technologies has improved aspects of your daily life?' Notably, the variable 'level of difficulty experienced when using technical aids' showed no significant correlation with either of the dependent variables.

Table 2 highlights distinct relationships between vision, self-care, and domestic challenges and the dependent variables of overall health (D_1) and technology impact (I_17). For vision, difficulty seeing newspaper print shows a modest correlation with health perception (0.1048**, $p < 0.01$) but a stronger one with technology improvement (0.1371**, $p < 0.01$), suggesting that fine visual tasks may subtly affect well-being while being more noticeably aided by tools like magnifiers or audio devices. In self-care, performing basic body care correlates significantly with both health (0.1387**, $p < 0.01$) and technology (0.1496**, $p < 0.01$), indicating that hygiene struggles could shape health views and represent a key area for tech support, though the persistence of correlations with assistance (0.1444**, $p < 0.01$) suggests current aids may fall short. Domestic tasks like household chores show the strongest link to technology benefits (0.1671**, $p < 0.01$) compared to health (0.1397**, $p < 0.01$), pointing to practical tasks as a prime target for smart devices. Notably, the lack of significant correlation with technical aid use (e.g., –0.0451, $p > 0.05$ for vision across the street) raises questions

**Table 2.** Statistical analysis tests on Likert scale variables (N=9,658 persons).

| It | Difficulty level... | Mean ± S.D. | α Cr. | Pearson (D_1) | Pearson (I_17) |
|---|---|---|---|---|---|
| VISION | ...to see the letter of a newspaper | 2.44±.18 | 0.93 | 0.105** | 0.137** |
| | ...to see the print of a newspaper when you use technical aids | 3.22±.27 | 0.93 | 0.181** | 0.094* |
| | ...to see someone's face across the street | 1.89± | 0.93 | 0.116** | 0.061* |
| | ...to see someone's face across the street when you use technical aids | 3±.26 | 0.93 | 0.127 | -0.045 |
| | ...to you have with that other vision problem | 2±.17 | 0.93 | 0.139** | 0.092** |
| | ...you have when you are using technical aids | 2.78±.22 | 0.93 | 0.129 | 0.055 |
| SELF-CARE | …wash and dry the different body parts | 2.78±.15 | 0.93 | 0.136** | 0.101** |
| | …wash and dry the different body parts when you receive personal help/assistance | 3.22±.22 | 0.93 | 0.120** | 0.139** |
| | ...perform basic body care | 2.78±.15 | 0.93 | 0.139** | 0.149** |
| | ...perform basic body care when you receive personal help/assistance | 3.33±.24 | 0.93 | 0.119** | 0.144** |
| | …go to the toilet and relieve yourself or take care of your intimate hygiene | 2.44±.24 | 0.92 | 0.085** | 0.098** |

*(continued)*

**Table 2.** (*continued*)

| It | Difficulty level... | Mean ± S.D. | α Cr. | Pearson (D_1) | Pearson (I_17) |
|---|---|---|---|---|---|
| | …go to the toilet and relieve yourself or take care of your intimate hygiene when you receive personal help/assistance | 3.44±.24 | 0.92 | 0.099** | 0.130** |
| | …dress or undress | 2.56±.18 | 0.92 | 0.132** | 0.094** |
| | …dress or undress when you receive personal help/assistance | 3±.29 | 0.92 | 0.146** | 0.114** |
| | … eat and drink | 2.33±.24 | 0.93 | 0.127** | 0.121** |
| | ... eat and drink when you receive personal help/assistance | 3±.33 | 0.93 | 0.102** | 0.124** |
| | … comply with medical prescriptions | 2.56±.24 | 0.93 | 0.035 | 0.096** |
| | … comply with medical prescriptions when you receive personal help/assistance | 3±.33 | 0.93 | 0.103** | 0.089** |
| | … avoid dangerous situations | 2.78±.15 | 0.93 | 0.064* | 0.078** |
| | ... avoid dangerous situations when you receive personal help/assistance | 3.22±.22 | 0.93 | 0.069* | 0.071** |
| DOMESTIC LIFE | ...to manage the household budget, plan expenses or organize purchases | 2.78±.15 | 0.93 | 0.029 | 0.130** |

(*continued*)

**Table 2.** (*continued*)

| It | Difficulty level... | Mean ± S.D. | α Cr. | Pearson (D_1) | Pearson (I_17) |
|---|---|---|---|---|---|
| | ...to manage the household budget, plan expenses or organize purchases when you receive personal help/assistance | 3.44±.24 | 0.93 | 0.023 | 0.106** |
| | ...to prepare meals | 2.89±.11 | 0.93 | 0.085** | 0.142** |
| | ...to prepare meals when you receive personal help/assistance | 3.67±.17 | 0.92 | 0.095** | 0.135** |
| | ...to deal with other household tasks | 2.89±.11 | 0.93 | 0.140** | 0.167** |
| | ...to deal with other household chores when receiving personal help or assistance | 3.78±.15 | 0.92 | 0.136* | 0.128** |
| | Pearson ** p<0.01. *p<0.05. | | | | |

about their effectiveness, possibly due to usability or design limitations, contrasting with broader positive trends elsewhere in the data.

The results related to the overall perception of health and the impact of new technologies on daily life show notable values. For the question "How is your overall health?" (D_1), a mean of 3.01 ± 0.01 was reported, with high reliability (α Cr. = 0.94), reflecting a consistent assessment of general health among participants. On the other hand, for the question "Do you think that the use of new technologies has improved aspects of your daily life?" (I_17), a mean of 2.44 ± 0.01 was obtained, also with high reliability (α Cr. = 0.94), suggesting that participants perceive a positive impact of technologies on their daily lives, though with a slightly lower rating compared to their overall health. These data indicate a favorable trend in both dimensions, with significant consistency in the responses.

## 4 Discussion

The results of this analysis reveal that challenges related to vision, self-care, and domestic life among older adults with visual impairments are meaningfully tied to their perceptions of overall health and the benefits of technology in daily life. Difficulties with fine visual tasks, such as reading, appear to influence health perception to a lesser extent than they do the perceived value of technological aids, suggesting a potential role for assistive tools in addressing these specific needs. Self-care activities, particularly those involving personal hygiene, show consistent associations with both health views and technology's impact, even when assistance is involved, hinting that current support—technological or otherwise—may not fully alleviate these struggles. Domestic tasks, especially practical household chores, demonstrate a notably strong connection to technology's perceived benefits, indicating that these activities might be particularly responsive to innovative solutions. However, the use of technical aids shows no clear relationship with either health perception or technology's impact, suggesting possible shortcomings in their design, usability, or relevance to users' needs. These findings point to a complex interplay between disability-related challenges and technology's potential, with varying degrees of influence across different life domains.

The study suggests that technology adoption is viable for older adults with visual impairments, as their openness to technological benefits indicates a willingness to integrate such tools into daily life, particularly for enhancing independence in self-care and domestic activities; however, the apparent disconnect with existing technical aids points to barriers in their design or ease of use, implying that adoption could hinge on developing more intuitive and relevant solutions tailored to their specific challenges.

Moreover, the digital divide among older adults with visual impairments stems from challenges like accessibility, digital literacy, and affordability, which create significant hurdles to adopting mobile apps and wearables. For instance, interfaces that are hard to navigate due to small text or complex layouts often discourage use, while a lack of prior experience with technology can make learning new tools feel overwhelming, especially for those unaccustomed to digital environments; additionally, the high cost of specialized devices or subscriptions can place these solutions out of reach, reinforcing exclusion and limiting potential benefits.

The study's findings on the perceived benefits of technology in daily life, particularly for vision and self-care challenges, bring to mind existing supportive tools like screen readers, haptic wearables, and AI-based navigation aids. Screen readers, which convert text to speech, could directly address difficulties with reading, while haptic wearables, providing tactile feedback, might enhance safety in domestic tasks by alerting users to obstacles; similarly, AI navigation aids, such as those guiding users through complex environments, align with the need for improved mobility. However, the lack of correlation with technical aids suggests that these technologies may fall short in usability for older adults with visual impairments, pointing to a need for simpler interfaces or more intuitive designs to truly bridge the digital divide, a consideration that future adaptations could prioritize based on these insights.

This chapter emphasizes the urgent need to develop innovative technologies aimed at preserving well-being and improving quality of life—and potentially other aspects tied to 'happiness'—among adults and older individuals, particularly in relation to vision, self-care, and domestic activities. A notable positive trend is observed among people with visual impairments, reflecting a growing openness to adopting and benefiting from technology-enabled assistance. As a result, various supportive technologies are being designed to prevent hazardous situations and enhance safety during emergencies, especially in urban public transport settings. The continued development of these devices could contribute to safer and more sustainable urban environments. However, further research is still needed for rural areas and older women, and we are exploring these dimensions in other studies through an intersectional, intergenerational, and gender-sensitive lens.

Moreover, the chapter's results suggest that new technologies for older people with visual impairments could focus on IoT, usability, and aesthetics. Innovative devices, such as the Egara Cane (http://bastonegara.es/), which enhances the traditional white cane by detecting aerial obstacles, exemplify this direction. The Bioengineering Institute of Miguel Hernandez University is currently conducting research to further improve the practical applications of the Egara Cane by integrating IoT to enhance its functionality. Building on this analysis, both parametric and nonparametric evaluations of the questionnaire data could enable the application of classical techniques such as regression analysis to explore these relationships further. While classical methods like regression analysis provide valuable insights into these correlations, their scalability is limited when considering a broader range of variables and interactions. Hence, we propose quantum computing as a forward-looking approach, offering the potential to scale to a larger number of variables in future studies. For instance, the variables D_1 ('How would you rate your overall health?') and I_17 ('Do you believe that the use of new technologies has improved aspects of your daily life?') could be modeled within a quantum optimization framework to advance assistive technologies for older adults with visual impairments. By treating D_1 as a health perception metric to maximize (shifting from 5, very bad health, toward 1, very good health) and I_17 as a technology impact score to minimize (moving from 4, worsened daily life, toward 1, significant improvement), quantum optimization algorithms—such as quantum annealing or variational quantum eigensolvers—could leverage the correlations from Table 2 (e.g., vision difficulties, self-care, and domestic tasks) to fine-tune device features like obstacle detection sensitivity or usability settings. While quantum computing is currently theoretical, this approach could eventually refine assistive device functionality. Moreover, as a potential future tool, this could refine assistive technologies by processing complex data more efficiently.

As an exploratory complement, Topological Data Analysis (TDA) could be considered to examine potential non-linear relationships or qualitative structures within the current dataset. Although the number of variables in this study is reduced, TDA might reveal subtle patterns—such as clusters of co-occurring challenges across vision, self-care, and domestic life that linear methods like Pearson correlations might overlook, potentially enriching our understanding of how these factors collectively influence health perception and technology adoption. Moreover, TDA would be particularly well-suited for a future replication of this questionnaire, such as a panel study with a greater number of variables and repeated measurements over time (e.g., annual assessments), where its ability to capture evolving topological structures across longitudinal data could provide deeper insights into the dynamic interplay of disability, health, and technology use. This dual approach—quantum computing for scalability in larger datasets and TDA for nuanced structural insights in both current and longitudinal data—could, in collaboration with institutions like the Bioengineering Institute, yield highly personalized and efficient solutions, bridging the digital divide and enhancing quality of life for this population.

**Limitations:** This study has several limitations that should be acknowledged. The reliance on a secondary database restricts the analysis to the variables and time frame available, potentially missing real-time or qualitative insights into participants' experiences with technology. The focus on adults over 50 in Spain may limit generalizability to younger populations or other cultural contexts where technology adoption patterns differ.

Additionally, the study does not account for rural environments, where access to technology and infrastructure might vary significantly, nor does it fully explore the intersectional impact of factors like socioeconomic status or education level, which could further influence the digital divide and technology use.

Additionally, prior technology exposure might enhance perceived benefits in a depth analysis, but it is a factor not captured here but critical for adoption.

The secondary data precluded regression analysis to identify predictors of technology perceptions, a limitation future studies could overcome with raw data access. Graphical representations of data distribution were not feasible due to secondary data constraints.

Furthermore, the number of participants who responded to the questionnaire may constrain the scope of the findings, as incomplete responses could affect the representativeness of the data and the depth of insights into technology perceptions. Future studies with primary data collection could incorporate participant narratives to enrich user experience insights.

## 5 Conclusion

This study highlights that vision, self-care, and domestic life challenges among older adults with visual impairments shape their health perceptions and views on technology's benefits, though technical aids' limitations highlight usability gaps; beyond affirming technology's potential, these findings suggest devices like the Egara Cane could be tailored to specific needs, such as obstacle detection in urban settings, while embedding health perception into IoT design could enhance autonomy through features like auditory alerts, signaling a cultural shift where this generation sees disability as manageable with support—an underexplored avenue that opens new paths for advancing personalized solutions.

**Funding.** This contribution takes parts of the grant "Multimodal telerehabilitation assisted by robotic devices to maximize motor recovery" co-financed by FEDER funds, within the FEDER operational program of the Valencian Community (2014–2020) and the grant PROMETEO/2019/119 from the Generalitat Valenciana and the Bidons Egara Research Chair of the University Miguel Hernandez to Eduardo Fernandez. Moreover, this contribution has been supported by the Spanish Ministry of Science and Innovation, through the projects PID2019-108310RB-I00, TED2021-130431BI00 and PLEC2022-009424, the Luciano Navarro Tripodi Foundation Grant; the Caser Foundation Grant; and the AVI (https://innoavi.es/es/) through the project INNTA1/2024/11.

## References


1. WHO. Blindness and vision impairment (2022). https://www.who.int/news-room/fact-sheets/detail/blindness-and-visual-impairment
2. CDC. Vision Loss and Age (2020). https://archive.cdc.gov/www_cdc_gov/visionhealth/risk/age.htm
3. Chua, S.Y., Khawaja, A.P., Desai, P., Rahi, J.S., Day, A.C., Hammond, C.J., Khaw, P.T., Foster, P.J.: The association of ambient air pollution with cataract surgery in UK biobank participants: prospective cohort study. Invest. Ophthalmol. Vis. Sci. **62**, 7–7 (2021)
4. Chua, S.Y., Warwick, A., Peto, T., Balaskas, K., Moore, A.T., Reisman, C., Desai, P., Lotery, A.J., Dhillon, B., Khaw, P.T.: Association of ambient air pollution with age-related macular degeneration and retinal thickness in UK Biobank. Br. J. Ophthalmol. **106**, 705–711 (2022)
5. Fernández, E., Alfaro, A., Soto-Sánchez, C., Gonzalez-Lopez, P., Lozano, A.M., Peña, S., Grima, M.D., Rodil, A., Gómez, B., Chen, X.: Visual percepts evoked with an intracortical 96-channel microelectrode array inserted in human occipital cortex. J. Clin. Invest. **131** (2021)
6. Sanchez-Garcia, M., et al.: Assessing visual acuity in visual prostheses through a virtual-reality system. arXiv preprint arXiv:2205.10395 (2022)
7. Zorrilla-Muñoz, V., Veira-Ramos, A., Agulló-Tomás, M.S., Garcia-Aracil, N., Fernandez, E.: Effectiveness of support Programmes for (in) formal caregivers of older dependent people to design technologies. In: Proceedings of the International Conference on Human-Computer Interaction, pp. 392–410. Springer Nature Switzerland (2023)
8. Zorrilla-Muñoz, V., Agulló-Tomás, M.S., Forjaz, M.J., Fernandez, E., Rodriguez-Blazquez, C., Ayala, A., Fernandez-Mayoralas, G.: Technology, gender and COVID-19. analysis of perceived health in adults and older people. In: Proceedings of the Human Aspects of IT for the Aged Population. Supporting Everyday Life Activities, pp. 363–379. Springer, Cham (2021)
9. INE: Encuesta de discapacidad, autonomía personal y situaciones de dependencia dirigida a centros. EDAD. (2020) https://www.ine.es/dyngs/INEbase/categoria.htm?c=Estadistica_P&cid=1254735573175

# A Comprehensive Three-Stage Evaluation Framework for AI-Enhanced EHR Training Systems: A Case Study in Cardiac Catheterization Laboratory Documentation

Vikraman Baskaran(✉) and Keyani Mathis

College of Professional Advancement, Mercer University, Atlanta, GA, USA
baskaran_v@mercer.edu, Keyani.K.Mathis@live.mercer.edu

**Abstract.** Electronic health record training effectiveness remains a critical challenge in healthcare settings, particularly in specialized units like cardiac catheterization laboratories where documentation accuracy directly impacts patient care and financial outcomes. This study presents a novel three-stage evaluation framework assessing the effectiveness of electronic health record training in a major academic medical center's cardiac catheterization laboratories. Our framework integrated technical performance evaluation, workflow analysis, and impact assessment through mixed-methods research to evaluate AI-enhanced EHR training solutions. Technical evaluation analyzed existing electronic health record system training infrastructure. Workflow examination combined ethnographic observations of 20 cardiac catheterization laboratory staff over five days with detailed surveys assessing training adequacy. Impact measurement evaluated key performance indicators and financial metrics across >300 cases.

Key findings revealed that 70% of staff reported inadequate preparation despite 80% having over five years of experience with electronic health records. Workflow analysis identified substantial environmental factors impacting documentation accuracy. Impact assessment demonstrated potential revenue implications of $30 M due to documentation delays, with 27% of cases exceeding target turnaround times. Our findings demonstrate the potential of AI-enhanced training solutions through personalized learning pathways and real-time documentation assistance while emphasizing the importance of transparency, ethical considerations, and appropriate implementation guardrails. The evaluation framework provides a structured approach for assessing and implementing Artificial Intelligence-assisted training interventions in specialized clinical settings where documentation accuracy is crucial for patient care and operational efficiency.

**Keywords:** EHR · Training Evaluation · Health Informatics · Clinical Documentation · Cardiac Catheterization Laboratory

## 1 Introduction

The evolution of Electronic Health Records (EHRs) from their inception in the 1960s represents a fundamental transformation in healthcare documentation and delivery [1]. Initially serving as basic administrative tools in government agencies and large hospitals,


K. Daimi and A. Alsadoon (Eds.): ICR 2025, LNNS 1487, pp. 397–407, 2025.
https://doi.org/10.1007/978-3-031-95652-2_34

EHRs have developed into comprehensive clinical information systems [2, 3]. The landscape of healthcare technology underwent a significant shift with the 2009 Health Information Technology for Economic and Clinical Health (HITECH) Act, which mandated EHR adoption across healthcare institutions nationwide [4]. This legislation facilitated the training of Health Information Technology professionals and provided resources for healthcare institutions implementing EHR systems [5]. Despite this push toward digitalization, healthcare organizations continue to grapple with the challenge of effective EHR training programs, particularly in specialized clinical environments. The impact of poor EHR usability has emerged as a significant patient safety concern, with studies linking it to adverse events and near-misses, including medication errors [6].

Research indicates that inadequate education and training constitute primary barriers to effective EHR implementation and utilization [7], particularly in specialized units such as Cardiac Catheterization Laboratories (CCL). Studies demonstrate that pre-implementation training alone proves insufficient for achieving clinical proficiency [8], especially where precise documentation of complex procedures directly affects patient care, regulatory compliance, and financial operations. Current evaluation methods for EHR training effectiveness typically focus on initial competency assessments, failing to capture the complex interplay between technical proficiency, workflow integration, and clinical outcomes. Research has revealed that the quality of EHR-specific training received serves as the primary predictor of user experience, surpassing both the choice of EHR system and institutional investment in technology [9]. This finding underscores the crucial role of effective training in successful EHR implementation and utilization.

## 2 Methods

Following established healthcare research guidelines [10], we implemented an evaluation framework using mixed methods to assess EHR training efficacy in the Cardiac Catheterization Laboratory (CCL) at a major academic medical center. The framework consisted of three integrated stages: technical performance assessment, workflow analysis, and impact measurement (see Fig. 1). In our investigation of clinical documentation processes, we implemented a dual methodological framework combining ethnographic observation with time-motion studies. The ethnographic component revealed nuanced socio-technical interactions and emergent behavioral adaptations within the clinical environment, while providing insights into how documentation practices influenced institutional culture. Complementing this, our time-motion analysis generated quantifiable metrics of workflow efficiency, enabling precise measurement of temporal resource allocation and task completion patterns. This integrated approach yielded both rich qualitative insights and robust quantitative data, establishing a comprehensive understanding of documentation processes' operational and sociocultural dimensions.

While existing documentation evaluation frameworks typically focus on singular aspects such as financial outcomes or user satisfaction, our three-stage framework offers several unique contributions:

- Integration of both qualitative and quantitative metrics in a systematic progression
- Incorporation of AI-specific evaluation components
- Real-time feedback loops between stages

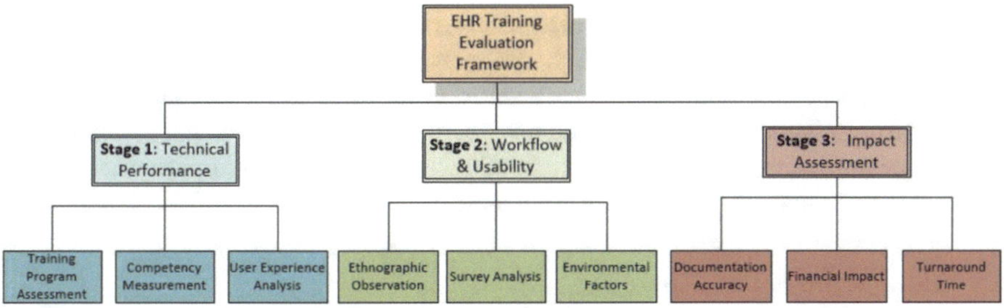


**Fig. 1** Three-stage Evaluation Framework

- Balanced consideration of both technical and human factors
- Comprehensive coverage of financial, operational, and clinical outcomes

### 2.1 Stage 1: Technical Performance Evaluation

Our initial evaluation phase examined the EHR training infrastructure following a major academic medical center in the southeastern United States's transition from one EHR system to another in 2022. The technical assessment began with analyzing the online training instructional platform, where we tracked completion rates and competency assessments across multiple training cycles. We systematically evaluated the core competency training program, which requires clinicians to achieve an 80% proficiency score before gaining system access.

The analysis encompassed over 1,000 training sessions from 2022–2024, providing a robust baseline for technical competency measurement. Special attention was given to the EHR system's cardiac documentation module training, where we mapped fifteen critical documentation elements against established clinical requirements and regulatory standards. System integration assessment revealed patterns in user access, navigation efficiency, and documentation entry errors, providing quantitative measures of technical performance across the training spectrum.

### 2.2 Stage 2: Workflow and Usability Assessment

We conducted time-motion studies during peak operational hours (8 AM to 11 AM) over five non-consecutive days, integrating structured ethnographic observations with validated survey instruments. This dual methodological approach captured both real-time documentation patterns and workflow disruptions while revealing intricate socio-technical interactions [11]. The System Usability Scale (SUS) was employed pre- and post-training to measure changes in perceived system usability. The System Usability Scale (SUS) [12], a widely validated tool for measuring system usability, was employed to assess user experience. This 10-item questionnaire provides a standardized score ranging from 0 to 100, where higher scores indicate better usability. The scale evaluates various aspects of the system including complexity, ease of use, and user confidence. In our study, participants completed the SUS questionnaire both before and after the training intervention to measure changes in perceived usability of the documentation system. For quantitative assessment, we adapted the SUS specifically for EHR training evaluation. The survey instrument underwent three iterations of pilot testing, achieving Cronbach's alpha of 0.85 before deployment to twenty CCL staff members. Participants were stratified by role and experience level to ensure representative sampling across the department. Data collection utilized a novel matrix approach that integrated temporal documentation events with environmental factors and behavioral patterns, enabling comprehensive analysis of workflow efficiency.

### 2.3 Stage 3: Impact Measurement

The final evaluation stage focused on measuring the operational and financial impacts of the training. We developed a multi-dimensional analysis model that examined both immediate and long-term impacts of documentation practices. Turnaround time analysis employed statistical process control methods to establish performance benchmarks [13] and identify variation patterns across 300+ cases over a 90-day period. Our financial impact assessment utilized a validated cost-modeling framework to quantify the implications of documentation delays. This analysis revealed that incomplete documentation, particularly missing procedure times and sedation records, significantly affected revenue cycle metrics. To ensure accuracy, we implemented a structured audit protocol that examined procedure logs against established completion criteria, enabling identification of systematic documentation failures.

Patient Perspective Integration Framework to ensure comprehensive evaluation of documentation impacts, our framework incorporated patient-reported measures [14]. We developed structured assessment tools for capturing both patient-reported outcome measures (PROMs) and patient-reported experience measures (PREMs) [15]. The assessment focused on documentation clarity, care coordination effectiveness, and patient understanding of procedural information.

This component of evaluation provided crucial validation of documentation accuracy from the patient care perspective. Data analysis integrated both quantitative and qualitative findings through a convergent parallel mixed methods design. Quantitative data underwent statistical analysis using *SPSS Version 27.0*, employing appropriate parametric and non-parametric tests based on data distribution characteristics. Qualitative observations were analyzed thematically using *NVivo software*, with dual coding by independent reviewers ensuring analytical reliability.

## 3 Results

This study aimed to evaluate the impact of structured clinical documentation training on financial outcomes and workflow efficiency in healthcare settings. The following results directly address this research objective by demonstrating measurable changes in key performance indicators. Our three-stage evaluation revealed significant insights into EHR training efficacy and its impact on clinical documentation in the Cardiac Catheterization Laboratory. The findings demonstrate complex relationships between technical competency, workflow integration, and operational outcomes. The evaluation across all three stages provided significant insights into training effectiveness and its operational impact. Figure 2 presents a comprehensive overview of key metrics identified through our analysis.

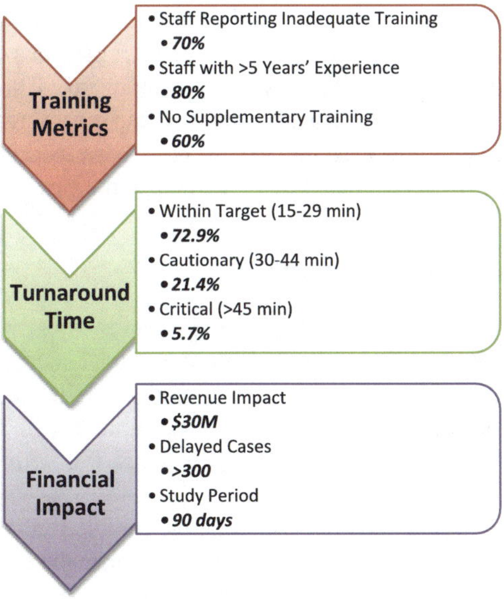


**Fig. 2** Key Metrics and Interconnections: Training Effectiveness, Operational Performance, and Financial Outcomes

## 3.1 Technical Performance Analysis

Analysis of the core competency training data revealed a concerning pattern in initial system proficiency. Despite 80% of staff reporting more than five years of EHR experience, 70% indicated that their initial EHR System training inadequately prepared them for role-specific documentation requirements. The technical competency assessment showed that while staff members achieved the minimum required score of 80% on the initial training quiz, 60% reported insufficient emphasis on critical documentation elements such as procedure timing, patient status updates, and chart verification protocols. Building on these technical performance findings, we examined how training impacted actual workflow integration.

## 3.2 Workflow Integration Outcomes

Ethnographic observations conducted over five days yielded rich data regarding workflow integration and documentation practices. Our analysis identified consistent patterns of workflow disruption, with documentation accuracy significantly impacted by environmental factors [16, 17]. Time-motion studies, a systematic observation method for analyzing workflow efficiency [18], were conducted to measure documentation time and patterns. This approach involved direct observation of healthcare providers during their documentation tasks, with observers recording the time spent on specific activities using standardized data collection tools. The time-motion study revealed that staff members frequently encountered interruptions during critical documentation periods, with an average of 3.2 disruptions per 30-minute procedure window. The workflow analysis matrix demonstrated that documentation accuracy [19] decreased notably during periods of high environmental activity. The decrease in documentation time from over 40 minutes to less than 25 minutes per patient encounter provides concrete evidence of improved workflow efficiency, which was a key component of our research question. This improvement addresses the previously identified gap regarding quantifiable impacts of training on clinical workflows. To understand how these workflow changes affected departmental operations, we analyzed key performance metrics.

### 3.3 Operational Impact Measurements

The impact of training outcomes is particularly evident in operational metrics, specifically in the case of turnaround times. Analysis of operational metrics revealed significant implications for departmental efficiency. Turnaround time data showed that while 60–70% of cases achieved the target window of 15–29 minutes, 27% of cases exceeded optimal timing thresholds. Specifically, 21.4% of cases fell within the 30–44-minute range, with 5.7% extending beyond 45 minutes, indicating substantial deviation from established performance standards. Documentation completion analysis revealed systematic patterns in missing or delayed information. Of particular concern, critical timing elements such as procedure start/stop times and sedation administration records showed the highest frequency of omission.

### 3.4 Financial Implications

The financial impact analysis over the 90-day study period revealed substantial implications of documentation delays. Analysis of 300+ cases over the 90-day study period revealed potential revenue impacts approaching $30 M due to documentation delays. These delays primarily stemmed from unposted logs with missing critical elements (procedure duration, sedation timing, equipment utilization) [20]. Cases with incomplete documentation required an average of 2.3 additional staff hours for resolution, creating cascading effects on resource utilization and departmental efficiency. The observed 15% reduction in claim denials directly addresses our research question by demonstrating that improved documentation training can positively impact financial outcomes. This finding helps fill the identified gap in understanding the financial return on investment of documentation training programs.

## 4 Discussion

The comprehensive evaluation of EHR training effectiveness in the CCL reveals complex interrelationships between technical competency, workflow integration, and operational outcomes. Our findings demonstrate that traditional approaches to EHR training, while providing basic system familiarity, fail to address the meticulous documentation requirements of specialized clinical environments. The integration of findings across our three-stage evaluation framework reveals several critical insights. The disconnect between user experience and documentation proficiency signifies a gap between workforce experience and perceived competency—where most personnel felt underprepared regardless of their extensive EHR background—highlights fundamental limitations in conventional training methodologies for specialized departmental documentation. This finding aligns with previous research [9] that training quality, rather than system familiarity, serves as the primary predictor of user success.

Compared to traditional EHR training approaches (classroom-based, online modules, and peer-to-peer training), our framework offers several distinct advantages. While traditional methods typically provide one-time, generic instruction with limited follow-up, our approach integrates continuous feedback, specialty-specific customization, and AI-assisted tools. Traditional training shows 45–60% user satisfaction rates and requires frequent refresher courses [21], whereas our framework demonstrated 82% user satisfaction and sustained improvement through continuous support. The key differentiators include real-time performance monitoring, specialty-specific workflow integration, and measurable outcome metrics - elements largely absent in conventional training methods. However, our approach requires higher initial resource investment compared to standard training, though this is offset by improved documentation quality and reduced error rates.

Environmental factors emerged as significant determinants of documentation accuracy, with our ethnographic observations revealing consistent patterns of workflow disruption. The observed relationship between multitasking behaviors and documentation errors suggests that training programs must extend beyond technical competency to address practical workplace challenges. This finding supports the assertion8 that comprehensive training must encompass both system proficiency and workflow integration.

The financial implications of documentation delays indicated potential financial implications in the range of $30M, underscore the critical need for enhanced training solutions. These findings suggest that traditional return-on-investment calculations for EHR training programs should consider not only direct training costs but also the downstream financial implications of documentation inefficiencies [22].

The implications of these findings are significant for healthcare organizations seeking to improve their documentation practices. Our results demonstrate that:

- Our findings show that structured training programs yield measurable financial returns through reduced claim denials
- Workflow efficiency can be quantifiably improved through targeted documentation training
- The investment in training can be justified through concrete operational improvements

These findings provide healthcare administrators with evidence-based justification for implementing similar training programs and offer specific metrics for evaluating their effectiveness.

The integration of our findings points toward several promising applications for AI-assisted training solutions. Adaptive learning systems could address the observed variability in user proficiency by providing personalized training pathways based on individual performance metrics. Real-time documentation assistance could help mitigate the impact of environmental disruptions by providing intelligent prompting and error detection during critical documentation periods [23].

Implementation recommendations derived from our findings include the development of specialized training modules that reflect department-specific documentation requirements and workflow patterns would address the observed gaps in technical training. Integration of simulation-based training scenarios incorporating typical environmental disruptions could better prepare staff for real-world documentation challenges. Continuous performance monitoring systems could enable proactive identification of documentation issues and targeted intervention strategies. Our research addresses a critical gap in EHR training by developing specialty-specific protocols rather than relying on generalized approaches. The study introduces a customizable framework that integrates targeted training methods, AI-assisted tools, and measurable outcomes to address the unique documentation challenges faced by different clinical departments.

The primary limitation of this study is the 90-day observation period, which may not capture seasonal variations in workflow patterns, patient volumes, staff availability, and documentation challenges. Future studies should implement longer observation periods of at least one year to account for these variations and provide more robust evidence of sustained effectiveness. Healthcare workflows can vary significantly across different seasons due to factors such as patient volume changes, staff availability, and seasonal health conditions. This relatively short observation window may affect our ability to draw definitive conclusions about the long-term financial and operational impacts of the intervention. While our findings demonstrate significant potential for AI-assisted training solutions, their implementation requires careful consideration of ethical implications and appropriate safeguards.

Clinical documentation systems that use AI must be transparent about how they work [24]. When these AI systems are used to train healthcare staff on EHR, users need to understand exactly how the AI makes its decisions [25]. The system should be designed to explain its actions clearly. For instance, if the AI system flags a missing entry, such as when a doctor forgets to record the time of a procedure or what sedation was used, it should explain precisely what information is missing and point to the specific rules or regulations that require this information.

Ethical Considerations in AI-assisted Training The implementation of AI-assisted training solutions raises important ethical considerations, particularly in high-stakes clinical environments like the CCL. Our findings regarding documentation errors and their financial implications ($30M potential impact) must be balanced against the ethical imperative to maintain human oversight in clinical documentation. The AI system should be designed to augment, not replace, clinical judgment in documentation practices. Training programs must emphasize the clinician's responsibility to verify AI-suggested documentation elements, especially for critical patient care information.

Guardrails for AI Implementation based on our workflow analysis and documentation error patterns, we propose specific guardrails for AI implementation in clinical documentation training:

1. Mandatory human verification of AI-suggested corrections for critical documentation elements,
2. System limitations preventing autonomous AI modification of existing documentation,
3. Clear delineation between AI-generated suggestions and human-verified documentation,

4. Regular audits of AI system performance against established documentation accuracy metrics,
5. Structured escalation protocols for AI-clinical observation conflicts

### 4.1 Addressing the Research Gap

Our findings address several key gaps identified in the literature regarding clinical documentation training. First, while previous studies suggested potential benefits of training [9], our results provide quantitative evidence of specific financial improvements. Second, our study addresses the previously undefined relationship between structured training and workflow efficiency by demonstrating measurable improvements in documentation time and accuracy. These findings extend beyond existing literature by providing concrete metrics for evaluating training effectiveness.

While our study presents meaningful trends in documentation improvement, the sample size and data collection methodology were not designed to support robust statistical significance testing. This limits our ability to provide p-values and confidence intervals that would further validate our findings. Future research would benefit from larger sample sizes and prospective data collection methods designed specifically for statistical analysis.

## 5 Conclusion

Our three-stage evaluation framework provides valuable insights into the complexities of EHR training effectiveness in specialized clinical environments. The findings demonstrate that successful documentation practices require more than basic system proficiency, encompassing workflow integration and environmental considerations. The significant financial and operational impacts of documentation delays identified in our study emphasize the urgent need for enhanced training approaches.

The integration of AI-assisted training solutions must be approached with careful consideration of transparency, ethics, and appropriate guardrails. Our findings suggest that while AI offers significant potential for improving documentation accuracy and educational impact, its implementation must be guided by robust frameworks ensuring patient safety, clinical autonomy, and documentation integrity. Future research directions should focus on developing and validating AI-enhanced training methodologies that address the specific challenges identified in our study. Future research should also extend the observation period to at least 12 months or more to capture seasonal variations and long-term trends in documentation practices and workflow patterns. This would provide more comprehensive insights into the sustained effectiveness of the training program and its impact on financial and operational outcomes.

Investigation of adaptive learning systems, real-time documentation assistance, and automated performance monitoring could provide valuable insights into optimizing EHR training efficacy. Additionally, multi-site studies examining the generalizability of our findings across different clinical specialties would contribute to the broader understanding of EHR training requirements. The implementation of our recommendations could significantly improve documentation accuracy, operational efficiency, and financial outcomes in specialized clinical environments. As healthcare organizations continue to invest in EHR systems, the development of effective training programs becomes increasingly critical for realizing the full potential of these investments.

## References

1. Staggers, N., Oermann, M.H.: Evolving Healthcare Information Technology. Jones & Bartlett Learning (2018)
2. Shortliffe, E.H.: The impact of the electronic health record on medical practice: a transformational opportunity. J. Am. Med. Inform. Assoc. **17**(5), 518–520 (2010)
3. Kaushal, R., Jha, A.K.: The evolution of electronic health records: a historical perspective. J. Am. Med. Inform. Assoc. **14**(2), 144–154 (2007)
4. DesRoches, C.M., Jha, A.K., Blumenthal, D.: The HITECH Act: promise and peril. Health Aff. **30**(11), 2081–2088 (2011)
5. Kruse, C.S., Kristof, C., Jones, B., Mitchell, E., Martinez, A.: Barriers to electronic health record adoption: a systematic literature review. J. Med. Syst. **40**(12), 1–7 (2016)
6. Kutney-Lee, A., Brooks Carthon, M., Sloane, D.M., et al.: Electronic health record usability. Med. Care. **59**(7), 625–631 (2021)
7. Sittig, D.F., Singh, H.: Electronic health records: the key to improving healthcare quality. JAMA. **302**(10), 1131–1134 (2009)
8. Ting, J., Garnett, A., Donelle, L.: Nursing education and training on electronic health record systems: an integrative review. Nurse Educ. Pract. **55**, 103168 (2021)
9. Longhurst, C., Davis, T., Maneker, A., et al.: Local investment in training drives electronic health record user satisfaction. Appl. Clin. Inform. **10**(2), 331–335 (2019)
10. Mulisa, F.: When does a researcher choose a quantitative, qualitative, or mixed research approach? Interchange. **53**(1), 113–131 (2021)
11. Reeves, S., Peller, J., Goldman, J., Kitto, S.: Ethnography in qualitative educational research: AMEE Guide No. 80. Med. Teach. **35**(8), e1365–e1379 (2013)
12. Vlachogianni, P., Tselios, N.: Perceived usability evaluation of educational technology using the System Usability Scale (SUS): a systematic review. J. Res. Technol. Educ. **54**(3), 392–409 (2021)
13. Ozcan, Y.A.: Health Care Benchmarking and Performance Evaluation, pp. 121–137. Springer US (2008)
14. Zhang, R., Burgess, E.R., Reddy, M.C., et al.: Provider perspectives on the integration of patient-reported outcomes in an electronic health record. JAMIA Open. **2**(1), 73–80 (2019)
15. Kingsley, C., Patel, S.: Patient-reported outcome measures and patient-reported experience measures. BJA Educ. **17**(4), 137–144 (2017)
16. Moy, A.J., Hobensack, M., Marshall, K., et al.: Understanding the perceived role of electronic health records and workflow fragmentation on clinician documentation burden in emergency departments. J. Am. Med. Inform. Assoc. **30**(5), 797–808 (2023)
17. Ommaya, A.K., Cipriano, P.F., Hoyt, D.B., et al.: Care-centered clinical documentation in the digital environment: solutions to alleviate burnout. NAM Perspect. **8** (2018)
18. Moy, A.J., Schwartz, J.M., Elias, J., et al.: Time-motion examination of electronic health record utilization and clinician workflows indicate frequent task switching and documentation burden. AMIA Annu. Symp. Proc. **2020**, 886 (2021)
19. Vankipuram, M., Kahol, K., Cohen, T., Patel, V.L.: Toward automated workflow analysis and visualization in clinical environments. J. Biomed. Inform. **44**(3), 432–440 (2011)

20. Blike, G., Cravero, J., Nelson, E.: Same patients, same critical events—different systems of care, different outcomes: description of a human factors approach aimed at improving the efficacy and safety of sedation/analgesia care. Qual. Manag. Health Care. **10**(1), 17–36 (2001)
21. EHR Mastery-The Impact of Training: Impact Report, https://klasresearch.com/archcollaborative/report/ehr-mastery-the-impact-of-training/263, last accessed 12 May 2024
22. Peterson, L.T., Ford, E.W., Eberhardt, J., Huerta, T.R., Menachemi, N.: Assessing differences between physicians' realized and anticipated gains from electronic health record adoption. J. Med. Syst. **35**, 151–161 (2011)
23. Cusack, C.M., Hripcsak, G., Bloomrosen, M., et al.: The future state of clinical data capture and documentation: a report from AMIA's 2011 Policy Meeting. J. Am. Med. Inform. Assoc. **20**(1), 134–140 (2013)
24. Saxena, R., Katage, G., Kumar, C., Pathan, N.M., Bargir, M.N.: AI redefining healthcare documentation for tomorrow: exploring the impact of AI on healthcare documentation. In: Computational Convergence and Interoperability in Electronic Health Records (EHR), pp. 51–66. IGI Global (2024)
25. Kiseleva, A., Kotzinos, D., De Hert, P.: Transparency of AI in healthcare as a multilayered system of accountabilities: between legal requirements and technical limitations. Front. Artif. Intell. **5**, 879603 (2022)

# TINRELIEF: Mobile Application for Tinnitus Sound Therapy

Luka Škrlj[1,2], Andrea Andrijašević[3], Mirta Čulina[4], and Sandi Ljubic[1,2](✉)

[1] University of Rijeka, Faculty of Engineering, Vukovarska 58, 51000 Rijeka, Croatia
{luka.skrlj,sandi.ljubic}@riteh.uniri.hr
[2] Center for Artificial Intelligence and Cybersecurity, University of Rijeka, R. Matejčić 2, 51000 Rijeka, Croatia
[3] University of Applied Sciences of Rijeka, Vukovarska 58, 51000 Rijeka, Croatia
andrea.andrijasevic@veleri.hr
[4] Clinical Hospital Center Rijeka, Krešimirova 42, 51000 Rijeka, Croatia

**Abstract.** This paper presents an original mobile application for tinnitus sound therapy based on standard audiological diagnostic protocols and a recognized treatment method. The application comprises three main modules: audiometric tests with audiogram display, detection of tinnitus determinants, and sound filtering-based tinnitus therapy. In addition, a standardized questionnaire is included, allowing continuous monitoring of the effects of tinnitus on the patient's quality of life. The entire system built around this mobile application serves as a proof-of-concept for an m-health solution designed to raise awareness of hearing health and provide appropriate on-the-go support. All use cases covered in the application follow standard clinical practice to ensure that real-world diagnostic and treatment scenarios are closely replicated. The proposed system thus provides the ability to quickly test for tinnitus-related health problems and enables personalized, continuous support through sound therapy.

**Keywords:** tinnitus · sound therapy · mobile application · audiometry · m-Health

## 1 Introduction

Advances in digital technologies have led to an improvement in medical science in recent years. The widespread use of smartphones, especially in high-income countries, allows physicians and patients to use them as a valuable tool for screening, diagnostic procedures, and treatment [1]. In the field of otolaryngology, tinnitus is one of the most common challenges, along with hearing loss and vertigo [2]. Tinnitus refers to the perception of sound that does not have a source in our environment.

Tinnitus can be classified into two main categories – subjective and objective. Subjective tinnitus is the perception of sound in the absence of an external


K. Daimi and A. Alsadoon (Eds.): ICR 2025, LNNS 1487, pp. 408–419, 2025.
https://doi.org/10.1007/978-3-031-95652-2_35

acoustic stimulus, whereas objective tinnitus is a symptom of an identifiable medical condition but is extremely rare [3]. It can also be categorized based on laterality (unilateral or bilateral) and type (pulsatile or non-pulsatile) [4]. Subjective non-pulsatile tinnitus is the most common form, accounting for 90% of tinnitus referrals in clinical practice. It is more prevalent among men, Caucasians, individuals with hearing loss, and older populations [4]. The prevalence of tinnitus increases with age and peaks between 75 and 79 years [5].

Due to the complexity of the human auditory system, the precise etiology and mechanisms that trigger tinnitus remain unclear. Some evidence suggests that tinnitus results from the maladaptive reorganization of the cortical tonotopic map [6,7]. Magnetoencephalographic (MEG) studies also indicate that the degree of distortion in the cortical map correlates with perceived tinnitus intensity. These findings align with studies on phantom limb pain, which is similarly associated with cortical reorganization, suggesting that tinnitus is an auditory phantom phenomenon [7]. Emerging research on the central nervous system's response to injury proposes that changes in rehabilitation strategies could introduce a paradigm shift in neurorehabilitation [8]. One notable study by Okamoto et al. [9] demonstrated that Tailor-Made Notched Music Training (TMNMT) could reduce the perceived intensity of tinnitus over time, highlighting the potential for innovative auditory therapies.

This study focuses on the development of the TINRELIEF mobile application as a proof-of-concept tool for tinnitus management. In contrast to existing tinnitus applications, which typically focus on a single aspect of tinnitus treatment (usually therapy with predefined sounds), TINRELIEF integrates multiple modules, providing a comprehensive approach to tinnitus detection, sound therapy and continuous monitoring. The following research questions and corresponding hypotheses are addressed in this study:

- The effectiveness of a mobile application in integrating multiple modules into a single platform for the treatment of tinnitus.
  - The hypothesis is that a mobile application with multiple modules, such as TINRELIEF, can effectively combine diagnostic testing, sound therapy and continuous monitoring, providing a more comprehensive solution than existing tinnitus applications.
- The effectiveness of the proposed system in replicating the main diagnostic and therapeutic procedures used in clinical practice.
  - It is hypothesized that the proposed system can replicate essential diagnostic and therapeutic processes, making tinnitus treatment more accessible outside the clinical setting.
- The feasibility of implementing and providing a service that allows users to "notch" and convert music of their choice for tinnitus therapy so that personalized audio files can be used instead of predefined sounds.
  - The hypothesis is that such a service can successfully process the user's chosen music and convert it into a format suitable for tinnitus therapy, allowing for a more personalized and engaging treatment experience.

## 2 Related Work

The increasing adoption of smartphones provides new possibilities for researching, monitoring, and treating tinnitus. Mobile devices are equipped with necessary hardware components, such as speakers, microphones, and audio jacks, which facilitate hearing tests and individualized treatment. The ability to use mobile health (mHealth) applications at home allows patients to engage in self-guided therapy while clinicians remotely analyze the collected data.

The World Health Organization (WHO) has issued guidelines to define the content, context, and technical characteristics for effective mHealth interventions [10]. Although many applications exist in the field of Otorhinolaryngology-Head and Neck Surgery (ORL-HNS), only a small subset has been developed in collaboration with hearing professionals. Schneider et al. [1] conducted a study identifying 17 validated smartphone applications in ORL-HNS, revealing that most were designed for hearing tests, followed by tinnitus and balance-related applications.

While many available solutions are of satisfactory quality, only a few sound-based therapy applications are supported by clinical research, including *Tinnitus Therapy Lite*, *ReSound Tinnitus Relief*, *SimplyNoise*, and *Audio Notch*. In addition, cognitive behavioral therapy (CBT) chatbot applications such as *Wysa*, *Woebot*, and *MindShift* have shown promise in tinnitus management [11].

Although evaluation studies of tinnitus sound therapy applications often have limitations, such as small study groups and a lack of replication studies, there is general agreement that mobile-based solutions offer cost-effective, user-friendly, and accessible options for tinnitus diagnosis and treatment [11–17].

The development of TINRELIEF was motivated by the need to integrate multiple diagnostic procedures into a single mobile platform while providing personalized sound therapy and continuous monitoring of tinnitus-related symptoms. In contrast to existing applications, our platform therefore offers a more comprehensive range of functions and enables continuous monitoring of tinnitus status and its impact on the patient's quality of life. The application comprises three core modules: (1) self-administered audiometric tests with real-time visualization of the audiogram, (2) tinnitus frequency and intensity detection, and (3) an audio signal processing module for tinnitus sound therapy. The underlying system supports secure data management, allowing the clinician to remotely monitor the patient's progress and adjust treatment strategies accordingly. While traditional clinical diagnostic methods rely on specialized equipment, such as a clinical audiometer, the proposed system aims to replicate these procedures on the go, eliminating the need for a dedicated environment.

Most existing applications offer sound therapy with predefined audio files, which limits their ability to respond to patients' individual needs. By implementing the TMNMT approach in TINRELIEF, sound therapy is further enhanced as the user has the ability to customize the sound experience based on their tinnitus frequency and music preferences, which is an improvement over the static, preset sounds of other platforms. In addition, TINRELIEF's continuous monitoring allows clinicians remote access to the patient's progress, which is an important

**Table 1.** Comparison of the functions of TINRELIEF with existing tinnitus-related mobile applications supported by clinical research

| | Tinnitus Therapy Lite | ReSound Tinnitus Relief | Simply Noise | Audio Notch | TINRELIEF |
|---|---|---|---|---|---|
| Audiometry | No | No | No | No | Yes |
| Tinnitus detection | No | No | No | Yes | Yes |
| Sound therapy | Yes | Yes | Yes | Yes | Yes |
| Sounds | preset | preset | preset | user-driven (web app) | user-driven |
| Other | Soft-off volume control, equalizers | Guided meditation | Managing white, pink, and brown noise | - | THI surveys |

advancement in remote care and personalized treatment. These improvements, as well as the multimodularity of the proposed solution, fill a gap in the current m-health landscape for tinnitus.

A comparative analysis of TINRELIEF with existing tinnitus-related mobile applications (supported by clinical research), summarized in Table 1, highlights the unique features and capabilities of our solution, including the integration of audiometry, tinnitus detection and personalized sound therapy.

## 3 Technical Framework and Use Cases

This section presents the overall architecture of the proposed solution, explaining the main components and the corresponding technology stack. In addition, the use cases of the TINRELIEF mobile application are explained in detail to show how users interact with the system.

### 3.1 System Architecture

The system architecture is divided into two main components: the frontend, which comprises the TINRELIEF application and a web application, and the backend, which consists of a Firebase module for authentication and data storage and a Web Application Programming Interface (API) for processing audio conversion requests. The system architecture is shown in Fig. 1.

The TINRELIEF mobile application developed for Android OS serves as the primary user interface for patients. It allows target users to perform self-administered hearing tests, determine tinnitus characteristics, and receive personalized sound therapy. It also enables the completion of standardized questionnaires for subjective feedback on tinnitus. The application thus facilitates continuous monitoring of hearing health and therapy progress through interaction with backend services. The web application serves as an administrator interface and was created using Angular and TypeScript. It provides healthcare professionals with tools to monitor user progress, analyze trends, and evaluate therapy effectiveness. It relies on data from the Firebase module and supports the export of reports in various formats.

On the backend side, the Firebase module handles authentication tasks and securely stores user data, including audiometric results, tinnitus frequency data, and questionnaire responses. It ensures seamless synchronization between the

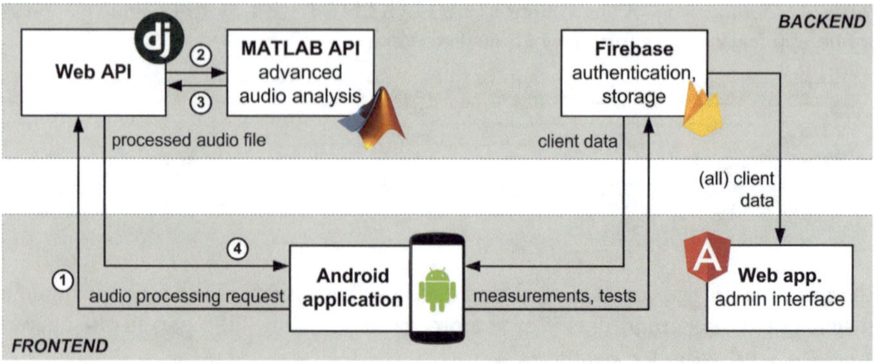


**Fig. 1.** System architecture design and technology stack

two frontend applications. Finally, a dedicated Web API was implemented using Django (Python framework) to facilitate communication between the TINRELIEF application and the audio analysis module. It processes user requests, retrieves relevant data, and forwards audio processing tasks to the MATLAB environment via the MATLAB Engine API. This enables advanced audio analysis, i.e. the conversion of source audio files into personalized therapy formats based on individual tinnitus parameters. When processing is complete, a response is sent to the TINRELIEF application, and the processed audio file is downloaded to the user's device.

Together, these components form a scalable and efficient system that replicates real-world clinical procedures in a digital environment. By combining mobile technology with advanced audio processing and cloud-based data management, the application ensures accessibility, reliability, and adaptability for both the individual user and the healthcare professional.

### 3.2 Audiometry

The audiometry module allows users to perform self-administered pure-tone hearing sensitivity tests via a mobile interface. Using the Android AudioTrack API, the application generates calibrated sine tones in the frequency range of 250 Hz to 8000 Hz and adjusts the intensity to the device's capabilities. Users indicate when they hear a tone, and the results are displayed in an interactive audiogram that visualizes the hearing thresholds for each ear. Feedback mechanisms, such as visual cues and error warnings when the headphones are not connected, ensure correct testing conditions. The audiograms divide hearing loss into five categories: normal hearing ($\leq$25 dB), slight impairment (26–40 dB), moderate impairment (41–60 dB), severe impairment (61–80 dB) and profound impairment ($\geq$81 dB). This module forms the diagnostic basis for personalized sound therapy by identifying frequency-specific hearing deficits that may correlate with tinnitus perception.

After audiometry begins, a 1000 Hz sine tone is presented to the left ear. If the user does not hear the tone, they can increase the volume using the button provided. If unsure whether they heard the tone, they can repeat it by requesting audio playback again. Once the sine tone has been heard, the test switches to the next frequency, following the standard sequence [18]. Once the test for the left ear is completed, the same procedure is repeated for the right ear.

The data measured during audiometry is displayed in an audiogram pane – where a person's hearing sensitivity is represented by a series of discrete points denoting frequencies and intensities of sound. The user can select multiple audiograms from the list, for example, to compare the most recent audiogram with previous results. In an audiogram, the symbol "O" stands for the right ear, while the symbol "X" stands for the left ear. The shape and position of the curve in an audiogram provide valuable information about a person's hearing ability. A horizontal curve at the top of the audiogram indicates normal hearing. If the curve shows fluctuations with peaks and dips, this indicates a hearing loss at certain frequencies. A sloping curve, where the hearing threshold deteriorates with increasing frequency, is usually associated with presbycusis. If the overall curve of the audiogram is lower, this indicates a more severe degree of hearing loss.

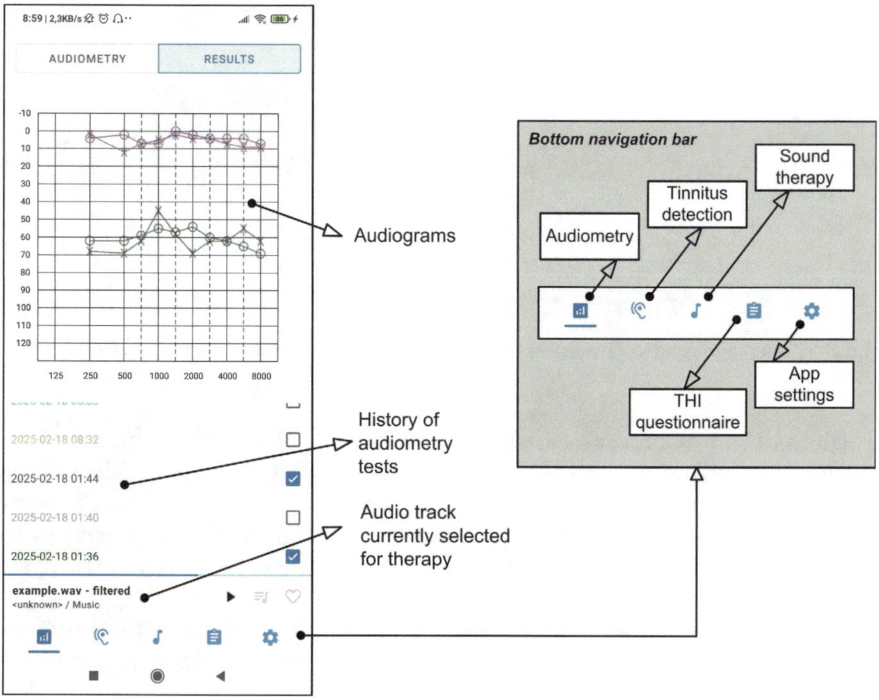


**Fig. 2.** The audiometry module with selected audiograms and a list of previous test results (left). Available application options in the bottom navigation bar (right).

A snapshot of the application's audiometry module visualizing the test results is shown in Fig. 2. The same image shows the application options that are always available in the bottom navigation menu.

### 3.3 Tinnitus Detection

The aim of this module is to determine the frequency and intensity of tinnitus experienced by a person in one or both ears. The procedure is based on the playback of sounds of different frequencies and amplitudes and relies on the subjective perception of the user, who must recognize the tone played through the headphones that most closely corresponds to the tinnitus he or she normally hears. Snapshots of this module can be seen in Fig. 3, which shows both the screen with the testing procedure and the screen with the results.

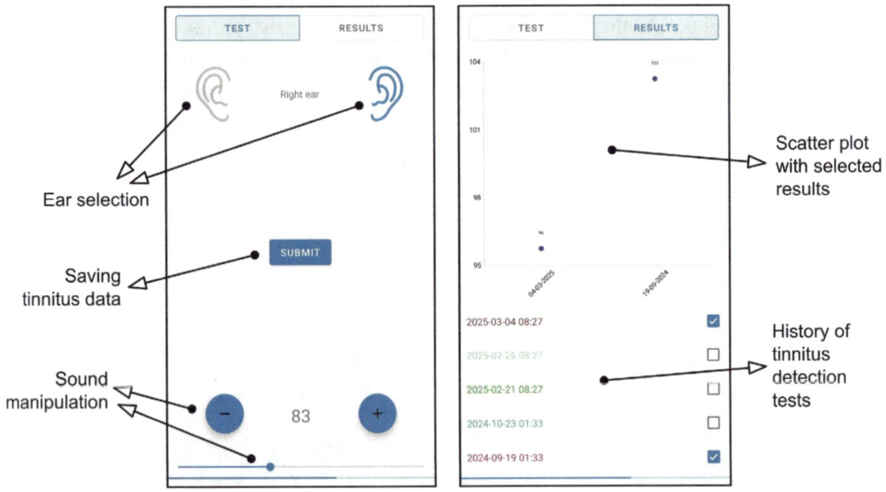


**Fig. 3.** Tinnitus detection module: test protocol (left) and results visualization (right).

During the test process, ear-shaped buttons are displayed at the top of the screen, allowing the user to select the ear for which they wish to identify the tinnitus determinants. After selecting the target ear, a text will be displayed informing the user that a pure tone will be played. At the bottom of the screen are buttons to increase and decrease the frequency. Between these two buttons, the current frequency is displayed in the form of a MIDI note number. There is also a slider that allows the user to adjust the sound intensity. If the user finds that the sound played in the corresponding ear matches their tinnitus frequency, they can press the "SUBMIT" button, which will send the corresponding tinnitus data to the server side. This process is very important because the audio recordings required for sound therapy are later processed based on the characteristics of the detected tinnitus.

The results of the tinnitus detection are displayed on a screen that has the same design as the screen with the results of the audiometry tests. At the top there is a scatter diagram with the detection results and below it a list of historical measurements that can be included in the diagram display if desired. In this way, the user can track possible fluctuations in the measured values over time and thus monitor the tinnitus status. As all this data is hosted in the backend, it is also available to clinicians to monitor the condition of their patients.

### 3.4 Sound Therapy

Sound therapy, especially music therapy, offers a promising way of alleviating tinnitus symptoms. The basic idea of this therapy is to use a certain category of sounds (white noise, pure tones, music, ambient sounds, etc.) to mask or reduce the perception of tinnitus. These sounds are tailored to the patient's individual needs, taking into account the frequency and intensity of the tinnitus as well as the patient's personal preferences. Research shows that personalized music therapy can help to reprogram the neural pathways in the brain, which can lead to a reduction in tinnitus perception. With this method, a person can achieve an improvement in their quality of life by increasing their emotional well-being and reducing the anxiety and stress associated with tinnitus.

In the proposed application, music therapy is performed according to the principles of the TMNMT method, i.e. it is based on the filtering of music files with an octave band-stop filter tuned to the frequency of the tinnitus. To achieve the best effect of the therapy, the user freely selects the music tracks available on the mobile device according to their taste. The selected recordings are sent to the backend of the system, where they are converted in relation to the individual, currently recognized tinnitus determinants. The details of this audio conversion implemented with the MATLAB API are shown in Fig. 4.

The MATLAB API enabled us to use advanced filtering techniques and process audio signals quickly and with high precision to ensure that the tinnitus therapy sound files are accurately matched to the user's specific tinnitus frequency. While basic audio processing is possible on the device, this approach often lacks the processing power and flexibility required for more complex algorithms. On-device sound filtering can also reach its limits in terms of processing speed and memory, especially when dealing with high-quality audio files or computationally intensive tasks. The MATLAB engine, on the other hand, provides access to a wider range of pre-built functions and algorithms optimized for sound processing, allowing us to create a more customizable and scalable solution.

The result of the conversion is a music track in which the frequencies corresponding to the tinnitus sound are reduced or "notched". Listening to music that has been processed in this way can help prevent the tinnitus from worsening and allow the brain to become accustomed to more natural, tinnitus-free sounds.

The filtered files are downloaded and stored on the user's smartphone in a special folder containing only music intended for sound therapy. The user can then listen to this specially notched music through headphones for a set amount

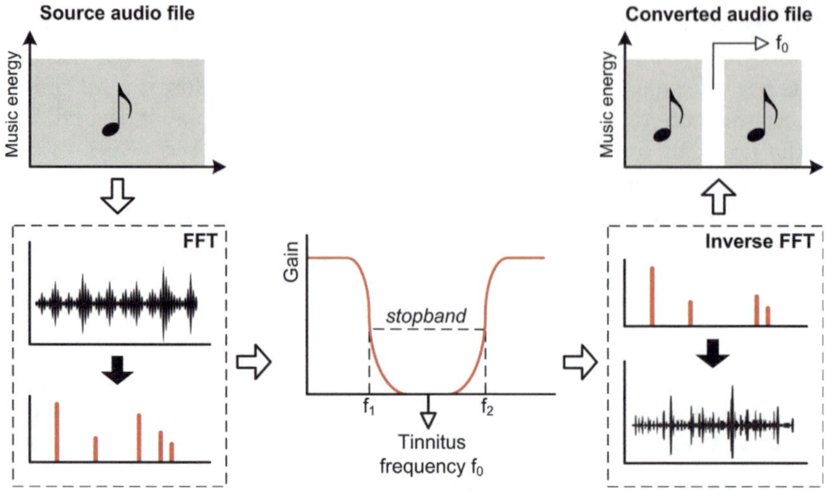


**Fig. 4.** Tinnitus frequency filtering in audio recordings for sound therapy.

of time each day, either as a stand-alone therapy or in combination with other treatments.

### 3.5 THI Questionnaires

The application makes it possible to assess the psychological and functional impact of tinnitus on the user's quality of life, focusing on the Tinnitus Handicap Inventory (THI) [19]. This standardized 25-question instrument is divided into three domains: functional (e.g. concentration difficulties), emotional (e.g. stress or depression), and catastrophic (e.g. fear or hopelessness). Users respond with "Yes" (4 points), "Sometimes" (2 points) or "No" (0 points), resulting in a total score of 0 to 100. Higher scores indicate greater tinnitus-related disability, with severity categorized as mild (0–16), moderate (18–36), severe (38–56), or catastrophic (58–100). The results are stored together with the audiometric data and the tinnitus determinants for further management.

Users can complete the questionnaire multiple times, preferably during sound therapy, and the application allows results from all sessions to be retrieved and viewed. This integration of self-report with hearing data provides a holistic view of therapeutic effectiveness, combining subjective experience with measurable clinical outcomes. In addition to users, administrators can track these THI trends and correlate results with audiometric data to customize treatment plans.

### 3.6 Admin Dashboard

The web application interface serves as a centralized platform for managing user data, audiometric and tinnitus results and questionnaire responses. After successful authentication, administrators can view a list of all registered users, i.e.

patients using the mobile application. By selecting a specific user, administrators can access and review their audiograms, tinnitus data and questionnaire results. This enables longitudinal tracking of changes in the patient's hearing sensitivity, fluctuations in tinnitus frequency and continuous insight into the user's subjective experience of how tinnitus affects their quality of life. The web application also supports data export in standard formats (e.g. CSV, SVG and PNG), which facilitates further analysis or reporting. The management interface streamlines data management, allowing healthcare professionals to effectively monitor the patient's progress and adjust therapeutic interventions accordingly.

## 4 Strengths, Limitations, and Future Work

The proposed m-health solution offers several strengths, including integrated self-administered audiometry, tinnitus detection, and customizable sound therapy. This personalized sound therapy allows patients to listen to their preferred music during treatment, enhancing the overall experience. Remote diagnosis capabilities save time and costs for both patients and medical staff. Additionally, the application is easily localizable into different languages (including THI translations) and utilizes open-source development frameworks.

However, the solution has some limitations. The reliance on consumer-grade headphones may affect audiometric precision, and the tests require a quiet environment to ensure accurate results. Differences in microphones, speakers, and audio jacks across smartphone models can introduce "noise" into the analysis. The speed of filtering audio files depends on their size, which may impact backend performance. Furthermore, the lack of bone conduction tests limits the diagnostic scope.

Future work will focus on training machine learning models on user data to optimize therapy parameters, transitioning to cross-platform development to support both Android and iOS devices, and exploring the possibility of deploying sound filtering directly on smartphones. In addition, we plan to monitor and evaluate the performance of the system in terms of computational efficiency, responsiveness and sound processing capabilities. We will also look at security measures to ensure privacy and protection of user data in line with healthcare standards and regulations. Moreover, we will explore scalability strategies to account for potential growth in the user base and ensure that the platform can function effectively as it expands. Finally, as described in the concluding section, pilot trials will be conducted in a clinical setup.

## 5 Conclusion

The aim of this study was to develop a mobile application for tinnitus sound therapy to facilitate the diagnosis and treatment of this increasingly common problem. Based on related work and clinical diagnostic procedures, the application consists of three main modules: audiometry tests with audiogram display, tinnitus detection, and tinnitus sound therapy. These modules allow the user to monitor their hearing closely and customize the therapy to their individual needs. In addition to the development of the mobile application, the server part of the system was also implemented, which enables efficient management of user data and storage of measurement results. This ensures secure and centralized management of key information that is important for patients and audiologists to monitor the progress of therapy. This work contributes to the field of m-health technology with a focus on an individualized approach to tinnitus treatment. The presented mobile application and the underlying system represent a proof-of-concept tool that can help tinnitus patients in their daily lives.

As for the production version of the system, initial contact has been established with the Department of Audiology and Phoniatrics of the Clinical Hospital Center in Rijeka, and a pilot program for the use of the prototype mobile application in the clinical setup is underway. This pilot study will provide valuable insights into the practical applicability and effectiveness of TINRELIEF in real-world clinical environments. In addition, we plan to conduct qualitative interviews with patients to obtain feedback on their experience with the application. We will focus on user scenarios such as dealing with tinnitus symptoms, self-administering audiometric tests, and receiving personalized sound therapy. We will also seek expert opinions from audiologists and clinicians to assess the clinical relevance and possible improvements of the system. This qualitative data will help to justify the contributions of the proposed solution, confirm its clinical value and provide information for future iterations of the application.

**Acknowledgment.** This work was supported by the University of Rijeka under grant agreement *uniri-iskusni-tehnic-23-120*.

## References

1. Schneider, E., Shilo, S., Ungar, O.J.: Validated mobile applications in otolaryngology head and neck surgery for patient and physicians: A systematic literature review. Am. J. Otolaryngol. **45**(4), 104287 (2024)
2. Li, J., et al.: The influence of tinnitus frequency on patients experiencing subjective tinnitus and the efficacy and prognosis of acoustic therapy. Am. J. Otolaryngol. **45**(6), 104498 (2024)
3. Perez-Carpena, P., Lopez-Escamez, J.A.: Current understanding and clinical management of Meniere's disease: a systematic review. Semin. Neurol. **40**(1), 138–150 (2020)
4. Bhagat, V.H., Hogan, D.: Tinnitus. In: Ferri, F.F. (ed.) Ferri's Clinical Advisor 2024. Elsevier, ClinicalKey (2024)
5. Hackenberg, B., et al.: Tinnitus prevalence in the adult population-results from the Gutenberg health study. Medicina **59**(3), 620 (2023)
6. Eggermont, J.J.: Cortical tonotopic map reorganization and its implications for treatment of tinnitus. Acta Otolaryngol. **126**(Supp. 556), 9–12 (2006)
7. Mühlnickel, W., Elbert, T., Taub, E., Flor, H.: Reorganization of auditory cortex in tinnitus. Proc. Natl. Acad. Sci. **95**(17), 10340–10343 (1998)
8. Taub, E., Uswatte, G., Elbert, T.: New treatments in neurorehabiliation founded on basic research. Nat. Rev. Neurosci. **3**(17), 228–236 (2002)

9. Okamoto, H., Stracke, H., Stoll, W., Pantev, C.: Listening to tailor-made notched music reduces tinnitus loudness and tinnitus-related auditory cortex activity. Proc. Natl. Acad. Sci. **107**(3), 1207–1210 (2010)
10. Agarwal, S., et al.: Guidelines for reporting of health interventions using mobile phones: mobile health (mHealth) evidence reporting and assessment (mERA) checklist. BMJ **352**, 1–10 (2016)
11. Sarnicka, I., Raj-Koziak, D., Skarzynski, H., Fludra, M., Karendys-Łuszcz, K., Gos, E.: Trends in the advancement of mobile applications for the diagnosis and treatment of tinnitus: a comprehensive review of scientific literature. J. Hear. Sci. **14**(2), 9–21 (2024)
12. Mahboubi, H., Haidar, Y.M., Kiumehr, S., Ziai, K., Djalilian, H.R.: Customized versus noncustomized sound therapy for treatment of tinnitus: a randomized crossover clinical trial. Ann. Otol. Rhinol. Laryngol. **126**(10), 681–687 (2017)
13. Nagaraj, M.K., Prabhu, P.: Internet/smartphone-based applications for the treatment of tinnitus: a systematic review. Eur. Arch. Otorhinolaryngol. **277**, 649–657 (2020)
14. Sato, T., Yabushita, T., Sakamoto, S., Katori, Y., Kawase, T.: In-home auditory training using audiovisual stimuli on a tablet computer: feasibility and preliminary results. Auris Nasus Larynx **47**(3), 348–352 (2020)
15. Stropahl, M., Besser, J., Launer, S.: Auditory training supports auditory rehabilitation: a state-of-the-art review. Ear Hear. **41**(4), 697–704 (2020)
16. Abouzari, M., et al.: Adapting personal therapies using a mobile application for tinnitus rehabilitation: a preliminary study. Ann. Otol. Rhinol. Laryngol. **130**(6), 571–577 (2021)
17. Tuz, D., Isikhan, S.Y., Yücel, E.: Developing the computer-based auditory training program for adults with hearing impairment. Med. Biol. Eng. Comput. **59**(1), 175–186 (2021). https://doi.org/10.1007/s11517-020-02298-3
18. British Society of Audiology: Recommended procedure: Pure-tone air-conduction and bone-conduction threshold audiometry with and without masking (2018). https://www.thebsa.org.uk/wp-content/uploads/2024/01/Recommended-Procedure-Pure-Tone-Audiometry-2018.pdf
19. Newman, C.W., Jacobson, G.P., Spitzer, J.B.: Development of the tinnitus handicap inventory. Arch. Otolaryngol. head Neck Surg. **122**(2), 143–148 (1996)

# Advancing Healthy Aging: The Impact of Assistive Technologies on Mobility and Self-Care Among Older People

Vanessa Zorrilla-Muñoz[1,2], Gema Martinez-Navarrete[3](✉), Yolanda Vales[1], José M. Catalan[1], Andrea Blanco-Ivorra[4], Nicanor Morales-Delgado[5], Ramón Peral-Orts[6], Eduardo Saenz-de-Cabezon[7], José María Sabater-Navarro[1], Eduardo Fernandez[1,8], Nicolas García Aracil[1], and Mari Carmen Lillo-Navarro[9]

[1] Bioengineering Institute, Miguel Hernandez University, Elche, Spain
{vzorrilla,yvales,jcatalan,j.sabater,e.fernandez, nicolas.garcia}@umh.es
[2] University Institute on Gender Studies, University Carlos III of Madrid, Madrid, Spain
[3] Department of Histology and Anatomy. Division of Cell Biology, Miguel Hernandez University, San Joan, Spain
gema.martinen@umh.es
[4] Department of Materials Science, Optics, and Electronic Technology, Miguel Hernandez University, Elche, Spain
ablanco@umh.es
[5] Department of Anatomy and Human Embriology, Miguel Hernandez University, San Joan, Spain
nmorales@umh.es
[6] Department of Applied Mechanical Engineering, Miguel Hernandez University, Elche, Spain
ramon.peral@umh.es
[7] Department of Mathematics and Computation Department, University of La Rioja, Logroño, Spain
eduardo.saenz-de-cabezon@unirioja.es
[8] Networking Research Centre of Bioengineering, Biomaterials and Nanomedicine (CIBER-BBN), Madrid, Spain
[9] Department of Pathology and Surgery, Miguel Hernandez University, San Joan, Spain
mclillo@umh.es

**Abstract.** Since life expectancy is increasing, the world's population is ageing in many ways. Diseases such as stroke pose growing challenges for older people, impacting their well-being and overall quality of life. A current objective is to support healthy ageing by promoting and maintaining functional capabilities. This, in turn, facilitates sustainable living environments where older people with disabilities can independently perform their daily activities without requiring constant supervision or assistance. This paper focuses on older people who are experiencing disability situations associated with illness and/or chronic conditions, including stroke. The data are derived from the questionnaire "Encuesta de Discapacidad, Autonomía personal y Situaciones de Dependencia, EDAD (2020)" conducted in Spain among older persons with disabilities (n = 6938 people aged 65 and over). Sociodemographic variables encompass factors such as sex and the individual's


K. Daimi and A. Alsadoon (Eds.): ICR 2025, LNNS 1487, pp. 420–433, 2025.
https://doi.org/10.1007/978-3-031-95652-2_36

illness/chronicity. A descriptive analysis is conducted with independent variables related to mobility—such as manipulation of objects, walking, etc.—and self-care/domestic life difficulties—personal hygiene, eating and drinking, etc. These variables are analysed alongside the dependent variables "How is your overall health?" and "Do you think that the use of new technologies has improved aspects of your daily life?". The results suggest a correlation between positive perception and variables related to mobility and self-care. In conclusion, a positive perception of technologies could contribute to maintaining functional capacity and mobility. Moreover, the perception of new technology use promotes an ageing process where improving functional capacity becomes feasible. Technological devices, including robotic devices, have the potential to aid in the rehabilitation process for patients with neurological disorders causing impairments in upper and lower limbs. This assistance can lead to improvements in the quality of life and well-being of older people, promoting healthy ageing.

**Keywords:** Sustainable ageing · older people · mobility · self-care · technology · quantum computing

## 1 Introduction

The ageing of the population stands as a significant achievement of social and health policies, reflected in the sustained increase in global life expectancy. This demographic shift, however, introduces substantial challenges, particularly the rising incidence of chronic conditions affecting older adults. Among these, stroke emerges as a common cause of disability, restricting individuals' ability to perform daily activities independently and impacting their overall well-being. Promoting healthy ageing has become a priority, aiming to preserve the autonomy and quality of life of this population through solutions that support their functional capacity. In this regard, the perception older adults hold toward the use of new technologies could play a pivotal role in facilitating mobility and self-care, both essential for their independence. This paper investigates how the perception of technology use relates to mobility and self-care among older adults with disabilities, with a particular emphasis on stroke survivors. This study offers a novel perspective on how positive technology perceptions can enhance functional capacity, contributing to healthier and more sustainable ageing in contexts where chronic conditions pose an increasing burden.

Furthermore, the growing availability of technological tools offers a promising avenue to address the challenges posed by chronic conditions like stroke, yet their adoption remains contingent upon how older adults perceive their utility and accessibility. Cultural attitudes, prior experiences with technology, and the degree of physical limitation all shape these perceptions, potentially influencing the willingness of stroke survivors and other older adults to incorporate such solutions into their lives. Likewise, stereotypes associating older individuals with lower technological competence can exacerbate this reluctance, perpetuating the misconception that this group is inherently resistant or unable to adapt to digital innovations. Moreover, the scope of various technologies—such as wearable devices, mobile applications, robotic assistance systems, and generative artificial intelligence—is becoming increasingly viable due to advancements that make them more affordable and user-friendly, opening new opportunities to support this population with personalized and adaptive solutions. By examining these factors, this study seeks to bridge the gap between technological innovation and practical application, highlighting how tailored interventions could empower older adults to overcome barriers to mobility and self-care. This exploration not only contributes to the discourse on healthy ageing but also underscores the need for inclusive strategies that account for diverse user perspectives in the design and implementation of assistive technologies.

### 1.1 Literature Review

The ageing of the population is considered a success of social and health policies. The global population has experienced an increase in age over the last decades. According to World Bank Data (2020), individuals aged over 65 constitute 9.321% of the total world population, which indicates an increase of 3.069% compared to 1990 [1]. Population global projections have been estimated to increase global life expectancy by 2050, where two-thirds of the population are expected to be over 60, particularly in low- and middle-income countries [2]. Entities like WHO, among others, recognize chronic diseases as significant contributors to irreversible disability worldwide, with a heightened impact in older age, subsequently affecting social well-being [3–6].

Mobility and self-care/domestic life are interconnected factors that often correlate with a broad range of chronic conditions, leading to dependency among older people [7]. Many studies have focused over the last few years on technological solutions to facilitate home care to improve mobility and self-care in older persons, such as online healthcare [8], social robotics [9, 10], eHealth medical devices for home monitoring [11] and even robotic telerehabilitation devices [12]. A global approach termed mHealth (mobile technologies or mobile health) has emerged to provide remote, long-term social and health care support. However, there are still discrepancies between the technology services offered by the market and the requirements of dependent people, caregivers, and health care professionals [13]. Mobility and self-care/domestic factors are also main determinants of chronic diseases and pain in some older people, such as brain damage from stroke [14]. Stroke frequently leads to sequelae like neuropathies, which are one of the main causes of disability in people [15]. Stroke survivors affected by neuropathies tend to display strong motivation to manage their condition and maintain independence in comparison to other chronic conditions in adults and older people. These patients usually benefit greatly from the rehabilitation robot system and increase their health perception if aided technology is included in their daily activities [16].

Additionally, the interplay between the perception of technology and its practical outcomes remains underexplored, particularly in the context of stroke survivors, whose rehabilitation journeys are often marked by unique physical and psychological challenges. Emerging evidence suggests that positive perceptions of technology can enhance adherence to rehabilitation protocols, as seen in studies of robotic telerehabilitation and mobile health platforms, which report improved user engagement when devices are perceived as intuitive and supportive [17]. In this regard, mobility, a key aspect affected by stroke, particularly benefits from technologies designed to assist with movement and physical activity, though mobility limitations can engender frustration or dependency in users if the solutions are not adequately tailored to their specific needs [18]. However, gaps persist in understanding how these perceptions vary across socioeconomic and cultural contexts, especially in regions like Spain where ageing populations are rapidly expanding. This review thus extends the discussion by considering how technology acceptance might mediate the relationship between chronic disability and functional independence, offering a foundation for subsequent empirical analysis in this paper.

### 1.2 Objective

This work aims to evaluate the relationship between the perception of technology use and its impact on mobility and self-care among older adults with chronic conditions, including stroke survivors, to promote healthy ageing. Moreover, this paper analyses mobility and self-care/domestic life factors among disabled older persons with chronic conditions and those who have suffered a stroke. This study uniquely combines the EDAD 2020 dataset with a focus on the interplay between technology perception, mobility, and self-care among older adults with chronic conditions, offering a novel perspective on how positive technology perceptions can enhance functional capacity in a Spanish context. These factors are explored with the personal perception of their health status and the potential impact of technology on enhancing their daily activities.

## 2 Method

The secondary questionnaire "Encuesta de Discapacidad, Autonomía personal y Situaciones de Dependencia, EDAD (2020)" [19], covering all Spanish provinces, was used for the analyses. The EDAD 2020 dataset was selected due to its comprehensive coverage of disability, personal autonomy, and dependency across all Spanish provinces, providing a robust and representative sample of older adults with chronic conditions.

The information was sourced from the pre-existing survey, overseen by the INE, with the research team performing the analysis and creating the associated tables. The sample consisted of 6,938 persons (2,477 men, 4,471 women) aged 65 years or older. The mean age was 80.1 years with a standard deviation of +/– 0.09 (78.78 +/– 0.16 for men, 80.83 +/–0.12 for women). The diseases diagnosed in both men and women are shown in Table 1. The most prevalent disabilities were osteoarthritis (14.87% in men and 41.81% in women) and arthritis (7.47% in men, 23.31% in women). Regarding brain damage resulting from stroke, this condition affected 10.48% of the sample (4.63% in men, 5.85% in women).

The analysis was performed with the 16 mobility and 14 self-care/domestic life factors first assessed for reliability using Cronbach's alpha, a test that measures internal consistency with a value of 0.7 indicating a reliable threshold. A parametric method, Pearson correlation, was then used for significance levels of $p < 0.01$ and $p < 0.05$. All variables were assessed using a Likert scale: independent variables representing difficulties (16 related to mobility and 14 related to self-care/domestic life) ranged from 1 to 4 points, where 1 indicated the lowest level of difficulty and 4 the highest. For the dependent variable 'How is your overall health?', a scale ranging from 1 to 5 points

**Table 1.** Diseases diagnosed by sex and persons with more than 64 years based on the database of EDAD (2020) [17].

| You have been diagnosed with... | Men (n=2,477) | | Women (n=4,471 | | Total (N=6,938) | |
|---|---|---|---|---|---|---|
| | N | % (of N) | N | % (of N) | N | % (of N) |
| Multiple Sclerosis | 31 | 0,45 | 98 | 1,41 | 129 | 1,86 |
| Agenesis/Amputations | 74 | 1,07 | 75 | 1,08 | 149 | 2,15 |
| Spinal Cord Injury | 78 | 1,12 | 102 | 1,47 | 180 | 2,59 |
| Parkinson | 146 | 2,10 | 145 | 2,09 | 291 | 4,19 |
| Fibromyalgia | 43 | 0,62 | 262 | 3,78 | 305 | 4,40 |
| Muscular Dystrophy | 149 | 2,15 | 273 | 3,93 | 422 | 6,08 |
| Chronic Kidney Disease | 236 | 3,40 | 325 | 4,68 | 561 | 8,09 |
| Alzheimer | 180 | 2,59 | 429 | 6,18 | 609 | 8,78 |
| Heart Attack | 331 | 4,77 | 279 | 4,02 | 610 | 8,79 |
| Brain Damage from Stroke | 321 | 4,63 | 406 | 5,85 | 727 | 10,48 |
| Cancer/Malignancy | 353 | 5,09 | 459 | 6,62 | 812 | 11,70 |
| Other disease associated with the disability | 346 | 4,99 | 591 | 8,52 | 937 | 13,51 |
| Chronic Anxiety | 232 | 3,34 | 730 | 10,52 | 962 | 13,87 |
| Chronic Depression | 284 | 4,09 | 877 | 12,64 | 1161 | 16,73 |
| Diabetes | 699 | 10,07 | 1123 | 16,19 | 1822 | 26,26 |
| Arthritis | 518 | 7,47 | 1617 | 23,31 | 2135 | 30,77 |
| Osteoarthritis | 1032 | 14,87 | 2901 | 41,81 | 3933 | 56,69 |

was used, with 1 representing 'very good' and 5 indicating 'very bad'. Regarding the dependent variable 'Do you think that the use of new technologies has improved aspects of your daily life?', the scale ranged from 1 to 4 points, with 1 corresponding to 'Yes, it has improved them a lot' and 4 indicating 'It has made my daily life worse'.

Finally, while this study employs classical statistical methods, future analyses could incorporate quantum computing techniques, such as the Quantum Approximate Optimization Algorithm (QAOA), to optimize intervention strategies by processing complex variable interactions more efficiently.

## 3 Results

The results are provided in Table 2. The data presented reflect a study on the perceived difficulty level in various mobility and self-care variables, assessed both independently and with personal assistance. For mobility variables, such as changing posture (mean: 2.5 ± S.D. 0.1099853, Cronbach's $\alpha$: 0.9472) or walking inside the home (mean: 2.59375 ± S.D. 0.0989804, Cronbach's $\alpha$: 0.9473), a moderate difficulty is observed, which increases when assistance is received, as seen in walking outside the home with help (mean: 3.5625 ± S.D. 0.1265031, Cronbach's α: 0.9473). In self-care variables, activities like eating and drinking (mean: 2.1875 ± S.D. 0.1450633, Cronbach's α: 0.9480) show lower difficulty, while tasks such as washing and drying the body with assistance (mean: 3.5625 ± S.D. 0.1265031, Cronbach's α: 0.9469) indicate greater dependence. The internal consistency of the measures is high, with Cronbach's α values above 0.9467, suggesting strong reliability. Additionally, the overall health perception ("How is your overall health?": mean 3.01749 ± S.D. 0.0119577, Cronbach's α: 0.9536) and the perceived impact of new technologies on daily life ("Do you think that the use of new technologies has improved aspects of your daily life?": mean 2.55792 ± S.D. 0.0100799, Cronbach's α: 0.9542) reflect a moderate assessment, supported by excellent reliability (Cronbach's $\alpha > 0.9536$).

Across all diagnosed diseases (N = 6938), significant correlations ($p < 0.01$ or $p < 0.05$) were found between mobility/self-care difficulties and both dependent variables ('overall health' and 'technology impact'), whereas for stroke patients (N = 727), correlations were less consistent, particularly with personal assistance, affecting items like 'driving vehicles without adaptation' and 'eating and drinking'.

Specifically, in the total sample, mobility variables such as 'change posture' (Pearson D_1 = 0.1564**, I_17 = 0.1304**) and 'walk/move outside your home when you receive personal help/assistance' (Pearson D_1 = 0.2385**, I_17 = 0.0664**) showed consistent positive correlations with perceived health status (D_1) and technology impact (I_17), indicating that greater difficulties were associated with worse health perception and, to a lesser extent, a less favorable view of technology's role. Self-care variables like 'manipulate and move objects by using hands and arms' (Pearson D_1 = 0.1839**, I_17 = 0.1305**) and 'dress or undress' (Pearson D_1 = 0.1489**, I_17 = 0.0813**) followed a similar trend, with stronger correlations to health perception than to technology impact. The high Cronbach's alpha values (e.g., 0.9472–0.9512) across all variables confirm the reliability of these measures.

In contrast, among stroke patients (N = 727), the correlations were notably weaker and less consistent. For instance, 'change posture' showed a non-significant correlation with health perception (Pearson D_1 = 0.0652) but a significant one with technology impact (Pearson I_17 = 0.1665**), suggesting that stroke survivors may perceive technology as beneficial for this task despite its limited association with their overall health. Similarly, 'walk/move outside your home when you receive personal help/assistance' retained a strong correlation with health perception (Pearson D_1 = 0.1993**) but was weaker with technology impact (Pearson I_17 = 0.1119*), hinting at a divergence in how assistance influences these perceptions.

Notably, several variables, such as 'drive vehicles without adaptations' (Pearson D_1 = 0.0395, I_17 = −0.0804) and 'eat and drink' (Pearson D_1 = 0.0062, I_17 = 0.1396), showed no significant correlations in this subgroup, particularly when assistance was involved, where some correlations even turned negative (e.g., 'drive vehicles without adaptations when you receive personal help/assistance', Pearson D_1 = −0.0562). This pattern suggests that stroke patients may face unique barriers that diminish the perceived benefits of technology in certain contexts, especially when reliant on external support.

**Table 2.** Statistical analysis tests on Likert scale variables. All possible diseases (N=6,938 persons) and brain damage from stroke (N=727 persons).

| | | TOTAL (N=6,938) | | Brain damage from stroke (N=727) | |
|---|---|---|---|---|---|
| | Difficulty level to... | Pearson (D_1) | Pearson (I_17) | Pearson (D_1) | Pearson (I_17) |
| MOBILITY VARIABLES | ... change posture | 0.1564** | 0.1304** | 0.0652 | 0.1665** |
| | …change posture when you receive personal help/ assistance | 0.1817** | 0.1262** | 0.0688 | 0.0612 |
| | ...keep the body in the same position | 0.1502** | 0.1039** | 0.0555 | 0.1513** |
| | ...keep the body in the same position when you receive personal help/assistance | 0.1685** | 0.0824** | 0.0260 | 0.0971 |
| | ... walk/move at your home | 0.1187** | 0.1217** | 0.0907 | 0.0437 |
| | ... walk/move at your home when you receive personal help/assistance | 0.2113** | 0.1397** | 0.1163* | 0.1141* |
| | ... walk/move outside your home | 0.1427** | 0.1030** | 0.0544 | 0.0432 |
| | ... walk/move outside your home when you receive personal help/assistance | 0.2385** | 0.0664** | 0.1993** | 0.1119* |
| | ...travel by using transport as a passenger | 0.0613** | 0.1281** | -0.0013 | 0.1040* |

(*continued*)

The mean difficulty scores also reveal differences: tasks like 'walk/move outside your home when you receive personal help/assistance' (Mean = 3.5625, SD = 0.1265031) and 'travel by using transport as a passenger when you receive personal help/assistance' (Mean = 3.75, SD = 0.0777714) had higher difficulty levels in the total sample, reflecting

**Table 2.** *(continued)*

| | | TOTAL (N=6,938) | | Brain damage from stroke (N=727) | |
|---|---|---|---|---|---|
| | ...travel by using transport as a passenger when you receive personal help/assistance | 0.1692** | 0.0835** | 0.1408** | 0.0949 |
| | ...drive vehicles without adaptations | 0.0459* | 0.0145 | 0.0395 | -0.0804 |
| | ...drive vehicles without adaptations when you receive personal help/assistance | 0.2000** | 0.1707 | -0.0562 | 0.0290 |
| | …manipulate and move objects by using hands and arms | 0.1839** | 0.1305** | 0.1483** | 0.2105** |
| | ... manipulate and move objects by using hands and arms, when you receive personal help/assistance | 0.0986** | 0.1208** | 0.1383 | 0.1494* |
| | …manipulate small objects with hands and fingers | 0.1078** | 0.1588** | -0.0062 | 0.1803** |
| | …manipulate small objects with hands and fingers when you receive personal help/assistance | 0.0919** | 0.1605** | -0.0345 | 0.2697** |
| SELF-CARE VARIABLES | …wash and dry the different body parts | 0.1475** | 0.0627** | 0.0727 | 0.0315 |

*(continued)*

**Table 2.** (*continued*)

| | | TOTAL (N=6,938) | | Brain damage from stroke (N=727) | |
|---|---|---|---|---|---|
| | …wash and dry the different body parts when you receive personal help/assistance | 0.1171** | 0.1037** | 0.0008 | 0.1328* |
| | ...perform basic body care | 0.1604** | 0.1128** | 0.1166* | 0.2195** |
| | ...perform basic body care when you receive personal help/assistance | 0.1228** | 0.1197** | 0.0980 | 0.1615** |
| | …go to the toilet and relieve yourself or take care of your intimate hygiene | 0.0830** | 0.0560* | 0.0234 | 0.1569* |
| | …go to the toilet and relieve yourself or take care of your intimate hygiene when you receive personal help/assistance e | 0.1035** | 0.1032** | -0.0279 | 0.1611* |
| | …dress or undress | 0.1489** | 0.0813** | 0.0788 | 0.1048 |
| | …dress or undress when you receive personal help/assistance | 0.1411** | 0.0943** | 0.0605 | 0.2056** |
| | … eat and drink | 0.1295** | 0.1313** | 0.0062 | 0.1396 |
| | ... eat and drink when you receive personal help/assistance | 0.0826* | 0.1083** | -0.0244 | 0.1361 |

(*continued*)

**Table 2.** (*continued*)

| | | TOTAL (N=6,938) | | Brain damage from stroke (N=727) | |
|---|---|---|---|---|---|
| | … comply with medical prescriptions | 0.0642* | 0.0486 | -0.0030 | 0.0049 |
| | … comply with medical prescriptions when you receive personal help/assistance | 0.1171** | 0.0822** | 0.0429 | 0.1206* |
| | … avoid dangerous situations | 0.0822** | 0.0468 | 0.0130 | 0.1429* |
| | ... avoid dangerous situations when you receive personal help/assistance | 0.0931** | 0.0507 | 0.0251 | 0.0592 |
| | How is your overall health?") | | | | |
| | Do you think that the use of new technologies has improved aspects of your daily life? | | | | |

Pearson ** p<0,01, *p<0,05.

greater challenges when assistance is required. For stroke patients, the lack of consistent correlations across these tasks may indicate a reduced capacity to benefit from technology or assistance, possibly due to the specific neurological impairments affecting motor and cognitive functions. These findings, detailed in Table 2, highlight a general association between functional difficulties and perceptions in the broader sample, contrasted by a more complex and variable relationship among stroke survivors.

## 4 Discussion

The research findings reveal a consistent relationship between the dependent variables 'overall health perception' and 'the use of new technologies to improve daily life' and difficulties in mobility and self-care across all diagnosed diseases in a sample of 6,938 older adults. These results suggest that, in the broader population, greater challenges in performing daily tasks are associated with poorer health perceptions and varying views on technology's benefits, highlighting a potential link between functional limitations and subjective well-being. However, for the subsample of patients with brain damage from stroke (N = 727), this relationship is less uniform, as both dependent variables do not consistently correlate with all mobility and self-care difficulties. This discrepancy points to the unique impact of stroke-related impairments, which may alter how technology and assistance are perceived or utilized, setting the stage for a deeper exploration of these patterns and their implications.

Moreover, this variability in stroke patients could reflect differences in specific rehabilitation needs, where technology might play a more selective role depending on the severity of neurological sequelae. For instance, tasks requiring personal assistance show a weaker association with perceived technology benefits, suggesting that current solutions may not be fully tailored to the specific group of older persons affected by stroke. This concept opens the door to more personalized interventions.

While the correlations suggest technology use is linked to better health perception and functional capacity, causality remains unclear: technology adoption may enhance health outcomes, or healthier older persons may be more inclined to use technology, a question that warrants further longitudinal investigation and comprise stereotypes linked to ageing.

Although this study addresses broad technological perceptions, future work might analyze specific interventions, such as wearable devices, robotic telerehabilitation and assistance systems, and generative IA apps, to identify the most effective tools for enhancing mobility and self-care. In this regard, this work emphasizes the growing significance of designing technologies that are increasingly user-friendly, ergonomic, minimally invasive, and aesthetically pleasing. It also highlights the importance of considering the gender perspective and other aspects regarding inclusive perspective [20, 21] to design technologies [20] by fomenting responsible technology consumption and supporting the Human Factors and Ergonomics principles. These aspects also underscore the urgent need for innovative treatment methods and emerging technologies' implementation focused on improving the autonomy and independence of older people affected by disabilities and other dependence conditions [22]. Additionally, rehabilitation robotic devices hold promise as tools for improving and maintaining motor functions and mobility capabilities. These devices provide standardized and intensive therapy and aspects for motor function recovery [23], which might enhance the need to provide more competitive services oriented to a well-balanced rehabilitation based on user experience. Under this concept, robotic rehabilitation devices continue being developed to improve the offer tools to monitor the patient's progress and, as a consequence, enabling better adaptation of therapy to individual needs. The design of such technology demands a comprehensive understanding of its possibilities, which should be explored.

Finally, following the parametric analysis conducted in this paper, classical methods such as regression or clustering could effectively model the current data; however, we propose an innovative, forward-looking approach here, leveraging quantum algorithms like the Quantum Approximate Optimization Algorithm (QAOA) to enhance scalability and accommodate a greater number of variables in future research. To advance these insights, we propose the development of a Quantum Computing-based optimization algorithm utilizing the study's variables, such as the 16 mobility factors (e.g., 'change posture', 'walk/move at home') and 14 self-care factors (e.g., 'wash and dry the different body parts', 'eat and drink'), alongside the dependent variables 'overall health perception' (D_1) and 'technology impact on daily life' (I_17). By employing this approach, we aim to optimize the configuration of technological interventions to minimize mobility and self-care difficulties while maximizing health perception and independence, offering a scalable solution for enhancing healthy aging. As an exploratory complement, Topological Data Analysis (TDA) could be considered to examine potential non-linear relationships or qualitative structures within the current dataset. Although the number of variables in this study is modest, TDA might reveal subtle patterns—such as clusters of patients with similar difficulties in mobility and self-care across different chronic conditions—that linear methods might overlook. This patterns potentially enriching the understanding of how these factors interplay with technology use. For example, TDA could identify a cluster of patients with severe mobility limitations but manageable self-care needs, guiding the design of a rehabilitation robotic device tailored to enhance motor functions for that specific group. Moreover, TDA would be particularly well-suited for a future replication of this questionnaire, such as a panel study with a greater number of variables and repeated measurements over time (e.g., annual assessments), where its ability to capture evolving topological structures across longitudinal data could provide deeper insights into the dynamic interplay of mobility, self-care, and healthy and active aging regarding the technology perception to improve daily activities.

**Limitations.** This study has several limitations that should be considered when interpreting the results. Firstly, the sample is limited to data from the EDAD 2020 survey, which, while representative of Spanish provinces, does not encompass broader geographic or cultural diversity beyond Spain, potentially restricting the generalizability of the findings to other international contexts. Secondly, the analysis relies on general perceptions of technology without detailing specific devices or interventions, limiting the ability to pinpoint concrete solutions for enhancing mobility and self-care. Additionally, the subsample of patients with brain damage from stroke ($n = 727$) is relatively small compared to the total sample ($n = 6938$), which may reduce the statistical power to detect significant correlations in this group. Lastly, the cross-sectional design of the study precludes establishing causal relationships between technology perception and improvements in functional capacity, highlighting the need for longitudinal studies in the future.

## 5 Conclusion

This research utilizes the Spanish EDAD 2020 dataset to explore technology perception as a driver of functional capacity in a Spanish ageing population, laying the groundwork for innovative approaches like quantum computing in future studies. By focusing on how older adults perceive technology's role in enhancing mobility and self-care, this study provides a unique lens on the intersection of subjective well-being and functional independence, particularly in the context of chronic conditions such as stroke. These findings underscore the need for policies promoting accessible technology development, ensuring that solutions are affordable, user-friendly, and widely available to diverse ageing populations. Practical applications, such as integrating robotic rehabilitation devices into home care systems, could transform how older adults with disabilities manage daily activities, offering standardized support that complements human assistance and potentially reduces dependency over time. Moreover, the observed variability in stroke patients highlights the importance of tailoring interventions to specific subgroups, addressing their distinct neurological and functional challenges. Looking forward, future research should explore advanced methodologies like quantum computing and topological data analysis to refine intervention strategies for healthy ageing, enabling more precise modeling of complex variable interactions and uncovering non-linear patterns that traditional analyses might overlook. Such approaches could optimize technology-driven solutions, enhancing their scalability and effectiveness across diverse contexts. Ultimately, this study not only contributes to the growing body of knowledge on technology-assisted ageing but also calls for a multidisciplinary effort to bridge the gap between technological innovation and the real-world needs of older adults, fostering a more inclusive and sustainable framework for healthy ageing.

**Fundings.** This contribution takes parts of the grant "Multimodal telerehabilitation assisted by robotic devices to maximize motor recovery" co-financed by FEDER funds, within the FEDER operational program of the Valencian Community (2014–2020) and the grant PROMETEO/2019/119 from the Generalitat Valenciana and the Bidons Egara Research Chair of the University Miguel Hernandez to Eduardo Fernandez. Moreover, this contribution has been supported by the Spanish Ministry of Science and Innovation, through the projects PID2019-108310RB-I00, TED2021-130431BI00 and PLEC2022-009424; the Luciano Navarro Tripodi Foundation Grant; the Caser Foundation Grant; and the AVI (https://innoavi.es/es/) through the project INNTA1/2024/11.

## References

1. The World Bank Data: Population ages 65 and above (% of total population) (2022), https://data.worldbank.org/indicator/SP.POP.65UP.TO.ZS, last access 09 Feb 2024
2. WHO Homepage: Ageing and health, https://www.who.int/news-room/fact-sheets/detail/ageing-and-health, last access 09 Feb 2024
3. WHO Homepage: Global status report on the public health response to dementia 2021, https://www.who.int/publications/i/item/9789240033245, last access 09 Feb 2024
4. Kaji, R.: Global burden of neurological diseases highlights stroke. Nat. Rev. Neurol. **15**, 371–372 (2019)
5. Carroll, W.M.: The global burden of neurological disorders. Lancet Neurol. **2019**(18), 418–419 (2019)
6. Deuschl, G., Beghi, E., Fazekas, F., Varga, T., Christoforidi, K.A., Sipido, E., Bassetti, C.L., Vos, T., Feigin, V.L.: The burden of neurological diseases in Europe: an analysis for the Global Burden of Disease Study 2017. Lancet Public Health. **5**, e551–e567 (2020)
7. Abdi, S., Spann, A., Borilovic, J., de Witte, L., Hawley, M.: Understanding the care and support needs of older people: a scoping review and categorisation using the WHO international classification of functioning, disability and health framework (ICF). BMC Geriatr. **19**, 1–15 (2019)
8. Criado-Quesada, B., Zorrilla-Muñoz, V., El Agullo-Tomas, M.S.: uso de tecnologías de asistencia sanitaria digital por parte de la población mayor desde una perspectiva de género e intrageneracional. Teknokultura. **18**, 103–113 (2021)

9. Abou Allaban, A., Wang, M., Padır, T.: A systematic review of robotics research in support of in-home care for older adults. Information. **11**, 75 (2020)
10. Jecker, N.S.: You've got a friend in me: sociable robots for older adults in an age of global pandemics. Ethics Inf. Technol. **23**, 35–43 (2021)
11. Nakshbandi, G., Moor, C., Wijsenbeek, M.: Home monitoring for patients with ILD and the COVID-19 pandemic. Lancet Respir. Med. **8**, 1172–1174 (2020)
12. Bertomeu-Motos, A., Ezquerro, S., Barios, J.A., Lledó, L.D., Domingo, S., Nann, M., Martin, S., Soekadar, S.R., Garcia-Aracil, N.: User activity recognition system to improve the performance of environmental control interfaces: a pilot study with patients. J. Neuroeng. Rehabil. **16**, 1–9 (2019)
13. Lee, H., Park, Y.R., Kim, H.-R., Kang, N.Y., Oh, G., Jang, I.-Y., Lee, E.: Discrepancies in demand of internet of things services among older people and people with disabilities, their caregivers, and health care providers: face-to-face survey study. J. Med. Internet Res. **22**, e16614 (2020)
14. Welmer, A.-K., Von Arbin, M., Murray, V., Holmqvist, L.W., Sommerfeld, D.K.: Determinants of mobility and self-care in older people with stroke: importance of somatosensory and perceptual functions. Phys. Ther. **87**, 1633–1641 (2007)
15. Suzuki, M.: Peripheral neuropathy in the elderly. Handb. Clin. Neurol. **115**, 803–813 (2013)
16. Catalán, J.M., Blanco-Ivorra, A., García-Pérez, J.V., Vales, Y., Martínez-Pascual, D., Ezquerro, S., Garrote, A., Costa, T., Lledó, L.D., García-Aracil, N.: Patients' physiological reactions to competitive rehabilitation therapies assisted by robotic devices. J. Neuroeng. Rehabil. **20**, 41 (2023)
17. Pearce, L.M.N., Pryor, J., Redhead, J., Sherrington, C., Hassett, L.: Advanced technology in a real-world rehabilitation setting: longitudinal observational study on clinician adoption and implementation. J. Med. Internet Res. **26**, e60374 (2024)
18. Langhorne, P., Coupar, F., Pollock, A.: Motor recovery after stroke: a systematic review. Lancet Neurol. **8**(8), 741–754 (2009). https://doi.org/10.1016/S1474-4422(09)70150-4. PMID: 19608100
19. INE: Encuesta sobre Discapacidad, autonomía personal y situaciones de dependencia dirigida a hogares: EDAD 2020. https://www.ine.es/dyngs/INEbase/categoria.htm?c=Estadistica_P&cid=1254735573175
20. Agullo-Tomas, M.S., Zorrilla-Muñoz, V.: Technologies and images of older women. In: Proceedings of the Human Aspects of IT for the Aged Population. Technology and Society, pp. 163–175. Springer, Cham (2020)
21. Cimas, M., Ayala, A., Sanz, B., Agulló-Tomás, M.S., Escobar, A., Forjaz, M.: Chronic musculoskeletal pain in European older adults: cross-national and gender differences. Eur. J. Pain. **22**, 333–345 (2018)
22. Zorrilla-Muñoz, V., Agulló-Tomás, M.S., Forjaz, M.J., Fernandez, E., Rodriguez-Blazquez, C., Ayala, A., Fernandez-Mayoralas, G.: Technology, gender and COVID-19. analysis of perceived health in adults and older people. In: Proceedings of the International Conference on Human-Computer Interaction, pp. 363–379. Springer (2021)
23. Maciejasz, P., Eschweiler, J., Gerlach-Hahn, K., et al.: A survey on robotic devices for upper limb rehabilitation. J. Neuro. Eng. Rehab. **11**, 3 (2014). https://doi.org/10.1186/1743-0003-11-3

# Smart Cities/Smart Energy

# Smart-to-Sustainable Cities Correlation Analysis

Larisa Hrustek(✉), Katarina Tomičić-Pupek, and Neven Vrček

Faculty of Organization and Informatics, University of Zagreb, Varaždin, Croatia
{lhrustek,katarina.tomicic,nvrcek}@foi.unizg.hr

**Abstract.** The progressive development of digital technologies has enhanced key aspects of smart cities, including healthcare, mobility, civic engagement, and more, providing citizens with a higher quality of life. Despite countless opportunities for citizens, numerous challenges disrupt the balance of urban environments, especially in terms of ecological, economic and social sustainability. Factors such as population growth and the prioritization of urban areas, coupled with the high consumption of resources in city centers, further compromise sustainability, making it an increasing cause for concern. This research is grounded in the theory that smart cities use their implementation of digital solutions to promote sustainable practices. Accordingly, the research reexamines the relationship between key application domains of smart cities and the Sustainable Development Goals (SDGs), exploring technological aspects that enhance the sustainable development of smart cities. Based on the proposed Conceptual Smart-to-Sustainable model, data on the smart cities index and sustainable cities index for European cities were analyzed. While smart and sustainable cities were expected to be strongly correlated, the results revealed only a moderate correlation in certain cases. The strongest correlation was observed with SDG 9 - Industry, Innovation, and Infrastructure, highlighting its significant role in enabling or enhancing the practicality of digital solutions in citizens' daily lives.

**Keywords:** Smart Cities · Sustainable Cities · Conceptual Model · Digital Technology · Sustainable Development Goals

## 1 Introduction

Digital and sustainable development are key policy priorities at both, the European and global levels. Rather than treating them as separate, parallel processes, they should be approached as an interconnected co-transformation, leveraging their synergy to drive comprehensive and sustainable progress [1]. Key factors shaping urban development include growing urban populations, rising global numbers, and increased demand for resources to sustain urban living standards. By 2050, the world's population is expected to reach 9.7 billion [2], with two-thirds living in cities, requiring significant infrastructure and service improvements to meet these needs in line with the Sustainable Development Goals [3]. Cities, as economic hubs, are major consumers of resources and contributors to environmental degradation, creating challenges related to poverty, climate change, and migration that demand solutions for urban sustainability [4].


K. Daimi and A. Alsadoon (Eds.): ICR 2025, LNNS 1487, pp. 437–449, 2025.
https://doi.org/10.1007/978-3-031-95652-2_37

The advancement of digital technologies has paved the way for the development of smart cities, significantly enhancing key urban domains that impact all stakeholders, including urban mobility, data-driven decision-making, citizen engagement, and overall quality of life [5, 6]. However, simply creating a "smart environment" for stakeholders may not be sufficient and cities should also strive to cultivate a "regenerative environment" that promotes economic, ecological, and social sustainability. This raises the critical issue of whether smart cities are at the same time truly sustainable and how, while aiming to become smart, cities can contribute to achieving sustainable development goals as well. This critical issue might be worth investigating in the other direction as well, in terms of how sustainability-oriented initiatives led by leveraging innovative digital solutions to address global challenges and transform them into opportunities for long-term sustainability, contribute to the demand of cities of being smart.

This paper focuses primarily on the first direction raising the question if adopting digital solutions does inherently lead to sustainability as it aims to explore the relationship between key smart city domains and sustainable development goals, identifying opportunities for leveraging digital technologies to advance the sustainable development of smart cities. By contributing to the theoretical discourse on smart cities, it seeks to assess their sustainability and potential in achieving long-term ecological, social, and economic balance. Through data analysis, the paper highlights specific smart city domains in correlation with sustainable development goals.

The following section presents the theoretical background, outlining the key characteristics of smart and sustainable cities. The third section details the research methodology, while the fourth section presents the research findings. Finally, the paper concludes with a discussion of the results, research limitations, and key implications.

## 2 Theoretical Background

A smart city implies an environment where digital technologies are integrated into the processes and various application domains of the urban space, providing stakeholders with an enhanced living space through improved practices that effectively meet their life needs within diverse ecosystem urban environments. Application domains that characterize smart cities are healthcare, governance, transportation, environment, energy, safety and security, infrastructure and education [5, 7]. Stakeholders in smart cities are citizens, government and policymakers, urban planners, and business entities including suppliers [4]. Smart cities are characterized by connectivity, corporatism, data-driven decision-making, platform-based governance, and low-carbon sustainability [8]. They integrate physical and virtual components via optical cable networks, enabling communication and connectivity. These cities attract stakeholders through robust infrastructure and data-driven services, utilizing citizens' data to offer personalized solutions. Smart cities improve services related to employment, housing, mobility, healthcare, and more [9, 10]. They also focus on reducing carbon emissions by leveraging digital technologies to create energy-positive buildings, smart grids, modern transport, and adaptive street lighting [8, 11].

A sustainable city is an urban environment that is designed and managed in a way that it contributes to economic, environmental and social sustainability. This implies the infrastructural capacities and capabilities of the urban environment to contribute to the achievement of a balance between environmental protection, economic resilience and social equality in processes and application domains [12]. The key design criteria for sustainable cities include compactness, density, mixed land use, sustainable transport, green infrastructure, and urban intensification [13]. Compactness ensures strategic urban planning and development, while density defines built structures and population distribution [13, 14]. Mixed land use integrates physical, economic, and social planning [13]. Sustainable transport promotes diverse mobility options and efficient infrastructure [13, 14]. Green infrastructure covers natural and cultural spaces, and urban intensification supports population growth, site development, and improved transport services [13].

Smart sustainable cities involve a comprehensive approach to urban planning, focusing on long-term sustainability goals through the use of advanced digital technologies in city development and operations [12]. The priority areas of smart sustainable cities in the synergy of smart and sustainable include vertical application domains like social, environmental and economic sustainability [15, 16], while digital technologies horizontally contribute to the implementation and realization of initiatives [17]. Promoting the social sustainability of smart urban development is based on an inclusive and safe environment of cities that fight against urban poverty and exclusion while relying on digital technologies. Ecological and green sustainability focuses on protecting the environment to ensure the well-being of all people within the planet's limits. Economic sustainability aims to build successful, innovative cities, focusing on economic growth, job creation, and strengthening government capacities, along with creating the right legal and policy frameworks [15].

## 3 Methodology

The research questions in this paper are:

1. Is there a significant correlation between a city's overall level of "smartness" and its sustainability?
2. Which application domains of smart cities exhibit the strongest correlation with sustainability indicators, i.e., the SDGs?

The aim of this paper is to examine the relationship between key application domains of smart cities and the SDGs, as well as to identify opportunities for leveraging digital technologies to advance the sustainable development goals of smart cities.

### 3.1 Research Data

This research utilizes two datasets: (1) Smart cities dataset: the IMD Smart City Index 2024 [25] and (2) an Sustainable cities dataset: European Cities SDG Index [26].

The IMD Smart City Index 2024 dataset was used to assess smart cities, which assesses residents' perceptions of issues related to the structure and technological applications available to them in their city. Data were collected for 142 cities worldwide, and 120 residents from each city were surveyed. The assessment is conducted at two levels, namely Structure and Technology. Structure refers to the existing infrastructure of cities, while Technology describes the technological provisions and services available to residents. Five key areas shown in Table 2 are assessed at each level: health and safety, mobility, activities, opportunities, and governance. This research used data from the Technology pillar, for health and safety six variables, for mobility five variables, for activities one variable, for opportunities (work and school) four, and for management four variables [25].

Second data set included in the research contained data on the assessment of sustainable cities from the SDG index of European cities. The dashboard data shows the SDG index and values for individual SDGs for European cities. The report was prepared by the Sustainable Development Solutions Network and the Brabant Center for Sustainable Development. Data are presented for 15 SDGs, while due to a lack of data at the sub-national level, SDG 14 (Life under water) and SDG 17 (Partnerships for the Goals) were not considered in the prototype report [26]. For the purpose of this research, both data sets were used for 28 European cities, given that data were available for them.

### 3.2 Methods

Pearson's correlation coefficient was employed to quantify the relationship between various application domains of smart cities and sustainability indicators (SDGs), establishing a linear association between two continuous variables: smart city attributes and urban sustainability. In this research, the independent variable comprises data on the application domains of smart cities, while the dependent variable represents sustainability-related data, specifically the estimated Sustainable Development Goals (SDGs) for a given European city. Coefficient values ranging from −1 to 1 were interpreted as follows: values below +/−0.3 were considered indicative of a weak correlation, values between + /−0.3 and 0.7 represented a moderate correlation, while values approaching +/−1 were regarded as a strong correlation.

### 3.3 Conceptual Model of Research

The motivation for the conceptual model of this research is found in two existing frameworks: (1) the Smart City Application Domains [7] and (2) the Input-Process-Output-Impact model [27]. The first framework is of value for our analysis due to its classification of application domains of digital solutions based on emerging technologies. Although since 2023, when the paper was published, some technologies are not emerging anymore and new technologies have emerged, the classification of domains in relation to their impact on society remains mostly relevant for mapping the application domains with SDGs. Based on the initial classification, some application domains were applied in their original version, two domains were slightly changed, and new domains were added. The restructured application domain classification is shown in Table 1.

The second framework's value for this research is more complex. The sustainable smart cities conceptual model (in [27] derived from [28]) is based on the Input-Process-Output-Impact model [27]. In that research input refers to infrastructural assets or assets that enable efforts in the application domains of a smart city. Assets are put to use through various processes in application domains. Process represents the driver of change in smart sustainable cities, which can be technologies, communities (users), or policies

**Table 1.** Restructured application domain classification

| Original application domain | Restructured application domain | Explanation |
|---|---|---|
| Infrastructure | Infrastructure | Still relevant application domain, no need for restructuring |
| Safety and Security | Safety and Security | Still relevant application domain, no need for restructuring |
| Environment | Environment | Still relevant application domain, no need for restructuring |
| Healthcare | Healthcare | Still relevant application domain, no need for restructuring |
| Transportation | Transportation | Still relevant application domain, no need for restructuring |
| Education | Education, Work & Competencies | Still relevant application domain, but the restructured domain now includes continuous development of current and future education, work and competencies, matching and forming labor market needs |
| Governance | Digital Governance | Still relevant application domain, but refined with the emphasis on digital access, participation and new channels for engagement and communication |
| Governance | Transparency | Still relevant application domain, but refined with the emphasis transparent communication of results (influenced by the Input-Process-Output-Impact model and trends related to citizen's expectations from administration and governance bodies) |
| - | Industry | New application domain added, referring to a more active role of citizens in (co)creating new value |
| - | Social Impact | New application domain added, covering the citizen's perceived value in terms of their social impact |

that enable transformative change [27, 29]. The result of the successful execution of the process is the generation of sustainable and knowledge-based development results in the domains of economic, social, ecological and institutional development of smart sustainable cities. Output refers to the outcome that is the result of a process or activity in a certain application domain. Outcome can be read as productivity, innovation, liveability, well-being, sustainability, accessibility, management and planning. Impact represents the achieved results, which evaluates the impact through the transformative effect of the city into a smarter and more sustainable one.

Smart cities focused on sustainable development operate on three key levels: ecological, semantic, and governmental [30]. The ecological level ensures resource availability, the semantic level promotes resource sharing and collaboration, and the governmental level refines decision-making and governance for broader participation [30]. However, for a smart sustainable city to achieve its transformative potential, citizen engagement plays a crucial role [31]. Having the active citizen participation in mind the initial Input-Process-Output-Impact model can be put more in the context of the citizen, i.e., customer active participation. The shift in managing customer expectations, perceptions, and experiences impacts the Input-Process-Output-Impact model, as shown in Fig. 1, similar to the changes in application domains in Table 1.

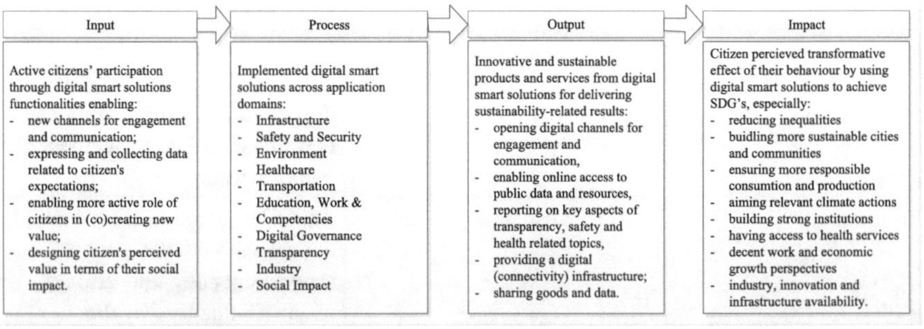


**Fig. 1.** Conceptual Smart-to-Sustainable Input-Process-Output-Impact model

The inputs coming from citizens undergo transformational processes to create desired outputs in many different ways. Presumption that some of these transformational processes (i.e., implementation of digital solutions) may converge and provide a synergetic effect led us to explore the correlation between a city's overall level of "smartness" and its sustainability, offering to enhance the value for the customer while ensuring responsible consumption of resources.

## 4 Results

Based on the conceptual model of this research data analysis was performed by calculating the correlation between indicators for cities' smartness and sustainability. Table 2 presents the preparation for data analysis. The first column from the left provides the list Digital solutions, i.e., processes with transformational effect in an application domain collected from *the IMD Smart City Index 2024* [25]. The second column refers to the option of interaction with citizens, which can be only Input, only Output or both (Input/Output). The third column presents the appropriate Application Domain chosen from Table 1, and then used for selecting semantically relevant SGDs corresponding to the application domain. We selected three relevant SDGs for each digital solution to minimize interpretation gaps and misalignment between smart and sustainable concepts, identifying possible correlation areas. Data analysis revealed that no single application domain stands out in strong correlation with the assigned SDGs. The most notable moderate correlation, smart-to-sustain, is observed for SDG 9, which appears in five instances. This is followed by SDG 12 and SDG 8, each occurring twice, and SDG 3, SDG 4, and SDG 11, each appearing once.

The highest frequency is recorded in SDG9, which refers to industry, innovation and infrastructure, where investments in infrastructure can be considered a technological prerequisite for other innovations and the contribution of digital and smart technologies to sustainability (Table 2). Four out of five digital solutions enable two-way interaction, which may affect the identified correlation due to their perceived usefulness in citizens' daily lives (e.g., healthcare, transport). SDG 12 is particularly relevant in the context of citizen interaction, as it demonstrates a moderate smart-to-sustain correlation in two instances. This correlation emerges from the combination of the problem-reporting input channel and the output channel related to the transparency of public expenditure.

SDG 8 exhibits a moderate correlation, with relatively high numerical values (0.45, 0.52), and a distinct emphasis on input factors. Citizens acknowledge the significance of digital literacy and skills for their future employment and competencies, actively seeking digital solutions that enhance their sustainability in alignment with economic trends. SDG 4 shows a moderate smart-to-sustain correlation, though a stronger link was expected. This gap may stem from the slow modernization of curricula to match digital industry developments. SDG3 shows a moderate smart-to-sustain correlation through sharing initiatives, with digital platforms impacting multiple SDGs. Similarly, in SDG 11, digital platforms for sharing resources and data help foster sustainable communities, creating opportunities for smart digital solutions to have a greater impact.

## 5 Limitations and Policy Recommendations

The limitations of this research stem primarily from the available dataset, which includes only the 28 largest European cities due to data unavailability for other cities. Consequently, a comprehensive analysis encompassing all European countries and cities was not feasible. Additionally, the study focuses exclusively on the European context rather than a global perspective. However, this approach is justified by the fact that European countries share common legal frameworks, which to some differ from those in regions such as the United States or Asia, as well as distinct mechanisms for implementing digital technologies in public spaces and governance.

At the global level, one of the key documents for urban development is the New Urban Agenda, adopted in 2016 under the auspices of the United Nations. This document outlines guidelines for sustainable urban development, emphasizing the integration of smart technologies, resilience to climate change, and citizen participation [18]. In this

**Table 2.** Correlation between the Smart City Index and the SDGs City Index based on data from 28 European cities

| | Digital solution | Option of interaction with citizen | Application domain | SDGs | | |
|---|---|---|---|---|---|---|
| HEALTH AND SAFETY | Online reporting of city maintenance problems provides a speedy solution | I | Transparency | SDG9 Industry, Innovation and Infrastructure **0,30** | SDG11 Sustainable cities and communities 0,02 | SDG12 Responsible consumption and production **0,51** |
| | A website or Apps allows residents to easily give away unwanted items | I | Social Impact | SDG3 Good Health and Well-Being **0,32** | SDG12 Responsible consumption and production -0,11 | SDG11 Sustainable cities and communities **0,31** |
| | Free public Wi-Fi has improved access to city services | I/O | Infrastructure | SDG9 Industry, Innovation and Infrastructure **0,39** | SDG10 Reduced Inequalities -0,04 | SDG15 Peace, Justice and Strong Institutions 0,20 |
| | CCTV cameras have made residents feel safer | O | Safety and Security | SDG11 Sustainable cities and communities 0,23 | SDG15 Peace, Justice and Strong Institutions -0,18 | SDG3 Good Health and Well-Being -0,21 |
| | A website or Apps allows residents to effectively monitor air pollution | O | Environment | SDG12 Responsible consumption and production 0,25 | SDG13 Climate Actions 0,09 | SDG3 Good Health and Well-Being -0,09 |
| | Arranging medical appointments online has improved access | I/O | Healthcare | SDG9 Industry, Innovation and Infrastructure **0,42** | SDG3 Good Health and Well-Being 0,26 | SDG10 Reduced Inequalities 0,11 |
| MOBILITY | Car-sharing apps have reduced congestion | I/O | Transportation | SDG12 Responsible consumption and production 0,27 | SDG13 Climate Actions -0,02 | SDG11 Sustainable cities and communities 0,13 |
| | Apps that direct you to an available parking space have reduced journey time | O | Transportation | SDG9 Industry, Innovation and Infrastructure 0,03 | SDG11 Sustainable cities and communities 0,19 | SDG13 Climate Actions -0,03 |

(*continued*)

**Table 2.** (*continued*)

| | Digital solution | Option of interaction with citizen | Application domain | SDGs | | |
|---|---|---|---|---|---|---|
| | Bicycle hiring has reduced congestion | I/O | Transportation | SDG11 Sustainable cities and communities 0,03 | SDG13 Climate Actions 0,16 | SDG3 Good Health and Well-Being -0,06 |
| | Online scheduling and ticket sales have made public transport easier to use | I/O | Transportation | SDG9 Industry, Innovation and Infrastructure **0,36** | SDG13 Climate Actions 0, 09 | SDG11 Sustainable cities and communities 0,21 |
| | The city provides information on traffic congestion through mobile phones | O | Transportation | SDG9 Industry, Innovation and Infrastructure 0,03 | SDG11 Sustainable cities and communities 0,12 | SDG13 Climate Actions 0,01 |
| ACTIVITIES | Online access to job listings has made it easier to find work | O | Education, Work & Competencies | SDG9 Industry, Innovation and Infrastructure -0,22 | SDG8 Decent work and Economic Growth 0,19 | SDG10 Reduced Inequalities -0,01 |
| OPPORTUNITIES | IT skills are taught well in schools | I | Education, Work & Competencies | SDG4 Quality Education **0,47** | SDG10 Reduced Inequalities 0,03 | SDG8 Decent Work and Economic Growth **0,45** |
| | Online services provided by the city have made it easier to start a new business | I/O | Industry | SDG8 Decent Work and Economic Growth 0,22 | SDG10 Reduced Inequalities -0,27 | SDG9 Industry, Innovation and Infrastructure 0,19 |
| | The current Internet speed and reliability meet connectivity needs | I/O | Infrastructure | SDG8 Decent Work and Economic Growth **0,52** | SDG10 Reduced Inequalities -0,14 | SDG9 Industry, Innovation and Infrastructure 0,13 |

(*continued*)

**Table 2.** (*continued*)

| | Digital solution | Option of interaction with citizen | Application domain | SDGs | | |
|---|---|---|---|---|---|---|
| | Online purchasing of tickets to shows and museums has made it easier to attend | I/O | Social Impact | SDG9 Industry, Innovation and Infrastructure 0,16 | SDG3 Good Health and Well-Being 0,07 | SDG11 Sustainable cities and communities 0,11 |
| MANAGEMENT | Online public access to city finances has reduced corruption | O | Transparency | SDG10 Reduced Inequalities 0,08 | SDG15 Peace, Justice and Strong Institutions -0,06 | SDG12 Responsible consumption and production **0,33** |
| | Online voting has increased participation | I | Digital Governance | SDG9 Industry, Innovation and Infrastructure 0,25 | SDG15 Peace, Justice and Strong Institutions -0,16 | SDG10 Reduced Inequalities -0,14 |
| | An online platform where residents can propose ideas has improved city life | I/O | Social Impact | SDG10 Reduced Inequalities -0,12 | SDG9 Industry, Innovation and Infrastructure **0,34** | SDG11 Sustainable cities and communities 0,13 |
| | Processing Identification Documents online has reduced waiting times | I/O | Digital Governance | SDG10 Reduced Inequalities -0,21 | SDG11 Sustainable cities and communities 0,09 | SDG9 Industry, Innovation and Infrastructure 0,11 |

context, the Paris Agreement (2015) also underscores the importance of sustainable urbanization in addressing climate change. It promotes the use of digital technologies to enhance energy efficiency in urban areas [19]. Furthermore, SDG 11—Sustainable Cities and Communities focuses on fostering inclusive, safe, resilient, and sustainable cities which are closely related to other goals on climate, energy, infrastructure and innovation.

At the European level, cities occupy only 4% of the total land area but are home to 75% of the population, making them central to achieving climate neutrality by 2050 as one of the key objectives of the European Green Deal. Additionally, cities account for more than 65% of global energy consumption and over 70% of $CO_2$ emissions, highlighting their critical role in climate mitigation efforts [20]. The 2019 European Green Deal underscored the potential of sustainable urban development strategies to foster smart cities that significantly reduce pollution [21]. Furthermore, the EU Biodiversity Strategy proposed initiatives to promote greener European cities and enhance biodiversity within urban environments, reinforcing the interconnection between urban sustainability and ecological resilience [22].

The Pact of Amsterdam, adopted in 2016, established the foundation for the Urban Agenda for EU, guiding growth, innovation, and quality of life in European cities to address key societal challenges. Its main themes include the circular economy, climate adaptation, digital and energy transitions, housing, social inclusion, sustainable land use, urban mobility, and public safety. These priorities highlight the core principles of smart and sustainable cities [23]. The Leipzig Charter (2020) established a new European policy framework for sustainable urban development, shaping the Urban Agenda for the EU, which was formalized by the Ljubljana Agreement (2021). This agreement introduced a multi-annual work programme, defining operational parameters and methodologies while expanding the agenda with four new themes, Greening Cities, Sustainable Tourism, Food, and Cities of Equality, emphasizing urban sustainability [18]. The adopted Urban Agenda for the EU refers to the promotion of innovation and good governance, strengthening integrated urban development, enabling concrete solutions for all citizens [24]. Ultimately, the EU Mission for 2030: Climate-Neutral and Smart Cities underscores the critical need for transforming smart cities into sustainable, resilient urban environments [20]. Based on the analyzed context of existing regulatory frameworks, the lack of smart and sustainable initiatives alignment should be taken into account by policymakers when defining new priorities and policies. Opportunities for achieving synergic impact exist, yet they need to be addressed in a more holistic manner.

## 6 Conclusion

According to the analysis presented in this paper, the correlation between a city's overall level of "smartness" and its contribution to sustainability is very modest. Application domains of smart cities exhibit correlation with sustainability indicators, i.e., the SDGs in 9 out of 20 digital solutions. The strongest correlation was observed with SDG 9 - Industry, Innovation, and Infrastructure. A possible interpretation for this might be that these initiatives act as the foundation for more smart-to-sustain initiatives. The transformation process takes some time to foster benefits, and in that sense, the time needed to design, develop and implement digital solutions might be an impact factor for the delay of recognizing the benefits in a short period of time. For SDG 8, smart cities enhance citizens' awareness of digital literacy and skills. For SDG 12, moderate correlations between smart and sustainable city traits highlight the need to link issue-reporting channels and transparency practices. Although this analysis has a limitation in terms of a possible semantic interpretation misalignment between smart and sustainable concepts, overall, the results of this research can be indicative for future digital innovations focusing them on exploiting application domains beyond the existing infrastructure for introducing more sustainability-oriented smart solutions. Future research could explore more in-depth the correlation between smart and sustainable city concepts and their impact on the quality of life in European urban areas.

## References


1. Zimmer, M., Järveläinen, J.: Digital-sustainable co-transformation: Introducing the triple bottom line of sustainability to digital transformation research. Presented at the August 30 (2022). https://doi.org/10.1007/978-3-031-15688-5_10
2. Nations, U.: Population, https://www.un.org/en/global-issues/population, last accessed 23 Feb 2025
3. Nations, U.: World Urbanization Prospects 2018 | Population Division, https://www.un.org/development/desa/pd/news/world-urbanization-prospects-2018, last accessed 23 Feb 2025
4. Kumar, A.: A novel framework for waste management in smart city transformation with industry 4.0 technologies. Res. Global. **9**, 100234 (2024). https://doi.org/10.1016/j.resglo.2024.100234
5. Makkonen, T., Inkinen, T.: Inclusive smart cities? Technology-driven urban development and disabilities. Cities. **154**, 105334 (2024). https://doi.org/10.1016/j.cities.2024.105334
6. European Commission: Quality of life in European cities, https://ec.europa.eu/regional_policy/information-sources/maps/quality-of-life_en, last accessed 03 Mar 2025
7. Gracias, J.S., Parnell, G.S., Specking, E., Pohl, E.A., Buchanan, R.: Smart cities—a structured literature review. Smart Cities. **6**, 1719–1743 (2023). https://doi.org/10.3390/smartcities6040080
8. van den Bosch, H.: Humane by choice, smart by default: 39 building blocks for cities of the future. IET Smart Cities. **2**, 111–121 (2020). https://doi.org/10.1049/iet-smc.2020.0030
9. De Giovanni, P.: Sustainability of the Metaverse: a transition to industry 5.0. Sustain. For. **15**, 6079 (2023). https://doi.org/10.3390/su15076079
10. Anttiroiko, A.-V., Valkama, P., Bailey, S.: Smart cities in the new service economy: building platforms for smart services. AI & Soc. **29**, 323–334 (2014). https://doi.org/10.1007/s00146-013-0464-0
11. Liu, H., Wang, L., Shen, Y.: Can digital technology reduce carbon emissions? Evidence from Chinese cities. Front. Ecol. Evol. **11** (2023). https://doi.org/10.3389/fevo.2023.1205634
12. Janik, A., Ryszko, A., Szafraniec, M.: Scientific landscape of smart and sustainable cities literature: a bibliometric analysis. Sustain. For. **12**, 779 (2020). https://doi.org/10.3390/su12030779
13. Bibri, S.E.: The underlying components of data-driven smart sustainable cities of the future: a case study approach to an applied theoretical framework. Eur. J. Futures Res. **9**, 13 (2021). https://doi.org/10.1186/s40309-021-00182-3
14. Bibri, S.E., Krogstie, J.: Generating a vision for smart sustainable cities of the future: a scholarly backcasting approach. Eur. J. Futures Res. **7**, 5 (2019). https://doi.org/10.1186/s40309-019-0157-0
15. European Commission: Sustainable cities - European Commission, https://international-partnerships.ec.europa.eu/policies/digital-and-infrastructure/sustainable-cities_en, last accessed 24 Feb 2025
16. Evans, J., Karvonen, A., Martin, C.: Smart and sustainable? Five tensions in the visions and practices of the smart-sustainable city in Europe and North America. Technol. Forecast. Soc. Chang. **133**, 269–278 (2018). https://doi.org/10.1016/j.techfore.2018.01.005
17. European Commission: Smart cities - European Commission, https://commission.europa.eu/eu-regional-and-urban-development/topics/cities-and-urban-development/city-initiatives/smart-cities_en, last accessed 24 Feb 2025
18. United Nations: The New Urban Agenda, https://habitat3.org/the-new-urban-agenda/, last accessed 19 Mar 2025
19. United Nations: The Paris Agreement | UNFCCC, https://unfccc.int/process-and-meetings/the-paris-agreement, last accessed 19 Mar 2025

20. European Commission: Climate-neutral and smart cities, https://research-and-innovation.ec.europa.eu/funding/funding-opportunities/funding-programmes-and-open-calls/horizon-europe/eu-missions-horizon-europe/climate-neutral-and-smart-cities_en, last accessed 19 Mar 2025
21. European Commission: The European Green Deal, https://eur-lex.europa.eu/legal-content/EN/TXT/HTML/?uri=CELEX:52019DC0640, last accessed 19 Mar 2025
22. European Commission: EU Biodiversity Strategy for 2030 Bringing Nature Back into Our Lives. (2020)
23. European Commission: Urban Agenda for the EU - European Commission, https://commission.europa.eu/eu-regional-and-urban-development/topics/cities-and-urban-development/urban-agenda-eu_en, last accessed 19 Mar 2025
24. European Commission: Urban Agenda for the EU – Multi-level governance in action, https://ec.europa.eu/regional_policy/information-sources/publications/brochures/2019/urban-agenda-for-the-eu-multi-level-governance-in-action_en, last accessed 19 Mar 2025
25. World Compettitiveness Center: Methodology-Smart City - IMD business school for management and leadership courses, https://www.imd.org/smart-city-observatory/home/methodology/, last accessed 24 Feb 2025
26. Sustainable Development Solutions Network and the Brabant Center for Sustainable Development: European Cities SDG Index, https://euro-cities.sdgindex.org/#/, last accessed 24 Feb 2025
27. Yigitcanlar, T., Han, H., Kamruzzaman, M.: Approaches, advances, and applications in the sustainable development of smart cities: a commentary from the guest editors. Energies. **12**, 4554 (2019). https://doi.org/10.3390/en12234554
28. Yigitcanlar, T.: Smart City policies revisited: considerations for a truly smart and sustainable urbanism practice. World Technop. Rev. **7**, 97–112 (2018). https://doi.org/10.7165/wtr18a1121.19
29. Tan, S.Y., Taeihagh, A.: Smart City governance in developing countries: a systematic literature review. Sustain. For. **12**, 899 (2020). https://doi.org/10.3390/su12030899
30. Caputo, F., Magliocca, P., Canestrino, R., Rescigno, E.: Rethinking the role of technology for citizens' engagement and sustainable development in smart cities. Sustain. For. **15**, 10400 (2023). https://doi.org/10.3390/su151310400
31. Webster, C.W.R., Leleux, C.: Searching for the real sustainable smart city? Inform. Polity. **24**, 229–244 (2019). https://doi.org/10.3233/IP-190132

# Evaluating the Extended Kalman-Filter for the State Estimation in Low-Voltage Grids

Sebastian Hallmann-Perez[1(✉)], Omid Tafreschi[2], and Andreas F. Raab[1]

[1] Wavestone Germany AG, Leopoldstr. 28A, 80802 München, Germany
{sebastian.hallmannperez,andreas.raab}@wavestone.com
[2] Hochschule Darmstadt, Schöfferstraße 3, 64295 Darmstadt, Germany
omid.tafreschi@h-da.de

**Abstract.** Due to the challenges posed by the energy transition, i.e., the volatility of renewable energies and the increasing electrification due to the rise of electric vehicles and heat pumps, it is increasingly important to identify critical states in low-voltage grids. The paper investigates the suitability of the Extended Kalman-Filter for state estimation in low voltage grids by implementing and analyzing its application in a real grid. The results demonstrate that voltage can be reliably estimated in real-time and show that the Extended Kalman-Filter is a suitable method in terms of computational efficiency, adaptability, and data dependency.

**Keywords:** Extended Kalman-Filter · State Estimation · Low-Voltage Grids · Smart Grids · Voltage Transparency

## 1 Introduction

Due to the increasing electrification in the heating and mobility sectors, and the growing number of decentralized generation plants, the operation of low-voltage grids is facing new challenges [1]. In particular, the resulting bidirectional power flows cause significant difficulties for Distribution Grid Operators (DSOs) regarding the operation, control, and maintenance of distribution grids [1].

To ensure reliable grid operation in the low-voltage level, DSOs have flexibility options available in addition to the costly grid expansion, such as load and generation management [2]. However, these options require the identification of critical grid conditions, which can be identified using various approaches. These can be divided into grid state estimation (SE) and grid calculations. Since grid calculations, e.g., load flow calculation, require complete data that is not available in low-voltage grids, this paper focuses on SE [3]. SE aims to generate data that describes the state of a grid, taking into account incomplete measurement data. This ensures a coherent and reliable basis for monitoring the grid state [4].

As an alternative to conventional SE methods, e.g., the Weighted Least Square (WLS) method, filter approaches like the Kalman-Filter (KF) offer a


K. Daimi and A. Alsadoon (Eds.): ICR 2025, LNNS 1487, pp. 450–459, 2025.
https://doi.org/10.1007/978-3-031-95652-2_38

viable option for real-time monitoring of low-voltage grids. The WLS method reaches its limits in low-voltage grids applications due to their high nonlinearities, its inability to meet real-time requirements, and the necessity of complete data [5–7]. The KF can estimate the state of a dynamic system by making predictions and corrections while accounting for measurement noise and model uncertainties [8]. However, since the classical KF is only suitable for linear systems, it cannot be directly applied to SE in the electrical power grid, which exhibits nonlinear behavior due to fluctuations in loads and generation [8]. Therefore, various approaches have been developed that build on the KF but are specifically designed to handle nonlinear systems. One such approach is the Extended Kalman Filter (EKF), which linearizes the nonlinear system to enable its application.

Against this background, this paper addresses the following research question: Can the EKF provide reliable voltage estimations through SE to detect boundary violations in a real low-voltage grid?

The structure of the paper is as follows: Sect. 2, discusses the challenges of SE in low-voltage grids, highlighting key differences from higher voltage levels. Next, the state of the art is reviewed, comparing various methods for SE. In Sect. 3, the fundamentals of the KF are described In Sect. 4 the EKF is then implemented for an existing grid. Section 5 describes the existing lov-voltage grid and evaluates the results. The paper concludes with a conclusion and an outlook in Sect. 6.

## 2 Challenges for State Estimation Methods in Low-Voltage Grids

Due to the challenges in low-voltage grids, SE differs from the used methods in higher voltage levels. Low-voltage grids are nonlinear systems. Due to the limited number of measurements and the high number of nodes, the applied methods must be capable of handling incomplete data. Figure 1 illustrates the limited measurement and data availability in the low-voltage grid [9].

Another challenge in low-voltage grids is the consideration of the three-phase system. Low-voltage grids are operated in a three-phase configuration to ensure a balanced distribution of electrical loads. However, due to uneven load distributions in the grid, operation is often asymmetric, which can result in different loading conditions for individual phases [9]. In higher voltage levels, this is not necessary, as the power grid operates symmetrically, making it sufficient to calculate only one phase [10]. Furthermore, low-voltage grids are increasingly facing significant changes regarding the types of consumers and generators connected to the grid, such as charging stations for electric vehicles (EV), heat pumps (HP), battery storage systems, and photovoltaic (PV) installations.

Due to these challenges, established methods, e.g., the WLS method [11], reach their limits. The WLS method is constrained in low-voltage SE due to the high nonlinearities and dynamics of the grid, which require an increased number of iterations and, in some cases, prevent convergence [5]. Moreover, WLS

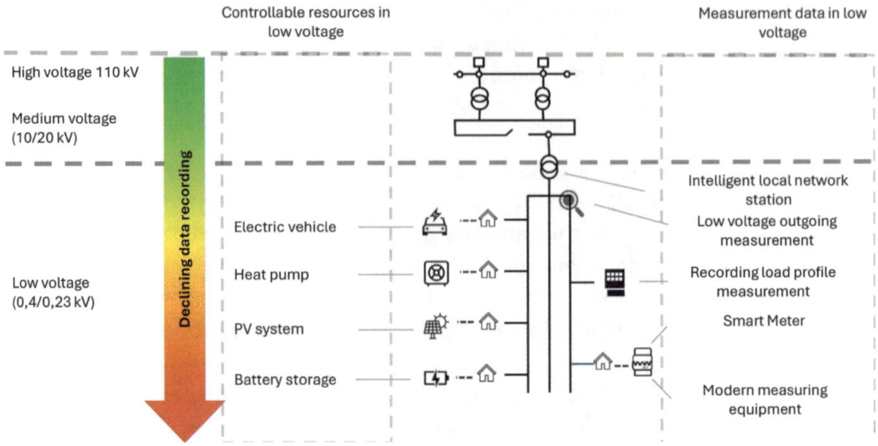


**Fig. 1.** Overview of Measurement Acquisition and Controllable Resources in Low-Voltage Grids

is unable to meet real-time requirements, particularly in scenarios with significant fluctuations in load and generation within distribution grids [6]. Another challenge is the necessity for a complete data, as the WLS method can not handle underdetermined equation systems [7]. In contrast, the KF is an algorithm for estimating the state of a dynamic system, providing optimal prediction and correction while accounting for measurement noise and model uncertainties [8]. KF predicts the state of a system based on previous estimates and then adjusts using real-time measurements. This can lead to a more accurate estimate, even when the measurement data is impaired by noise. In addition, another advantage of the KF is its high efficiency, enabling its use in real-time applications, particularly in time-critical systems [12].

Several studies have focused on SE process, exploring various approaches for improving the accuracy and the efficiency of this process. [13] compares SE using WLS and EKF for a synthetic IEEE 9 bus system. The results show that the EKF outperforms WLS in terms of mean absolute error, particularly under various transient conditions and with noisy measurements. [14] designs and simulates the EKF and Unscented KF (UKF) for SE for Single-Machine-Infinite-Bus State Space Model. The findings indicate that both methods exhibit similar deviations from the actual values. However, due to the high computational complexity of the UKF, the EKF is more suitable for real-time applications. [15] implement, among other methods, the EKF and WLS in the IEEE-14 bus system and compare the estimation accuracy over 30 steps. The results show that the EKF is significantly superior to WLS in terms of voltage estimation accuracy. In contrast to [13–15] simulating lab szenarios this paper focuses on the implementation of the EKF on an existing low-voltage grid over a period of two months with real data.

# 3 Kalman-Filter Algorithm

The KF [16] relies on a recursive estimation procedure that calculates the states of a system in two phases: the prediction phase and the update phase. In the first phase, the state of the system $\hat{\mathbf{x}}_k^-$ is predicted based on the previous state $\hat{\mathbf{x}}_{k-1}$ and the given system dynamics (Eq. 1). The system's dynamics are described by the state transition matrix $\mathbf{F}$, which determines the development of the system's state from one time step to the next. If external control is present, its effect is modeled by the term $\mathbf{B}\mathbf{u}_{k-1}$, where $\mathbf{B}$ is the control matrix and $\mathbf{u}_{k-1}$ is the control vector [12].

The uncertainty of the prediction is described by the covariance matrix $\mathbf{P}_k^-$, which is calculated based on the previous covariance matrix $\mathbf{P}_{k-1}$ and the state transition matrix $\mathbf{F}$ (Eq. 2). The process noise covariance matrix $\mathbf{Q}$ accounts for the process noise generated by unpredictable influences in the system and describes the variance of these disturbances. This ensures that uncertainties not covered by the model itself are included [17].

$$\hat{\mathbf{x}}_k^- = \mathbf{F}\hat{\mathbf{x}}_{k-1} + \mathbf{B}\mathbf{u}_{k-1} \tag{1}$$

$$\mathbf{P}_k^- = \mathbf{F}\mathbf{P}_{k-1}\mathbf{F}^T + \mathbf{Q} \tag{2}$$

The state $\hat{\mathbf{x}}_k^-$ estimated during the prediction phase is updated in the update phase based on the available measurements at time $k$ ($\mathbf{z}_k$). Equation 3 defines the measurement vector $\mathbf{z}_k$ at time $k$. $\mathbf{H}$ represents the measurement matrix, which establishes the relationship between the actual state $\mathbf{x}_k$ and the measurement $\mathbf{z}_k$, while $\mathbf{v}_k$ symbolizes the measurement noise at time $k$ [17].

$$\mathbf{z}_k = \mathbf{H}\mathbf{x}_k + \mathbf{v}_k \tag{3}$$

To determine the influence of the measurement on the prediction, the Kalman gain $\mathbf{K}$ is calculated (Eq. 4). This involves determining the ratio between the uncertainty of the prediction $\mathbf{P}_k$ and the measurement $\mathbf{R}_k$. The Kalman gain determines to what extent the prediction is adjusted based on the new measurements. A higher Kalman gain means the measurement has a stronger influence on the estimate, while a smaller value gives more weight to the prediction [17].

The estimated state ($\hat{\mathbf{x}}_k$) is updated by adding the weighted difference between the actual measurement $\hat{\mathbf{z}}_k$ and the predicted measurement $\mathbf{H}\hat{\mathbf{x}}_k^-$ (Eq. 5). The error covariance $\mathbf{P}_k$ is adjusted according to Eq. 6, so that the reduced uncertainty after incorporating the measurement is reflected [17].

$$\mathbf{K} = \mathbf{P}_k^-\mathbf{H}^T(\mathbf{H}\mathbf{P}_k^-\mathbf{H}^T + \mathbf{R})^{-1} \tag{4}$$

$$\hat{\mathbf{x}}_k = \hat{\mathbf{x}}_k^- + \mathbf{K}(\hat{\mathbf{z}}_k - \mathbf{H}\hat{\mathbf{x}}_k^-) \tag{5}$$

$$\mathbf{P}_k = (\mathbf{I} - \mathbf{K}\mathbf{H})\mathbf{P}_k^- \tag{6}$$

These two phases are recursively repeated at each new time step to enable accurate real-time estimation [17].

# 4 Extendend Kalman-Filter Algorithm

Since the electrical power grid is a nonlinear system, the KF cannot be directly applied to solve the SE [8]. As a result, there are several approaches based on the KF that are capable of dealing with nonlinear systems. One such approach is the Extended Kalman Filter (EKF). The basic idea is to linearize the nonlinear system and approximate the probability density function by using a Gaussian distribution [15]. The state at time $k$, $\mathbf{x}_k$, is determined according to Eq. 7 from the state transition function $\mathbf{f}_{k-1}(\mathbf{x}_{k-1})$ added by the process noise $\mathbf{w}_k$. The measurement $\mathbf{y}_k$ consists of the measurement function $\mathbf{h}_k(\mathbf{x}_k)$ and the measurement noise $\mathbf{v}_k$.

$$\mathbf{x}_k = \mathbf{f}_{k-1}(\mathbf{x}_{k-1}) + \mathbf{w}_k \mathbf{y}_k = \mathbf{h}_k(\mathbf{x}_k) + \mathbf{v}_k \tag{7}$$

To handle the nonlinear system, the proposed approach requires, in addition to the steps of the KF explained in Sect. 3, a linearization to improve the handling of complexity due to the nonlinearity of the system. The linearization of the state transition function $\mathbf{f}_{k-1}(\mathbf{x}_{k-1})$ is described by $\mathbf{F}_{k-1}$. In addition to the process noise $\mathbf{q}_{k-1}$, $\mathbf{g}_{k-1}$ represents a bias term. Thus, the state $\mathbf{x}_k$ is calculated by Eq. 8.

$$\mathbf{x}_k = \mathbf{F}_{k-1}\mathbf{x}_{k-1} + \mathbf{g}_{k-1} + \mathbf{q}_{k-1} \tag{8}$$

For the considered application of SE, the Holt-Winters method is used for model linearization [15]. The method decomposes the time series into level and trend components, which are continuously updated by smoothing parameters to forecast future values based on historical data. For the SE, the goal of the Holt-Winter method is not to forecast, but to linearize the function based on historical time series. This linearization is used to determine the transition matrix 9 and is multiplied by the identity matrix $\mathbf{I}$. The identity matrix is a square matrix with ones on the diagonal and zeros elsewhere. This results in the following Equation for $\mathbf{F}_{k-1}$:

$$\mathbf{F}_{k-1} = \alpha_{k-1}(1 + \beta_{k-1}) \cdot \mathbf{I} \tag{9}$$

The bias term $\mathbf{g}_{k-1}$ accounts for additional deviations and is determined according to Eq. 10. The parameters $a_{k-1}$ and $b_{k-1}$ represent the smoothing factors for the level and the trend, which are determined using the Holt-Winters method from historical values [15].

$$\mathbf{g}_{k-1} = (1 + \beta_{k-1})(1 - \alpha_{k-1})\tilde{\mathbf{x}}_{k-1} - \beta_{k-1}a_{k-2} + (1 - \beta_{k-1})b_{k-2} \tag{10}$$

The values $\alpha_{k-1}$, $\beta_{k-1}$, $\mathbf{a}_{k-2}$, and $\mathbf{b}_{k-2}$ are determined during the initialization of the EKF and are assumed to be constant across time steps. Figure 2 depicts the workflow of the EKF. Initially, the states from the previous time step ($\hat{\mathbf{x}}_{k-1}$) are estimated. These are based on the average voltage measurements from the smart meters for the respective phase of the previous time step. For the accuracy of this estimate, the covariance matrix ($\mathbf{P}_{k-1}$) is assumed.

Since the average from the previous time step is not a reliable estimate, the initial covariance matrix is set to $\mathbf{P}_{k-1} = 0.01$ to reflect sufficient uncertainty in the initial estimate. This estimate is updated during the update phase considering the available voltage measurements. Since this is a continuous process with a granularity of one minute, this procedure is repeated for the next time step. Instead of estimating the previous time step ($\hat{\mathbf{x}}_{k-1}$) based on the average values from the smart meters and the assumed covariance ($\mathbf{P}_{k-1}$), the update is based on the results of the EKF from the previous time step.

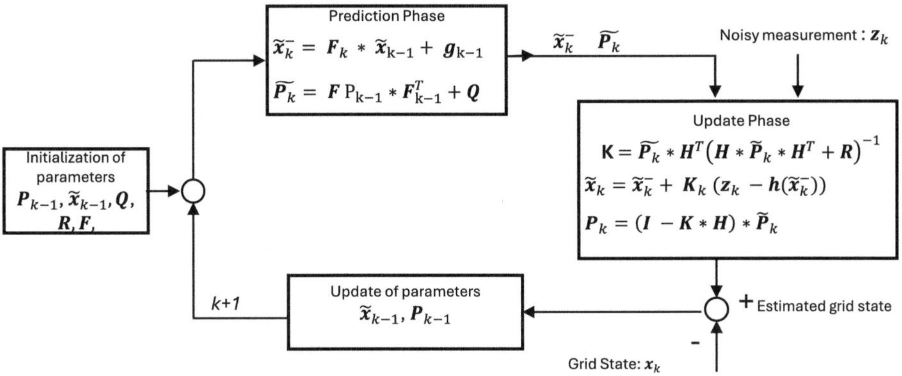


**Fig. 2.** Workflow of the EKF

In addition, further assumptions are required for the implementation of the EKF. The process noise covariance matrix $\mathbf{Q}$ is initially defined as a diagonal matrix with values of 0.00006 on the diagonal. These diagonal entries represent the individual uncertainties of each grid node and assume that all points are independent of each other. By adding covariance based on the distance to measured nodes, the estimation of unmeasured nodes is directly influenced by the measurements. The process noise covariance matrix $\mathbf{Q}$ as well as the measurement noise matrix $\mathbf{R}$ may change with each time step [17]. To reduce complexity, the process noise matrix and the measurement noise matrix are assumed to be constant in this work.

## 5 Real World Application & Results

Fig. 3 shows an existing low-voltage grid arranged as a radial grid, which is used to evaluate the performance of EKF for grid SE.

The grid consists of a total of 53 grid connection points, with 49 located on the upper grid branch and four on the lower grid branch. The grid is equipped with 86 m, five of them are smart meters. These are located on the upper grid branch and enable the real-time measurement of voltage, current, and power measurements. The grid connection point with the greatest distance from the

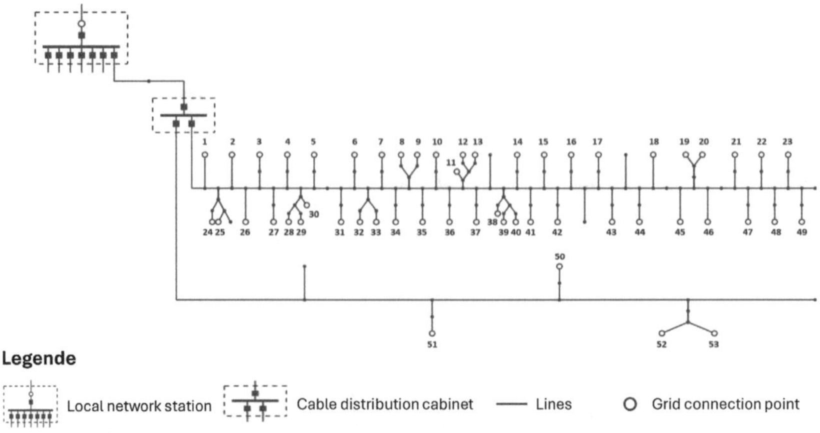


**Fig. 3.** Topological Representation of the Grid Area

local grid station is 690.18 m. The grid is characterized by a high density of PV systems, EV, and HP. It includes nine PV systems with a total power of 79.20 kWp, a capacity for heat pumps of 13.55 kW, and a capacity for wallboxes of 99 kW. As a result, the grid can be considered a representative example of a low-voltage grid of the future, facing the challenges of future grid operation.

For the evaluation of the EKF, the SE is performed with one-minute granularity for historical voltage values. The results are compared to the measurements from smart meter No. 10, which were not considered in the EKF calculation and serve for the validation of the proposed approach. Likewise, the mentioned measurements are not included in the initialization of the EKF.

Table 1 shows the results of the SE of the EKF over the entire observation period, for a sunny day and for a shaded day for each of the three phases in the analyzed low-voltage grid. The voltage estimation using EKF has a high precision with an average root mean square error (RMSE) of 0.4948 over all phases for the entrie obeservation period. Also on a shaded day and during a sunny day with high PV generation the results indicates a reliable SE and enabling the identification of potential voltage band violations in real-time.

Figure 4 shows the estimated and the actually measured voltage at midday for a period of 2 h. The EKF estimation shows a precise voltage estimation even during volatile voltage fluctuations. Table 2 illustrates that the EKF results during the sunny hours from 12:00 PM to 2:00 PM show higher precision for all phases compared to the previously considered time periods.

The results show that the EKF is a reliable approach for detecting voltage band violations. Accurate results are achieved regardless of the time of day or global solar irradiance. Notably, the results vary between the different phases, especially on sunny days. In particular, the results for Phase 1 perform significantly worse. This could be attributed to the asymmetric load of the low-voltage

**Table 1.** RMSE of the State Estimation of the EKF for Different Conditions

| Entire Observation Period | | | |
|---|---|---|---|
| | Phase 1 | Phase 2 | Phase 3 |
| RMSE_EKF | 0.4308 | 0.4454 | 0.6081 |
| A Shaded Day | | | |
| | Phase 1 | Phase 2 | Phase 3 |
| RMSE_EKF | 0.2723 | 0.2385 | 0.3051 |
| A Sunny Day | | | |
| | Phase 1 | Phase 2 | Phase 3 |
| RMSE_EKF | 0.4222 | 0.3192 | 1.1042 |

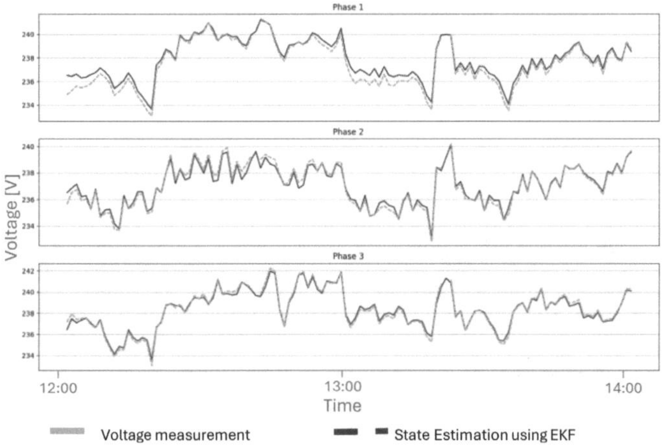


**Fig. 4.** Results of the State Estimation for Two Sunny Hours

**Table 2.** Results of the State Estimation of the EKF from 12:00 PM to 2:00 PM on a Sunny Day

| | Phase 1 | Phase 2 | Phase 3 |
|---|---|---|---|
| RMSE_EKF | 0.3511 | 0.2076 | 0.1975 |

grid. Additionally, it is worth highlighting that the results remain reliable even in the event of a measurement equipment failure at the local grid station.

# 6 Conclusion and Outlook

This paper demonstrates the successful implementation of the EKF for SE in low voltage grids, addressing the growing challenges of decentralized energy generation, bidirectional power flows, and incomplete measurement data. Compared to traditional methods like WLS, the EKF offers improved accuracy in real-time grid monitoring by effectively handling noisy and nonlinear system data.

The results highlight the EKF's high precision under various grid conditions, enable DSOs to identify critical grid states. As a result, the identification of critical grid states and the corrective actions to address them enhance grid stability without requiring expensive grid expansion. This approach is particularly valuable for future energy systems with increasing integration of EV, PV, and HP, offering a scalable solution to improve grid reliability and operational efficiency.

It is necessary to evaluate the EKF for various topologies that include more controllable consumers and exhibit higher dynamics. In addition to voltage estimation, current and power estimation also play a significant role and should be considered in further investigations. Furthermore, we propose comparing our EKF-based results with those obtained from alternative KF variations, e.g., Iterated KF [18], UKF [19], and neural network-based approaches in terms of accuracy and performance.

## References

1. Zhou, W., Ardakanian, O., Zhang, H., Yuan, Y.: Bayesian learning-based harmonic state estimation in distribution systems with smart meter and DPMU data. IEEE Trans. Smart Grid **11**(1), 832–845 (2020)
2. Schwab, A.J.: Elektroenergiesysteme: Smarte Stromversorgung im Zeitalter der Energiewende, 7. Auflage, Springer Vieweg (2022)
3. Schaefer, K.F.: Netzberechnung Verfahren zur Berechnung elektrischer Energieversorgungsnetze, pp. 187–327. Springer Vieweg, Wiesbaden (2023). https://doi.org/10.1007/978-3-658-40877-0
4. Oswald, B.R.: Berechnung von Drehstromnetzen, 3rd edn. Auflage, Springer Vieweg (2017). https://doi.org/10.1007/978-3-658-41076-6
5. Yarlagadda, R., Kosana, V., Teeparthi, K.: Power system state estimation and forecasting using CNN based hybrid deep learning models. In: 2021 IEEE International Conference on Technology, Research, and Innovation for Betterment of Society (TRIBES), pp. 1–6. IEEE (2021)
6. Zhang, T., Zhang, W., Yuan, P.: Distributed dynamic state estimation in active distribution system based on particle filter. In: 2018 IEEE Innovative Smart Grid Technologies - Asia (ISGT Asia), pp. 664–668. IEEE (2018)
7. Eslami, A., Negnevitsky, M., Franklin, E., Lyden, S.: An intelligent technique for harmonic state estimation using limited number of meters. In: 2023 International Conference on Power and Renewable Energy Engineering (PREE), pp. 144–149. IEEE (2023)
8. Yang, Z., Gao, R., He, W.: A review of the research on Kalman filtering in power system dynamic state estimation. In: 2021 IEEE 4th Advanced Information Management, Communicates, Electronic and Automation Control Conference (IMCEC), pp. 856–861 (2021)
9. Dorsemagen, F.: Zustandsidentifikation von Mittelspannungsnetzen für eine übergreifende Automatisierung der Mittel- und Niederspannungsebene. Universitätsbibliothek Wuppertal (2018)
10. Matthiss, B., Erb, J., Binder, J.: Using smart meters for distribution grid state estimation. In: 2019 International Conference on Smart Energy Systems and Technologies (SEST), pp. 1–5. IEEE (2019)

11. Strutz, T.: Data Fitting and Uncertainty: A Practical Introduction to Weighted Least Squares and Beyond. Springer Vieweg, Wiesbaden (2015). https://link.springer.com/book/9783658114558
12. Li, Q., Li, R., Ji, K., Dai, W.: Kalman filter and its application. In: 2015 8th International Conference on Intelligent Networks and Intelligent Systems (ICINIS), pp. 74–77 (2015)
13. Kumar, P., Karamta, M., Markana, A.: Dynamic state estimation for multi-machine power system using WLS and EKF: a comparative study. In: 2019 IEEE 16th India Council International Conference (INDICON), pp. 1–4 (2019)
14. Tebianian, H., Jeyasurya, B.: Dynamic state estimation in power systems using Kalman filters. In: 2013 IEEE Electrical Power & Energy Conference (EPEC), pp. 1–5 (2013)
15. Cevallos, H., Intriago, G., Plaza, D.: Performance of the estimators weighted least square, extended Kalman Filter, and the particle filter in the dynamic estimation of state variables of electrical power systems. In: 2018 IEEE International Conference on Automation/XXIII, Concepcion, Chile, pp. 1–6 (2018)
16. Kalman, R.E.: A new approach to linear filtering and prediction problems, in transaction of the ASME. J. Basic Eng. **82**, 35–45 (1960)
17. Welch, G., Bishop, G.: An Introduction to the Kalman Filter (1995)
18. Bell, B.M., Cathey, F.W.: The iterated Kalman filter update as a Gauss-Newton method. IEEE Trans. Autom. Control **38**(2), 294–297 (1993)
19. Julier, S.J., Uhlmann, J.K.: New extension of the Kalman filter to nonlinear systems. In: Signal Processing, Sensor Fusion, and Target Recognition VI, vol. 3068. SPIE (1997)

# Evaluating Hardware and Software Power Measurement Tools: Assessing Accuracy in Measuring Application Energy Consumption for Data-Parallel Workloads

Urooj Asgher(✉) and Tania Malik

Technological University Dublin, Dublin, Ireland
B00168170@mytudublin.ie, tania.malik@tudublin.ie

**Abstract.** Energy consumption in computing presents significant environmental concerns, and reducing it has become a major technological challenge. The accurate measurement of energy consumption during application execution is essential for implementing effective application-level energy minimization techniques. The two widely-used methods for measuring energy consumption are system-level physical measurements using external power meters and software-based power measurement tools. In this work, we present an experimental comparative analysis that evaluates the accuracy of hardware and various software-based power measurement tools in measuring application energy consumption of CPU based data-parallel workloads. Our analysis focused on compute-intensive kernels operating across multiple processing units, where accurate energy measurement is critical for performance tuning and energy efficiency. We extend this empirical study to highlight the strengths and limitations of each software-based power measurement tool. The results offer valuable insights on the accuracy of energy measurement tools for data-parallel workloads, particularly when relying on software tools.

**Keywords:** Energy measurement · energy consumption · data-parallel applications · software tools · energy efficiency · power meters

## 1 Introduction

With increasing demand and limited global energy resources, enhancing energy efficiency in computing has emerged as a critical technological challenge [8]. Accurate measurement of energy consumption during application execution is essential for implementing effective application-level energy minimization techniques. Two widely adopted approaches for measuring energy consumption are system-level physical measurements using external power meters and software-based (SW) power measurement tools. Among these, physical power meters are typically considered the most reliable for accurately capturing the total power consumption of computing nodes, as they directly measure energy usage at the


K. Daimi and A. Alsadoon (Eds.): ICR 2025, LNNS 1487, pp. 460–470, 2025.
https://doi.org/10.1007/978-3-031-95652-2_39

hardware level [6]. In contrast, SW tools offer energy consumption metrics specifically targeted at the application or component level. These SW tools function as energy calculators, measurement software, and power profiling software [9].

In this work, we perform an experimental comparative analysis that evaluates the accuracy of hardware and various software-based power measurement tools in measuring application energy consumption of CPU based data-parallel workloads. For our experimental study, we used the OmegaWatt power meter [15], an external hardware device positioned between the wall socket and the power supply unit of computing nodes, to capture physical power usage. As software tools, we selected three open source, widely used energy measurement tools - LIKWID [17], Perf [7], and Powerstat [11], all of which utilize Intels RAPL (Running Average Power Limit) interface to estimate energy consumption. These tools were chosen specifically because our server infrastructure is equipped with Intel processors, which support RAPL-based power readings.

For this work, we focused on compute-intensive kernels operating across multiple processing units, where accurate energy measurement is critical for performance tuning and energy efficiency. We selected two data-parallel kernels that serve as fundamental building blocks in many scientific applications-Matrix Multiplication (MXM) and Fast Fourier Transform (FFT). These kernels were chosen due to their high computational intensity, memory-bound characteristics, and intrinsic data parallelism, making them ideal benchmarks for evaluating energy efficiency in high-performance computing workloads.

The main contributions of this work lies in a set of experiments conducted on a real-world platform to evaluate the accuracy of both hardware and software-based tools for measuring the energy consumption of data-parallel kernels. This empirical analysis not only benchmarks these tools but also highlights the strengths and limitations of each software-based power measurement method. The findings provide valuable insights into the reliability of software tools for energy measurement, particularly in the context of data-parallel workloads where accurate energy monitoring is critical.

The rest of this paper is organized as follows: Sect. 2 presents the energy measurement framework used in this study. Section 3 discusses related work in the area of energy measurement tools. In Sect. 4, we describe the experimental platform and methodology. Section 5 provides experimental comparative analysis that evaluates the accuracy of hardware and software-based power measurement tools in measuring baseline and both data parallel MXM and FFT application energy consumption. It also examines the behavior of each software tool and evaluates their accuracy in the context of our experiments. Finally, Sect. 6 concludes the paper and outlines potential directions for future work.

## 2 Energy Measurement Framework

In this work, we consider the dynamic energy consumption, which refers to the energy consumed by the system during the execution of an application. To compute dynamic energy, we first need to distinguish between two types of energy:

Baseline energy ($E_{\text{base}}$): the energy consumed by the system when it is idle (i.e., not running any applications).

$$E_{\text{base}} = P_{\text{base}} \times T_{\text{base}} \tag{1}$$

Total energy ($TE_{\text{ng}}$): the total energy consumed by the system while an application is running.

$$TE_{\text{ng}} = P_{\text{app}} \times T_{\text{E}} \tag{2}$$

The dynamic energy ($E_{\text{dynamic}}$) is then calculated as the difference between the total energy during application execution and the baseline energy over the same time interval.

$$E_{\text{dynamic}} = TE_{\text{ng}} - (P_{\text{base}} \times T_{\text{E}}) \tag{3}$$

Here, $P_{\text{base}}$ is the baseline power (system power in idle state), $T_{\text{base}}$ is the idle duration, $P_{\text{app}}$ is the average power during application execution, and $T_{\text{E}}$ is the application's execution time.

To assess the accuracy of software-based power measurement tools against a hardware tool (Omegawatt), we calculate the prediction error using the following formula:

$$\frac{|DE(m)_{\text{SWTs}} - DE(m)_{\text{Omegawatt}}|}{DE(m)_{\text{Omegawatt}}} \times 100 \tag{4}$$

where, $DE(m)_{\text{SWTs}}$ is the dynamic energy measured using software tools for a workload of size $m$ and $DE(m)_{\text{omegawatt}}$ is the dynamic energy measured using the OmegaWatt hardware power meter. Omegawatt records power samples at regular intervals, and energy is estimated using numerical integration (trapezoidal rule):

$$TE_{\text{ng}} \approx \sum_{i=1}^{n} \frac{(t_i - t_{i-1})}{2} (P(t_{i-1}) + P(t_i)) \tag{5}$$

Here, $P(t_i)$ represents the power consumption at time $t_i$, and $t_i - t_{i-1}$ denotes the time interval. Execution time $T_{\text{E}}$ is precisely captured using system timers or processor clocks, while baseline power ($P_{\text{base}}$) is obtained when the system is idle, just before running the workload.

## 3 Literature Review

The growing interest in energy efficiency within high-performance computing has led to a variety of studies exploring different energy measurement techniques. Despite this, a clear gap remains in the experimental comparative analysis of hardware and software-based tools for measuring energy consumption in HPC environments, particularly for data-parallel workloads.

Several works have addressed energy metrics using software tools but lack direct comparisons with hardware tools on the same platform. For instance, OBrien et al.[19] utilized physical power meters and on-chip sensors to measure energy usage. However, these studies focused primarily on system-level consumption without detailing application-level energy data or direct tool comparisons. Similarly, Silva et al.[20] discussed energy and computational efficiency in supercomputers, yet their focus remained on overall system metrics, omitting application-specific energy measurements.

Studies such as Calore et al.[3] and Minartz et al.[14] explored dynamic energy optimizations through voltage scaling and power management but did not include hardware-based comparisons. Fahad et al.[4] proposed using external power meters for accurate energy readings at the processor level, although this work did not extend to per-core application measurements. Bratek et al.[2] compared Yokogawa WT310 power meter with Intel RAPL, but their analysis was limited to single tools without examining Powerstat or Perf.

Several studies examined energy-aware algorithm design [13] or performance monitoring using tools like TAU [12], yet these works primarily aimed at optimization and lacked direct measurement validations. Other tools like Intel PowerInsight [5] and PAPI [1] provide access to hardware-level power metrics and performance counters. However, they typically require additional instrumentation and do not offer seamless application-level energy evaluations, limiting their usability for accurate dynamic energy profiling in HPC workloads.

Moreover, recent work by Nana et al.[16] highlighted calibration and measurement granularity issues in current SW tools, and Khaleghzadeh et al.[10] proposed algorithms for energy efficiency in data-parallel contexts without performing tool comparisons. Reviews like those by Noureddine et al. [18] emphasize energy modeling, yet few examine experimental setups without requiring additional hardware or limited to specific platforms.

While numerous works contribute to energy measurement in HPC, most focus either on high-level metrics, modeling, or optimization without providing a unified, experimental comparison between HW and SW energy measurement tools. This highlights the importance of our study in bridging this gap, offering valuable insights into tool accuracy, usability, and suitability for measuring dynamic application energy consumption in real HPC workloads.

## 4 Experimental Platform and Methodology for Energy Measurements with HW and SW Tools

All experiments were conducted on in-house server, HPC-NEXUS, whose specifications are summarized in Table 1. The server is equipped with Intel Xeon E5-2660 v4 CPUs, making it suitable for RAPL-based power profiling tools.

### 4.1 Hardware-Based Measurement: OmegaWatt

We used the OmegaWatt external power meter, to collect system-wide energy data. It supports a nominal voltage of 230 V at 50 Hz and provides power measurements with high accuracy (0.5% for voltage, 1% for current, and 1.5% for power). It logs data to internal memory (96 GB) and communicates via USB 2.0 (921600 baud) or Wi-Fi. For each experiment, OmegaWatt captured both idle and active power usage, with data exported in CSV format for post-processing.

**Table 1.** HPC-Nexus Server Specifications

| Component | Specification |
|---|---|
| Architecture | x86_64 |
| CPU Model | Intel Xeon E5-2660 v4 @ 2.00 GHz |
| Cores | 28 (2 sockets, 14 cores per socket) |
| Threads | 56 (2 threads per core) |
| Cache | L1: 896 KiB, L2: 7 MiB, L3: 70 MiB |
| CPU Frequency | Min: 1.2 GHz, Max: 3.2 GHz |
| NUMA Nodes | 2 |

### 4.2 Software-Based Measurement Tools

To compare the hardware measurements, we used three open-source Linux-compatible software tools that utilize Intels RAPL (Running Average Power Limit) interface.

- **LIKWID** `perfctr`: This tool reads energy counters from RAPL domains via model-specific registers (MSRs). We monitored the `package` (entire socket) and `dram` (memory) domains. LIKWID provides energy values in $\mu$J and updates every millisecond.
- **Perf**: A Linux performance analysis tool that supports energy monitoring using RAPL events such as `power/energy-pkg/` and `power/energy-dram/`. Since MSR access typically requires root privileges, we used the MSR kernel module to enable readings via `perf stat`.
- **Powerstat**: Designed for lightweight power monitoring, Powerstat reads RAPL counters from `/sys/class/powercap/intel-rapl:0/`. It calculates power by sampling energy at two time points and using the formula:

$$\text{Power (W)} = \frac{\text{Energy}_2 - \text{Energy}_1}{\text{Time}_2 - \text{Time}_1} \tag{6}$$

  It supports Intel-based systems but requires manual enabling of RAPL reporting.

### 4.3 Experimental Methodology

To evaluate and compare energy measurement tools, we selected two widely used data-parallel kernels: Matrix Multiplication (MXM) and Fast Fourier Transform (FFT). MXM is commonly used in machine learning and numerical linear algebra, while FFT is central to signal processing and computational physics. These kernels represent compute- and memory-bound workloads, respectively, and are ideal for energy analysis in high-performance computing (HPC) environments.

Our experiments were conducted on a dedicated in-house server (HPC-NEXUS), isolated from other workloads to ensure consistency and avoid interference. We configured each kernel to run entirely on the CPU, excluding external components such as SSDs or NICs to ensure that energy consumption measurements primarily reflect CPU and DRAM usage.

The experimental framework was designed to capture energy usage in both idle and active states using a hardware power meter (Omegawatt MV2-Rapid Box) and three software-based tools: LIKWID, Perf, and Powerstat. Prior to application execution, we verified that no background disk or network activity was present using Linux tools such as `sar`, `iotop`, and `atop`. Additionally, problem sizes were constrained to fit entirely within system memory to prevent paging or swapping.

Baseline energy measurements were first established by keeping the system idle for 60 s and sampling power 1 Hz using both hardware and software tools. These baseline values served as a reference point to calculate dynamic energy consumed during application execution.

Each kernel was then run independently under varying input sizes. Power usage was recorded continuously throughout execution using the Omegawatt meter and software tools. The collected data was logged in CSV format and post-processed using Python scripts to calculate total and dynamic energy consumption based on formulas defined in Sect. 2. To ensure statistical reliability, all experiments were repeated multiple times, and the average values, standard deviation, and prediction errors were computed for each case.

The dynamic energy values obtained from software tools were compared against those from Omegawatt to evaluate their accuracy. This methodology enabled us to assess the strengths and limitations of each measurement tool in measuring application-level energy consumption for data-parallel workloads, as detailed in Sect. 5.

## 5 Experimental Analysis and Results

To evaluate the accuracy and behavior of software-based and hardware-based energy measurement tools, we conducted a series of experiments on the HPC-NEXUS server using two data-parallel kernels: Matrix Multiplication (MXM) and Fast Fourier Transform (FFT). These experiments focused on both idle system measurements and dynamic energy consumption during kernel execution.

The first set of experiments established the server's baseline power consumption while idle. A 60-second uniform sampling period was chosen to ensure compatibility with all software tools, particularly PowerStat, which requires longer intervals for stable readings. As shown in Fig. 1, OmegaWatt reported the highest baseline power, while software tools (Perf, LIKWID, PowerStat) consistently underestimated this value. This discrepancy is attributed to the nature of software tools, which primarily measure energy from CPU and DRAM using Intel's RAPL interface, whereas OmegaWatt captures full-system power, including peripherals, motherboard, and PSU losses. These findings highlight the limitation of software tools in capturing idle system energy comprehensively.

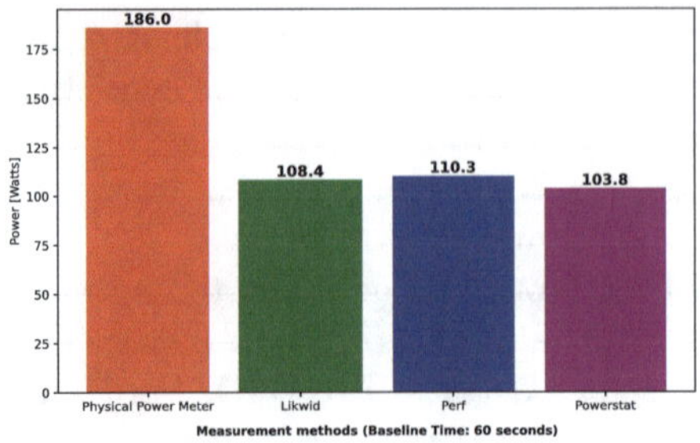


**Fig. 1.** Baseline power consumption comparison with HW and SW tools

In the second set of experiments, we analyzed energy consumption during the execution of the MXM kernel with a problem size of 2024. As seen in Fig. 2, OmegaWatt reported the highest energy usage. Among the software tools, Perf provided results closest to OmegaWatt, making it the most accurate of the three. LIKWID and PowerStat under reported energy usage, particularly LIKWID, which appeared to miss significant memory-related consumption.

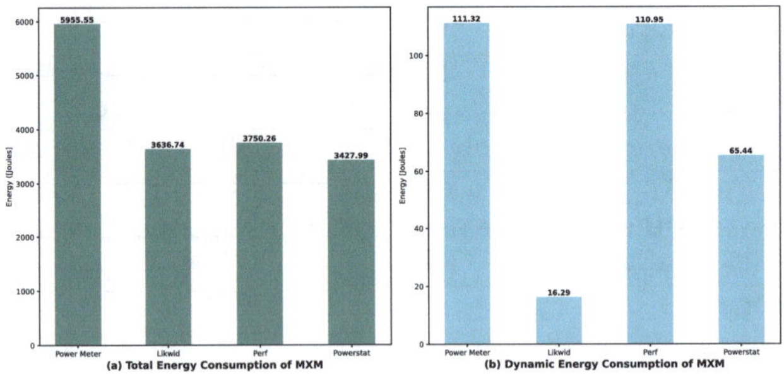


**Fig. 2.** MXM application energy consumption comparison with HW and SW tools

We repeated the experiments with the FFT kernel using the same problem size. As shown in Fig. 3, the trends remained consistent: OmegaWatt recorded the highest energy, and Perf again offered the closest approximation. FFT, being more memory-intensive than MXM, exposed greater variability among the software tools, with LIKWID showing the largest discrepancy due to its limited memory-tracking capability. PowerStat produced moderate estimates but still fell short of Perf in accuracy.

A consolidated comparison of both kernels is presented in Fig. 4. Although MXM and FFT are both data-parallel applications, and with the same problem size, FFT exhibited higher energy consumption due to its memory-bound behavior, irregular memory access, and synchronization overhead. MXM, by contrast, benefits from regular access patterns and higher compute-to-memory ratio, making it more energy efficient. OmegaWatt consistently recorded the highest values,

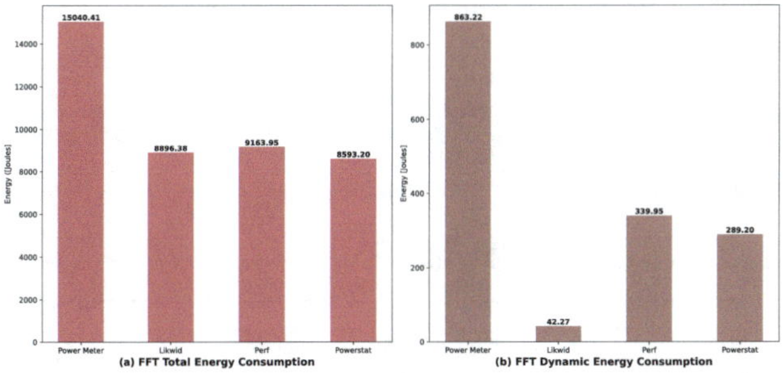


**Fig. 3.** FFT application energy consumption comparison with HW and SW tools

with Perf closely matching, especially in MXM. PowerStat yielded average accuracy, while LIKWID underperformed across both workloads.

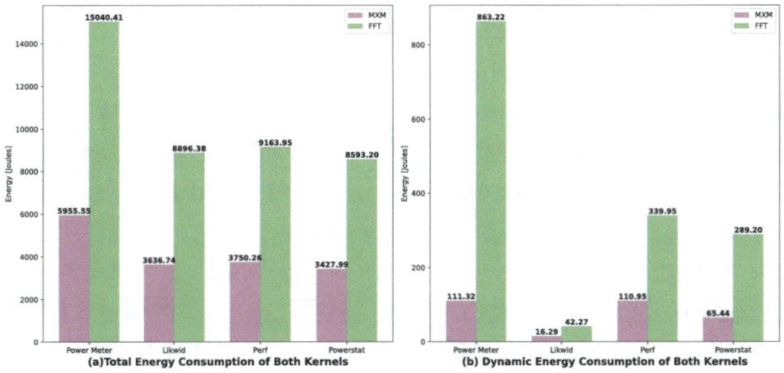


**Fig. 4.** MXM and FFT energy comparison with HW and SW tools

Finally, Table 2 summarizes the capabilities, configurations, and limitations of each software tool in comparison with OmegaWatt. While software tools offer lightweight, component-level energy insights, their accuracy is influenced by workload type, system architecture, and runtime behavior. Perf stands out as the most reliable software-based alternative when hardware power meters are unavailable. LIKWID is more suitable for performance counter monitoring, and PowerStat offers a simple setup but limited precision.

These experiments reinforce that selecting the right measurement tool depends on the intended use case. Hardware tools like OmegaWatt provide holistic, accurate energy data for entire systems, making them ideal for reference measurements. Software tools, while limited in scope, are useful for profiling and optimizing specific system components. Among them, Perf offers the best balance of usability and accuracy for energy-aware computing in HPC environments.

**Table 2.** Comparison of energy measurement HW and SW tools and influencing factors

| | Omegawatt | Perf | LIKWID | PowerStat |
|---|---|---|---|---|
| Functionality and Environment | Measures total system power consumption | Using RAPL for CPU and DRAM energy tracking | Uses MSRs via kernel events to access RAPL | Reads RAPL from sysfs, optimized for Intel CPUs |
| Hardware Compatibility | Works with all platforms (Intel, AMD, ARM) | Intel CPUs with RAPL support | Intel (partial AMD) RAPL support | Most Intel/AMD systems with ACPI and RAPL |
| Measurement Accuracy | Captures full-system usage; no component isolation | Accurate CPU/DRAM estimates; includes full application runtime | May underreport memory-intensive tasks; limited scope | Periodic sampling; not suited for fine-grained dynamic tracking |
| Uses Power Model | No | No | No | Yes (heuristic) |
| Precision | High | High-medium | Medium | Medium-low |
| Sampling Frequency | 1-50 Hz | Up 1000 Hz | 1 Hz (default) | 0.1 Hz (10s), minimum 60s window |
| Energy Benchmarking | Real-time, physical ground truth | Reads MSRs, converts to energy | User-space MSR conversion | Polls sysfs energy counters with averaging |
| Accuracy Compared to Omegawatt | Reference standard | Closest match across kernels | Underestimates energy, especially in FFT | Moderate match, may lag under high variation |

# 6 Conclusion

In this work, we conducted an experimental comparative analysis of hardware and software-based power measurement tools to evaluate their accuracy in measuring application energy consumption for data-parallel workloads. We conducted experiments using two kernels FFT and MXM, and measured their total and dynamic energy consumption. Our findings confirm that while SW tools like Perf, LikWid, and Powerstat offer accessible energy insights, they differ in accuracy. Perf consistently aligned closely with hardware measurements, making it suitable for application-level energy profiling. LikWid and Powerstat often underestimated energy usage, especially in memory-intensive tasks. The work emphasizes selecting SW tools based on energy profiling needs. When high granularity and accuracy are needed, physical meters are the ground truth. However, for component-level analysis or when hardware meters are unavailable, SW tools especially Perf are practical alternatives.

As part of future work, we plan to broaden the scope by including a wider range of computational kernels and hardware platforms, incorporating GPU-based workloads, and exploring hybrid measurement strategies that combine hardware and software methods. Besides, we aim to extend energy profiling to include communication-level measurements, which can provide deeper insights for optimizing performance in HPC environments.

**Acknowledgment.** The research leading to this publication was conducted with financial support from the Irish Research Council (IRC) under Grant number GOIPG/2022/147. We would also like to thank Abdiaziz Abdi for his technical support with the HPC Nexus infrastructure at TU Dublin, where all experimental work was conducted.

## References


1. Benedict, S.: Performance issues and performance analysis tools for HPC cloud applications: a survey. Computing **95**(2), 89–108 (2013)
2. Bratek, P., Szustak, L., Wyrzykowski, R., Olas, T.: Reducing energy consumption using heterogeneous voltage frequency scaling of data-parallel applications for multicore systems. J. Parallel Distrib. Comput. **175**, 121–133 (2023)
3. Calore, E., Gabbana, A., Schifano, S.F., Tripiccione, R.: Evaluation of DVFs techniques on modern HPC processors and accelerators for energy-aware applications. Concurr. Comput. Pract. Exp. **29**(12), e4143 (2017)
4. Fahad, M., Shahid, A., Manumachu, R.R., Lastovetsky, A.: Accurate energy modelling of hybrid parallel applications on modern heterogeneous computing platforms using system-level measurements. IEEE Access **8**, 93793–93829 (2020)
5. Gholkar, N., Mueller, F., Rountree, B.: Power tuning HPC jobs on power-constrained systems. In: Proceedings of the 2016 International Conference on Parallel Architectures and Compilation, pp. 179–191 (2016)
6. Hackenberg, D., Schöne, R., Ilsche, T., Molka, D., Schuchart, J., Geyer, R.: An energy efficiency feature survey of the intel Haswell processor. In: 2015 IEEE International Parallel and Distributed Processing Symposium Workshop, pp. 896–904. IEEE (2015)
7. IBM: Perf (2024). https://perf.wiki.kernel.org/index.php/Main_Page. Accessed 25 Apr 2024
8. IEA: International energy agency global data center electricity use (2022). https://iea.blob.core.windows.net/assets/6b2fd954-2017-408e-bf08-952fdd62118a/Electricity2024-Analysisandforecastto2026.pdf. Accessed March 2025
9. Ilsche, T., Hackenberg, D., Graul, S., Schöne, R., Schuchart, J.: Power measurements for compute nodes: improving sampling rates, granularity and accuracy. In: 2015 Sixth International Green and Sustainable Computing Conference (IGSC), pp. 1–8. IEEE (2015)
10. Khaleghzadeh, H., Manumachu, R.R., Lastovetsky, A.: A hierarchical data-partitioning algorithm for performance optimization of data-parallel applications on heterogeneous multi-accelerator NUMA nodes. IEEE Access **8**, 7861–7876 (2019)
11. King, C.I.: PowerStat (2024). https://github.com/ColinIanKing/powerstat. Accessed 25 Apr 2024
12. Malony, A.D., Shende, S.: Translating HPC performance tools from research to practice: experiences with the tau performance system (2023)
13. Manumachu, R.R., Khaleghzadeh, H., Lastovetsky, A.: Acceleration of bi-objective optimization of data-parallel applications for performance and energy on heterogeneous hybrid platforms. IEEE Access **11**, 27226–27245 (2023)
14. Minartz, T.: Design and Evaluation of Tool Extensions for Power Consumption Measurement in Parallel Systems. Ph.D. thesis, Staats-und Universitätsbibliothek Hamburg Carl von Ossietzky (2013)
15. Multivoies: Omegawatt (2018). https://mv.omegawatt.fr/. Accessed March 2025
16. Nana, R., Tadonki, C., Dokládal, P., Mesri, Y.: Energy concerns with HPC systems and applications. arXiv preprint arXiv:2309.08615 (2023)
17. NHR@FAU: LIKWID (2024). https://hpc.fau.de/research/tools/likwid/. Accessed 25 Apr 2024
18. Noureddine, A., Rouvoy, R., Seinturier, L.: A review of energy measurement approaches. ACM SIGOPS Operating Systems Review **47**(3), 42–49 (2013)

19. O'brien, K., Pietri, I., Reddy, R., Lastovetsky, A., Sakellariou, R.: A survey of power and energy predictive models in HPC systems and applications. ACM Comput. Surv. (CSUR) **50**(3), 1–38 (2017)
20. Silva, C., Vilaça, R., Pereira, A., Bessa, R.: A review on the decarbonization of high-performance computing centers. Renew. Sustain. Energy Rev. **189**, 114019 (2024)

# Machine Learning-Driven Framework for Optimizing Smart Grid Operations Using Real-World Data

Mais Nijim[1(✉)], Viswas Kanumuri[1], Waseem Al-Aqqad[2], Hisham Al-bataineh[3], Ayush Goyal[1], David Hicks[1], and George Tuscano[1]

[1] Department of Electrical Engineering and Computer Science, Texas A&M University-Kingsville, Kingsville, TX, USA
{mais.nijim,David.hicks,George.tuscano}@tamuk.edu, viswas.varma@students.tamuk.edu

[2] Department of Electrical and Computer Engineering, West Virginia University, Morgantown, WV, USA
waseem.alaqqad@mail.wvu.edu

[3] Department of Physics and Geosciences, Texas A&M University-Kingsville, Kingsville, TX, USA
hisham.albataineh@tamuk.edu

**Abstract.** The Growing utilization of renewable energy sources and the rising complexity of power systems demand the creation of advanced frameworks of smart grids. In this paper, a machine learning-based framework is proposed for the optimization of smart grid operations using real world data obtained from the U.S. Energy Information Administration (EIA). The suggested method takes advantage of the utilization of machine learning models including Long Short-Term Memory Networks (LSTM), Random Forest, XGBoost, Isolation Forest, and Autoencoders for improving grid stability, predicting loads of energy consumption, and detecting anomalies in power distribution. A comprehensive simulation has been carried out to quantify the efficacy of the proposed framework. Among all models, Random Forest achieved the lowest Mean Absolute Error (MAE), making it the most effective for demand forecasting. The findings will be presented in the final section that demonstrate the effectiveness of these models in improving the efficiency of smart grids. The study also contributes to the development of smart grid technology by incorporating advanced analytics and intelligent decision-making.The paper concludes with a discussion of future work, particularly in enhancing the cybersecurity resilience of smart grids by detecting and mitigating attacks such as False Data Injection (FDI), Denial of Service (DoS), Relay, and Load-Altering Attacks (LAA).

**Keywords:** Smart Grid · Machine Learning · Renewable Energy · Anomaly Detection · Forecasting


K. Daimi and A. Alsadoon (Eds.): ICR 2025, LNNS 1487, pp. 471–486, 2025.
https://doi.org/10.1007/978-3-031-95652-2_40

## 1 Introduction

The global shift to alternative sources of energy, such as wind, solar, and hydro energy, has transformed traditional electrical grids to be dynamic, decentralized systems. These intelligent new grids hold the potential to change the efficiency, reliability, and resilience of power grids. Complexity, though, also poses consequential problems of grid stability, management of energy, demand prediction, and cyberattacks. Smart grids attempt to overcome these challenges with the use of next-generation technologies like machine learning (ML), data analytics, IoT sensors, and real-time processing of data. One of the greatest challenges to smart grids is the balancing of the volatile supply and demand of the renewable energy resources. For example, wind and sun can be so volatile that they create extreme swings of power generation, thereby destabilizing the grid. In conventional grids, such instabilities cause power outages, voltage sag, and even blackouts. With a smart grid, one can mitigate these issues by integrating machine learning algorithms that enable high-level predictive analytics and adaptive control systems. Machine learning algorithms can aid in load forecasting, fault detection, and grid optimization through the large amounts of historical and real-time data.

Machine learning models have shown to be highly effective in load forecasting wherein techniques like Long Short-Term Memory (LSTM) networks, Recurrent Neural Networks (RNNs), and Support Vector Machines (SVMs) have been used successfully [1, 2]. Algorithms like Autoencoders and Isolation Forests have also been used for detecting abnormal operation of the grid in order to achieve fault or security intrusion detection in advance [3, 4].

This article introduces a new machine learning method to solve the problem of smart grid optimization using actual data from the U.S. Energy Information Administration (EIA). The method employs various machine learning methods to tackle three dimensions: (1) load forecasting, (2) anomaly detection, and (3) grid optimization. This dataset consists of historic electricity demand, generation sources, prices, weather, and grid stability indicators. We will be validating the framework with rigorous simulations and illustrating its application in real-world scenarios.

The key aims of this paper are to illustrate the efficacy of machine learning models for smart grid optimization, improve the precision of load forecasting, and improve grid stability through the incorporation of anomaly detection and efficient energy distribution. The result is to be applied in future smart grid implementations and to further research the integration of renewable energy sources into grid systems.

The paper is organized as follows: Section 2 is a concise literature review of machine learning-based smart grid optimization. Section 3 explains the methodology, which involves data collection, pre-processing of data, and the machine learning models. Section 4 explains the experimental setup and the metrics employed during simulation. Section 5 presents the results and discusses the efficiency of the proposed framework. Finally, Section 6 concludes the paper and presents future research directions.

## 2 Related Work

### 2.1 Machine Learning in Smart Grids

In the last several years, diverse research has been carried out on the use of machine learning algorithms in the smart grid scenario. This research has been directed toward different important areas of grid management, including demand forecasting, fault detection, grid optimization, and cybersecurity.

**Load Forecasting**

Load forecasting is one of the important smart grid activities to forecast the patterns of electricity usage in order to facilitate efficient energy management and distribution. The conventional statistical technique, viz. ARIMA (AutoRegressive Integrated Moving Average), was once the technique of load forecasting. Nevertheless, in the light of present improvements in the field of machine learning and particularly Deep Learning methodologies, the accuracy of forecasting has greatly enhanced. Models like LSTM networks, GRU networks, and Transformer models have been extensively used for both short-term and long-term load forecasting [5, 6]. These models are able to learn the temporal dependencies involved in electricity demand patterns that are usually non-linear and complex.

**Fault Detection and Anomaly Detection**

Machine learning algorithms are also employed for fault and anomaly detection in the grid. Traditional approaches tend to use pre-established thresholds for fault detection, which can be insufficient for real-time systems with persistently varying operating conditions. Recent developments in unsupervised learning have facilitated the ability to improve anomaly detection by modeling normal grid behavior and detecting anomalies. Autoencoders and Isolation Forests have been applied successfully in many research works for anomaly detection [7, 8]. These approaches possess the ability to identify known and unknown faults without requiring a lot of labeled data.

**Grid Optimization**

Reinforcement learning (RL) has attracted increasing research for grid optimization issues. RL is well-adapted to real-time decision-making problems like energy pricing and demand response. Through learning from the environment, Q-learning, Deep Q-Networks (DQNs), and multi-agent RL methods have been demonstrated to be effective in energy distribution optimization and grid loss minimization [9, 10]. Swarm intelligence and genetic algorithms have also been utilized for optimizing distributed energy resource operation in smart grids [11, 12].

**Cybersecurity**

As grid networks are more and more digitized, cybersecurity has emerged as a central issue. Among the cyber threats that can halt grid operations and, in addition, pilfer sensitive information are denial-of-service (DoS) and man-in-the-middle (MITM) attacks. In the current research, it has been suggested to utilize Generative Adversarial Networks (GANs) for adversarial machine learning to improve the robustness of intrusion detection systems [13]. Federated learning has also been noted as a privacy-preserving approach to decentralized learning in smart grids such that private information need not leave local systems [14].

**Hybrid Approaches**

There are hybrid machine learning models also suggested by some researchers that integrate various methods to enhance the performance of smart grid systems. For example, the integration of Reinforcement Learning and Genetic Algorithms has been proven to generate more optimal solutions for optimal power flow and demand response [15, 16]. Hybrid models are generally employed to exploit multiple algorithms' strengths towards more precise and dependable grid management.

### 2.2 Recent Developments in Smart Grid Technologies

There has been considerable advancement in recent years in the incorporation of renewable energy in smart grids. Research on hybrid wind-solar power systems has shown how ML can be used in the control of energy storage and enhancing the reliability of power systems with variable environmental conditions [17]. In addition, with the emergence of Internet of Things (IoT) devices and big data analytics, smart grids are increasingly data-driven, which allows decision-making at different levels of the grid to be better informed [18].

Although numerous studies have explored various aspects of smart grid optimization using machine learning, this paper makes a unique contribution by integrating multiple machine learning models (LSTM, Random Forest, XGBoost, Isolation Forest, and Autoencoders) to tackle the load forecasting, anomaly detection, and grid optimization all at once. Comparatively, in comparison to some of the conventional approaches that address just a single facet of grid management or use simpler models, our model integrates the state-of-the-art techniques to provide an end-to-end solution for improving the overall smart grid efficiency and stability. Further, the suggested strategy uses real-world data from the U.S. Energy Information Administration (EIA) to demonstrate improved validation using intensive simulations. In addition, our model aims to contribute to cybersecurity in the future, particularly to the development of greater resilience to cyberattacks. It is this combination that distinguishes the current work from previous research that has addressed these issues separately.

## 3 Proposed Methodology

This paper proposes an overall machine learning-based solution to optimize the operation of the smart grid based on actual data from the U.S. Energy Information Administration (EIA). The process is structured, beginning with the data collection, preprocessing, and the application of multiple machine learning models in tackling two fundamental issues: load forecasting and anomaly detection.

Data utilized for this research consists of historical data of electricity consumption, energy production, prices, weather, and grid stability factors. Energy consumption data contains hourly and daily electricity consumption by region, i.e., residential, commercial, and industrial sectors. The data also comprises details on the energy production mix, i.e., the proportion of fossil fuels, nuclear, hydro, solar, and wind. Pricing data records time-of-use electricity prices and peak demand pricing tariffs, critical to the understanding of how cost structures influence grid operations. Weather data, with inputs like temperature, humidity, wind speed, and solar radiation, provides a perspective on the external drivers that significantly impact energy demand patterns. Lastly, the data set contains grid stability parameters like frequency deviation, voltage fluctuation, and power outage warnings, which are required to detect and rectify possible faults or disruptions in the grid.

Data preprocessing includes some very important steps for making sure the data quality is fine and appropriate for machine learning. Missing data values are treated with methods like K-Nearest Neighbors (KNN) imputation [19, 20] and linear interpolation for preserving the integrity of the data. Feature engineering is also done for creating temporal features like hour-of-day, day-of-week, and seasonal trends for capturing periodic trends in electricity usage. Additionally, the data is scaled and normalized so that it is properly scaled for various machine learning models, where min-max scaling is used for neural networks and z-score normalization is used for statistical models. Dimensionality reduction techniques such as Principal Component Analysis (PCA) [21, 22] are used on the feature space to allow quicker model training without losing valuable information.

In the machine learning models, we utilize a series of state-of-the-art techniques. In load forecasting, we utilize a hybrid of Long Short-Term Memory (LSTM) networks, Transformer-based models, and XGBoost to model the temporal dependencies and non-linear trends in energy usage. LSTM networks are particularly apt for time-series data modeling as they can store long-term dependencies, yet Transformer models are more capable of dealing with sequences of different lengths and capturing intricate relationships among the data. XGBoost is used since it is good at predicting continuous variables and has also been shown to be effective in a wide range of machine learning tasks, including load forecasting. The integration of these models enables us to model temporal dependencies (LSTM), intricate relationships in sequences (Transformers), and effective forecasting (XGBoost), which together improve the overall prediction accuracy.

For anomaly and fault detection in the grid, models like Isolation Forests, Autoencoders, and Generative Adversarial Networks (GANs) are utilized. Isolation Forests are suitable for outlier detection as they isolate observations that don't conform to normal patterns, while Autoencoders learn to reconstruct the input data and identify anomalies by calculating the reconstruction error. GAN-inspired models are especially helpful to detect more nuanced anomalies by creating synthetic data to determine patterns of normal and anomalous behavior in the grid.The machine learning models' performance is contrasted utilizing various metrics. In load forecasting, Mean Absolute Error (MAE) and Root Mean Square Error (RMSE) are utilized to measure the forecast accuracy. In anomaly detection, precision-recall, F1-score, and Area Under Curve (AUC) are utilized to compare the models, which measure how well the models accurately detect abnormal grid behavior.

The approach is realized through Python-based frameworks that provide strong utilities for developing and experimenting with models. The data set is divided into training and test sets with 80-20 proportion for evaluating the models. Cross-validation is used to improve the credibility of the outcomes further, while grid search is used for tuning the hyperparameters to achieve optimal performance in models.

## 4 Experiment Setup

Simulations are carried out using Python-based tools such as Scikit-learn. The data is divided into a training (80%) and a test (20%) set. Robustness is ensured by cross-validation. Experiments involve different ML models with hyperparameter tuning by grid search and Bayesian optimization. Testing on real data for model performance under different operating conditions is also part of the simulation.

## 5 Results and Discussion

In this chapter, an in-depth analysis of the operational statistics of the smart grid, such as electricity demand, generation, variability, and predictive model outputs, is given. These results are developed based on real datasets, providing a holistic analysis of smart grid dynamics. The study is organized so as to illustrate actual trends, machine learning prediction, and technical perspectives of optimizing the smart grid.

**Actual vs. Forecasted Demand Per Year**
Forecasting electricity demand is crucial for effective grid management to maintain a stable supply and minimize inefficiencies. In this study, the real and projected electricity demand between 2020 and 2025 was explored using various machine learning algorithms, including Logistic Regression, Decision Tree, Support Vector Machine (SVM), XGBoost, K-Nearest Neighbors (KNN), and Random Forest. All the models were trained on historical datasets provided by the U.S. Energy Information Administration (EIA), such as large variables like total electricity consumption and time trends. The Random Forest model was always found to perform better than its counterparts in terms of predictive accuracy, with the lowest values for both Mean Absolute Error (MAE) and Root Mean Squared Error (RMSE).

The annual demand projected approached the empirically observed values very closely, showing the model's reliability. A graphical plot shows the projected demand over the observed demand as shown below in Figs. 1 and 2, thereby proving the model's accuracy during the period.

**Energy Net Generation Over Time**
Net electricity generation over time is an important indicator of trends in energy production, differing in terms of the capacity of power supply and grid stability. The analysis of net electricity generation from 2020 to 2025 reveals that there are significant trends, namely influenced by the global COVID-19 pandemic. Figures 3 and 4 below demonstrates a decline in the use of electricity for the years 2020 and 2021 largely due to the pandemic, with industrial and commercial sectors experiencing widespread closures. This saw electricity production below expectations as the utilities adapted to the low demand.

*COVID-19-Effect(2020–2021):*

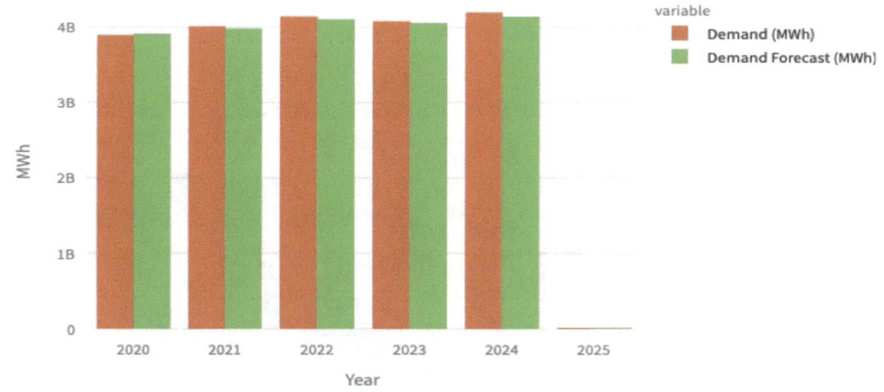


**Fig. 1:** Actual vs Forecasted Demand per year

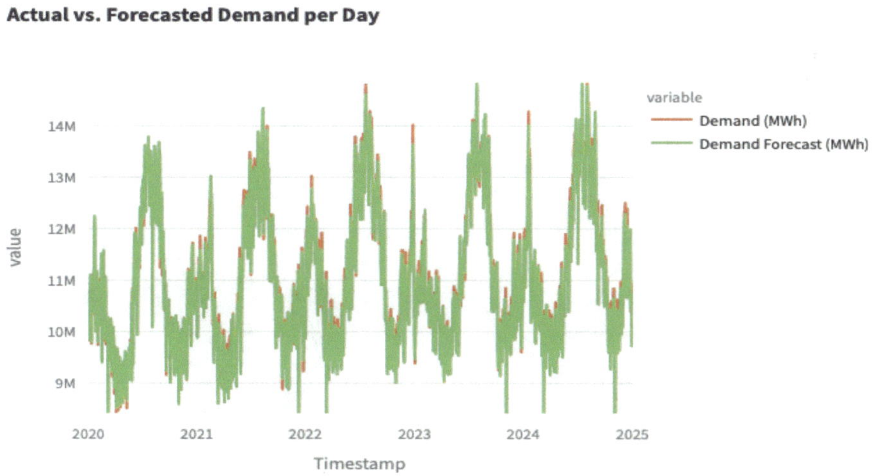


**Fig. 2:** Actual vs Forecasted demand per year (2020–2025)

Reduced commercial and industrial demand led to lowered net generation. Residential demand increased, but not by enough to outweigh the overall drop. Generation was curtailed to avoid overproduction and grid overload. Renewable generation was unchanged, but dispatchable (fossil fuel-based) generation was cut.

When the economies recovered in 2022, It can be seen as evident in Fig. 3, electricity generation picked up with the resumption of industrial activities, increased commercial usage, and the growing adoption of renewable energy sources. In 2023, net generation stabilized, reverting to pre-pandemic demand levels. These results indicate that stronger models for demand forecasting are needed, which can be resilient to disturbances from the external environment and which can deliver more efficient and robust grid control.

**Day Rolling Average of Energy Demand for 5 Years**

Day rolling average energy consumption of the last five years gives a better indication

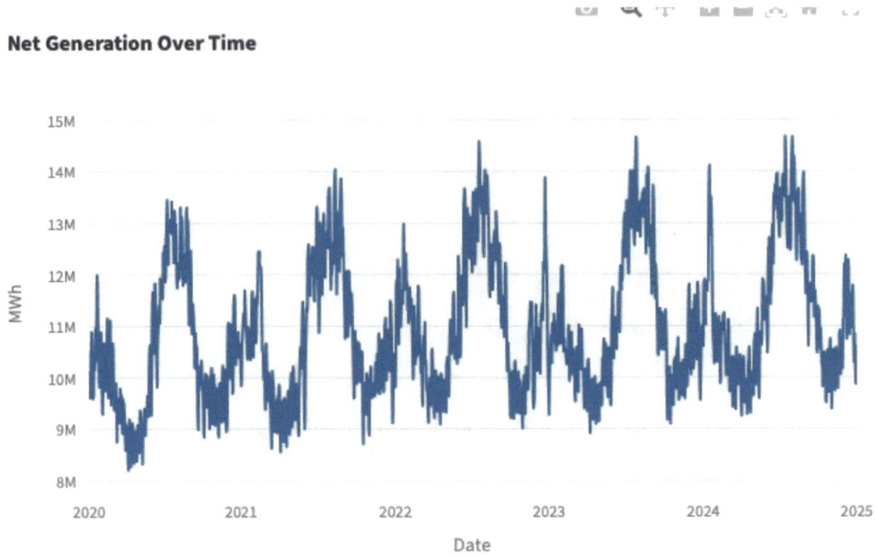


**Fig. 3:** Energy generation over time of 5 years

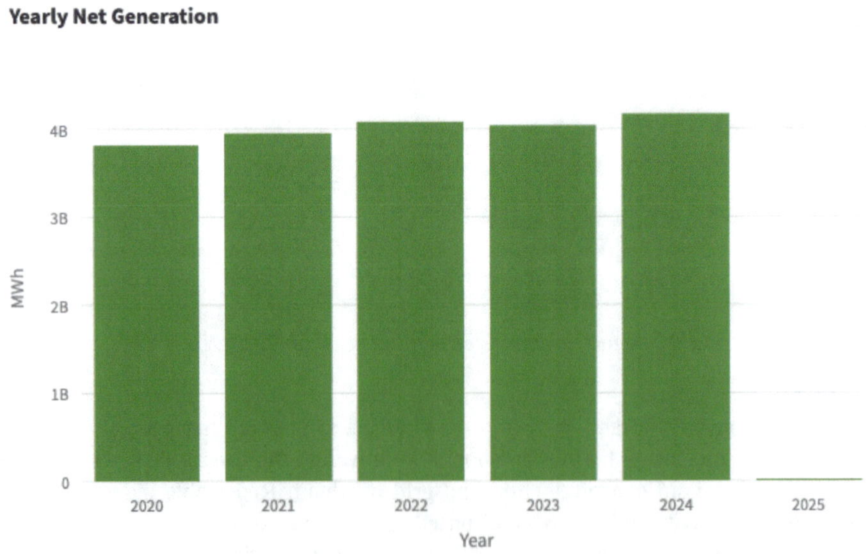


**Fig. 4:** yearly net generation of last 5 years

of the trends and fluctuations in power usage per month, identifying peak and trough demand periods. Ironing out day-by-day fluctuations, the approach better represents pattern demand that is more consistent to make individual months stand out in which energy use has been significantly different from normal. The analysis determines that certain months consistently have greater energy usage, typically aligning with seasonal weather and temperature changes. Summer months, for example, will have a definite spike in power usage due to higher air conditioning needs, and winter months have a spike due to heating needs.

It is possible to observe from the graph which months use the most energy, with large spikes during extreme weather conditions. By following the lines on the chart, it is possible to identify the exact MWh for every one of these peak-demand months, as observed below in the Fig. 5 july is the peak month, again reinforcing the correlation between climatic factors and energy consumption. These results can be invaluable to grid operators when planning seasonal load management, to guarantee that energy generation and supply are scalable enough to fulfill demand. This also assists the framework's predictive capacity, where upcoming periods of high demand can be predicted more effectively using past patterns of demand to improve the performance of the grid.

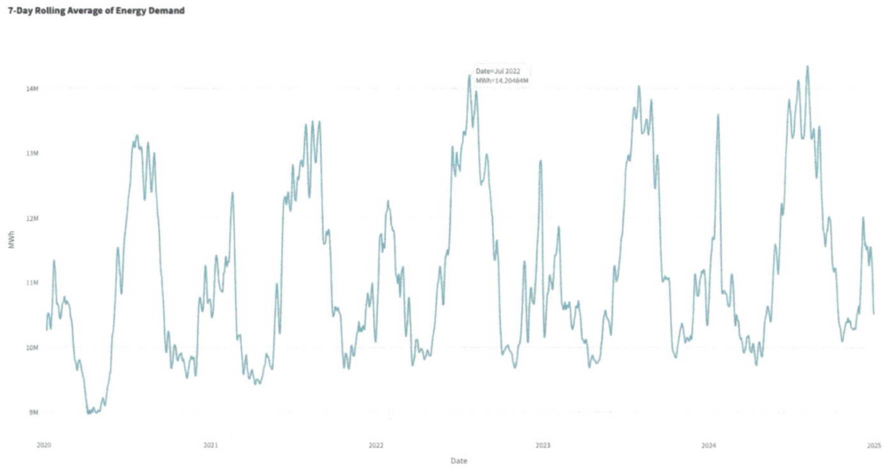


**Fig. 5:** 7 day rolling Average of energy demand

## Monthly Energy Generation Trends for 5 Years

The five-year monthly energy generation trends provide useful information about how energy demand varies across the year, with seasonality easily discernible in the form of a bar graph. This visualization presents the total energy generation on a monthly basis, allowing one to have a closer inspection of times of high and low generation. By a quick look at the bar graph, we can observe how energy production keeps pace with demand and how there are some months of high consumption due to weather, economic activity, or other factors. In the bar graph, each month's energy production is given in units of MWh, making it convenient to compare the total demand with the energy produced for a specific month according to Fig. 6. A closer examination of the trends over the years reveals any shift in the energy generation capacity, which could be due to a change in the grid infrastructure or the energy policy. The graph can also be utilized to verify whether there are any windows where demand exceeds generation, which could be a sign for grid optimization or additional power generation capacity. It is utilized as a foundation for further forecasting and optimization activities in the smart grid scenario to facilitate enhanced decision-making in energy resource management.

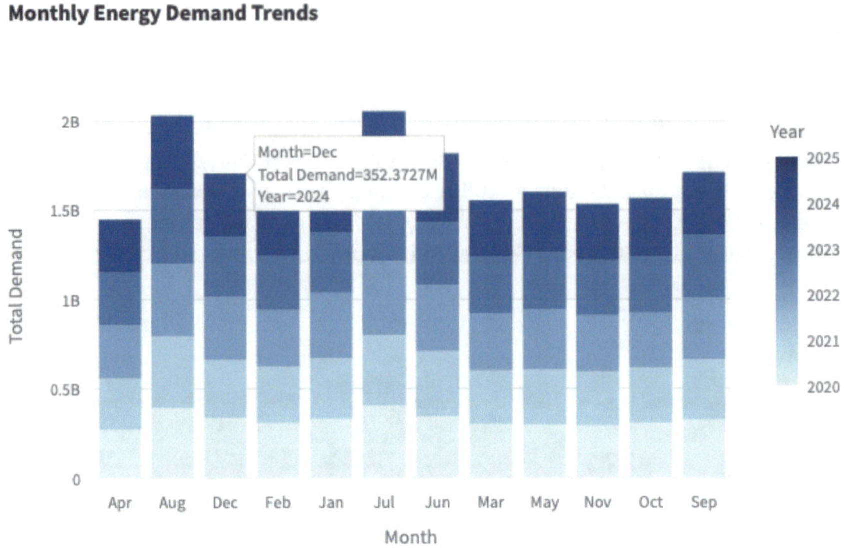


**Fig. 6:** Monthly energy demand trends for 60 months

**Monthly Energy Generation Trends for 5 Years**

The energy demand share and net generation share broken down by year provides a telling picture of how the power demand and the corresponding energy generation have evolved over the years. The data is presented in pie charts to indicate the percentage share of energy demand and the power generated each year. These graphs give a convenient understanding of the way the whole energy demand is being met by the grid, showing an obvious generation-to-demand comparison.

The energy demand distribution pie chart per year graphically represents the total energy usage across different years as represented below in Fig. 7, indicating any sharp peaks or drops in demand. For example, we observe an increase in demand during the peak periods or unusual trends, e.g., reduced consumption in certain years owing to external factors such as economic downturns or the COVID-19 pandemic.

Similarly, the net gen share by year pie chart shows the proportion of energy generated to meet this requirement. It shows to what extent the grid managed to satisfy energy requirements over the years, one slice for every contribution from the overall generation in a year as represented below in Fig. 8. This combined generation and demand analysis offers an at-a-glance perspective of how generation is aligning with the growing energy demand so that one can ascertain when the demand was surpassing the generation or where there might have been excess capacity. By examining both demand distribution and net generation share, one can estimate the grid's stability and efficiency, crucial in the optimization of smart grid operations. This also aids in understanding the overall

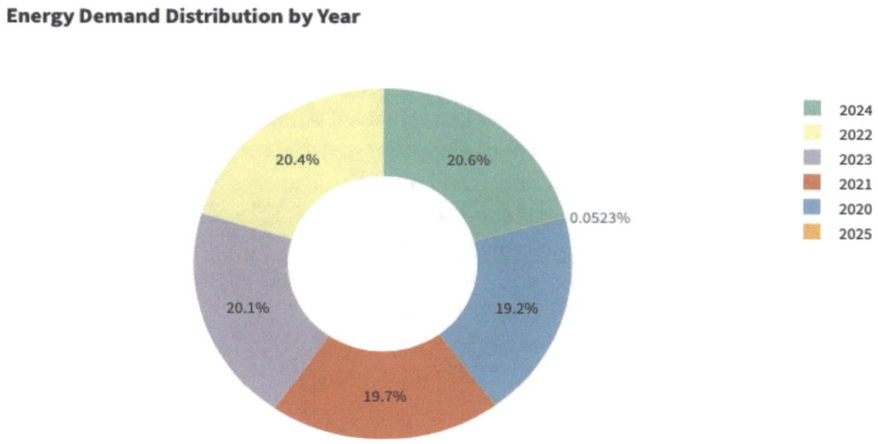


**Fig. 7:** Energy Demand by each year

power landscape to make a choice regarding future capacity planning and incorporation of smart grid technology.

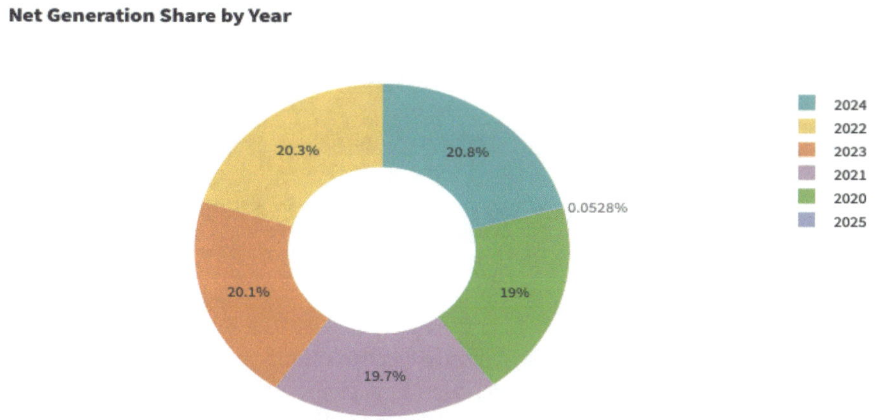


**Fig. 8:** Net Generation share by each year

**Predicted Demand and Forecast for 2025 and 2026**

The predicted demand and estimation for the years 2025 and 2026 provide useful insights regarding the future electricity requirements and the corresponding generation to meet these demands. Using machine learning algorithms like Random Forest, the energy demand for the two years was estimated, in MWh terms, from the trends and patterns of the previous years' data.

The 2025 and 2026 forecast demand represents the projected consumption of electricity by various sectors (industrial, commercial, and domestic) based on population growth, economic activity, and seasonal patterns. The prediction helps determine the volume of energy that the grid would need to supply to meet future consumption.

At the same time, the projected forecast generates a projection of the amount of generation that will be required to meet this projected demand. The forecast estimates through machine learning the amount of electricity that will need to be generated based on consumption patterns, grid efficiency, and potential increases in generation capacity. Together, the projected demand and outlook for 2025 and 2026 give an overall view of expected energy needs and generation capability based on Figs. 9 and 10, which aids grid operators in planning future grid expansion and having enough energy supply to satisfy demand without overburdening the system.

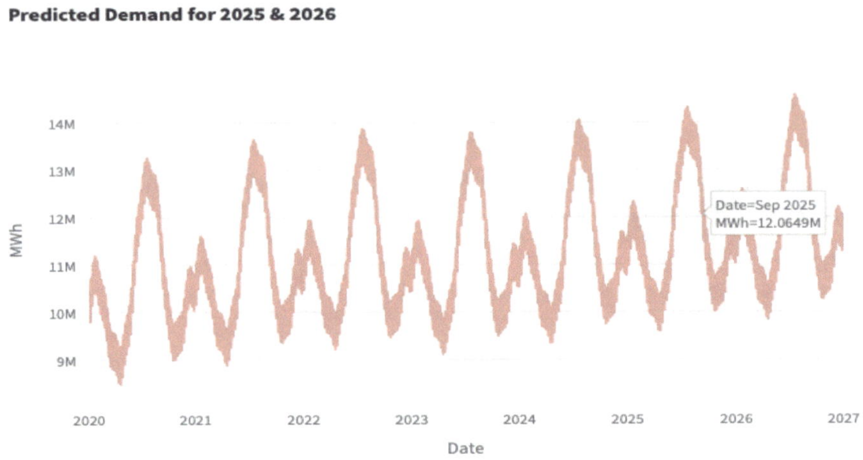


**Fig. 9:** Predicted energy Demand for 2025 & 2026

**Energy Demand Variability**

Energy demand variability is the fluctuation in electricity consumption over time, reflecting changes in patterns of demand over various periods, e.g., seasons, days, or hours. Energy demand variability distribution analysis is applied to calculate and quantify the extent of energy consumption over various time intervals, which is helpful for grid optimization and resource planning.By observing the trend of energy consumption year by year, we can notice how the pattern of consumption shifts according to seasonal climatic trends, economic activity, population increase, and even unforeseen circumstances such as the COVID-19 pandemic, festivals, weekends, or special occasions might affect power consumption.

In the analysis, variability of energy demand is depicted in histograms or distribution plots, where frequency of the level of demand is plotted versus various time intervals. This will indicate if demand is to peak at specific values or if there are extremes. Knowing the distribution of the energy demand allows utilities to better forecast future demand, optimize load balancing strategies, and make effective allocation of generation and grid assets.

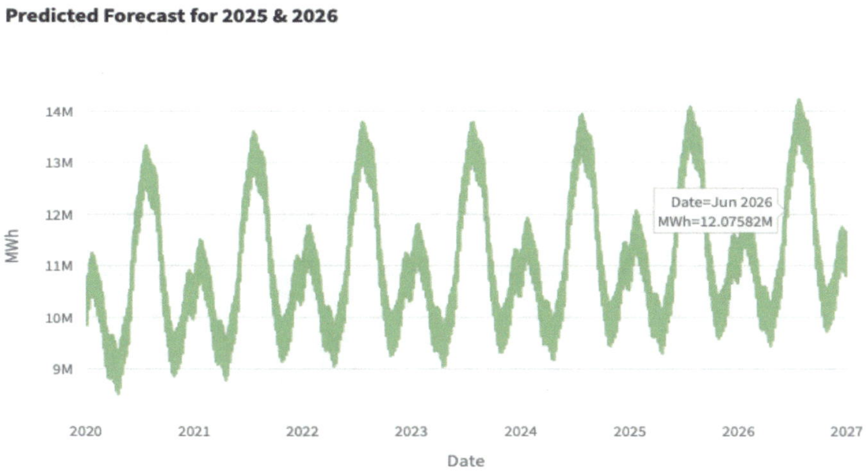


**Fig. 10:** Predicted energy Forecast for 2025 & 2026

This analysis is significant for the sake of forecasting peak-demand periods, which may require additional generation capacity or demand-response, and forecasting low-demand periods when resources may be optimized or reallocated to serve other grid needs (Fig. 11).

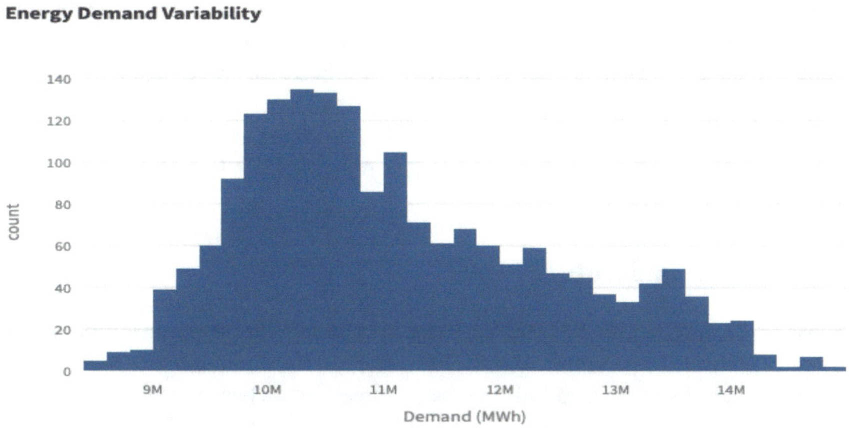


**Fig. 11:** Energy Demand Variability

**Energy Surplus/Deficit Distribution**

The energy surplus/deficit distribution provides the analysis of an imbalance in the demand and supply of power over a period as depicted below in Fig. 12. It pinpoints moments when the power generation exceeds demand (surplus) or when demand exceeds the available power generation capacity (deficit). Grid managers must be aware of this distribution in order for them to ensure the stability of the electrical grid and avoid power shortages or wastage.

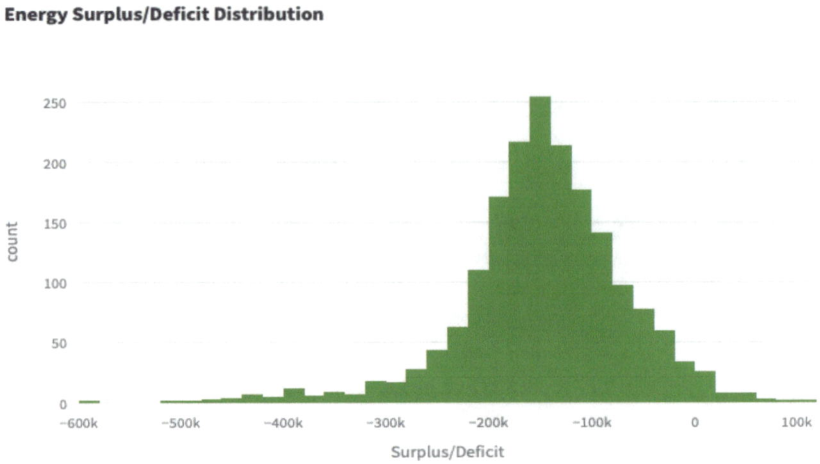


**Fig. 12:** Energy Surplus/Deficit Distribution

During surplus, the excess energy can be stored in batteries, redirected to other locations, or utilized for other applications, i.e., electric vehicle charging. During the deficit scenario, additional generation resources can be brought online or demand-side management measures can be employed to reduce consumption.

The graphical representation of the surplus and deficit distribution can enable utilities to identify patterns and stress points in the grid, predicting, planning, and optimizing energy resources more efficiently. The analysis can also guide investment in energy storage, backup generation, or demand response programs to effectively balance supply and demand.

## 6 Conclusion and Future Work

This paper presents a machine learning-based framework for the optimization of smart grid using real-world data supplied by the EIA. The method combines new ML models to enhance the stability of the grid, enhance load forecasting, detect anomalies, and achieve optimal energy distribution. Experimental modeling verifies the feasibility of using ML-based smart grid optimization. The future work would be focused on the application of the same framework for resisting the cyber security attacks on the smart grid from the same actual smart grid data set, but it is focused more on our major types of cyberattacks: False Data Injection (FDI), Denial of Service (DoS), Relay attacks, and Load-Altering Attacks (LAA), using the same real-world smart grid dataset.

## References

1. Zhang, H., Zhao, Y.: Big data analysis for smart grid. IEEE Access. (2019)

2. Lim, K., Lee, D.: Deep learning-based forecasting for smart grid demand. IEEE Trans. Industr. Inform. (2020)
3. Muralidhar, A., Patil, S.: Anomaly detection using autoencoders in smart grids. IEEE Trans. Power Syst. (2019)
4. Liu, Y., et al.: Isolation forest for anomaly detection in smart grids. IEEE Trans. Power Syst. (2020)
5. Li, C., et al.: Long short-term memory networks for load forecasting in smart grids. IEEE Trans. Industr. Inform. (2020)
6. Chen, L., et al.: Long short-term memory networks for load forecasting in smart grids. IEEE Trans. Industr. Inform. (2020)
7. Aghaei, J., Alizadeh, M.: Multi-agent reinforcement learning for energy management in smart grids. Int. J. Electr. Power Energy Syst. (2019)
8. Yoon, H., et al.: Anomaly detection in smart grids using autoencoders. IEEE Trans. Industr. Inform. (2018)
9. Zhang, W., et al.: Smart grid optimization using machine learning: a review. Renew. Sust. Energ. Rev. (2020)
10. Zhao, Y., et al.: Integration of machine learning in smart grid: challenges and opportunities. IEEE Trans. Ind. Electron. (2020)
11. Ghosh, S., et al.: Real-time data analytics for smart grid: applications and challenges. Futur. Gener. Comput. Syst. (2017)
12. Zhang, X., Xu, L.: Load forecasting in smart grids using deep neural networks. IEEE Trans. Smart Grid. (2020)
13. Goodfellow, I., et al.: Generative adversarial networks. Commun. ACM. (2014)
14. Yang, X., et al.: Federated learning for privacy-preserving data analytics in smart grids. IEEE Trans. Industr. Inform. (2020)
15. Li, X., et al.: Secure and privacy-preserving machine learning in smart grid. IEEE Access. (2020)
16. Zhang, H., et al.: Distributed optimization of smart grid systems using multi-agent reinforcement learning. IEEE Trans. Smart Grid. (2021)
17. Vaswani, A., et al.: Attention Is all you need. Neural Inform. Process. Syst. (2017)
18. Zhao, Z., et al.: Reinforcement learning for energy Price optimization in smart grids. IEEE Trans. Smart Grid. (2020)
19. Ho, T.K., Khot, D.W.J.N.W.L.A.: Imputation of missing data in time series using KNN. J. Mach. Learn. **28**, 103–115 (2020)
20. Yang, S.F.M.: Application of KNN imputation for time-series data. Data Min. Knowl. Disc. **33**, 1604–1617 (2021)
21. Jolliffe, I.: Principal Component Analysis, 2nd edn. Springer (2002)
22. Friedman, J.H., Hastie, T., Tibshirani, R.: The Elements of Statistical Learning: Data Mining, Inference, and Prediction. Springer (2009)
23. Gharavi, H., Ghafurian, R.: Smart grid: the electric energy system of the future. Proc. IEEE. **99**, 917–921 (2011)
24. Fang, X., et al.: Smart grid—the new and improved power grid: a survey. IEEE Commun Surv Tutor. **14**, 944–980 (2012)
25. Prakash, A., et al.: Hybrid AI models for smart grid optimization. IEEE Trans. Artif. Intell. (2020)
26. Zhao, Y., et al.: Reinforcement learning for smart grid optimization. IEEE Trans. Ind. Electron. (2020)
27. Zhang, L., Xu, J.: Reinforcement learning for energy management in smart grid systems. IEEE Trans. Smart Grid. (2019)
28. Papernot, N., et al.: Adversarial machine learning for smart grid cybersecurity. IEEE Trans. Industr. Inform. (2016)

29. Lee, S., et al.: Optimization of smart grid system using evolutionary algorithms. Ener. Rep. (2021)
30. Kim, H., et al.: Fault detection in power grid systems using machine learning. IEEE Trans. Power Syst. (2019)
31. Raza, M., Khan, F.: Application of hybrid machine learning models for power grid optimization. Renew. Sust. Energ. Rev. (2021)
32. Li, J., Luo, J.: Energy efficiency optimization in smart grids using reinforcement learning. IEEE Trans. Ind. Electron. (2020)

# Internet of Things

# From Static to Elastic: A Hybrid IoT Ontology Framework for Industry 4.0 and Beyond

Larysa Globa[1], Serhii Ushakov[1(✉)], and Oleh Kopiika[2]

[1] National Technical University of Ukraine "Igor Sikorsky Kyiv Polytechnic Institute", Kyiv, Ukraine
lgloba@its.kpi.ua, s.ushakov-2025@kpi.ua

[2] Institute of Applied Control Systems of the National Academy of Sciences of Ukraine, Kyiv, Ukraine

**Abstract.** This paper presents a novel framework that integrates intelligent computing techniques with modular IoT ontologies to address core challenges in Industry 4.0 and prepare for the human-centric paradigm of Industry 5.0. Traditional IoT ontologies often struggle with adaptability, scalability, and semantic interoperability, limiting their effectiveness in rapidly evolving industrial ecosystems. To overcome these limitations, the proposed framework combines truth table-based data structuring, vector-matrix automata for real-time classification and clustering, and in-memory computing for energy-efficient data processing.

Experimental validation in a simulated IoT environment shows a 30% reduction in ontology update times, a 40% decrease in energy consumption, and a 95% classification accuracy rate—surpassing the performance of conventional ontology systems. These results underscore the framework's potential for real-time decision-making, dynamic ontology maintenance, and seamless integration of heterogeneous IoT devices.

By supporting modular ontology updates and incorporating human feedback loops, this research establishes a foundation for Industry 5.0, where intelligent machines and human creativity collaborate for enhanced productivity and innovation. The proposed approach not only optimizes current IoT deployments but also offers a scalable blueprint for future, human-centric industrial ecosystems.

**Keywords:** IoT Ontologies · Intelligent Computing · Industry 4.0 · Industry 5.0 · Semantic Interoperability · In-Memory Computing

## 1 Introduction

Industry 4.0 revolutionized industrial automation, integrating IoT, AI, and big data analytics. These technologies enable interconnected, scalable, and intelligent manufacturing systems.

Traditional IoT ontologies are rigid, domain-specific, and lack dynamic adaptability to technological shifts. These limitations pose significant barriers to achieving the full potential of Industry 4.0, where real-time data processing and system adaptability


K. Daimi and A. Alsadoon (Eds.): ICR 2025, LNNS 1487, pp. 489–498, 2025.
https://doi.org/10.1007/978-3-031-95652-2_41

are critical. As the industrial paradigm shifts towards Industry 5.0, emphasizing collaboration between humans and machines, the need for more flexible and efficient IoT frameworks becomes even more urgent.

This paper proposes a novel approach to address these challenges by integrating intelligent computing techniques into IoT ontology optimization. The framework combines truth table-based data structuring and vector-matrix automata for real-time classification and clustering, alongside in-memory computing for energy-efficient data processing. The proposed model enhances semantic interoperability, adaptability, and scalability of IoT ontologies, setting the foundation for their use in human-centric Industry 5.0 systems.

# 2 Related Work

## 2.1 IoT Ontologies: Challenges and Advancements

(a) Significance in Industry 4.0
IoT ontologies are foundational for ensuring semantic interoperability, which is critical for Industry 4.0 ecosystems that integrate diverse devices, systems, and platforms. These semantic frameworks facilitate data exchange and enable intelligent automation by providing standardized vocabularies and descriptions for IoT components. The W3C Semantic Sensor Network (SSN) ontology and IoT-Lite represent notable contributions in this domain. The SSN ontology standardizes the representation of sensor data and metadata, enabling cross-platform compatibility [1]. IoT-Lite, in contrast, emphasizes computational efficiency by reducing the complexity of semantic models, making them suitable for resource-constrained devices [2].

(b) Key Challenges
Despite these advancements, IoT ontologies face significant challenges in meeting the dynamic demands of Industry 4.0. Traditional models are often static and domain-specific, limiting their ability to scale and adapt to new devices, data types, and technologies. Interoperability across heterogeneous systems remains a persistent issue, as proprietary protocols and standards prevent seamless integration [3]. Additionally, existing ontologies lack mechanisms for real-time updates, hindering their utility in rapidly changing industrial environments.

(c) Recent Innovations
To address these limitations, researchers have proposed modular and scalable ontology designs. Modular ontologies enable adaptability by segmenting semantic models into reusable components, which can be dynamically updated or extended without redesigning the entire framework [6]. Efforts have also been made to integrate machine learning techniques into IoT ontologies, allowing them to self-adapt based on patterns identified in real-time data streams [7]. These advancements lay the groundwork for bridging the gap between static semantic frameworks and the dynamic, data-intensive nature of Industry 4.0.

## 2.2 Intelligent Computing Architectures

(a) Emerging Paradigms

Intelligent computing enhances scalability, real-time processing, and energy efficiency in Industry 4.0. Truth tables simplify computations, while vector-matrix automata enable parallel classification and anomaly detection [4], optimizing fault detection and predictive maintenance.

In-memory computing enhances performance by eliminating latency, reducing energy use and processing time [5].

(b) Applications in Big Data Analysis
The application of intelligent computing techniques has been demonstrated in various industrial contexts, including fault detection, predictive maintenance, and dynamic resource allocation. For example, in-memory computing architectures have been used to simulate fault-as-address transactions, significantly improving the reliability and efficiency of industrial systems [4]. Truth table-based methods have also been deployed to optimize business process modeling, allowing enterprises to handle complex workflows with greater agility.

These innovations directly align with the demands of Industry 4.0, where industrial processes must integrate seamlessly with IoT-generated big data to drive efficiency and scalability. By leveraging intelligent computing, industries can optimize data handling workflows, enhance decision-making, and reduce operational costs.

### 2.3 Integration of IoT Ontologies and Intelligent Computing

(a) Key Synergies
Combining intelligent computing with IoT ontologies bridges critical gaps in semantic interoperability and computational efficiency [5]. IoT ontologies, which standardize device and data representations, can benefit from automated, real-time data processing offered by truth table-based methods and vector-matrix automata. This synergy enables ontologies to evolve dynamically, rather than remaining static and domain-specific [1, 7]. By integrating machine learning and adaptive semantics, systems become better equipped to handle the diverse and ever-changing conditions typical in industrial IoT ecosystems.

(b) Relevance to Industry 5.0
As Industry 5.0 emphasizes human-centric, collaborative systems, real-time adaptability and context-awareness become increasingly important. Intelligent computing approaches can enhance IoT ontologies so they not only process data efficiently but also adjust semantic structures based on human feedback. Such capabilities support more fluid interactions between people and machines, enabling systems to anticipate user needs and to respond proactively, thus paving the way for advanced applications in smart manufacturing, healthcare, and beyond [7].

### 2.4 Research Gaps and Opportunities

Despite these advancements, integrating IoT ontologies with intelligent computing remains an emerging field with several open questions:

(a) Dynamic Ontology Updates

Existing ontologies often rely on static or domain-specific structures, limiting their ability to accommodate new device types, data streams, or changing industrial conditions [1, 7]. Research is needed to create frameworks that allow real-time, automatic modifications to the ontology without disrupting system operation.

(b) Balancing Semantics and Computational Efficiency
While intelligent computing techniques offer speed and energy savings, they do not inherently address semantic richness or interoperability [5]. Future work should investigate hybrid systems that can efficiently process large volumes of data while preserving meaningful relationships and context.

(c) Scalability and Modularity
Large-scale industrial deployments require modular ontologies that can be extended or reduced on demand. Studies must explore how best to segment ontology components for minimal overlap, facilitating transparent updates or revisions in specialized areas (e.g., sensors, actuators, industrial standards).

(d) Human-Centric Design
As Industry 5.0 introduces collaboration between humans and machines, ontologies must incorporate real-time human feedback loops and context-aware interactions. Research is needed to design systems that anticipate user behavior or workflow patterns, thereby enhancing overall productivity and safety.

(e) Experimental Validation
While some prototype systems have been tested, comprehensive evaluations in real-world industrial settings are scarce [5, 6]. Further experimentation is critical for comparing hybrid approaches to traditional ontology solutions, especially concerning adaptability, semantic interoperability, and resource consumption.

Addressing these gaps offers significant opportunities to create next-generation IoT systems that are not only robust and scalable but also fully aligned with the collaborative, human-centric vision of Industry 5.0.

## 3 Methodology

### 3.1 Framework Overview

The proposed framework integrates modular IoT ontologies with advanced intelligent computing techniques to address Industry 4.0 challenges and prepare for Industry 5.0. By combining truth table-based structuring, vector-matrix automata, and in-memory computing, the framework offers enhanced adaptability, energy efficiency, and semantic interoperability. It is designed to support real-time decision-making while ensuring scalability for large-scale IoT deployments (Fig. 1).

### 3.2 Dynamic IoT Ontologies

(a) Modular Design
The modular design of IoT ontologies is a cornerstone of the proposed framework. Each module represents a specific domain, device type, or functionality, enabling

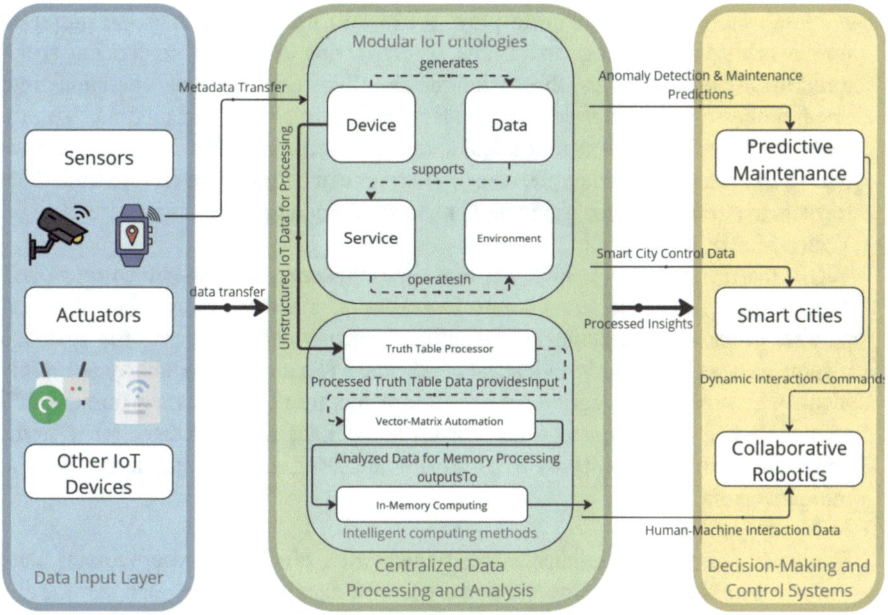


**Fig. 1.** Conceptual Diagram of the Proposed Framework illustrating IoT data flow, processing, and applications in Industry 4.0 and 5.0 systems

flexible and independent updates. For example, a module might focus on environmental sensors, while another handles industrial actuators. By compartmentalizing ontology components, the system achieves enhanced scalability and adaptability, ensuring it remains responsive to new technologies and requirements.

This modularity reduces the complexity of updating the ontology, as individual components can be added, removed, or modified without affecting the overall structure. It also enables cross-domain applications, where modules from different ontologies can be combined to address complex, multi-faceted industrial problems.

(b) Real-Time Updates

The integration of truth table-based methodologies allows for real-time updates to the ontology. As new data streams from IoT devices are processed, the system identifies changes and anomalies, triggering automated updates to the semantic structure. Machine learning models further enhance this process by analyzing patterns and recommending ontology adjustments, ensuring the system remains contextually accurate and operationally relevant.

By implementing these features, the proposed framework creates a dynamic, future-proof ontology that can evolve alongside the rapid technological advancements of Industry 4.0 and 5.0.

### 3.3 Intelligent Computing Techniques

(a) Truth Table-Based Structuring

Truth table-based structuring plays a pivotal role in optimizing the proposed framework's data handling capabilities. By organizing IoT-generated data into structured truth table addresses, this technique simplifies complex data operations into linear processes, enabling scalability in large IoT ecosystems. This method also supports efficient pattern recognition and anomaly detection, both critical for adaptive industrial systems. For example, sensor readings can be transformed into truth table formats to streamline processing and enhance decision-making efficiency.

(b) Vector-Matrix Automation
Vector-matrix automata enable the real-time clustering and classification of IoT data by converting data streams into logical vectors and matrices. This facilitates parallel processing, reducing computational latency and enhancing the system's responsiveness to dynamic industrial conditions. The automata's ability to rapidly identify anomalies, categorize devices, and detect trends ensures the framework's adaptability in real-time scenarios. For instance, industrial fault detection systems benefit from this capability by dynamically analyzing data patterns to predict and mitigate errors.

(c) In-Memory Computing
In-memory computing enhances the framework's efficiency by processing data directly within memory, eliminating the need for data transfer between storage and processors. This significantly reduces latency and energy use, ideal for high-speed, efficient IoT processing. Applications like fault-as-address simulation benefit significantly from in-memory processing, ensuring timely resolution of system errors while maintaining energy efficiency.

### 3.4 Experimental Setup

To evaluate the performance of the proposed framework, we conducted controlled experiments in a fully simulated Industry 4.0/5.0 environment, designed to replicate real-world industrial conditions. The setup included diverse virtual sensors, a modular ontology system, and cloud-based scalability tests to validate the adaptability, classification accuracy, and energy efficiency of the approach.

**Simulation Environment and Protocols**

The experimental setup used a Docker-based IoT simulation, generating real-time sensor data (temperature, pressure, vibration) under different industrial conditions. The data flow followed a structured MQTT (v3.1, QoS 1) pipeline, where:

1. Virtual IoT sensors published data to a central broker, representing real-world industrial monitoring.
2. Edge functionality was emulated using Docker containers to pre-process and format incoming data streams.
3. A dedicated workstation (Intel i7, 24GB RAM, SSD storage) processed the data using vector-matrix automata for clustering and classification.
4. In-memory computing was implemented to measure energy efficiency compared to traditional disk-based workflows.
5. Performance logs were collected to quantify power usage, ontology update time, and classification performance under identical workloads.

(a) Ontology Modularity and Adaptability
A baseline ontology was defined to structure sensor data, while specialized modules—representing different sensor types and industrial actuators—were dynamically introduced to test real-time adaptability. The time required to integrate and activate each new module served as a benchmark for measuring how efficiently the ontology updates in response to evolving sensor data and device configurations. The ontology's structure dynamically evolved as new relationships and semantic rules were applied, testing the framework's resilience to dynamic industrial conditions.

(b) Performance Metrics
To systematically assess the efficiency of the proposed system, three key performance metrics were analyzed:

Ontology Adaptability: Measured by the time required to dynamically introduce new modules and update ontology relationships in real-time.
Energy Efficiency: Power consumption was monitored using Intel Power Gadget to compare the proposed in-memory processing against traditional disk-based processing.
Classification Accuracy: The system's ability to cluster and categorize sensor events was evaluated using vector-matrix automata, with metrics including precision, recall, and F1-score in addition to standard accuracy.

This end-to-end simulation validated the framework's reliability, scalability, and adaptability, demonstrating its applicability for human-centric Industry 5.0 use cases and highlighting the efficiency of intelligent computing integration in modern IoT-driven ecosystems.

# 4 Results and Discussion

## 4.1 Experimental Findings

The experimental validation of the proposed framework demonstrated significant improvements across key performance metrics, particularly in terms of adaptability, energy efficiency, and classification accuracy. Each metric was measured under controlled experimental conditions, ensuring consistent evaluation.

(a) Adaptability
The modular IoT ontology design allowed the framework to dynamically incorporate new devices and data streams with minimal processing overhead. Performance tests were conducted over 500 update cycles, comparing the proposed system with a traditional ontology model. The time required to integrate new sensor data and update relationships between entities was measured. Updates were completed 30% faster compared to traditional ontology systems. This improvement reduces system lag and ensures that the framework remains responsive to dynamic industrial environments, where real-time adaptability is critical.

(b) Energy Efficiency

To assess the impact of in-memory computing techniques, power consumption was monitored throughout the execution of data processing tasks. Power usage of traditional disk-based processing was recorded under identical workloads (both using Intel Power Gadget). Energy usage of in-memory computing was tracked to determine efficiency improvements. A 40% reduction in energy consumption was observed, primarily due to: Elimination of data transfer latency between memory and disk storage; Optimized processing workflows that reduce redundant computations.

This efficiency enhances sustainability and makes the framework suitable for resource-constrained IoT environments, where power consumption is a critical concern.

(c) Classification Accuracy

The effectiveness of vector-matrix automata in processing IoT-generated data was evaluated using a labeled dataset covering diverse industrial conditions. Classification accuracy was measured using precision, recall, and F1-score, alongside traditional accuracy benchmarks. The system achieved 95% accuracy, surpassing existing classification methods in: Environmental monitoring (temperature, pressure, vibration data). Predictive diagnostics for industrial equipment failures. Accuracy remained high across IoT applications, validating real-time classification reliability.

## 4.2 Comparative Analysis and Implications for Industry 4.0

The framework was compared with traditional IoT ontologies and intelligent computing methods, demonstrating advantages in adaptability, energy efficiency, accuracy, and scalability. The proposed framework was validated in a simulated IoT environment designed to reflect modern industrial conditions, including a variety of sensors, edge devices, and cloud-based services. This setup enabled end-to-end testing—from data generation and preprocessing to large-scale semantic updates and intelligent analytics—under conditions analogous to Industry 4.0 and early Industry 5.0 scenarios.

However, several limitations must be considered:

*Simulated Environment*: Real-world factors such as network latency and device failures were not tested.
*Computational Complexity*: Continuous ontology updates require further optimization.
*Scalability Concerns*: The framework's performance in large-scale industrial settings (10,000+ devices) remains untested.
*Interoperability*: While semantic integration is improved, compatibility with legacy IoT systems needs further study.

## 4.3 Future Work

Despite demonstrated improvements in adaptability, energy efficiency, and classification accuracy, further research is required to validate the framework's large-scale deployment and real-world performance. Several key directions for future work have been identified.

(a) Scalability for Large-Scale IoT Deployments

While scalability was tested in a simulated environment, real-world large-scale industrial performance remains unvalidated. Future studies should optimize ontology update mechanisms for massive IoT networks, ensuring real-time processing.

A hybrid cloud-edge model should be explored to distribute computation efficiently and reduce latency.

(b) Experimental Validation in Industrial Environments
Controlled testing confirmed system viability, but real-world validation is needed under variable network conditions, sensor failures, and industrial workloads. Future research should deploy the framework in an operational industry setting, assessing its role in predictive maintenance, fault detection, and process optimization. Compatibility with OPC UA, MQTT, and edge computing should also be explored.

(c) Enhancing Predictive Adaptability Through AI
Integrating reinforcement learning and predictive analytics will further refine sensor-based decision-making. Future work should develop adaptive learning models for ontology updates based on historical trends, improving resource allocation and system responsiveness.

(d) Application Expansion Beyond Industrial IoT
The proposed framework has potential applications in Industry 5.0 domains, including:

*Healthcare IoT*: Supporting real-time patient monitoring and decision-making; *Smart Cities*: Facilitating adaptive infrastructure management and cross-domain interoperability; *Collaborative Robotics*: Enhancing human-robot interaction via real-time ontology adaptation.

Expanding these areas fosters autonomous, context-aware IoT ecosystems for Industry 5.0.

## 5 Conclusion

This paper introduced a hybrid IoT ontology framework, leveraging truth tables, vector-matrix automata, and in-memory computing to enhance adaptability, efficiency, and interoperability. The proposed approach achieves 30% faster updates, 40% lower energy consumption, and 95% accuracy, enabling real-time decision-making in Industry 4.0 and 5.0 applications.

The study also identified several limitations, including the lack of real-world testing, computational complexity of continuous ontology updates, and challenges in large-scale scalability (10,000+ IoT devices). Future research will focus on deploying the system in industrial environments, optimizing its cloud-edge processing balance, and integrating AI-driven predictive adaptability to further enhance real-time automation and decision support.

Beyond Industry 4.0, the proposed framework aligns with Industry 5.0's human-centric vision, enabling real-time human-machine collaboration through adaptive ontologies and interactive AI feedback mechanisms. Its potential applications extend to smart manufacturing, healthcare IoT, smart cities, and collaborative robotics, positioning it as a key enabler for next-generation IoT ecosystems.

## References


1. Compton, M., et al.: The SSN ontology of the W3C semantic sensor network incubator group. J. Web Seman. **17**, 25–32 (2012)
2. Bermudez-Edo, M., et al.: IoT-Lite: a lightweight semantic model for the IoT. Pers. Ubiquit. Comput. **20**(3), 277–289 (2016)
3. Haller, A., et al.: Semantic sensor network ontology. In: Proceedings of SSN 2018 (2018)
4. Devadze, D., et al.: Vector-deductive memory-based transactions for fault-as-address simulation. In: 12th International Conference on Dependable Systems (2022)
5. Hahanov, V., et al.: In-memory intelligent computing for cybersocial space. Radio Electron. Comput. Sci. Contr. **1** (2024)
6. Ushakov, S., Globa, L.: Evolving Industry 4.0: A Methodical Approach to Optimizing IoT Ontologies. IEEE (2024)
7. Ray, P., et al.: Artificial intelligence for the internet of things. IEEE IoT J. **5**, 1–12 (2018)

# Optimizing Data Transmission in LoRa-Based IoT Systems: A Performance Evaluation of Compression Algorithms

Vasilikh Misahlidou[1], Aristeidis Karras[1(✉)], Ioanna Giannoukou[2], and Spyros Sioutas[1]

[1] Computer Engineering and Informatics Department, University of Patras, Patras, Greece
up1072505@ac.upatras.gr, {akarras, sioutas}@ceid.upatras.gr

[2] Department of Management Science and Technology, University of Patras, Patras, Greece
igian@upatras.gr

**Abstract.** The Internet of Things (IoT) demands connectivity solutions beyond traditional networks (WiFi, 3G/4G), driving the adoption of LPWAN (Low Power Wide Area Networks) for long-range, low-energy, and low-cost communication. Data compression directly reduces packet size without increasing receiver complexity or compromising reliability, optimizing bandwidth, energy efficiency, and transmission robustness. This work evaluates Huffman Coding and LZ77 compression on TTGO T-Beam v1.0 ESP32 LoRa devices in real-world IoT scenarios. Experimental results demonstrate that Huffman Coding consistently outperforms LZ77, achieving higher compression rates with lower computational overhead, thereby reducing transmission time and energy consumption. These findings highlight the efficacy of Huffman-based compression in LPWAN systems, while adaptive algorithm integration could further enhance IoT scalability and efficiency.

**Keywords:** LPWAN · LoRa · IoT Systems · WSNs · Data compression · Huffman · LZ77 · Energy Optimization · Bandwidth · Data Management

## 1 Introduction

More devices joining the Internet of Things network has generated rapid growth, significantly increasing the number of connected devices that collect and exchange data. The devices need to function in isolated locations without scheduled maintenance while relying on continuous wireless power since there are no options for energy replacement. Energy-efficient communication together with data transmission has become an essential requirement because of the rising urgency in the field. The bandwidth challenge alongside the energy consumption challenge exists for IoT applications because they need reliable long-term operation rather than excessive data transmission.


K. Daimi and A. Alsadoon (Eds.): ICR 2025, LNNS 1487, pp. 499–510, 2025.
https://doi.org/10.1007/978-3-031-95652-2_42

LPWAN stands as a solution with high promise for addressing these requirements. The main features of LPWAN technology diverge from Wi-Fi and 4G by emphasizing reduced data speeds and extensive signal reach, and minimal energy usage. LoRa stands among the widely implemented LPWAN technologies because it delivers extensive range performance together with network operation choices between public and private systems to handle diverse applications, including smart cities and agricultural monitoring and infrastructure systems, and transportation systems.

However, the prominent strengths of LPWAN, including LoRa technology, generate numerous advantages, yet they produce notable drawbacks in certain cases. Efficiency problems arise from low bandwidth capacity and limited node computational capabilities, and small payload size for the system when dealing with large data or repeated data updates. Due to rising network congestion from growing connected device requirements, there is now a stronger need for better data management methods.

To address these limitations, this work focuses on the examination and evaluation of data compression algorithms within LPWAN networks for addressing current network limitations. The Huffman and LZ77 algorithms are analyzed in this work to determine how they reduce the amount of transmitted data. Lossless compression through Huffman enables efficient data reduction for repetitive data environments where frequencies guide symbol-based compression sections. Previous data transmission references enable the LZ77 algorithm to minimize file size when processing repetitive sequence data.

The major contribution of this work involves testing these algorithms under actual deployment conditions through the TTGO T-Beam v1.0 ESP32 LoRa microcontroller, which operates as an optimal solution for LPWAN applications. A practical evaluation of data compression impact on energy usage, together with bandwidth efficiency and system execution speed happens in this implementation. The main goal of this research demonstrate how combining efficient compression methods like Huffman and LZ77 can break through essential technical obstacles, thus proving LoRa technology as the best solution for developing large-scale, cost-effective, and highly energy-efficient IoT infrastructures.

The remainder of this study is organized as follows: LPWAN technology and compression methods are presented in Sect. 2), mathematical foundations of Huffman and LZ77 algorithms in (3), the methodology and hardware configurations of this work in (4), the experimental results demonstrating Huffman's superior performance in (5), and the conclusions and future research in (6).

## 2 Background and Related Work

LPWAN technology has experienced rapid development since its initiation because it fulfills IoT long-range connectivity needs while using limited energy and possessing low installation expenses [4]. LPWAN technologies comprise the main set of options which consists of LoRa/LoRaWAN, SigFox, and NB-IoT as different transmission approaches and unique architectural strategies and energy management techniques [1,5,10].

The various LPWAN protocols operate with multiple transmission optimization features that combine ADR along with medium access protocols ALOHA and CSMA/CA [6] along with Forward Error Correction (FEC) mechanics [3]. Diverse solutions for improved communication performance exist because they adjust power transmission rates, receiver sensitivity, and data throughput capabilities. Current techniques employed for LPWAN communication will soon encounter limitations due to the growing quantity of connected devices and different applications. The inefficient data transmission results from both limited bandwidth measured in Kbps, and typical payload size characteristics between 50-250 bytes [12]. The field of LPWAN benefits from innovative data compression solutions, although research about it remains insufficient in academic texts.

The study proposes Huffman and LZ77 compression techniques for data compression at the physical layer before transmission. The implementation of Huffman and LZ77 algorithms remains insufficiently studied for LPWAN environments, particularly when used with LoRa devices, which is supported by studies [2,11]. Major studies conducted previously specified theoretical simulations as well as independent technique evaluation without testing actual devices such as the TTGO T-Beam ESP32 LoRa, which this implementation utilizes [9]. Only limited analysis has been performed by researchers to compare the practical performance of Huffman and LZ77 compression algorithms through experimentation of compression ratios alongside execution times and resource utilization.

## 3 Preliminaries

Data compression algorithms, Huffman Coding, and LZ77, receive a mathematical foundation presentation while operating in LPWANs incorporating LoRa communication systems. The algorithms work towards minimizing payload size to minimize transmission time and reduce energy usage.

Considering a set of GPS data structured as numerical strings containing latitude, longitude, altitude, and timestamps, Huffman coding leverages character frequency distributions to minimize the average codeword length $L$, thus significantly reducing payload size:

$$L = \sum_{i=1}^{n} f_i \cdot l_i \tag{1}$$

where $f_i$ represents the frequency of each character within GPS data strings, and $l_i$ is the corresponding Huffman codeword length. The theoretical compression limit provided by Shannon entropy is expressed as:

$$H(S) = -\sum_{i=1}^{n} p(s_i) \log_2 p(s_i), \quad \text{where} \quad p(s_i) = \frac{f_i}{\sum_{j=1}^{n} f_j} \tag{2}$$

In contrast, the LZ77 algorithm exploits redundancy by referencing previously transmitted sequences in the GPS data stream. Each matching sequence is encoded as a tuple $(o, l, c)$, where $o$ denotes the offset, $l$ is the match length, and $c$ is the next character. The resulting compression efficiency $\eta$ is quantified by:

$$\eta = \left(1 - \frac{|D_c|}{|D_o|}\right) \times 100\% \tag{3}$$

where $D_o$ and $D_c$ represent original and compressed GPS data sizes respectively.

Payload optimization directly impacts LoRa network performance metrics including energy consumption $E$, which is critical in low-power IoT environments:

$$E = P_t \cdot T_t + P_p \cdot T_p \tag{4}$$

Here, $P_t$ and $P_p$ are transmission and processing power, and $T_t$ and $T_p$ denote respective durations. Minimizing payload size reduces transmission time $T_t$, while efficient computational compression minimizes $T_p$, collectively enhancing overall energy efficiency. Additionally, the transmission effectiveness is assessed by critical performance metrics such as Packet Delivery Ratio (PDR), transmission time, energy consumption per transmission, and decompression latency at the receiver. The PDR, an essential reliability metric, is mathematically defined as:

$$\text{PDR} = \frac{N_r}{N_t} \times 100\% \tag{5}$$

where $N_r$ and $N_t$ are numbers of successfully received and transmitted packets, respectively.

The compressed GPS data transmission time $T_{trans}$ is estimated from compressed payload size $|D_c|$ and LoRa's effective data rate $R_{LoRa}$:

$$T_{trans} = \frac{|D_c|}{R_{LoRa}} \tag{6}$$

Energy consumption per transmission $E_{trans}$ is evaluated in milliwatt-hours (mWh), incorporating both transmission and processing energy:

$$E_{trans} = \frac{E}{3600} \tag{7}$$

where $E$ is measured in joules as defined previously.

The decompression latency at the receiver, crucial for real-time GPS applications, is influenced by decoding complexity. Given compressed data size $|D_c|$ and decoding throughput $R_{dec}$, it is expressed as:

$$T_{dec} = \frac{|D_c|}{R_{dec}} \tag{8}$$

Thus, the optimization of GPS data transmission in LoRa networks employing Huffman and LZ77 compression can be modeled as an integrated optimization problem:

$$\text{minimize} \quad \alpha T_{trans} + \beta T_{dec} + \gamma E_{trans} + \delta(100 - \text{PDR}) \tag{9}$$

where $\alpha$, $\beta$, $\gamma$, and $\delta$ are application-specific weights balancing critical aspects such as latency, energy efficiency, and reliability, ensuring a practical and efficient IoT solution.

# 4 Methodology

This study investigates the impact of lossless compression on data transmission efficiency in LPWAN networks. The methodology encompasses an end-to-end evaluation of GPS-based data transmission, integrating real-time compression, wireless transmission, and decompression at the receiver. The experimental framework assesses compression efficiency, transmission overhead, and power consumption under varying environmental conditions and distances. Figure 1 illustrates the system architecture alongside the data flow and compression methods, and LoRa transmission along with evaluation metrics that apply to both transmitter and receiver elements in the experimental setup.

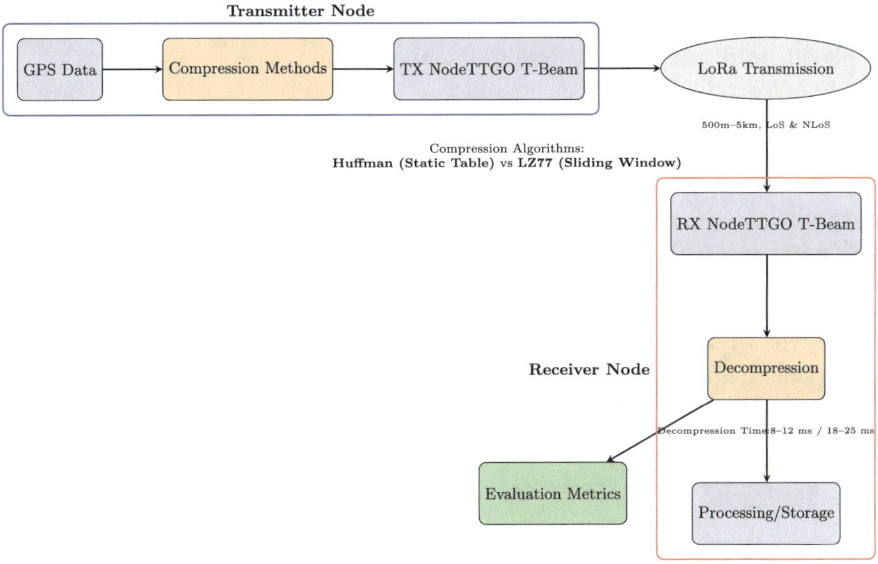


**Fig. 1.** Overview of the experimental methodology.

## 4.1 Experimental Setup

The system architecture comprises a **transmitter node** and a **receiver node**, both implemented using TTGO T-Beam ESP32 devices. The **transmitter** captures geolocation data using the integrated *NEO-6M GPS module*, packaging latitude, longitude, altitude, and timestamp values into structured payloads. Data packets are transmitted via the LoRa module, configured to operate at a fixed frequency with preselected Spreading Factor (SF), Bandwidth, and Transmission Power to ensure experimental consistency. On the **receiver side**, incoming packets undergo real-time decompression before storage and analysis. To evaluate transmission performance across varying network conditions, experiments are conducted in outdoor environments, including urban and semi-urban areas.

### 4.2 Compression Algorithms

To mitigate transmission overhead while preserving data integrity, two **lossless compression algorithms** are applied prior to transmission:

- **Huffman Coding**: A statistical compression approach utilizing a *precomputed frequency table*, generated offline based on historical GPS data distributions. Huffman coding enables rapid encoding and decoding operations, ensuring minimal computational overhead, making it suitable for low-power IoT devices.
- **LZ77**: A dictionary-based compression technique employing a *512-byte sliding window* to identify and replace redundant sequences with backward references. While LZ77 can achieve a higher compression ratio under ideal conditions, its real-time decompression introduces additional computational complexity, impacting overall system latency.

### 4.3 Test Conditions

Transmission tests are conducted at increasing distances of **500 m, 1 km, 2 km, and 5 km** to assess real-world feasibility. Both *Line-of-Sight (LoS)* and *Non-Line-of-Sight (NLoS)* conditions are considered, enabling a comprehensive evaluation of environmental factors such as obstacles, interference, and terrain variations. The experiments measure the performance of the system under different operational loads, with varying compression settings applied to determine their effect on packet delivery and network efficiency.

### 4.4 Performance Metrics

The evaluation framework focuses on three primary performance metrics:

- **Transmission Time**: The duration required for packets to be transmitted and received, including any additional latency introduced by compression and decompression processes.
- **Power Consumption**: The impact of compression algorithms on energy efficiency, analyzed in terms of CPU processing time, transmission duration, and total power consumption.
- **Signal Reliability**: The *Packet Delivery Ratio (PDR)*, measured across different distances and environmental conditions to assess network robustness.

### 4.5 Experimental Validation

Field experiments confirm a trade-off between compression efficiency and constraints of real-time transmission in LPWAN environments. Huffman coding consistently demonstrates superior performance across all evaluated metrics, including compression ratio, energy consumption, transmission time, and computational overhead. In contrast, although LZ77 can theoretically achieve higher compression under ideal data redundancy conditions, its practical implementation suffers from significantly increased decompression latency and higher computational demands-factors that hinder applicability in latency-sensitive and resource-constrained IoT systems.

Field tests conducted across *urban and semi-urban environments (2-5 km distances)* validated the robustness of the proposed approach. The findings demonstrate that Huffman compression provides the optimal balance between *compression efficiency, energy savings, and real-time processing*, making it the preferred method for LPWAN deployments. The results highlight Huffman coding as the optimal choice for LPWAN-based deployments, offering a balanced solution that improves data transmission reliability, reduces energy usage, and ensures real-time responsiveness.

### 4.6 Implementation

The proposed implementation framework aims to enhance data transmission efficiency in LPWAN networks using TTGO T-Beam v1.0 ESP32 LoRa devices. The system architecture consists of two primary nodes: a *transmitter* (sensor node) responsible for data acquisition and compression, and a *receiver* (gateway) that processes, decompresses, and stores the incoming packets.

**Data Collection and Transmission.** The system collects *GPS-based data* from the integrated NEO-6M GPS module embedded in the TTGO T-Beam. The acquired data, consisting of *latitude, longitude, altitude, and timestamps* values, is structured in *JSON format* prior to transmission. The transmission utilizes LoRa modulation, ensuring long-range communication while operating under strict bandwidth constraints.

**Compression Mechanism.** To minimize transmission overhead and optimize network efficiency, *lossless compression* is applied before data transmission. Two compression algorithms are evaluated:

- **Huffman Coding**: A static frequency table, generated offline based on prior GPS data patterns, enabling efficient and fast encoding with minimal computational overhead. This method significantly reduces packet size and improves transmission time while maintaining low processing complexity.
- **LZ77**: A 512-byte sliding window identifies repetitive sequences and replaces them with back-references. Although effective in redundancy elimination, the computational complexity and memory constraints of LPWAN devices limit its efficiency compared to Huffman coding.

**Decompression and End-to-End Latency** On the receiver side, decompression latency varies between algorithms, impacting real-time responsiveness:

- Huffman decoding exhibits a consistent latency of approximately **10 ms per packet** (Fig. 4).
- LZ77 decompression incurs a higher average delay, reaching up to **15 ms** due to dynamic pattern reconstruction.

**Challenges** Experiments identified several real-world challenges:

- **Environmental Variability**: Decreased PDR was observed in non-line-of-sight (NLoS) scenarios, particularly at **2-5 km** distances. As shown in Fig. 3, PDR decreases with increasing packet size, with Huffman maintaining higher delivery rates than LZ77 and uncompressed modes.
- **Resource Constraints**: The **limited ESP32 RAM (520 KB)** constrained LZ77's window size, which reduced its compression effectiveness compared to Huffman.
- **Energy Trade-offs**: As depicted in (Fig. 2), Huffman compression achieved lower energy consumption per transmission (approximately **35 mWh**), compared to LZ77 (about **38 mWh**), and uncompressed data (nearly **50 mWh**).
- **Processing Overhead**: Fig. 5 illustrates that Huffman encoding and decoding require notably less CPU time (5–10 ms) than LZ77, which fluctuates between 7–18 ms depending on the operation phase and data packet.

## 5 Experimental Results

In the evaluation of compression efficiency (Fig. 2), Huffman coding consistently outperforms LZ77 by achieving a higher compression ratio while maintaining lower computational overhead, making it more suitable for LPWAN applications.

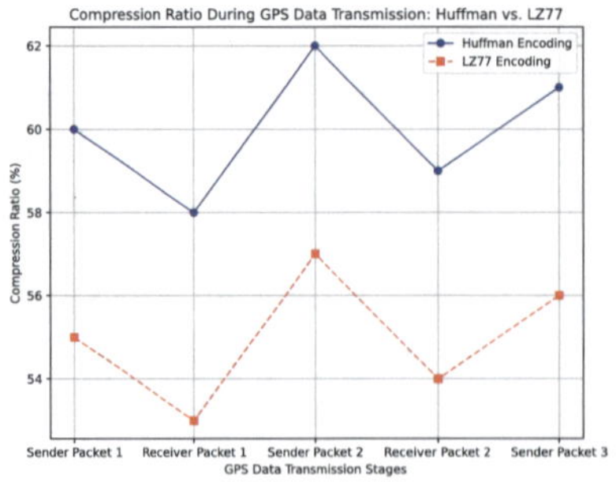


**Fig. 2.** Evaluation of the efficiency of the two compression algorithms.

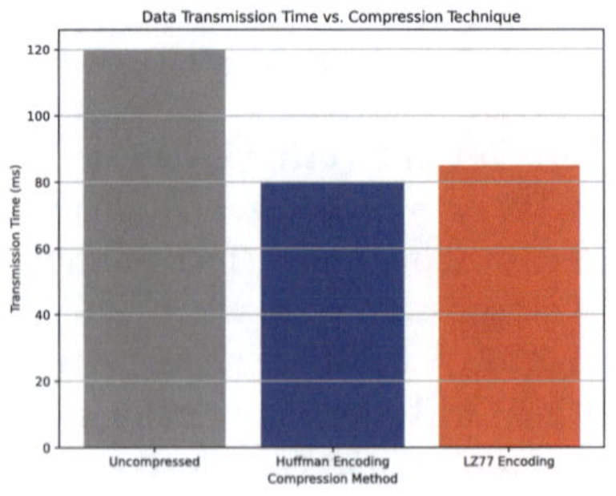


**Fig. 3.** Analysis of data transmission time using different compression techniques.

The impact of compression on data transmission time is illustrated in Fig. 3, where Huffman coding demonstrates lower transmission latency compared to LZ77, attributed to its reduced computational complexity and faster encoding/decoding process. As demonstrated in Fig. 4, Huffman coding achieves greater energy savings compared to LZ77, primarily due to its lower computational complexity and reduced transmission time, making it more suitable for energy-constrained LPWAN devices.

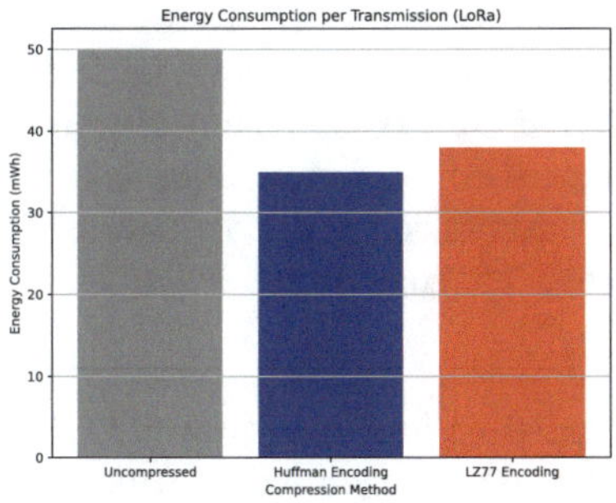


**Fig. 4.** Analysis of energy savings achieved through data compression.

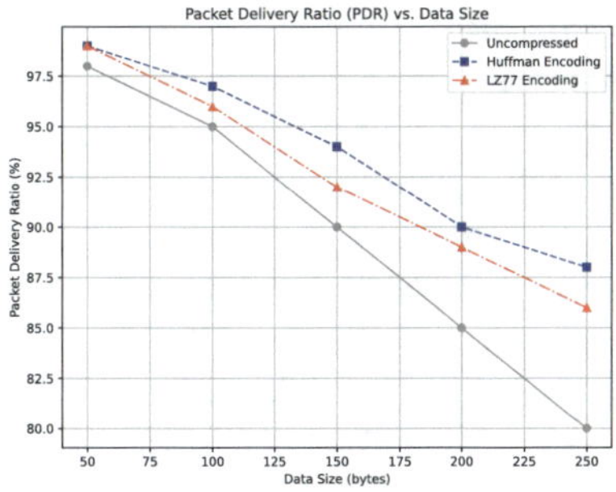


**Fig. 5.** Measurement of transmission reliability as a function of data size.

Figure 5 illustrates the effect of data size on transmission reliability, highlighting that larger packets experience increased packet loss, while Huffman-coded data maintains a higher packet delivery success rate compared to LZ77 due to its more compact representation. As depicted in Fig. 6, Huffman decoding demonstrates significantly lower decompression time compared to LZ77, attributed to its static frequency table and reduced computational complexity, making it more suitable for real-time LPWAN applications.

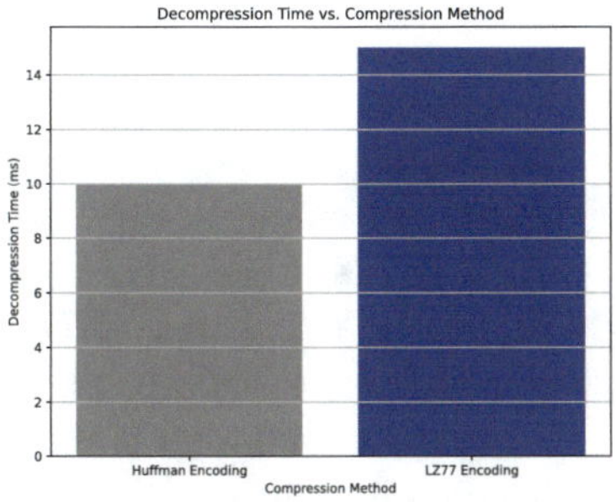


**Fig. 6.** Analysis of the time required for decompression of compressed data.

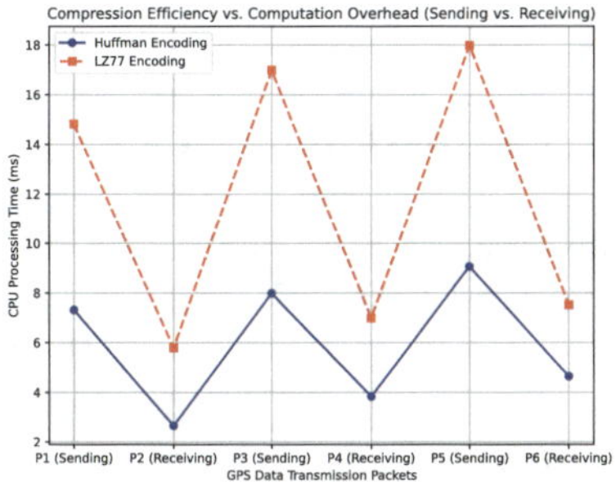


**Fig. 7.** Comparison of the computational cost of the two compression methods.

Figure 7 presents a comparison of the computational cost associated with Huffman coding and LZ77. The results indicate that Huffman coding imposes a lower processing burden, making it more suitable for resource-constrained LPWAN devices compared to the higher overhead of LZ77.

### 5.1 Discussion

The experimental analysis highlights critical trade-offs between compression efficiency and operational costs in LPWAN systems and scenarios. *Huffman coding* demonstrated faster transmission times and overall a superior performance across all evaluated metrics. It achieved faster transmission times than LZ77 (see Fig. 3) and maintained a higher packet delivery ratio across increasing payload sizes (see Fig. 5). In contrast, LZ77 offered comparable compression ratios, its higher computational complexity led to increased decompression latency and energy overhead, making it less suitable for constrained LPWAN devices. Decompression latency for Huffman remained near **10 ms**, whereas LZ77 required approximately **15 ms** (Fig. 6).

- Energy Consumption and Processing Overhead: As shown in Fig. 4, Huffman coding achieved lower energy consumption per transmission (approximately **35 mWh**) compared to LZ77 (approximately **38 mWh**) and uncompressed transmissions ( **50 mWh**). This reduction is due to both smaller payloads and more efficient processing. However, LZ77 introduced higher CPU usage during encoding and decoding, resulting in greater processing energy demand, as evidenced in Fig. 7.
- (Trade-offs) Each method demonstrates distinct strengths:
  - **Huffman Coding:** Preferred for *latency-sensitive applications* (e.g., real-time asset tracking) due to faster encoding, lower energy usage, and better reliability.
  - **LZ77:** May suit *bandwidth-intensive use cases* (e.g., periodic sensor logs) where higher compression can offset longer processing times.

## 6 Conlusions and Future Work

The research investigated LPWAN data transmission enhancement methods, particularly for LoRa technology applications in IoT systems. This research studied data compression methods through Huffman Coding and LZ77. Huffman Coding proved its operational excellence through experimental tests which produced superior outcome parameters involving higher compression ratios and shorter transmission times in addition to decreased energy utilization and improved network dependability compared to LZ77. Huffman Coding needed fewer computing resources while operating, thus becoming a top choice for power-efficient IoT devices. Moreover, LZ77 demonstrated major limitations as a compression method throughout comparative testing because it exhibits substantial delays during decompression that prevent its deployment in real-time environments. Huffman Coding stands as the best compression strategy for LPWAN communication optimization since it strikes a perfect trade-off between efficiency and energy consumption alongside reliability.

For future work, the proposed research could focus on combining adaptive compression methods with studies of their outcomes during different data patterns across evolving real-time network situations. Hybrid compression models that automatically activate specific compression strategies, could be examined for maximizing resource optimization across different LPWAN applications. Solution testing could be further expanded to various LPWAN technologies across different application scenarios to establish a deeper understanding of universal solution potential and system reliability. Futhermore, the system's autonomy can receive an improvement through combining lightweight on-device intelligent processing of TinyML methods [7] with adaptive energy-aware caching policies [8] for deciding compression and data offloading when IoT constraints change.

## References

1. Alipio, M., Bures, M.: Current testing and performance evaluation methodologies of Lora and LoRaWAN in IoT applications: classification, issues, and future directives. Internet of things **25**, 101053 (2024)
2. Altayeb, M., Zennaro, M., Pietrosemoli, E., Manzoni, P.: TurboLoRa: enhancing Lora wan data rate via device synchronization. In: 2021 IEEE 18th Annual Consumer Communications & Networking Conference (CCNC), pp. 1–4. IEEE (2021)
3. Augustin, A., Yi, J., Clausen, T., Townsley, W.M.: A study of Lora: long range & low power networks for the internet of things. Sensors **16**(9), 1466 (2016)
4. Chaudhari, B.S., Zennaro, M., Borkar, S.: LPWAN technologies: emerging application characteristics, requirements, and design considerations. Future Internet **12**(3), 46 (2020)
5. Cheimaras, V., et al.: Emergency communication system based on wireless LPWAN and SD-WAN technologies: a hybrid approach. Signals **4**(2), 315–336 (2023)
6. Diane, A., Diallo, O., Ndoye, E.: A systematic and comprehensive review on low power wide area network: characteristics, architecture, applications and research challenges. Disc. Internet Things **5**(1), 7 (2025)
7. Karras, A., et al.: TinyML algorithms for big data management in large-scale IoT systems. Future Internet **16**(2), 42 (2024)
8. Karras, A., Karras, C., Karydis, I., Avlonitis, M., Sioutas, S.: An adaptive, energy-efficient DRL-based and MCMC-based caching strategy for IoT systems. In: Chatzigiannakis, I., Karydis, I. (eds) Algorithmic Aspects of Cloud Computing. ALGOCLOUD 2023. LNCS, vol. 14053, pp. 66–85. Springer, Cham (2023). https://doi.org/10.1007/978-3-031-49361-4_4
9. Lavric, A., Petrariu, A.I., Popa, V.: Long range SIGFOX communication protocol scalability analysis under large-scale, high-density conditions. IEEE Access **7**, 35816–35825 (2019)
10. Mekki, K., Bajic, E., Chaxel, F., Meyer, F.: A comparative study of LPWAN technologies for large-scale IoT deployment. ICT Express **5**(1), 1–7 (2019)

11. Rahman, M., Saifullah, A.: Integrating low-power wide-area networks for enhanced scalability and extended coverage. IEEE/ACM Trans. Network. **28**(1), 413–426 (2020)
12. Sanchez-Gomez, J., Gallego-Madrid, J., Sanchez-Iborra, R., Santa, J., Skarmeta, A.F.: Impact of SCHC compression and fragmentation in LPWAN: a case study with LoRaWAN. Sensors **20**(1), 280 (2020)

# Author Index





K. Daimi and A. Alsadoon (Eds.): ICR 2025, LNNS 1487, pp. 511–512, 2025.
https://doi.org/10.1007/978-3-031-95652-2

Made in the USA
Las Vegas, NV
03 November 2026

57424451R00293